RESIDENTS HANDBOOK OF PEDIATRICS

Seventh Edition

THE HOSPITAL
FOR SICK CHILDREN
TORONTO, CANADA

RESIDENTS HANDBOOK OF PEDIATRICS

Seventh Edition

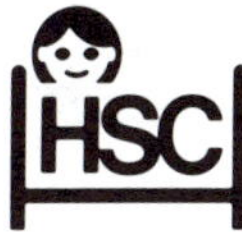

THE HOSPITAL
FOR SICK CHILDREN
TORONTO, CANADA

WILLIAM H. ABELSON, M.D.
R. GARTH SMITH, M.B., B.S.

1987
B.C. DECKER INC • Toronto • Philadelphia

Publisher

B.C. Decker Inc
3228 South Service Road
Burlington, Ontario   L7N 3H8

B.C. Decker Inc
320 Walnut Street
Suite 400
Philadelphia, Pennsylvania   19106

Sales and Distribution

United States
and Possessions

The C.V. Mosby Company
11830 Westline Industrial Drive
Saint Louis, Missouri   63146

Canada

The C.V. Mosby Company, Ltd.
5240 Finch Avenue East, Unit No. 1
Scarborough, Ontario   M1S 4P2

United Kingdom, Europe
and the Middle East

Blackwell Scientific Publications, Ltd.
Osney Mead, Oxford OX2 OEL, England

Australia

Harcourt Brace Jovanovich
30–52 Smidmore Street
Marrickville, N.S.W. 2204
Australia

Japan

Igaku-Shoin Ltd.
Tokyo International P.O. Box 5063
1-28-36 Hongo, Bunkyo-ku, Tokyo 113, Japan

Asia

Info-Med Ltd.
802–3 Ruttonjee House
11 Duddell Street
Central Hong Kong

South Africa

Libriger Book Distributors
Warehouse Number 8
"Die Ou Looiery"
Tannery Road
Hamilton, Bloemfontein 9300

South America
(non-stock list
representative only)

Inter-Book Marketing Services
Rua das Palmeriras, 32
Apto. 701
222-70 Rio de Janeiro
RJ, Brazil

RESIDENTS HANDBOOK OF PEDIATRICS   ISBN 1–55664–002–1

Library of Congress catalog card number: 87-70933

10   9   8   7   6   5   4   3   2

CONTRIBUTORS

WILLIAM H. ABELSON, M.D., F.R.C.P.(C)

> Formerly, Chief Resident, Department of Pediatrics; Currently, Fellow, Division of Infectious Diseases, The Hospital for Sick Children, Toronto, Ontario

Epidemiology

GLENN B. BERALL, B.Sc., M.D.

> Clinical Fellow, Division of Clinical Nutrition, Department of Pediatrics, The Hospital for Sick Children, Toronto, Ontario

Nutrition

SCOTT M. BRYSON, M.Sc.Phm., M.P.S.

> Associate Professor, University of Toronto Faculty of Pharmacy; Coordinator, Therapeutic Drug Monitoring, Department of Pharmacy, The Hospital for Sick Children, Toronto, Ontario

Formulary

J. RAYMOND BUNCIC, M.D., C.M., F.R.C.S.(C)

> Associate Professor, Ophthalmology, University of Toronto Faculty of Medicine; Staff Neuro-ophthalmologist, Eye Clinic, The Hospital for Sick Children, Toronto, Ontario

Ophthalmology

GERARD J. CANNY, M.D., F.R.C.P.(C)

> Assistant Professor, Pediatrics, University of Toronto Faculty of Medicine; Staff Physician, Division of Chest Diseases, Department of Pediatrics, The Hospital for Sick Children, Toronto, Ontario

Respirology

CLYDE T. CAVE, M.B., B.S., D.C.H., F.R.C.P.(C)

> Clinical Fellow, University of Toronto Perinatal Complex, Women's College Hospital, Toronto, Ontario

Adolescent Care
Behavioral Pediatrics

SUNIL J. DESAI, M.B., Ch.B., D.C.H., M.R.C.P.(Eng),
F.R.C.P.(C)

Pediatric Hematology Fellow, McMaster University Medical
Centre, Hamilton, Ontario
Hematology and Oncology
Procedures

JOHN J. DOYLE, M.D., F.R.C.P.(C)

Clinical Fellow, Division of Hematology/Oncology, The
Hospital for Sick Children, Toronto, Ontario
Hematology and Oncology

LEE DUPUIS, M.Sc.Phm.

Lecturer, University of Toronto Faculty of Pharmacy;
Coordinator, Drug Information Service and Education,
Department of Pharmacy, The Hospital for Sick Children,
Toronto, Ontario
Formulary

GIAN EGGER, B.Sc., M.D.

Senior Fellow, Division of Cardiology, The Hospital for Sick
Children, Toronto, Ontario
Cardiology

ROBERT M. EHRLICH, M.D., F.R.C.P.(C)

Professor, Pediatrics, University of Toronto Faculty of
Medicine; Chief, Division of Endocrinology, The Hospital
for Sick Children, Toronto, Ontario
Endocrinology

GRAHAM ELLIS, Ph.D., M.R.C.Path., D.A.B.C.C.

Associate Professor, Clinical Biochemistry, University of
Toronto Faculty of Medicine; Assistant Biochemist, Depart-
ment of Biochemistry, The Hospital for Sick Children,
Toronto, Ontario
Laboratory Reference Values

MOHAMMED FADLALLAH FAROUQ, M.B., B.Ch.

Clinical Fellow, Division of Infectious Diseases, The Hospi-
tal for Sick Children, Toronto, Ontario
Infectious Diseases
Procedures

DARCY FEHLINGS, M.D.

Associate Resident, Department of Pediatrics, The Hospital for Sick Children, Toronto, Ontario

Nutrition

LAURA A. FINLAYSON, M.D., F.R.C.P.(C)

Lecturer in Dermatology, Dalhousie University Faculty of Medicine; Active Staff, Dermatology, Victoria General Hospital and Consultant Staff, Dermatology, Izzak Walton Killam Hospital for Children, Halifax, Nova Scotia

Dermatology

VITO FORTE, M.D., F.R.C.S.(C)

Assistant Professor, Otolaryngology, University of Toronto Faculty of Medicine; Staff Otolaryngologist, The Hospital for Sick Children, Toronto, Ontario

Otolaryngology

LESLIE GABAY, M.B., B.S., F.R.C.P.(C)

Fellow, Division of Endocrinology, The Hospital for Sick Children, Toronto, Ontario

Gastrointestinal and Liver Disorders
Procedures

LEE ANN GALLANT, M.D., F.R.C.P.(C)

Lecturer, Department of Pediatrics, University of Toronto Faculty of Medicine; Associate Staff, Department of Pediatrics, The Hospital for Sick Children, Toronto, Ontario

Metabolic Disease

MARK L. GREENBERG, M.B., Ch.B., F.R.C.P.(C)

Associate Professor, Pediatrics, University of Toronto Faculty of Medicine; Senior Staff Physician, Division of Hematology/Oncology, The Hospital for Sick Children, Toronto, Ontario

Approach to the Pediatric Patient

ANNE MARIE GRIFFITHS, M.D., F.R.C.P.(C)

Assistant Professor, Pediatrics, University of Toronto Faculty of Medicine; Staff Physician, Division of Gastroenterology, Department of Pediatrics, The Hospital for Sick Children, Toronto, Ontario

Gastrointestinal and Liver Disorders

ROBIN P. HUMPHREYS, M.D., F.R.C.S.(C), F.A.C.S.

Associate Professor, Departments of Surgery and Anatomy, University of Toronto Faculty of Medicine; Staff Neurosurgeon, Department of Surgery, The Hospital for Sick Children, Toronto, Ontario

Neurology and Neurosurgery
Procedures

INGRID JARVIS, M.D., F.R.C.P.(C)

Staff Physician and Clinical Associate, Division of Dermatology, The Hospital for Sick Children, Toronto, Ontario

Dermatology
Procedures

DOUGLAS H. JOHNSTON, D.D.S., Dip.Paed.

Associate in Dentistry, University of Toronto Faculty of Medicine; Head, Division of Pediatric Dentistry, The Hospital for Sick Children, Director, Dentistry, Bloorview Childrens Hospital, and Consultant, Dentistry, Hugh MacMillan Medical Centre, Toronto, Ontario

Dentistry

MARK S. KORSON, M.D.

Formerly, Senior Pediatric Resident, The Hospital for Sick Children, Toronto, Ontario; Currently, Clinical Fellow in Genetics and Metabolism, Children's Hospital Medical Center, Boston, Massachusetts

Laboratory Reference Values

IVAN KRAJBICH, M.D., B.Sc., F.R.C.S.(C)

Lecturer, Department of Surgery, University of Toronto Faculty of Medicine; Staff Orthopaedic Surgeon, The Hospital for Sick Children, Toronto, Ontario

Orthopaedics

LEO LEVIN, M.D., F.R.C.P.(C)

Senior Fellow, Division of Nephrology, The Hospital for Sick Children, Toronto, Ontario

Nephrology
Procedures

DAUNE L. MacGREGOR, M.D., F.R.C.P.(C)

Associate Professor, Pediatrics, University of Toronto
Faculty of Medicine; Staff Physician, Division of Neurology,
Department of Pediatrics, The Hospital for Sick Children,
Toronto, Ontario

Neurology and Neurosurgery

HARRIET L. MacMILLAN, M.D., F.R.C.P.(C)

Chief Resident, Department of Child Psychiatry, The
Hospital for Sick Children, Toronto, Ontario

Behavioral Pediatrics

MICHAEL A. McGUIGAN, M.D., C.M., F.A.A.P., ABMT

Assistant Professor, Pediatrics and Pharmacology, University
of Toronto Faculty of Medicine; Medical Director, Poison
Information Centre, The Hospital for Sick Children,
Toronto, Ontario

Poisoning

MARCELLINA MIAN, M.D., F.R.C.P.(C)

Assistant Professor, Pediatrics, University of Toronto Faculty
of Medicine; Director, SCAN Program and Staff Pediatrician,
Outpatient Department, The Hospital for Sick Children,
Toronto, Ontario

Behavioral Pediatrics

ANTHONY J. O'CONNELL, M.B., B.S., F.F.A.R.A.C.S.

Formerly, Chief Critical Care Fellow, Pediatric
Intensive Care Unit, The Hospital for Sick Children,
Toronto, Ontario; Currently, Staff Intensivist, The Children's
Hospital, Camperdown, New South Wales, Australia

Emergencies

PATRICIA C. PARKIN, B.Sc., M.D.

Chief Resident, Department of Pediatrics, The Hospital for
Sick Children, Toronto, Ontario

Formulary

MERCER C. RANG, M.B., B.S., F.R.C.S.(Eng), F.R.C.S.(C)

Assistant Professor, Pediatrics, University of Toronto Faculty
of Medicine; Staff Physician, Division of Gastroenterology,
Department of Pediatrics, The Hospital for Sick Children,
Toronto, Ontario

Orthopaedics

CAROL A. REDMOND, M.D., F.R.C.S.(C)
Research Fellow, Department of Pediatric Gynecology, The Hospital for Sick Children, Toronto, Ontario
Gynecology

JOHN J. REISMAN, B.A., M.D., F.R.C.P.(C)
Clinical Fellow, Division of Chest Diseases, The Hospital for Sick Children, Toronto, Ontario
Respirology
Procedures

EVE A. ROBERTS, M.D., F.R.C.P.(C)
Assistant Professor, Pediatrics and Medicine, University of Toronto Faculty of Medicine; Staff Physician, Department of Pediatrics, Division of Gastroenterology, The Hospital for Sick Children and Associate Staff, Toronto General Hospital, Toronto, Ontario
Gastrointestinal and Liver Disorders

JAY D. ROSENFIELD, M.D., F.R.C.P.(C)
Senior Fellow, Developmental Pediatrics, The Hospital for Sick Children, Toronto, Ontario
Growth and Development

PETER G. RUMNEY, M.D., C.C.F.P.
Senior Resident, Department of Pediatrics, The Hospital for Sick Children, Toronto, Ontario
Gynecology

RAYFEL SCHNEIDER, M.B., B.Ch.
Chief Resident, Department of Pediatrics, The Hospital for Sick Children, Toronto, Ontario
Allergy and Immunology
Rheumatology

DONNA SECKER, B.Sc., R.P.Dt.
Dietitian-Nutritionist, Department of Food Services, The Hospital for Sick Children, Toronto, Ontario
Nutrition

CHRISTOPHER A. SIDES, M.B., Ch.B., F.F.A.R.C.S.

Formerly, Associate Chief Critical Care Fellow, Pediatric
Intensive Care Unit, The Hospital for Sick Children,
Toronto, Ontario; Currently, Senior Anesthetic Registrar,
Royal Infirmary, Leeds, England

Emergencies

R. GARTH SMITH, M.B., B.S., F.R.C.P.(C)

Formerly, Chief Resident, Department of Pediatrics, The
Hospital for Sick Children; Currently, Clinical Neonatology
Fellow, University of Toronto Perinatal Complex, Women's
College Hospital, Toronto, Ontario

Neonatology
Ophthalmology
Procedures

RICARDO A. SUPERINA, M.D., C.M., F.R.C.S.(C)

Assistant Professor, Surgery, University of Toronto Faculty of
Medicine; Attending Surgeon, The Hospital for Sick
Children, Toronto, Ontario

Procedures
Surgery

PAUL K. SWAN, M.B., B.S., F.F.A.R.A.C.S.

Formerly, Chief Critical Care Fellow, Pediatric Intensive Care
Unit, The Hospital for Sick Children, Toronto, Ontario;
Currently, Staff Intensivist, Princess Margaret Hospital for
Children, Perth, Western Australia

Emergencies

INGRID TEIN, M.D., F.R.C.P.(C)

Clinical Fellow, Neurology, Department of Pediatrics, The
Hospital for Sick Children, Toronto, Ontario

Neurology and Neurosurgery

MARGARET W. THOMPSON, Ph.D., F.C.C.M.G.

Professor, Medical Genetics and Pediatrics, University of
Toronto Faculty of Medicine; Senior Staff Geneticist, The
Hospital for Sick Children, Toronto, Ontario

Genetics

LEA VELSHER, M.D., C.M., F.R.C.P.(C)

Clinical Fellow, Department of Genetics, The Hospital for
Sick Children, Toronto, Ontario
Genetics

JENTIEN VERMAAT, M.B., Ch.B., F.R.C.P.(C)

Consultant Pediatrician, Scarborough Grace General
Hospital, Scarborough, Ontario
Nephrology
Fluids and Electrolytes

ROBERT D. WAGMAN, M.D., F.R.C.S.(C)

Fellow, Pediatric Ophthalmology, The Hospital for Sick
Children, Toronto, Ontario
Ophthalmology

RONALD M. ZUKER, M.D., F.R.C.S.(C), F.A.C.S.

Assistant Professor, Surgery, University of Toronto Faculty of
Medicine; Head, Division of Plastic
Surgery and Director of the Burn Unit, The Hospital for
Sick Children, Toronto, Ontario
Plastic Surgery

PREFACE

Many changes have occurred since the previous (6th) edition of the *Residents' Handbook of Pediatrics*, which appeared about eight years ago. Rapid advances in pediatric diagnostic and therapeutic measures rendered obsolete much of the information contained in the previous edition, and with the shift in pediatric residency training programs toward more subspecialty exposure and less toward primary care, an up-to-date, easily comprehensible and readily available source of information is in great demand.

The current seventh edition of the *Handbook* addresses the need for a pocket-sized, practical volume for individuals involved in the management of general and acute pediatric problems; it provides an extensive formulary (of which we are particularly proud!), an excellent procedures section, plus sufficient practical details regarding the diagnosis and the management of both common and emergency problems.

We have changed the presentation by alphabetizing chapter headings to make information more easily accessible. The use of illustrations is extensive, and a new feature is the use of color plates. The chapter format has been modified to facilitate rapid extraction of useful information in emergency situations by means of using short succinct syntax, bold print, and indentation. We have also tried to include "warning signs" intended to avert potential disaster.

Despite the increased content, we have succeeded in preserving the handy, practical size (characteristic of previous editions) which could easily replace present volumes now carried in the labcoat pocket or purse. Subsequently, we anticipate revisions every three to four years.

W.H. Abelson, M.D., F.R.C.P.(C)
R.G. Smith, M.B., B.S., F.R.C.P.(C)

ACKNOWLEDGEMENTS

There were many individuals whose assistance and encouragement were invaluable to those of us involved in the writing and production of this *Handbook*: Erwin Gelfand, Stanley Read, Chaim Roifman, Stephen Feanny, Barry Zimmerman (Allergy and Immunology), Eudice Goldberg (Adolescent Care), Rose Geist (Behavioral Pediatrics), Richard Rowe, Robert Freedom, David Malkin (Cardiology), Lionel Boxall (Dermatology), Denis Daneman (Endocrinology), Gerald Arbus, William Balfe, Diane Hebert, Michèlle Farine (Nephrology and Fluid and Electrolytes), Gary Tithecott (Gynecology), Alvin Zipursky, Mark Greenberg, Ronald Murphy (Hematology and Oncology), Ronald Gold, Jay Keystone, Christine Newman (Infectious Diseases), Joseph Clarke (Metabolism), Jonathan Hellmann, Martin Skidmore, Arne Ohlsson, Haresh Kirpalani, Geoffrey Sherwood (Neonatology), Paul Pencharz, David Kenny, Alvina Hills and the Department of Food Services (Nutrition), Michael O'Keefe (Ophthalmology), Ronald Laxer (Rheumatology), Robert Filler (Surgery), Desmond Bohn, John Edmonds (Emergencies), Annette Poon, Martin Petric (Laboratory Reference Values), Daniel Goldstein, Michelle Brill-Edwards (Formulary), and all other senior staff and heads of departments who gave their valuable time and experience.

We would also like to thank Mr. Alex Wright and the staff of the Visual Education Department and Eva McGrath and her long-suffering employees in the wordprocessing department of The Hospital for Sick Children, Toronto. Special thanks to Mrs. Sharon Bain for her contribution of patience and secretarial assistance that eased the "growing pains" associated with this publication.

Last, but by no means least, we are most grateful to the publisher Brian Decker whose confidence in us and contagious enthusiasm helped erase incipient doubts which may have arisen in the early stages; to Barbara Brown for overseeing the writing of this book, her department for their editorial and proofreading effort; and to Dennis Boyes and the production staff who ably guided the book to publication.

NOTICE

FOREWORD

What blood tests should be ordered on an infant who is admitted with severe unexplained anemia? What is a rational approach to the management of status epilepticus in a child? How should hypernatremic dehydration be managed and what complications might occur? What is the dosage of drug X and what side-effects require close monitoring? *The Residents' Handbook of Pediatrics* does not serve as a miniature pediatric textbook nor is it intended to be a "cookbook" to replace a logical problem solving approach to a condition or to a specific disorder. The *Handbook* has been designed to act as a guide to the diagnosis and management of the myriad of pediatric disorders that present in the office setting, the clinic or emergency room, and on the hospital wards. The *Handbook* has been condensed into a reference source that is pocket-sized and appropriately organized and indexed. There are helpful tables, graphs, nomograms, and current data which will assist the physician in the investigation and management of the child with a medical problem.

The *Handbook* will be of interest to the medical student, house officer, subspecialty trainee, and the pediatrician and family physician. Many chapters will be useful to nurses, psychologists, social workers, and to other disciplines that frequently interact with children.

The *Handbook* was written and edited almost completely by our senior pediatric residents with guidance and helpful suggestions from the attending staff. Each chapter from the previous edition of eight years ago was rewritten to introduce new material and discard outdated information. This edition of *The Handbook* has several new chapters that are important to the practice of pediatrics today; these include adolescent medicine, psychosocial issues, and a section on epidemiology. Finally, the Formulary underwent an extensive revision and provides concise and informative guidelines for drug management in the pediatric population.

The residents who worked together to produce this *Handbook* realize that there are many ways to investigate and treat a child. Thus, the *Handbook* is not intended to be the final answer or the only approach to a specific question or disorder confronting the student or physician. I want to congratulate the house staff and faculty advisors on their wonderful achievement in putting together this splended publication.

Robert H.A. Haslam, M.D., F.R.C.P.(C)

CONTENTS

I

INTRODUCTION

Approach to the Pediatric Patient

The fun and excitement of clinical medicine derives from the challenge it poses to one's problem solving skills. With expanding skills and knowledge, clinical judgment and insight are invoked in the context of helping other humans. When these other humans are children, the process is particularly rewarding.

Since the process of diagnosis and management is rather like solving a mystery, a strategy for processing the clues necessary for problem solving must be generated. The components of this strategy include: history taking, physical examination, formulation, and management—investigation, treatment and follow-up.

HISTORY TAKING

The purpose of soliciting a complete history in clinical medicine is to enable the interviewer, by the end of the history taking, to generate hypotheses as to the disease process(es) with which the patient presents. The intent is not to be able to put a name to a disease, but rather to be able to generate several working postulates for the process causing symptoms. Once this is achieved, the physical examination can become a focused endeavor that attempts to confirm or eliminate each of the proposed hypotheses.

A second objective of history taking is to allow the examiner a window on the interaction between the child and his care givers and an insight into the impact of the child's health problem on his living circumstances. This requires evaluation and definition of the family structure and function and observation of the interaction with the family members present. The illness of a child may impose particular stress on a family when the illness is chronic or when the family is fragmented.

The history taking process thus ought to encompass two sequences of inquiry:

A Series of Questions Precipitated by Already Elicited Information

These questions derive from defining the reason for attendance at the doctor or hospital, i.e., the main complaint. For example, if the patient's main complaint is headache, knowing and understanding the pathophysiology of headache will suggest a series of specific questions, such as where in the head the headache is situated, whether it is worse when standing or when lying, and so on. The answers to these questions will spawn new questions, and thus following a line of questioning is rather like following a series of sign posts along a trail. In your questioning, view each question as a branch point in a decision making tree. Should the answer to any given question be affirmative, it ought to be followed by an appropriate set of questions that expand the affirmative answer. If, on the other hand, the answer is negative, an option has been eliminated, and a new set of questions will be required. Thus in following the sequential trail, a wide range of questions, based on a knowledge of pathophysiology, are asked, and in the process, a sequential narrowing of options and postulates is achieved.

A Contextual Set of Questions

These questions attempt to place the child in the context of his prior history, his family, his behavioral and social milieu, his drug-chemical milieu, and his developmental milieu. Such questions are crucial, since much influence is exerted upon the child by his milieu and vice versa, and much interaction occurs between developmental, behavioral, and physical facets.

The following areas must be inquired into in depth:

- Pregnancy and birth history
- Neonatal history
- Feeding history
- Developmental milestones, including specific questioning about fine and gross motor development, social development, language development, and cognitive development. Vision and hearing ought to be included under developmental questioning.
- Immunizations
- Allergies
- Current medications
- Family history, including details of parental age and health, siblings and miscarriages, consanguinity, and occupations
- Previous medical history
- Review of systems. This should be brief but comprehensive enough to cover the major symptoms in all the organ systems.
- Social history—e.g., who cares for the child, day care, school context.

At the completion of an adequate history taking, a working formulation of the patient's disease process ought to be possible. It is in the elicitation of a superior history that a superior clinician can be identified.

PHYSICAL EXAMINATION

The physical examination must always be a comprehensive physical examination that seeks to elicit all physical abnormalities regardless of whether they are immediately relevant. However, the history will have highlighted areas of particular concern and interest that will need to be examined with greater attention than others.

Pediatric patients are different. At certain ages children naturally exhibit apprehension with strangers, and make that evident. They may also have had previous frightening contacts with health care professionals, and be anxious. Overcoming this reluctance is part of the fun of pediatrics. Spending a little time establishing a comfortable relationship with the child enhances the accuracy of the examination immeasurably by allowing a calm and systematic evaluation of both physical findings and developmental status. It will also afford you the unique personal satisfaction that a responsive child can give.

The completeness of the examination varies with the acuteness of the child's illness. It is appropriate to focus rapidly on the relevant major systems in an acutely ill child and equally appropriate to proceed more slowly and in different order in an elective patient.

Before laying hands on the patient, spend some time observing. Look at the degree of illness, acuteness or chronicity of illness, parent-child interaction, and cleanliness and other indicators of social well-being. Then proceed to examine in a systematic fashion. It is best to order the examination to permit most of it to occur while the child is calm and not crying—it is very difficult to evaluate the abdomen of a wailing child. Thus, the examination of ears and throat in a baby, and the rectal examination in an older infant, should be deferred until the end of the examination.

Each individual examiner will develop his own preferred order of examination, but a suggested sequence for the examination is as follows:

- General features
    1. Absence or presence of respiratory distress
    2. Cyanosis or pallor
    3. State or hydration and perfusion
    4. Nutritional status

5. Bodily proportion; i.e., is there abdominal distention, symmetry of the chest, obvious deformities?
6. Are there dysmorphic features, either specific (e.g., Down syndrome) or nonspecific?
7. Is the child in pain?
8. Is the child behaving in an age appropriate fashion?

- Record the vital signs—blood pressure, pulse, respiratory rate.
- In all patients, height, weight, and state of pubertal development must be recorded. Height and weight should be plotted on the appropriate growth curve. Head circumference should be recorded and plotted for infants.
- Begin at the head, and conduct an examination appropriate to age. In an infant the status of the fontanelles is necessary. Palpation of the cervical lymph node chains and thyroid and auscultation of the carotid vessels are more important in the older child.
- Inspect the chest, looking for accessory muscle activity, abdominal retractions, and abnormal cardiac pulsations. Then palpate, percuss, and auscultate the chest and heart.
- Inspect the abdomen, feel the femoral pulses, and examine the genitalia in a young child. Then palpate the abdomen. Palpating the abdomen in a younger child requires gentleness and patience rather than pressure and haste. Feel systematically for the liver, spleen, kidneys, and any unusual masses. Auscultate the abdomen for bowel sounds and bruits.
- Turn the child over and inspect the back.
- In the younger child, inspect the perineum at this stage. In the older child, defer this until the end of the examination.
- Conduct a formal neurologic examination, including cranial nerves, peripheral nervous system, and a concurrent cognitive evaluation.

Formal examination of the fundi should take place; it may be helpful with the young infant to have the mother hold the child over her shoulder for this. A formal developmental evaluation ought to be done in all children, but might be comfortably deferred until the end of the examination. In the neonatal period, evaluation of specific neonatal reflexes must be carried out.
- Musculoskeletal examination: This must include an evaluation of the range of motion of all joints and the degree of development and strength of all muscle groups. If the child is old enough to walk, an evaluation of gait must be made. Examination of the hips is particularly important in the first year of life, and of the spine in the preadolescent and adolescent.
- Evaluation of the ears, nose, and throat.

FORMULATION

At the conclusion of the physical examination, definition of positive findings and important negative findings is essential. Summarize the relevant positive historical and physical findings, and proceed to postulate possible processes that might account for the child's complaints. This requires the development of a "differential diagnosis." A differential diagnosis should consider the process(es) that might account for the child's symptoms, and then define the specific disease entities that might account for the disordered process. The list of possible processes should be founded on positive findings from the history and physical examination.

The intent of a differential diagnosis is not to generate an exhaustive list of possibilities, but rather to generate a prioritized list of potential diseases in order to facilitate investigation and management.

Some children may have more than one or even

many problems. A list of these different problems should be made, in order to permit planning for the management of different problems. However, your thinking should be focused by listing the problems and their postulated causal processes, in order of priority. Less active problems can be listed and considered separately.

MANAGEMENT

Investigation

Most children require further investigation. Investigation should not be an undirected attempt to order as many tests as possible, but rather a focused and sequential investigation based on the hypotheses laid out. Under certain circumstances, such as the comatose patient, a broad spectrum of preliminary investigations will be needed immediately, but in most patients a well thought-out sequence of investigations is appropriate.

Treatment and Follow-Up

Treatment and follow-up depend on the conclusions derived from the investigation and must be tailored to the individual patient.

Following the type of structured strategy outlined above will ensure fun in your practice of pediatrics, and optimal care for your patients.

II

SYSTEMS

1 ADOLESCENT CARE

ADOLESCENT ISSUES: INTERVIEWING AND EXAMINING ADOLESCENTS

- Interacting with patients who are going through this traditionally turbulent stage differs somewhat from physician-patient interactions in the remainder of the pediatric population.
  1. Some things to be aware of during the interview
     - Clarify the patient's perception of his problem; this may be quite different from his parents' perceptions. The adolescent should be spoken to alone at some time.
     - Establish a sense of confidentiality with the patient, and discuss clear limits regarding your interactions with the family (exceptions: suicidal and homicidal ideation)
     - Listen to what the patient is saying
     - Be aware of nonverbal clues, such as body language or emotional displays
     - Be aware of the presenting complaint being used as a "ticket to enter," e.g., a means of bringing some other concern to your attention
     - Be aware of a "ticket to exit," e.g., using the chief complaint as a way of getting out of a no longer desirable activity, such as competitive sports
  2. Discomfort in dealing with the following subjects is as much a reflection of the physician's attitude as of the patient's attitude. Some issues to be sure to discuss (acronym from Neinstein) are as follows:

- H = *home*, including relations with parents, family responsibilities, family stresses, independence
- E = *education*, including present performance in school and career goals
- A = *activities*, including special interests, relationships with friends
- D = *drugs*, including smoking, alcohol
- S = *sexuality*, (Table 1–1)

TABLE 1–1 Important Issues in Adolescent Sexual History

Age of first sexual experience
Type of sexual activity (e.g., masturbation, intercourse, "petting")
Frequency of activity, number of sexual partners
Sexual orientation (e.g., homosexual, heterosexual)
Feelings related to sexual activity (e.g., guilt, peer pressure, degree of enjoyment)
Awareness and use of contraceptive methods
Awareness of sexually transmitted diseases

3. Specifics to include in the physical examination
   - Growth parameters
   - Sexual maturity rating (Tanner stage)—see p 223–225, developmental section
   - Assessment of thyroid (p 117–118)
   - Assessment of scoliosis (p 544)
   - Minor skin imperfections such as mild acne may assume considerable importance at this age, and your patient will probably appreciate the opportunity to discuss this
   - A pelvic examination in sexually active females, including an explanation of the procedure and the advantages of regular examinations
   - Breast examination: Be sure to explain gynecomastia if present in a male or the importance of self-examination in a female

- Testicular examination in males
4. Some laboratory tests to consider
    - CBC—iron deficiency is not uncommon in adolescence (p 255)
    - Establishing the presence of rubella anti-bodies in girls could prevent a later trage-dy of a congenitally infected infant. (A full immunization history should be obtained.)
    - Sexually active females—Pap smear, VDRL, and cultures for gonorrhea, chlamydia, and trichomonas should be done routinely
    - Sexually active males—VDRL and cultures when indicated
    - In "street kids," consider screening for hepatitis and HIV-I antibodies

EATING DISORDERS

Anorexia Nervosa

General Considerations

- Anorexia nervosa is a syndrome of self-starvation (with a relentless pursuit of thinness) in an attempt to exert some form of control. The diagnosis is based on DSM-III criteria (modified)
    1. Refusal or inability to maintain a normal body weight
    2. Loss of >25% of original body weight (may be less in pediatric population)
    3. Distorted body image
    4. Intense fear of weight gain or becoming fat
    5. No known medical or psychiatric cause for weight loss
- Anorectics may be subtyped into
    1. Bulimic anorectics (generally with more premorbid personality disturbance and intrafamilial tension)
    2. Restrictive anorectics (pure dieters)
- Most anorectics are female, though the number of affected males is apparently increasing

- Previously largely confined to the affluent, the disorder now affects *all* social classes and ethnic groups

Bulimia

- Bulimia may be a syndrome distinct from anorexia nervosa, characterized by secretive binge eating followed by self-induced vomiting, fasting, or use of laxatives or diuretics. The diagnosis is based on DSM-III
  1. Recurrent episodes of binge eating
  2. At least three of the following
     - Consumption of high calorie, easily ingested food during a binge
     - Termination of binging by abdominal pain, sleep, or vomiting
     - Secretive eating during a binge
     - Repeated attempts to lose weight
     - Frequent weight fluctuation of >4.5 kg
  3. Awareness of abnormal eating pattern and fear of not being able to stop voluntarily
  4. Depressed mood after a binge
  5. Not due to anorexia nervosa or any physical disorder

Clinical Features

- See Table 1–2

TABLE 1–2 Some Clinical Features of Anorexia Nervosa and Bulimia

	Anorexia	*Bulimia*

Psychologic
  High achievers with average or above average intelligence
  Perfectionistic
  Low self-esteem
  Distorted perceptions (especially body image)		

TABLE 1–2 Some Clinical Features of Anorexia Nervosa and Bulimia

	Anorexia	Bulimia
Behavioral	Increasingly desperate pursuit of thinness	Self-induced vomiting
	Preoccupation with food, calories, and exercise	Secretive overeating
	Decreased sexual interest	Sexually active
	Denial of weight problem	Distressed by symptoms
General	Hypothermia and cold intolerance	
	Dry skin	
	Lanugo, easy bruising	
Gastrointestinal	Slowed gastric emptying	Acute gastric dilation
	Constipation	Esophagitis, Mallory-Weiss syndrome
Cardiovascular	Bradycardia, dysrhythmias	Possible ipecac poisoning
	Hypotension	
Hematologic	Pancytopenia	
Metabolic	Features of dehydration	Hypochloremic, hyponatremic, metabolic alkalosis (may be secondary to vomiting, diuretics, or laxatives)
	Elevated carotene level	
Endocrine	Amenorrhea	Menstrual irregularities
	Growth retardation (if prolonged starvation during growth spurt)	
	"Senile" vaginitis	
	Partial diabetes insipidus	
	Euthyroid sick syndrome (TSH level normal; T_4 level normal or low; T_3 level low)	
	GH level normal or high (somatomedin C level low)	
	Estradiol-testosterone levels low	
	Basal FSH and LH levels low	

Management

- Best accomplished by a team
- Medical surveillance to detect severe physiologic upsets and intervene
- Individual psychotherapy to explore ways of coping and developing insight
- Family therapy and supportive counseling to assist family members in their efforts to help
- Dietitian—counseling to try to keep diet balanced and ensure appropriate caloric content

Exogenous Obesity

- Exogenous obesity is excessive weight attained usually because of increased caloric consumption with or without reduced physical activity. It is generally regarded as significant when
  1. Persistently >2 standard deviations (SDs) above ideal weight for height
  2. Triceps or subscapular skinfold thickness >85–90th percentile for age and sex
     - Long-term risks possibly include
       1. Hypertension
       2. Type II diabetes mellitus
       3. Early death
       4. Polycythemia

Management

- Supervised, balanced reducing diet combined with graded exercise program and supportive psychotherapy (behavior modification)

ABNORMAL GROWTH

General Considerations

- Growth takes on a special significance in adolescence, both for the parents (who worry about their child's "normality") and for the teenager (who feels different from his peers)

- Occasionally the complaint is of excessive growth, especially in girls, but most frequently short stature is the cause for concern
- Most cases of short stature in adolescence are the result of either constitutional delay of puberty or familial short stature. However, each case must be individually assessed.
- Some important preliminary steps include
  1. Establish that the case in question *does* fall more than 2 SDs below the mean (or <3rd percentile), by plotting on a standard growth chart (see p 210–217)
  2. If available, try to plot growth velocity from serial height values previously recorded. Remember that peak height velocity in girls occurs ~ 1½–2 yr earlier than in boys. Normal growth velocity is >5 cm/yr.
  3. Inquire about growth and sexual development of both parents. Measure both parents' height and calculate midparental height*
  4. Inquire about and look for any indication(s) of chronic disease or dysmorphism
  5. Birth weight and neonatal history (e.g., prematurity, small for gestational age) should be sought
  6. Establish sexual maturity rating (see p 223–225, developmental section)
  7. Establish detailed dietary history
- Determine whether short stature is associated with delayed or normal sexual development (Table 1–3)

* Midparental height is calculated by plotting the same-sex parent's height on the same height chart as the patient's height and then plotting the other parent's height (± 12.5 cm depending on sex of patient) on the same chart. For example, if the patient is a boy, 12.5 cm is *added* to the maternal height before plotting it, whereas if the patient is a girl, 12.5 cm is *subtracted* from the father's height. The midparental height is then the midpoint between both plotted points, which is the average predicted adult height of the child.

Short Stature With Delayed Sexual Development	Short Stature Without Delayed Sexual Development
Constitutional short stature Hypopituitarism, hypothyroidism, Cushing syndrome, Turner syndrome, Prader-Willi syndrome ± Chronic illness	Familial or genetic short stature Intrauterine growth retardation Chondrodystrophies—disproportionate short stature ± Chronic illness

- Constitutional growth delay is suggested by the following:
  1. Height at birth often normal, falling to 3rd percentile or below by age 2–3 yr and then running parallel to but below the 3rd percentile
  2. Consistent prepubertal growth velocity of $\geq$4–5 cm/yr
  3. Delayed adolescence often with a positive family history of similar delay while attaining normal adult height
  4. Height age = bone age < chronologic age
  5. Males >> females
- Familial short stature suggested by
  1. Consistent growth (normal velocity) < 3rd percentile
  2. Positive family history of short stature
  3. Final stature is short
  4. Height age < bone age = chronologic age
  5. Normal pubertal age

Management

- Investigations
  1. First line (after full history and physical

examination)
  - CBC and ESR
  - Urinalysis $\pm$ renal function
  - Bone age
  - Thyroid function (T_4, TSH)
  - Karyotype (in all females to rule out Turner's syndrome, especially if associated with delayed puberty)

2. Second line (as indicated)
  - Specific endocrinologic investigations (e.g., GH) best done by endocrinologist
  - GI series (consider inflammatory bowel disease)
  - Skull films or head CT scan

- Therapy
  1. Appropriate treatment of any identifiable organic cause (rare)
  2. Often psychologic counseling and support, along with a clear explanation of the reason for growth delay and probable outcome, are all that is required
  3. Selected cases of constitutional growth delay in boys can be treated with androgen (e.g., testosterone enanthate) to accelerate growth and sexual maturation after consultation with endocrinologist
  4. Follow-up at 6 mo intervals, or preferably more frequently

SUBSTANCE ABUSE

General Considerations and Clinical Features

- Includes unapproved use of licit drugs (medications, ethanol) as well as illicit or "street" drugs (most commonly cannabis products, hallucinogens)
- There is no pathognomonic clinical presentation; maintain a high index of suspicion
- Risk factors include
  1. Excessive alcohol use by one or both parents or strong family history of alcoholism

2. Increased availability of alcohol or drugs in home environment
   3. Early peer choices relevant to drug use or deviant behavior
   4. Significant parental conflicts
   5. Early childhood alienation from family and community structure (e.g., poor academic performance or school attendance)
   6. Inconsistent parenting style $\pm$ verbal, physical, or sexual abuse
- Be suspicious of accuracy of history (e.g., inappropriate fears by parents, denial by patient)
- Indirect clues include
   1. Deterioration in family relationships and school or athletic performance
   2. Law breaking and change of friends may also occur
   3. Lack of interest in appearance and personal hygiene
- Multiple functional complaints may be a sign of drug abuse
- Signs and symptoms of specific toxins (e.g., pinpoint pupils with opiates) may be present
- Areas to explore
   1. Number, frequency, amount, duration of use
   2. Peer group and factors influencing drug use
   3. Degree of disruption in family, academic, athletic, work, and social lives
   4. Family history of substance abuse or psychiatric disorders
   5. Solitary or group use of drugs (former at greatest risk)
   6. Physical or psychologic dependence

Management

- Physical examination generally not very helpful (occasionally thrombophlebitis or skin inflammation occurs at injection sites—"track marks"). Irritation of mucous membranes may lead to nose bleeds in cocaine users (or "red eyes" if

the conjunctival sac is used for absorption).
- Laboratory identification of drugs often is not *useful* (depending on timing of sample in relation to most recent drug use, rate of metabolism). It is sometimes possible to identify active substances or their metabolites in serum, (e.g., ethanol, opiates) or urine (e.g., cannabis).
- Liver function tests (AST, ALT) may be abnormal in up to 40% of heroin abusers
- There are no clear-cut successful treatment regimens. Helpful resources may include
  1. Support groups for patients or family
  2. Frequent individual counseling
  3. Specially interested friends, school teachers
- Involvement with substances may be a response to some underlying stress or psychopathologic disorder that needs to be identified and resolved before the symptom of substance abuse can be eradicated
- Hospitalization may be required for patients with medical complications (e.g., endocarditis) or withdrawal problems
- Counseling about the relationship between substance abuse and accidents needs to be given to all adolescents

CONTRACEPTION

- See p 245, gynecology section

SEXUALLY TRANSMITTED DISEASES

- See p 341, infectious diseases section

DEPRESSION AND SUICIDE

- See p 31 and 33, behavioral pediatrics section

SEXUAL ABUSE

- See p 35 and 249, behavioral and gynecology sections

Suggested Reading

1. Daniel WA. Adolescence. I. Medical aspects. Pediatr Ann 1986; 15(10):entire volume.
2. Daniel WA. Adolescence. II. Psychosocial aspects. Pediatr Ann 1986; 15(11):entire volume.
3. Neinstein LS. Adolescent health care—a practical guide. Baltimore: Urban and Schwarzenberg, 1984.

2 ALLERGY AND IMMUNOLOGY

IMMUNOLOGY

Immunodeficiency Disorders (IDDs)

General Considerations

- IDDs are characterized by an increased susceptibility to infection. This may present as:
  1. Recurrent pyogenic infections in different
  sites or more than one severe pyogenic
  infection, e.g., meningitis, osteomyelitis
  2. Prolonged infection with a poor response to
  antibiotics
  3. Unusually severe infections
  4. Infection with unusual organisms, e.g.,
  Pneumocystis carinii, Aspergillus
  5. Illness following live virus vaccination, e.g.,
  MMR
- IDDs may be primary or secondary. Secondary
immunodeficiency is more common.
  Causes of secondary immunodeficiency:
  1. Malignant disease, e.g., leukemia, lymphoma
  2. Immunosuppressive agents, e.g., antineoplastic drugs, corticosteroids, radiation
  3. Infections, e.g., HIV-I (see p 20)
  4. Hematologic disorders, e.g., sickle cell
  disease
  5. Metabolic disorders, e.g., diabetes mellitus,
  severe uremia, galactosemia
  6. Nutritional deficiencies, e.g., protein-calorie
  malnutrition
  7. Protein-losing states, e.g., nephrotic syndrome, protein-losing enteropathy
  8. Splenectomy
  9. Prematurity

TABLE 2–1 Classification of Primary Immunodeficiency Disorders

Predominant B cell defects
  Common variable immunodeficiency
  X-linked agammaglobulinemia
  Transient hypogammaglobulinemia of infancy
  Immunodeficiency with increased IgM (XL)*
  IgA deficiency

Predominant T cell defects
  DiGeorge syndrome
  Cartilage-hair hypoplasia
  Chronic mucocutaneous candidiasis
  Purine nucleoside phosphorylase deficiency

Combined T and B cell defects
  Severe combined immunodeficiency (AR or XL)*
  Severe combined immunodeficiency with adenosine deaminase (ADA) deficiency
  Combined immunodeficiency with immunoglobulins (Nezelof syndrome)
  Ataxia-telangiectasia (AR)*—↓IgA
  Wiskott-Aldrich syndrome (XL)*—↑IgA, ↑IgE, ↓IgM

Neutrophil disorders
  Defective production
    Cyclical neutropenia
    Aplastic anemia
    Kostmann's syndrome
    Schwachman-Diamond syndrome
  Disorders of cell movement
    Lazy leukocyte syndrome
    Hyperimmunoglobulin E syndrome
  Disorders of phagocytosis
    Actin dysfunction
  Defective microbicidal activity
    Chronic granulomatous disease
    Chédiak-Higashi syndrome (defective degranulation)

Deficiency of complement components
  Early components (C1-C4)—associated with collagen vascular disease
  Late components (C5-C9)—associated with Neisseria infection

* XL = X-linked inheritance; AR = Autosomal recessive inheritance.

Clinical Features

- Nonspecific features
  1. Failure to thrive
  2. Chronic diarrhea, often with malabsorption
  3. Absence of lymph nodes and tonsils (though patient may have lymphadenopathy)
  4. Hepatosplenomegaly
  5. Persistent candidiasis
  6. Family history of collagen vascular disorder, early infant deaths, or increased susceptibility to infection
- Specific features: see Table 2–2

Differential Diagnosis

- Specific exclusions to be made include
  1. Allergy, e.g., asthma, allergic rhinitis
  2. Foreign body associated with infection, e.g., aspirated foreign body, central venous line
  3. Cystic fibrosis
  4. Integumentary defects, e.g., ciliary abnormalities
  5. Infection with resistant organisms
  6. Continuous reinfection, e.g., contaminated water supply

Management

- Investigations
  1. Screening tests: see Table 2–2
  2. Further investigations
     - Should be done in consultation with pediatric immunologist or infectious disease specialist
     - Should be done if there is an abnormality detected on screening tests or if there is convincing clinical evidence of an IDD, even if screening test results are normal

- Treatment
  1. General measures
     - Antibiotics:
       a. Prophylactic, e.g., co-trimoxazole with neutropenia or post splenectomy
       b. Therapeutic
     - Immunizations:
       a. Avoid live vaccines in T cell and B cell disorders and some secondary IDDs (e.g., generalized malignant disease and immunosuppressive agents, including corticosteroids). Live vaccines can be given when there are neutrophil and complement disorders.
       b. Active immunization with pneumococcal vaccine, e.g., prior to splenectomy or in sickle cell disease
       c. Passive immunization with gamma globulin, especially after exposure to varicella (B cell, T cell, and some of the secondary IDDs)
     - Avoid contact with infectious diseases
     - Caution with blood transfusions
       a. Selective IgA deficiency: require washed packed cells to avoid anaphylaxis
       b. T cell defects: require irradiated blood products to prevent graft versus host reaction
     - Family studies and genetic counseling: prenatal diagnosis is available for some primary IDDs utilizing amniocentesis or fetal blood sampling
  2. Specific therapy
     - Gamma globulin replacement for B cell defects
     - Bone marrow transplantation for T cell and combined defects

TABLE 2–2 Clinical and Laboratory Differentiation of the Major Immunodeficiency Syndrome Subgroups

Immune Deficiency	B Cell (Antibody) Defects	T Cell (Cellular) Defects	Neutrophil Disorders	Complement Deficiencies
Relative incidence*	50%	30% 10% cellular 20% combined	18%	2%
Infecting organisms	Common pyogenic organisms, e.g., pneumococcus, H. influenzae	Bacteria, fungi, viruses, protozoa, mycobacteria	Staphylococcus, gram negative organisms, fungi	Bacteria (Neisseria with C6, C7, and C8 deficiency)
Common sites and types of infection	Skin, sinopulmonary, middle ear	Candidiasis of skin, mucous membranes and nails; pneumonitis; enteritis	Skin, lymph nodes, liver (abscess), lung, bone, periodontal, perirectal	Meningitis, disseminated gonococcal infection
Specific features	Tetany, congenital heart disease, unusual facies—DiGeorge syndrome Ataxia, telangiectasia of skin and conjunctivae—ataxia-telangiectasia Eczema, thrombocytopenia (with petechiae and bleeding)—Wiskott-Aldrich syndrome		Delayed umbilical cord detachment (>3 wk) Partial oculo-cutaneous	Associated autoimmune disorders

	Short limb dwarfism; fine, light colored hair—cartilage-hair hypoplasia		albinism—Chédiak-Higashi syndrome	
Screening tests[†]	1. Quantitative immunoglobulins: IgG, IgM, IgA (see p 759 for normal values) 2. Antibody levels: diphtheria, tetanus, polio, rubella 3. Isohemagglutinins: anti-A, anti-B—useful >6 mo 4. Schick test	1. Lymphocyte count: $<1.5 \times 10^9$/L (<1500/mm^3) 2. CXR for thymic shadow (<1 yr) 3. Delayed hypersensitivity skin tests, e.g., Candida, PPD, tetanus toxoid—less reliable <1 yr	1. Neutrophil count: $<1.5 \times 10^9$/L (<1500/mm^3)—must be repeated 2. IgE level 3. Bone marrow aspirate if persistent neutropenia 4. NBT test (nitroblue tetrazolium reduction)	1. Total hemolytic complement (CH$_{50}$) 2. C3, C4

* Excludes asymptomatic IgA deficiency. IgA deficiency occurs in ~ 1:400 individuals.
† Screening tests: CBC to be done in all cases. Neutrophil and complement studies if convincing history of IDD with normal T and B cell function. HIV-I serology in high risk groups for AIDS.

Immunoglobulins

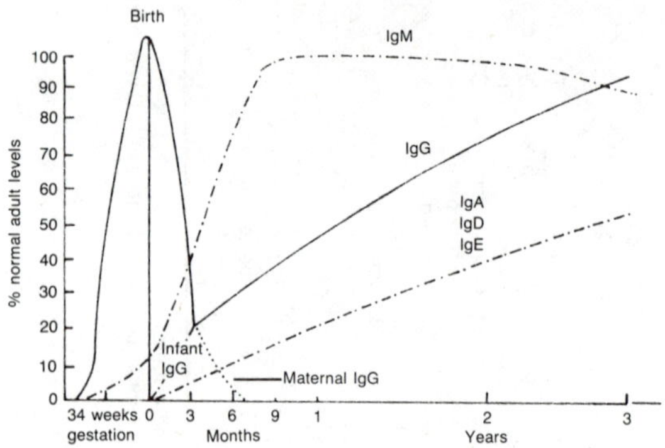

Figure 2–1   Changes in serum immunoglobulin levels in late fetal life and early childhood. (From Stern CM. Immunology. In: Godfrey S, Baum JD, eds. Clinical paediatric physiology. Oxford: Blackwell, 1979:22.)

Acquired Immunodeficiency Syndrome (AIDS)

General Considerations

- AIDS is caused by the human immunodeficiency virus, type I (HIV-I), having an incubation period of 1 mo to several years. It is *NOT* transmitted by casual contact.

Pediatric Risk Groups for AIDS

- Adolescents (same as for adults)
    1. Homosexual or bisexual males
    2. Persons who received blood or blood products (especially prior to November, 1985; since November, 1985, all blood donors in Canada have been screened for antibody to HIV-I)

3. Intravenous drug users
4. Sexual contacts of persons with HIV-I infection or persons from groups at increased risk for infection
5. Persons from areas where HIV-I infection or AIDS is endemic, e.g., equatorial Africa, Haiti
- Younger children
  1. Newborns and infants of a parent who has AIDS or who is a member of a high risk group
  2. Children receiving blood or blood products

Clinical Features

- There are three categories of infection with HIV-I:
  1. AIDS case. This is defined by
     - Presence of an opportunistic disease such as
       a. *Pneumocystis carinii* pneumonia
       b. Kaposi's sarcoma
       c. Chronic lymphoid interstitial pneumonitis (confirmed histologically)
     - Presence of at least one of the following:
       a. Serum antibody to HIV-I
       b. Low number of T helper cells
       c. Low ratio of T helper to T suppressor cells
     - Exclusion of the following:
       a. Congenital infections, e.g., toxoplasma or herpes simplex in the first month of life or cytomegalovirus in the first 6 mo of life
       b. Primary and secondary immunodeficiency disorders
  2. AIDS related complex (ARC)—nonspecific symptoms occurring in individuals in high risk groups
     - Lymphadenopathy
     - Weight loss or failure to thrive
     - Parotid swelling

- Increased susceptibility to infection
- 5–20% of adults with ARC develop AIDS over a 3 yr period, but the risk of progression to AIDS in children is unknown
3. Antibody to HIV-I in asymptomatic individuals
   - HIV-I can be found in the blood and body fluids of most antibody positive individuals, and therefore they are potentially infectious, but only by intimate sexual contact or through blood or blood products.

Management

- Precautions in caring for patients infected with HIV-I are the same as those for infection with hepatitis B.

ALLERGY

General Considerations

- Atopy may be defined as an increased tendency to form IgE antibodies to common environmental allergens
- Anaphylaxis: see p 661

Clinical Features

- Allergies in childhood commonly manifest as asthma, allergic rhinitis, atopic dermatitis, urticaria, and various forms of food reactions
- Symptoms suggestive of an allergic disorder:
  1. Eczema
  2. Seasonal rhinorrhea or conjunctivitis, associated with itching
  3. Sneezing, rhinorrhea, conjunctivitis, or edema shortly after contact with animals
  4. Immediate development of hives, swelling, or abdominal symptoms after ingestion of a specific food
  5. Cough (with or without wheezing) that is

prolonged, following an upper respiratory
tract infection
- A history of allergy in immediate family
  members—an important predictor of allergy in
  the child

Investigations

- Confirmation of allergic disorder
  1. WBC: eosinophilia of $>5\%$ or $>0.25 \times 10^9$/L (>250/mm^3)
  2. Smear of nasal secretions or bronchial mucus for eosinophils
  3. Serum IgE: if elevated, may be associated with an allergic disorder
- Identification of the cause
  1. These tests can be interpreted only in the context of the allergy history
     - Skin testing
       a. A sensitive technique for the detection of specific IgE antibodies
       b. Antihistamines should be withheld 24–48 hr prior to skin testing because they may blunt a wheal and erythema reaction (moderate corticosteroid therapy will not interfere with this reaction)
       c. Prick or scratch tests should always be tried first, since they are more specific, safer, less painful, and easier to perform than intradermal tests
       d. When the prick test is negative despite a history that strongly implicates a particular allergen in producing a patient's symptoms, intradermal tests may be done
       e. Skin testing should be carried out with common allergens implicated by the history (rather than a whole battery of tests)
       f. Skin tests (especially intradermal) may cause anaphylaxis in highly sensitive individuals

TABLE 2–3 Antigens Useful for Skin Testing*

Allergic Disorders	Antigens
Asthma Allergic rhinitis Allergic conjunctivitis	Pollens House dust House dust mites Molds Animal danders
Drug sensitivity	Penicillin Cephalosporins
Insect sting allergy	Insect venoms
Food reaction	Fish, nuts, peanuts, eggs (when these cause immediate and obvious reactions)

* Skin tests are less useful in identifying the specific allergens responsible for eczema, urticaria, angioedema, and other food reactions, such as those involving fruits and vegetables.

- Radioallergosorbent test (RAST)
  a. This is an in vitro test for the detection of specific IgE antibodies
  b. Particularly useful for life threatening hypersensitivity reactions and in patients with extensive dermatitis or severe dermatographia
  c. Not adequate for precluding anaphylactic sensitivity to penicillin (no available RAST for the minor determinants)
  d. Limited value for detecting insect venom allergy
- Challenge testing
  a. Useful for sensitivities to drugs, foods, and various biologic products, such as vaccines, insulins, and heterologous sera
  b. Associated with a risk of anaphylaxis and therefore should be undertaken with caution in a hospital

Treatment

- General measures
  1. Education—early recognition of an allergic reaction and early medical consultation
  2. Avoidance of allergens
     - Environmental, e.g.
       a. Minimize house dust
       b. Prohibit smoking in the home
       c. With pollen allergy, have air conditioner that recirculates the air within the home
     - Drugs—use of alternative antibiotics
     - Household pets—if there is clear evidence of allergy to a pet, it should be removed unless there is a compelling psychosocial reason that it should stay
  3. EpiPen Jr. or Anakit with instructions about its use. Epinephrine is the acute treatment of any allergic reaction with systemic symptoms such as stridor, breathing difficulty, or swelling of the tongue.
  4. Medic Alert bracelet
- Specific measures
  1. Allergic rhinitis
     - Antihistamines
     - Sympathomimetics: oral (e.g., pseudoephedrine), intranasal (for short-term use only, to avoid rebound vasodilation)
     - Intranasal steroids e.g., beclomethasone for symptoms resistant to antihistamine and decongestant therapy
     - Intranasal cromoglycate sodium (cromolyn sodium) for prophylaxis
     - Immunotherapy
  2. Insect allergy
     - Large local reaction: ice and elevation; antihistamines; immunotherapy *not* indicated
     - Systemic reaction, e.g., laryngeal, respiratory, or cardiovascular symptoms: if skin testing for venom specific IgE is positive,

venom immunotherapy is indicated (highly protective).
3. Penicillin allergy

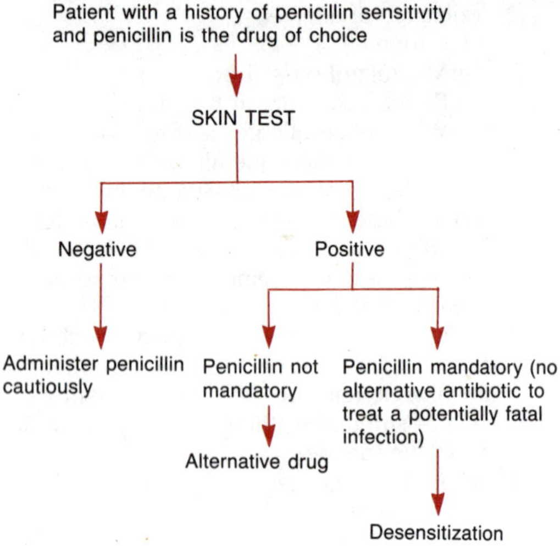

Figure 2–2 Management of suspected penicillin sensitivity.

- Skin testing must be performed immediately prior to penicillin therapy. It is not a valid predictor of sensitivity months or years later.
- Both the major and minor determinants must be tested
- Desensitization
  a. Oral regimen begins with 10^{-6} of the usual dose of the specific penicillin to be used and gradually increases
  b. Be prepared to treat anaphylaxis
  c. Avoid premedication with antihistamines and corticosteroids so as not to mask an early reaction

d. Once penicillin has been discontinued for >48 hr, the patient is no longer considered desensitized
- Other penicillins: Sensitivity to penicillin is a contraindication to use of any of the semisynthetic analogues of penicillin.
- Cephalosporins: If sensitivity to penicillin has been confirmed by skin testing, cephalosporins should be avoided. If skin testing has not been performed, the risk of a reaction to cephalosporins is unknown.

4. Food reaction
   - Elimination diets should be avoided in infants and toddlers because attention to nutrition is of paramount importance
   - If there is a readily identifiable reaction to a specific food, this can be eliminated, with appropriate substitution when necessary

5. For the specific management of the following conditions, refer to the pages indicated:
   - Asthma: see p 606
   - Anaphylaxis: see p 661
   - Atopic dermatitis: see p 83
   - Urticaria: see p 101

Hereditary Angioedema
General Considerations and Clinical Features

- Should be differentiated from allergic disorders
- Episodic attacks of localized subcutaneous edema, which is nonpitting, painless, and not associated with itching or inflammation
- Mucous membrane involvement may result in laryngeal edema, which may be fatal, or severe abdominal pain
- Episodes usually last 2–3 days
- Episodes may follow exercise, trauma, or emotional stress or may be associated with extremes of temperature and menstruation
- May be inherited as an autosomal dominant disorder

Management

- Investigations
  1. Low C4 with normal C3 (C4 remains low even between acute episodes)
  2. Low C1 esterase inhibitor level (level may be normal in 15%, but enzyme activity is always low)
- Treatment
  1. Acute: symptomatic; tracheotomy may be required
  2. Long-term: Stanozalol has limited usefulness in children because of androgenic side effects

Suggested Reading

Immunology

1. Jones JJ, Fulginiti VA. Recurrent bacterial infections in children. Pediatr Rev 1979; 1:99–108.
2. Rogers MF. AIDS in children: a review of the clinical, epidemiologic and public health aspects. Pediatr Infect Dis 1985; 4:230–236.
3. Stiehm RE. Clinical and laboratory evaluation of the child with suspected immunodeficiency. Pediatr Rev 1985; 7:53–61.

Allergy

4. Ellis EF, ed. Symposium on pediatric allergy. Pediatr Clin North Am 1983; 30(5):(entire issue).
5. Sher TH. Penicillin hypersensitivity—a review. Pediatr Clin North Am 1983; 30:161–176.
6. Subcommittee of the Allergy Section, Canadian Pediatric Society. Skin testing for allergy in children. Can Med Assoc J 1983; 129:828–830.
7. Zimmerman B, et al. Allergy in pediatrics. Can Fam Phys 1985; 31:1071–1074.

3 BEHAVIORAL PEDIATRICS

This section is subdivided into two subsections. The first deals with a general approach to pediatric psychiatric issues and the second, with child abuse.

CHILD PSYCHIATRY

General Considerations

- Psychiatric difficulties may present as
    1. A physical symptom reflecting an emotional disturbance, such as depression, anxiety, or unidentified stress or a psychosocial issue within the child or within the family
    2. Psychological factors complicating physical diseases or disorders
    3. Psychological reactions to medical drug treatment
    4. Behavioral problems on the hospital wards
    5. Problems at school (e.g., conduct disorder, attention deficit disorder [ADD])
    6. Disturbances of social interaction (e.g., autism, ADD)
- The chief complaint presented to pediatricians by the child or parent is estimated to be a behavioral or learning problem in 20–60% of the cases
- Any patient who presents with an "apparent" psychiatric symptom should be approached with the medical model
- A mental status examination should be carried out (Table 3–1)

Somatoform Disorders

General Considerations and Clinical Features

- The essential features of this group of disorders

1. Appearance
   Behavior—minor (e.g., nail biting, eye blinking) and major (psychomotor retardation)
   Speech—vocabulary (intelligence?), receptive and expressive
   Thought—form, content
   Perception—e.g., hallucinations—visual (organic brain syndrome) and auditory (schizophrenia)
   Mood—subjective (what they say), objective (what you see)

2. Sensorium (especially in acute or chronic brain syndromes)
   Orientation—person, place, time
   Memory—recent, long-term
   Attention and concentration
   Intelligence (general information, vocabulary)
   Judgment (patient's)
   Insight (why does he think he is ill?)

are physical symptoms suggesting a somatic disorder for which there are no demonstrable organic findings and for which there is positive evidence that the symptoms are linked to psychological factors or conflicts
- The following features should be sought
  1. The patient's prior use of symptoms as a psychological defence
  2. The presence of a significant emotional stress prior to onset of symptoms
  3. Evidence that the symptom is being used to solve a conflict, thereby achieving secondary gain

Acute Psychoses

General Considerations and Definitions

- Psychoses are conditions in which the patient's ability to care for himself and to distinguish reality from fantasy is severely impaired
- These include
  1. Infantile autism: A developmental disorder characterized by an inability to develop rela-

tionships with people, a delay in speech acquisition, and the presence of repetitive and stereotyped play activities
   2. Organic psychoses: May be associated with illnesses such as hypothyroidism, herpes simplex encephalitis, and systemic lupus erythematosus, to name a few. A wide variety of drugs may cause psychotic features, including such commonly used drugs as steroids, digitalis, and anticholinergic drugs (look for disorganization of sensorium).
   3. Functional psychoses: The main illnesses in this group are the schizophrenias and major affective disorders. They may begin in child-hood, but do so most often during the preadolescent or adolescent period. The onset may be as early as age 7 yr.

Management

- Any psychotic child needs to be assessed immediately by a member of the psychiatry team.

School Refusal

General Considerations/Management

- Definition: persistent nonattendance at school (originally termed "school phobia")
- A serious cause for educational concern
- The urgent aspect of this condition is that the child must be returned to school immediately or the situation will worsen
- If this is not possible with the help of a pediatrician, the child and family should be seen by a psychiatry consultant ASAP

Depression

General Considerations and Clinical Features

- Definition: depression is a disorder of mood

often described, e.g., as sad or hopeless, and associated with social withdrawal, numerous somatic complaints, cognitive changes, significantly low self-esteem, and feelings of worthlessness

- Depression may occur in children, with the frequency increasing in adolescence
- May occur transiently as part of normal mood swings or in reaction to short-lived situational episodes, may be persistent in response to chronic situational stress, or may be a true affective disorder
- In a depressed child or adolescent, manifestations of depression may be evident in the patient's thinking, behavior, affect, and body functioning (Table 3–2)

TABLE 3–2 Some Features of Depression in Childhood and Adolescence

Psychologic	Behavioral
Sad or despondent mood	School refusal or changes in performance
Negative self-esteem or poor self-image	Loss of interest in usual activities
Hopelessness, helplessness, and loneliness	Acting out, e.g., truancy, running away, petty crimes
Physical	crimes
Sleep disturbances	Sexual promiscuity
Eating disturbances (weight loss or obesity)	Hypochondriasis
Headaches, chronic fatigue	Substance abuse
Menstrual irregularities	Suicidal gestures
Gastrointestinal disturbances	

- Predisposing or precipitating factors include
  1. Family history of affective disorders
  2. Significant loss (real or imagined), such as divorce of parents, death of friend or relative, physical illness, or rejection by a boy- or girlfriend.
  3. Family conflicts or poor communication

  4. Discrepancy between self-perception and
     parental or self-expectations
  5. Learning disabilities
  6. Concerns related to peer relationships and
     sexuality

Management

- Treatment must be individualized in response to
  the degree of depression and its etiology
- Modalities include age appropriate supportive
  counseling, individual or family psychotherapy,
  and antidepressant medication

Suicide

General Considerations

- Suicide is one of the three major causes of
  teenage mortality; unsuccessful attempts are
  many times (~20–40 times) more common
- Males are more likely to succeed in suicide;
  females are more likely to attempt
- Every suicide gesture *must* be treated as a
  genuine emergency, with a full assessment not
  only of the physical effects of the attempt, but
  also of the precipitating factors, and arrangements made for follow-up and on-going
  treatment

Management

- This acute medical emergency is managed in
  the classic manner of
  1. Attending first to the condition itself, then
  2. The predisposing factors
  3. The complications, and finally
  4. Follow-up
- The management of the condition depends
  largely on the method used in attempting
  suicide
  1. Poisonings and overdoses are most frequently
     associated with females and suicidal gestures
  2. Firearms, explosives, and suffocation by hang-

ing or drowning are more likely to be used by males and represent a *non*-gesture
    3. Other methods include jumping from a high place and self-mutilation, which may cause bone or soft tissue damage
- Although it is not possible to identify the particular individual who will attempt suicide, the following *risk factors* should alert one to the possibility of a suicidal attempt, and should also be addressed in the treatment of any patient who has attempted suicide:
    1. Environment
        - Home
            a. History of broken family or family discord
            b. Recent loss of a significant person
            c. Alcoholic parents
            d. History of suicide in the family
        - School
            a. Change in performance
            b. Withdrawal from usual activities
    2. Individual
        - Changes in behavior—either increasing social isolation or an increase in daredevil or delinquent behavior
        - Substance abuse
        - Prior suicidal gesture or expression of desire to commit suicide (attempts by shooting or jumping are at higher risk than those by ingestion or cutting)
- Complications of an attempt include
    1. Success (i.e., death)
    2. Side effects of method used, e.g., drug effect
    3. Recurrence
    4. Changes in inter-relationships with peers and family
- Every suicide attempt managed in hospital requires a formal assessment by a psychiatrist. In addition, arrangements must be made for
    1. Medical treatment of any effects resulting from the current attempt

2. An assessment of the risk of reattempting, so
   that a decision can be made whether to
   hospitalize
3. Assessment of family, peer, and other existing
   support systems
4. Assessment of the individual's coping
   abilities
5. Identification of precipitating factors and plan
   of intervention as to how these may be
   changed
6. Identification of individuals or services that
   will be involved in follow-up. N.B. It is
   essential that those services expected to
   become involved be notified and be agree-
   able prior to the patient's discharge.

Child Abuse

General Considerations

- Definitions
   1. Physical injury or deprivation of nutrition,
      care, or affection in circumstances indicating
      that such injury or deprivation is not
      accidental
   2. Age inappropriate sexual encounter between
      a child and another individual
- Children may be the victims of more than one
  type of abuse

Management

- Investigations
   1. Assessment (see also Table 3–3)
      - History
         a. Allegations made by or on behalf of the
            child
         b. Guardian(s): social risk factors, substance
            abuse, mental health, present crisis; his-
            tory of sexual or physical abuse in
            guardian
         c. Child: development, past injuries, illness,

or accidental poisoning, behavior
  d. Presenting complaint: contradictory or no
     explanation; circumstances of the injury
     and home management of same (? inap-
     propriate)
- Physical examination: *must be conducted
  with patience and sensitivity*
  a. Complete examination is essential
  b. Plot heights and weights on appropriate
     charts
  c. Examine fundi of infants; check for
     retinal hemorrhages
  d. Examine genitalia and anus. Do internal
     examination only if specific indications.
     Do not use restraining measures: If the
     child will not cooperate, defer the exami-
     nation or enlist the help of a sub-
     specialist.
  e. Document all visible trauma—size,
     shape, color, and location
  f. Record child's behavior and reactions
- Laboratory investigations
  a. Suspected physical abuse
     - Hematology—rule out blood dyscrasia
     - Skeletal survey or bone scan in young
       children—record location and age of
       fractures and rule out metabolic bone
       disease
  b. Alleged sexual abuse (see also p 249)
     - Forensic specimen—some jurisdictions
       use sexual assault evidence kit
     - Specimen for sexually transmitted
       diseases
     - Pregnancy test
  c. Color photography. Record obvious
     trauma—important legal documentation.
- Treatment and further management
  1. Most jurisdictions have laws requiring profes-
     sionals to report *suspected* child abuse to the
     appropriate authorities *without delay*
  2. Admit for treatment or protection if indicated

TABLE 3–3 Child Abuse Indicators*

Physical	*Behavioral*

1. Injuries not explained by history given
2. General care and nutrition
    Inadequate clothing
    Poor hygiene
    Failure to thrive
    Inadequate medical attention
3. Bruises and welts
    On face, back, buttocks, thighs
    At different stages of healing
    In the shape of an instrument or hand
4. Burns
    Cigarette burns, especially multiple burns
    Immersion burns
    In the shape of an instrument
    Rope burns
5. Fractures
    To skull or facial structure
    Multiple, particularly at different stages of healing
    Spiral fractures
6. Retinal hemorrhages
7. Genitourinary
    Pregnancy
    Sexually transmitted diseases
    Abnormal dilation of orifices
	CHILD:
	1. Extreme wariness of parents and adults in general
	2. Extremes of behavior, e.g., aggressiveness, withdrawal, compliance, fearfulness
	3. Pseudomature behavior
	4. Self-destructive behavior, including suicide threats or attempts
	5. Changes in school performance
	6. Running away from home
	7. Sexual acting out or age inappropriate sexual knowledge
	8. Functional complaints, particularly abdominal pain
	
	GUARDIANS:
	1. Poor self-control, seem under stress
	2. Not responsive to child's needs
	3. History of physical or sexual abuse as a child
	4. Single parent, particularly if young and without support systems
	5. Substance abuse
	6. Mental illness

* While almost any physical or behavioral symptoms can be the result of child abuse, those listed are indicators that, particularly in combination, should raise the suspicion of the examining physician.

3. Treat injuries as indicated
4. Obtain necessary consultations, e.g., social work, psychiatry
5. Protection assessment to be carried out by appropriate authorities
6. Disposition to be planned with joint medical and social input

Suggested Reading

1. Daniel WA. Adolescence II. Psychosocial aspects. Pediatr Ann 1986; 15(11) (entire volume).
2. Fontana VJ. Child abuse and neglect. Pediatr Ann 1984; 13(10) (entire volume).
3. Neinstein LS. Adolescent health care—a practical guide. Baltimore: Urban and Schwarzenberg, 1984.
4. Rutter M, Hersov L. Child and adolescent psychiatry. 2nd ed. Oxford: Blackwell Scientific Publications, 1985.
5. Steinhauer PD, Rae-Grant Q. Psychological problems of the child in the family. 2nd ed. Toronto: Macmillan, 1983.

4 CARDIOLOGY

ABBREVIATIONS

AI	aortic insufficiency
AS	aortic stenosis
ASD	atrial septal defect
AVM	arteriovenous malformation
CAVSD	complete atrioventricular septal defect
CHB	congenital heart block
CHD	congenital heart disease
CHF	congestive heart failure
CMP	cardiomyopathy
CMV	cytomegalovirus
CRF	chronic renal failure
EFE	endocardial fibroelastosis
HLHS	hypoplastic left heart syndrome
ICP	intracranial pressure
IDM	infant of a diabetic mother
IHSS	idiopathic hypertrophic subaortic stenosis
MR	mitral regurgitation
MS	mitral stenosis
PA	pulmonary atresia
PAPVR	partial anomalous pulmonary venous drainage
PDA	patent ductus arteriosus
PFC	persistent fetal circulation
PS	pulmonary stenosis
RDS	respiratory distress syndrome
SBE	subacute bacterial endocarditis
SSS	sick sinus syndrome
SVT	supraventricular tachycardia
TA	tricuspid atresia
TAPVR	total anomalous pulmonary venous drainage
D-TGA	transposition of great arteries
L-TGA	corrected transposition of great arteries
TMI	transient myocardial ischemia
ToF	tetralogy of Fallot
VPB	ventricular premature beats
VSD	ventricular septal defect
VT	ventricular tachycardia

CYANOSIS (INFANT)

Differential Diagnosis

- Causes of peripheral cyanosis
  1. Acrocyanosis (autonomic)
  2. Sepsis
  3. Cold
  4. Polycythemia
- Causes of differential cyanosis
  1. Pink arms and blue legs:
     - Coarctation + PDA
     - PFC
     - HLHS + PDA
  2. Blue arms and pink legs: TGA + aortic arch interruption + PDA
- Causes of central cyanosis (PO_2 <50)
  1. PO_2 >50 but ↓ O_2 saturation = methemoglobinemia
  2. Hyperoxic test: (see Chapter 17, p 408)
     - PO_2 <100:CHD with R→L shunt
     - PO_2 >100
       a. Noncyanotic CHD + CHF
       b. Sepsis
       c. CNS lesion
       d. Hct >70
       e. Hypoglycemia
       f. Primary lung disease

CONGESTIVE HEART FAILURE

General Considerations

- Definition: a clinical syndrome in which the heart is unable to pump enough blood to meet the needs of the body or to dispose of venous return adequately, or a combination of both.

Differential Diagnosis

- Newborn: See Table 17–11 (p 411)
- Child:
  1. Rheumatic heart disease
  2. Endomyocardial disease (CMP)
  3. Endocarditis
  4. Anemia
  5. Dysrhythmias

Clinical Features and Investigations

- General features
  1. Tachycardia, tachypnea
  2. Gallop rhythm, weak pulse
  3. Failure to thrive
  4. Cardiomegaly
  5. Sweaty (cold sweat)
- Left sided failure (pulmonary congestion)
  1. Tachypnea
  2. Exertional dyspnea
  3. Orthopnea
  4. Wheezing, crackles
- Right sided failure (systemic congestion)
  1. Hepatomegaly
  2. Puffy eyelids
- Chest x-ray:
  1. Cardiomegaly
  2. ±Pulmonary venous congestion
- Electrocardiogram: not usually helpful in diagnosis of CHF

Management

- General measures
  1. Sitting up to relieve respiratory distress
  2. Humidified oxygen, 40–50% (monitor arterial blood gas levels)
  3. Digitalis should be given, except in presence of IHSS, complete heart block, or tamponade (see below)

4. ±Morphine sulfate, 0.1–0.2 mg/kg/dose SC q4h prn (may depress respiration)
- Digoxin
  1. Total digitalization dose (see Formulary)
     - Severe congestive heart failure demands initial IV administration. Early failure in less distressed infants can be treated orally. All patients should be switched to oral therapy as soon as feasible.
       Note: IV dosage is only 70–80% of amount used orally
     - One third stat, one third in 6 hr, and one third in another 8 hr
  2. Maintenance dose (see Formulary)
  3. Special situations
     - Myocarditis or myocardiopathy, e.g., rheumatic, viral, thalassemia, myocardial ischemia
       a. Use half the digitalization dose plus one half to one third the maintenance dose
       b. Monitor with ECG and serum digoxin levels
     - Renal failure
       a. Reduce dose
       b. Monitor with serum digoxin level (keep below 2.5 nmol/L [2.0 μg/L]) and electrocardiogram
     - Pulmonary edema
       a. Lasix, 1.0 mg/kg IV—slowly in 5–10 min
       b. Morphine, 0.2 mg/kg SC; maximal dose, 10 mg
       e. Digoxin: digitalize IV
       f. Oxygen
     - Digoxin monitoring (levels)
       a. After first five doses (and at least 6 hr after previous dose)
       b. In presence of CRF
       c. In presence of drugs that ↑ digoxin levels, e.g., quinidine, amiodarone
- Diuretics
  1. Acutely: furosemide (Lasix), 1 mg/kg/dose IM or IV (watch for ↓ K+)

2. Chronically: hydrochlorothiazide-
spironolactone (Aldactazide, Novospirozine),
1 mg/kg/dose PO q12h
- Vasodilators: captopril (see Formulary)

ELECTROCARDIOGRAPHY

General Considerations

**TABLE 4–1   Lead Placement for
Electrocardiography**

Lead	Positioning of Electrodes[*]
I	RA–LA
II	RA–LL
III	LA–LL
AVR	RA
AVL	LA
AVF	LE
V_1	4th RIC at RSB
V_2	4th LIC at LSB
V_3	Between V_2 and V_4
V_4	5th LIC at midclavicular line
V_5	5th LIC at anterior axillary line
V_6	5th LIC at midaxillary line
V_3R	V_3 on right chest
V_4	V_4 on right chest
V_7	Posterior axillary line

[*] RA = right arm; LA = left arm; LL = left leg; RIC = right intercostal space; LIC = left intercostal space; RSB = right sternal border; LSB = left sternal border.

Modified from Park MK. Pediatric cardiology for practitioners. Chicago: Year Book, 1984:36 and from Garson A Jr. The electrocardiogram in infants and children. Philadelphia: Lea & Febiger, 1983:32.

- Analyze ECG systematically: rate, rhythm, axis,
chamber enlargement, and strain-infarction (unusual in pediatrics; ST/T changes)
1. Rate: estimated by dividing 300 by number
of large squares (each 0.2 sec) between each
QRS, assuming regular rhythm. For normal
rates, see Table 4–2.

TABLE 4–2 Vital Signs in Pediatrics*

1. Acceptable Heart Rates in Pediatrics****

	Awake	Asleep	Exercise/Fever
Newborn	100→180	80→160	<220
1 wk→3 mo	100→220	80→200	<220
3 mo→2 yr	80→150	70→120	<200
2→10 yr	70→110	60→ 90	<200
>10 yr	55→ 90	50→ 90	<200

2. Respiratory Rates (Breaths/Minute) of Normal Children, of Both Sexes, Sleeping and Awake[†]

Age	Sleeping			Awake			Mean Difference Between Sleeping and Awake
	No.	Mean	Range	No.	Mean	Range	
6–12 mo	6	27	22–31	3	64	58–75	37
1–2 yr	6	19	17–23	4	35	30–40	16
2–4 yr	16	19	16–25	15	31	23–42	12
4–6 yr	23	18	14–23	22	26	19–36	8
6–8 yr	27	17	13–23	28	23	15–30	6
8–10 yr	19	18	14–23	19	21	15–31	3
10–12 yr	11	16	13–19	17	21	15–28	5
12–14 yr	6	16	15–18	7	22	18–26	6

* For normal blood pressures in children see nephrology section, page 445-450.
** From Adams FH, Emmanoulides GC, eds. Moss' heart disease in infants, children and adolescents. 3rd ed. Baltimore: Williams and Wilkins, 1983:729.
† From Kendig EL, Chernick V, eds. Disorders of the respiratory tract in children. Philadelphia: WB Saunders, 1983.

2. Rhythm
   - Check for P before each QRS
   - Check for QRS after each P
   - Measure PR interval (see Table 4–4)
   - Measure QRS interval (see Table 4–3)
   - Measure QT (calculate QTc):

   $$\text{corrected QT (QTc)} = \frac{\text{measured QT}}{\sqrt{R-R \text{ interval}}}$$

   QTc $>0.425 =$ long QT syndrome
   - Differential diagnosis of long QT syndrome
   a. Drugs, e.g., quinidine
   b. Electrolyte disturbances, e.g., $\downarrow K^+$,
      $\downarrow Ca^{2+}$,
      $\downarrow Mg^{2+}$
   c. CNS damage
   d. Myocarditis
   e. Jervell-Lange-Nielsen syndrome (long QT plus congenital deafness)
   f. Romano-Ward syndrome (long QT, normal hearing, autosomal dominant)
3. Axis determination (check lead I and AVF)
4. Chamber enlargement (Table 4–5)
5. ST/T changes

TABLE 4–3   QRS Duration (Sec) in V_5

Age	Minimum	2%	Mean	98%	Maximum
<1 day	0.018	0.031	0.051	0.075	0.078
1–2 days	0.030	0.032	0.048	0.066	0.069
3–6 days	0.027	0.031	0.049	0.068	0.072
1–3 wk	0.036	0.036	0.053	0.080	0.084
1–2 mo	0.033	0.033	0.053	0.076	0.084
3–5 mo	0.027	0.032	0.054	0.080	0.081
6–11 mo	0.030	0.034	0.054	0.076	0.081
1–2 yr	0.033	0.038	0.056	0.076	0.078
3–4 yr	0.039	0.041	0.057	0.072	0.078
5–7 yr	0.042	0.042	0.059	0.079	0.090
8–11 yr	0.039	0.041	0.062	0.085	0.087
12–15 yr	0.027	0.044	0.065	0.087	0.099

From Garson A Jr. The electrocardiogram in infants and children. Philadelphia: Lea & Febiger, 1983:397.

TABLE 4–4   Summary of Normal Values

Age Group	*Heart Rate (BPM)	Frontal Plane QRS Vector (degrees)	PR Interval (sec)	†Q III (mm)‡	†Q V_6 (mm)	RV_1 (mm)	SV_1 (mm)	R/S V_1	RV_6 (mm)	SV_6 (mm)	R/S V_6	*$SV_1 + RV_6$ (mm)	†$R + S$ V_4 (mm)
< 1 day	93–154 (123)	+ 59 to – 163 (137)	.08–.16 (.11)	4.5	2	5–26 (14)	0–23 (8)	.1–U (2.2)	0–11 (4)	0–9.5 (3)	.1–U (2.0)	28	52.5
1–2 days	91–159 (123)	+ 64 to – 161 (134)	.08–.14 (.11)	6.5	2.5	5–27 (14)	0–21 (9)	.1–U (2.0)	0–12 (4.5)	0–9.5 (3)	.1–U (2.5)	29	52
3–6 days	91–166 (129)	+ 77 to – 163 (132)	.07–.14 (.10)	5.5	3	3–24 (13)	0–17 (7)	.2–U (2.7)	.5–12 (5)	0–10 (3.5)	.1–U (2.2)	24.5	49
1–3 wk	107–182 (148)	+ 65 to + 161 (110)	.07–.14 (.10)	6	3	3–21 (11)	0–11 (4)	1.0–U (2.9)	2.5–16.5 (7.5)	0–10 (3.5)	.1–U (3.3)	21	49
1–2 mo	121–179 (149)	+ 31 to + 113 (74)	.07–.13 (.10)	7.5	3	3–18 (10)	0–12 (5)	.3–U (2.3)	5–21.5 (11.5)	0–6.5 (3)	.2–U (4.8)	29	53.5
3–5 mo	106–186 (141)	+ 7 to + 104 (60)	.07–.15 (.11)	6.5	3	3–20 (10)	0–17 (6)	.1–U (2.3)	6.5–22.5 (13)	0–10 (3)	.2–U (6.2)	32	61.5
6–11 mo	109–169 (134)	+ 6 to + 99 (56)	.07–.16 (.11)	8.5	3	1.5–20 (9.5)	.5–18 (4)	.1–3.9 (1.6)	6–22.5 (12.5)	0–7 (2)	.2–U (7.6)	32	53
1–2 yr	89–151 (119)	+ 7 to + 101 (55)	.08–.15 (.11)	6	3	2.5–17 (9)	.5–21 (8)	.05–4.3 (1.4)	6–22.5 (13)	0–6.5 (2)	.3–U (9.3)	39	49.5
3–4 yr	73–137 (108)	+ 6 to + 104 (55)	.09–.16 (.12)	5	3.5	1–18 (8)	.2–21 (10)	.03–2.8 (.9)	8–24.5 (15)	0–5 (1.5)	.6–U (10.8)	42	53.5
5–7 yr	65–133 (100)	+ 11 to + 143 (65)	.09–.16 (.12)	4	4.5	.5–14 (7)	.3–24 (12)	.02–2.0 (.7)	8.5–26.5 (16)	0–4 (1)	.9–U (11.5)	47	54
8–11 yr	62–130 (91)	+ 9 to + 114 (61)	.09–.17 (.13)	3	3	0–12 (5.5)	.3–25 (12)	0–1.8 (.5)	9–25.5 (16)	0–4 (1)	1.5–U (14.3)	45.5	53
12–15 yr	60–119 (85)	+ 11 to + 130 (59)	.09–.18 (.14)	3	3	0–10 (4)	.3–21 (11)	0–1.7 (.5)	6.5–23 (14)	0–4 (1)	1.4–U (14.7)	41	50

* 2–98% (mean)   † 98th percentile   ‡ mm at normal standardization   U = undefined (S wave may equal zero)
From Garson A Jr. The electrocardiogram in infants and children. Philadelphia: Lea & Febiger, 1983:404.

TABLE 4–5   Criteria for Chamber Enlargement (Hospital for Sick Children)

RVH

1. R in V_1 20 mm or more at all ages
2. S in V_6 0–7 days 14 mm, 8–30 days 10 mm, 1–3 mo 7 mm, 3 mo–16 yr 5 mm (or more)
3. R/S ratio in V_1 0–3 mo 6.5, 3–6 mo 4.0, 6 mo–3 yr 2.4, 3–5 yr 1.6, 6–15 yr 0.8 (or more)
4. T positive in V_1 if R/S more than 1.0

LVH

1. S in V_1 more than 20 mm at all ages
2. R in V_6 20 mm or more
3. Secondary T inversion in V_5 or V_6
4. Q 4 mm or more in V_5, V_6, or V_7

Right Atrial

1. Peaked P waves 3 mm or more in any lead

Left Atrial

1. Bifid P in any lead
2. P duration of more than 0.09 sec
3. Late inversion of P in V_1 of more than 1.5 mm

Combined Ventricular

Direct evidence of RVH + LVH or RVH + (a) q of 2 mm or more in V_5 or V_6 (b) inverted T in V_6 (after + 've in right chest leads)

From Davignon A, et al. Normal ECG standards for infants and children. Ped Cardiol 1979; 1:123–131.

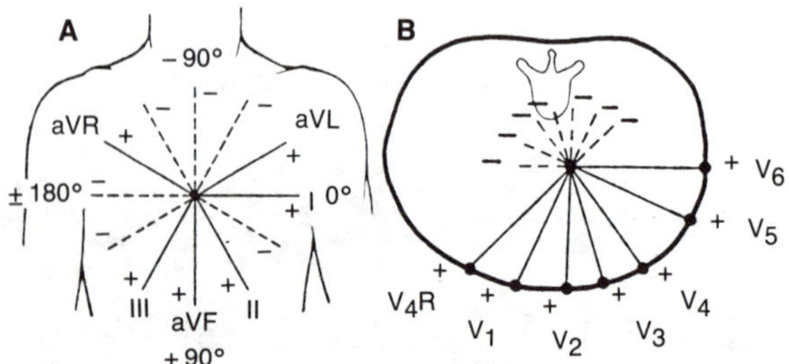

Figure 4–1   Hexaxial (*A*) and horizontal (*B*) reference systems. (From Park MK, Guntheroth WG. How to read pediatric ECGs. 2nd. ed. Chicago: Year Book, 1987.)

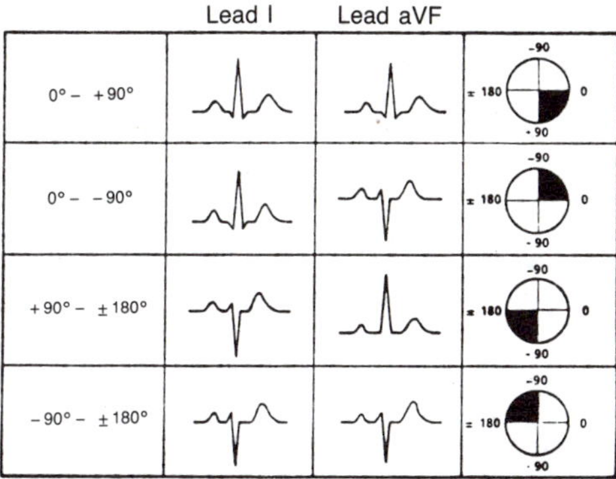

Figure 4–2 Locating quadrants of mean QRS axis from leads I and aVF. (From Park MK, Guntheroth WG. How to read pediatric ECGs. 2nd. ed. Chicago: Year Book, 1987.)

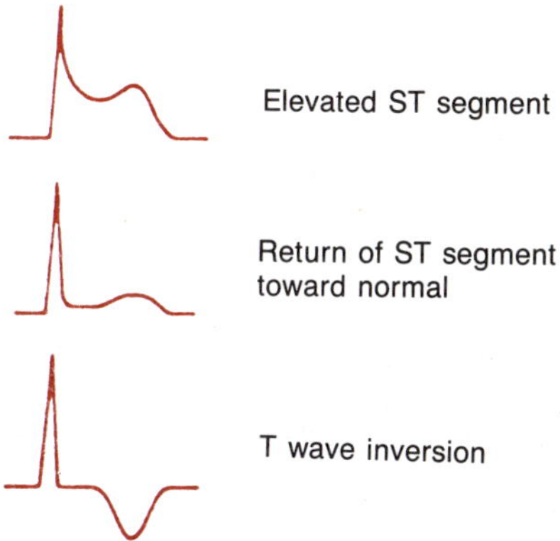

Figure 4–3 Time dependent changes of ST segment and T wave in pericarditis. (From Park MK, Guntheroth WG. How to read pediatric ECGs. 2nd. ed. Chicago: Year Book, 1987.)

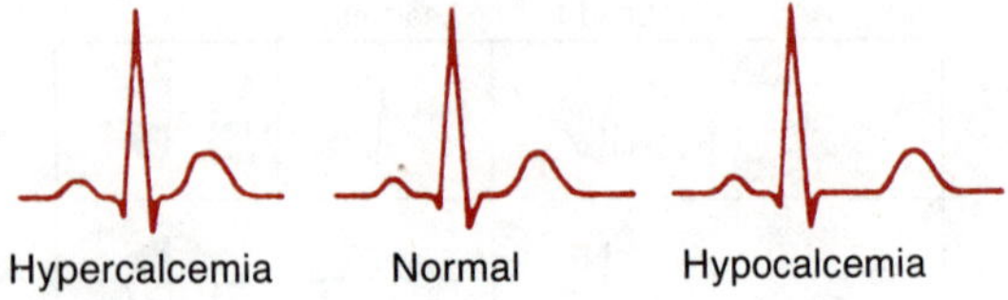

Figure 4–4 ECG findings in hypercalcemia and hypocalcemia. (From Park MK, Guntheroth WG. How to read pediatric ECGs. 2nd. ed. Chicago: Year Book, 1987.)

SERUM K

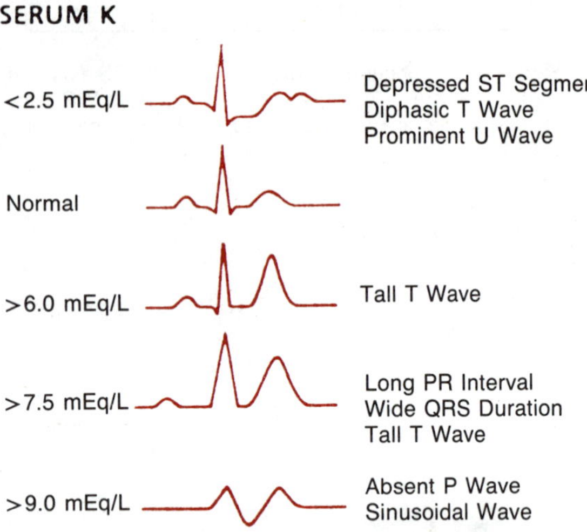

Figure 4–5 ECG findings in hypokalemia and hyperkalemia. (From Park MK, Guntheroth WG. How to read pediatric ECGs. 2nd ed. Chicago: Year Book, 1987.)

DYSRHYTHMIAS AND THEIR MANAGEMENT

- Do 12 lead ECG if not in extremis, and consult

cardiology team, if possible, for conditions requiring "special" management (marked with *).

Rhythm Originating in Sinus Node

Regular Sinus Rhythm

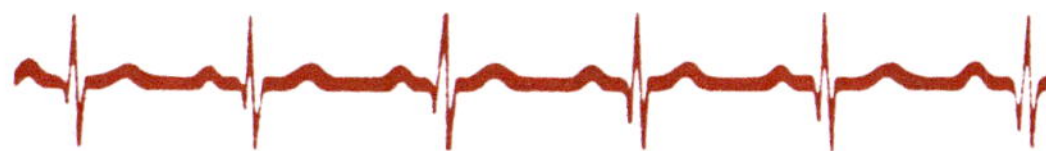

Figure 4–6 Regular sinus rhythm. (From Park MK, Guntheroth WG. How to read pediatric ECGs. 2nd. ed. Chicago: Year Book, 1987.)

Sinus Tachycardia

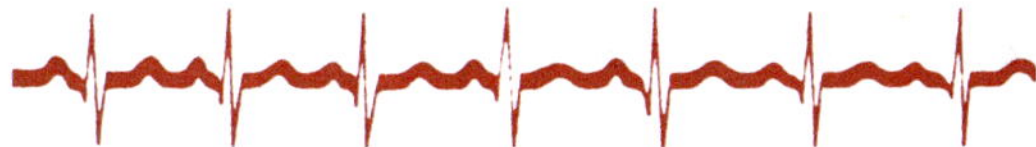

Figure 4–7 Sinus tachycardia. (From Park MK, Guntheroth WG. How to read pediatric ECGs. 2nd. ed. Chicago: Year Book, 1987.)

Causes

- Anxiety, fever, hypovolemia, shock, anemia, CHF, catecholamines

Treatment

- Treat underlying cause

Sinus Bradycardia

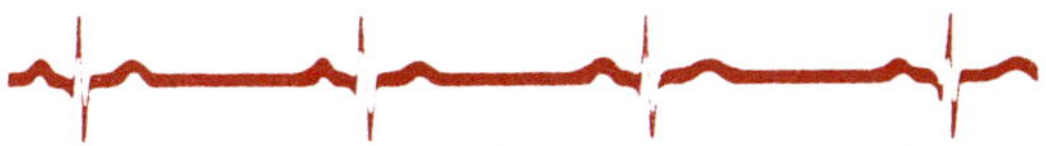

Figure 4–8 Sinus bradycardia. (From Park MK, Guntheroth WG. How to read pediatric ECGs. 2nd. ed. Chicago: Year Book, 1987.)

Causes

- Normal athletes, vagal stimulation
- ↑ ICP, hypothyroidism, hypothermia, hypoxia, hyperkalemia
- Digitalis, beta blockers

Treatment

- Treat underlying cause

Sinus Arrhythmia

- Normal variation with respiration

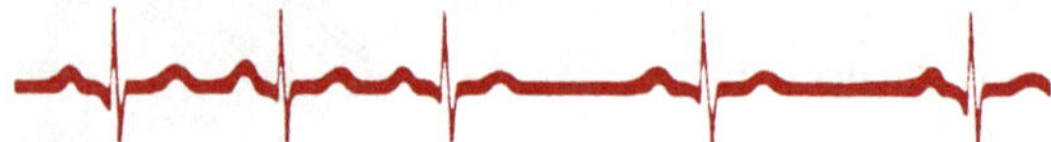

Figure 4–9 Sinus arrhythmia. (From Park MK, Guntheroth WG. How to read pediatric ECGs. 2nd. ed. Chicago: Year Book, 1987.)

Sinus Pause

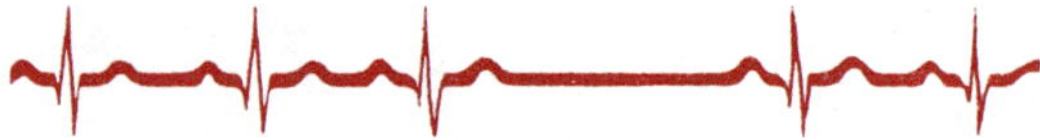

Figure 4–10 Sinus pause. (From Park MK, Guntheroth WG. How to read pediatric ECGs. 2nd. ed. Chicago: Year Book, 1987.)

Causes

- ↑ Vagal tone, hypoxia, digitalis toxicity, sick sinus syndrome (SSS)

Treatment

- Withhold digitalis; pacemaker may be required for SSS

Ectopic Atrial Rhythm

Atrial Premature Beat

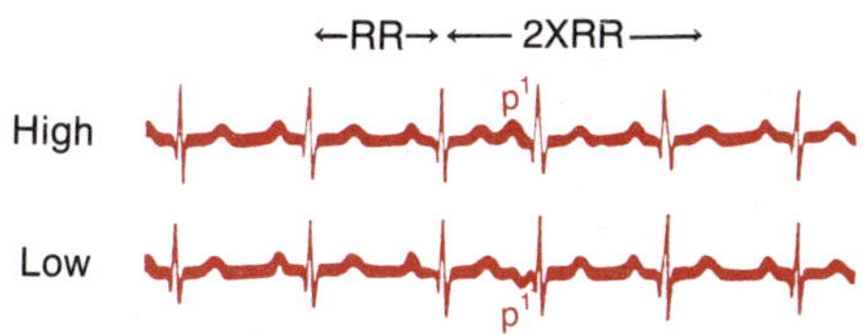

Figure 4–11   Atrial premature beat. (From Park MK, Guntheroth WG. How to read pediatric ECGs. 2nd. ed. Chicago: Year Book, 1987.)

- Ectopic focus

Causes

- Normal variation, post cardiac surgery, digitalis toxicity

Treatment

- Withhold digoxin

Wandering Pacemaker

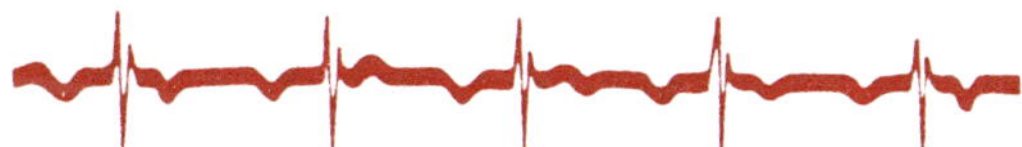

Figure 4–12   Wandering pacemaker. (From Park MK, Guntheroth WG. How to read pediatric ECGs. 2nd. ed. Chicago: Year Book, 1987.)

- Normal variation

Atrial Tachycardia*

(Supraventricular Tachycardia, SVT)

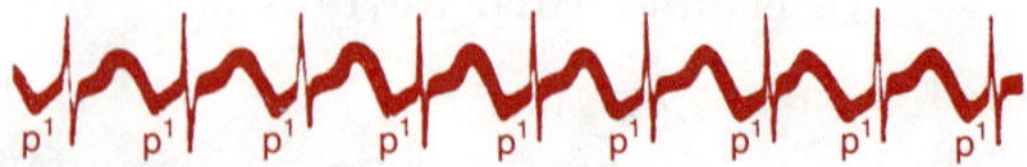

Figure 4-13 Atrial tachycardia. (From Park MK, Guntheroth WG. How to read pediatric ECGs. 2nd. ed. Chicago: Year Book, 1987.)

- \> 200/min

Causes

- Idiopathic in ~ 50%
- Wolf-Parkinson-White syndrome in ≃ 25% (delta waves seen only after conversion to sinus rhythm)
- Some congenital heart defects (Ebstein's anomaly, single ventricle, L-TGA)

Treatment

- If in CHF:
    1. Vagal maneuvers (ice bag on face most effective); *avoid eyeball pressure*
    2. DC cardioversion (synchronized), 0.5 joule/kg initially
    3. Overdrive pacing (esophageal or transvenous) when this sophisticated procedure is available, done by a cardiologist
    4. May need bicarbonate if acidotic
- If no CHF:
    1. Vagal maneuvers
    2. Phenylephrine, 0.01–0.1 mg/kg IV push (to double BP)
    3. Edrophonium, 0.2 mg/kg IV over 2–3 min; repeat in 15–30 min (keep atropine nearby)
    4. Verapamil, 0.15 mg/kg IV over 2–3 min; repeat in 15–30 min (watch for ↓ myocardial performance → hypotension)
    5. DC cardioversion (synchronous), 0.5 joule/kg
    6. *Do not use Verapamil or digoxin without cardiology consultation*

Atrial Flutter*

- Heart rate often >250/min

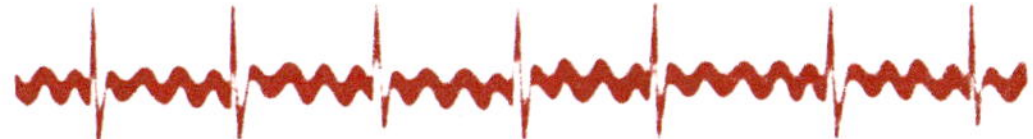

Figure 4-14 Atrial flutter. (From Park MK, Guntheroth WG. How to read pediatric ECGs. 2nd. ed. Chicago: Year Book, 1987.)

Causes

- CHD with dilated atria
- Myocarditis
- Digitalis toxicity

Treatment

- Digitalize if not due to digitalis toxicity
- DC cardioversion
- Quinidine to prevent recurrence

Atrial Fibrillation*

- Heart rate often >300/min

Rapid Ventricular Response

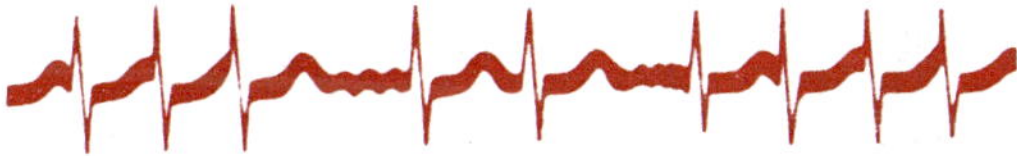

Slow Ventricular Response

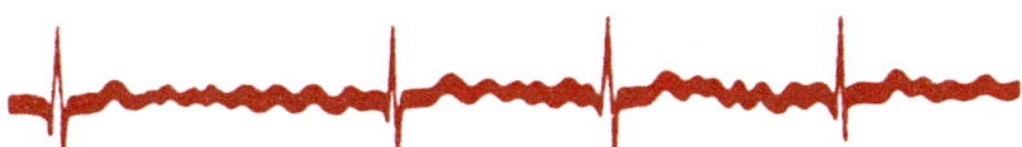

Figure 4-15 Atrial fibrillation. (From Park MK, Guntheroth WG. How to read pediatric ECGs. 2nd. ed. Chicago: Year Book, 1987.)

Causes

- Structural heart disease with dilated atria

- Myocarditis
- Digitalis toxicity
- Thyrotoxicosis, especially after infancy

Treatment

- As in flutter

Nodal Rhythms

Nodal Premature Beat

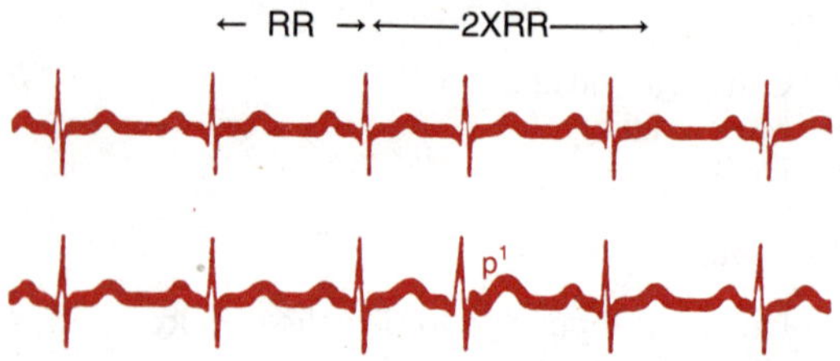

Figure 4–16 Nodal premature beat. (From Park MK, Guntheroth WG. How to read pediatric ECGs. 2nd. ed. Chicago: Year Book, 1987.)

Causes

- Idiopathic
- Post cardiac surgery
- Digitalis toxicity

Treatment

- Withhold digitalis

Sinus Pause and Nodal Escape Beat

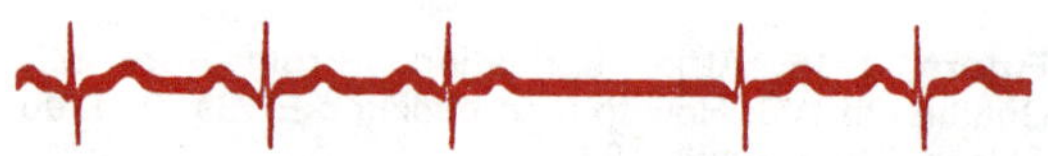

Figure 4–17 Sinus pause and nodal escape beat. (From Park MK, Guntheroth WG. How to read pediatric ECGs. 2nd. ed. Chicago: Year Book, 1987.)

Causes

- Normal variation, or
- Post Mustard or Senning operation (see p 68 and 69)

Treatment

- None

Nodal Tachycardia

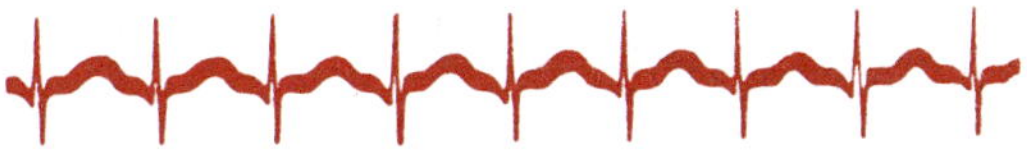

Figure 4–18 Nodal tachycardia. (From Park MK, Guntheroth WG. How to read pediatric ECGs. 2nd. ed. Chicago: Year Book, 1987.)

Causes

- Same as in atrial tachycardia

Treatment

- None if rate <150/min
- Quinidine

Ventricular Rhythms

Ventricular Premature Beat (VPB)

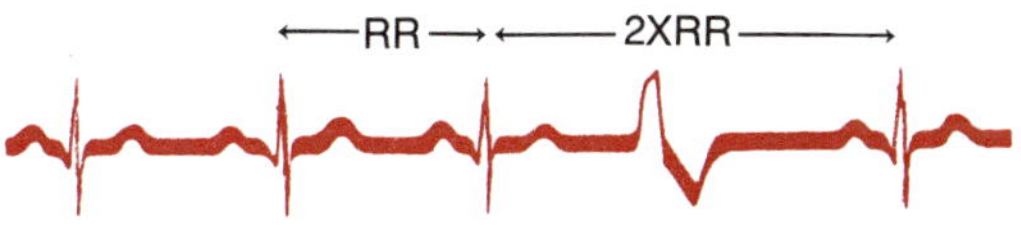

Figure 4–19 Ventricular premature beat. (From Park MK, Guntheroth WG. How to read pediatric ECGs. 2nd. ed. Chicago: Year Book, 1987.)

Causes

- Normal variation, myocarditis, long QT syn-

drome, CHD, post cardiac surgery, digitalis
toxicity
- Secondary to catecholamines, caffeine, am-
phetamines

Diagnosis

- Usually benign if VPBs ↓ or disappears with
exercise
- Significant if
  1. ↑ with activity
  2. Multifocal, especially couplets
  3. Underlying CHD
  4. Symptomatic

Treatment

- IV lidocaine, 1 mg/kg/dose followed by 10–50
μg/kg/min infusion
- Propranolol, quinidine, phenytoin, or procainamide (consult cardiology)

Ventricular Tachycardia (VT) *

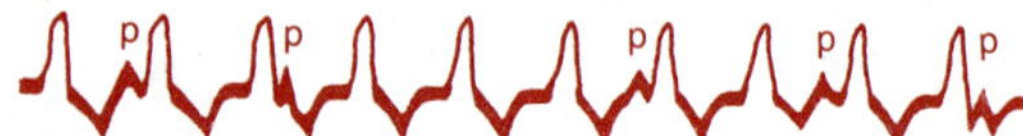

Figure 4–20   Ventricular tachycardia (or SVT with aber-
rant ventricular conduction). (From Park MK, Guntheroth
WG. How to read pediatric ECGs. 2nd. ed. Chicago: Year
Book, 1987.)

Causes

- As in VPBs

Treatment

- If symptomatic, DC cardioversion (syn-
chronized), 2 joules/kg
- Lidocaine, 1 mg/kg/dose IV over 1–2 min; then
10–50 μg/kg/min infusion
- Procainamide, 1 mg/kg/dose IV push q5 min for

up to 15 doses may be tried
- Correct blood gas levels or electrolyte disorders
- Recurrence prevented by propranolol, quinidine, phenytoin

Ventricular Fibrillation[*]

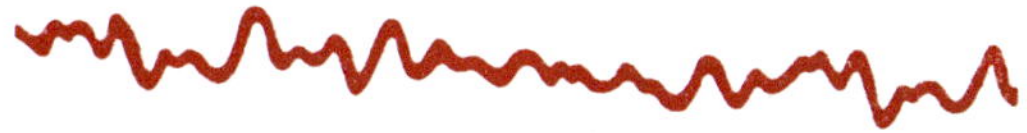

Figure 4–21 Ventricular fibrillation. (From Park MK, Guntheroth WG. How to read pediatric ECGs. 2nd. ed. Chicago: Year Book, 1987.)

Causes

- Postoperative, severe hypoxia, hyperkalemia, digoxin or quinidine toxicity, myocarditis, myocardial infarction, catecholamines, anesthetics

Treatment

- CPR
- DC cardioversion (asynchronous), 2 joules/kg
- Bretylium tosylate, 5 mg/kg IV push, in refractory cases (watch for hypotension; avoid in digoxin toxicity)

Heart Block

First Degree AV Block

- Check PR interval

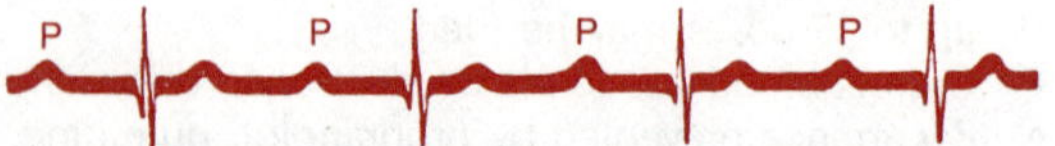

Figure 4–22 First degree AV block. (From Park MK, Guntheroth WG. How to read pediatric ECGs. 2nd. ed. Chicago: Year Book, 1987.)

Causes

- In some normal children
- Acute rheumatic fever
- Cardiomyopathies
- CHD (ASD, Ebstein's anomaly, CAVSD)
- Post cardiac surgery
- Digitalis toxicity

Treatment

- None unless digitalis toxicity

Second Degree AV Block

Mobitz I (Wenckebach) block

Causes

- In some normal children
- Myocarditis
- Cardiomyopathy
- Myocardial infarction
- CHD, post heart surgery
- Digitalis toxicity

Treatment

- Treat underlying cause

Mobitz II block (e.g., 2:1, 3:1, 4:1)

Causes

- Same as in type I

Treatment

- Treat underlying cause
- Occasionally pacemaker required

Mobitz Type I
(Wenckebach Phenomenon)

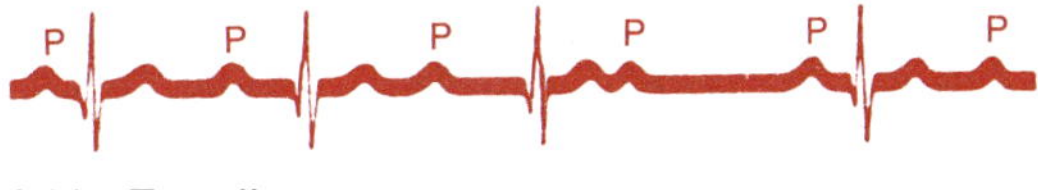

Mobitz Type II

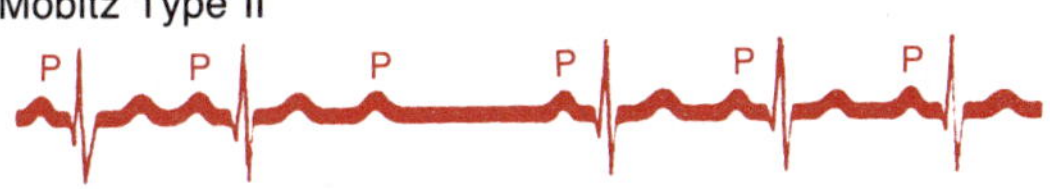

2:1 AV Block

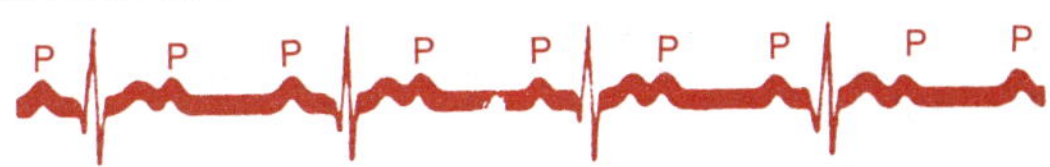

Figure 4–23 Second degree AV block. (From Park MK, Guntheroth WG. How to read pediatric ECGs. 2nd. ed. Chicago: Year Book, 1987.)

Complete (Third Degree) AV Block

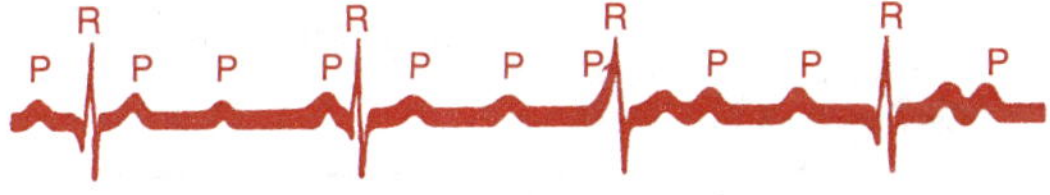

Figure 4–24 Complete (third degree) AV block. (From Park MK, Guntheroth WG. How to read pediatric ECGs. 2nd. ed. Chicago: Year Book, 1987.)

Causes

- Congenital AV block
  1. Idiopathic, maternal lupus, or mixed connective tissue disease
  2. L-TGA

- Acquired AV block
  1. Cardiac surgery
  2. Myocarditis
  3. Post MI

Treatment

- None in asymptomatic congenital complete HB (but if rate <55/min, Holter and consider pacemaker)
- Atropine or isoproterenol pending
- Transvenous pacing
- Permanent pacing

ELECTROCARDIOGRAM RELATED ELECTROLYTE DISTURBANCES

TABLE 4–6 Electrocardiogram Related Electrolyte Disturbances

Hyperkalemia	Tall, narrow, "tented" T waves
	Widening QRS complexes
	Wide flattened P waves
	Ectopic rhythms and intraventricular block
Hypokalemia	↑QTc interval with broad flat T wave
	ST segment depression
	T wave flattened or inverted
	U wave
	Ectopic beats, supraventricular-ventricular
Hypercalcemia	Short QTc interval
	Myocardial irritability
	↑PR interval, QRS duration, ± AV block
Hypocalcemia	↑QTc interval
Hypomagnesemia	↑QTc interval

Modified from Park MK. Pediatric cardiology for practitioners. Chicago: Year Book, 1984:250.

DRUG RELATED ECG CHANGES

- Digoxin
  1. Therapeutic effect
     - ↑ PR interval
     - ↓ QTc interval

- • ST segment changes opposite to QRS complex
    - • ↓ T wave amplitude
  2. Toxicity
    - • Bradycardia
    - • Various degrees of AV block
    - • *Any* type of arrhythmia
- Quinidine
  1. Therapeutic effect
    - • ↓ P wave amplitude
    - • Slight PR interval prolongation
    - • ↑ QRS duration—correlates with drug level
    - • ↑ QTc interval—correlates with drug level
  2. Toxicity
    - • Significant ↑ of PR interval
    - • ↑ QRS duration ≥ 50% over initial duration
    - • Sinoatrial or AV block
    - • Multifocal PVCs

ENDOCARDITIS

General Considerations

- Acute endocarditis
  1. Rare
  2. Secondary to septicemia (*S. aureus* most common organism)
  3. Preexisting heart disease not required
  4. Most common post cardiac surgery or in IV drug abusers
  5. Mortality > 50%
- Subacute endocarditis
  1. Usually in children > 2 yr with underlying cardiovascular abnormalities ± prosthetic materials in heart; infection starts with bacteremia, even transient (occurs in > 50% of dental procedures)
  2. All forms of congenital heart disease except secundum ASD predispose to SBE; most frequently infected are those with VSD, tetralogy of Fallot, and aortic stenosis

3. 90% of cases involve *Streptococcus viridans,
Streptococcus faecalis,* and *Staphylococcus
aureus*

Clinical Features

- Insidious onset of fever, fatigue, pallor, ↓
  appetite
- New or changed heart murmur in many patients
- Fever in 80%
- Splenomegaly in 70%
- Microemboli to skin in 50% (petechiae on skin,
  mucous membranes, and conjunctivae most
  common)
- Emboli to other organs in 50%
  1. Pulmonary emboli in VSD, tetralogy of Fallot
  2. CNS emboli in left sided lesion
  3. Hematuria, renal failure

Management

- Investigation
  1. Blood cultures—at least three taken from
     separate sites in 24 hr, *using strict* aseptic
     technique, *prior* to starting antibiotics. More
     cultures may be necessary if patient has
     received antibiotics during preceding 2 wk.
  2. CBC, differential, ESR (? left shift with ↑ ESR),
     urea, creatinine
  3. Urine microscopy (microscopic hematuria in
     30%)
  4. 2D-ECHO (? vegetations)
- Treatment
  1. Prior to culture results
     - Penicillin, 6–20 million U/day IV in six
       divided doses

       or

     - Cloxacillin, 100 mg/kg/day IV in six divided
       doses

       and

  - Streptomycin, 20 mg/kg/day IM in one or two divided doses
2. Organism isolated dictates any changes in antibiotics, to be given parenterally 4–6 wk

Follow-Up

- ~ 90% cure for *S. viridans*
- ~ 50% cure for *S. aureus*
- *Prevention:* see Formulary, p 878–879

MYOCARDITIS

Causes

- Most commonly viral infection: coxsackie A and B, rubella, varicella, CMV, herpes, enterovirus, adenovirus, influenza
- Acute rheumatic fever (p 67)
- Collagen vascular disease
- Kawasaki disease (p 72)

Clinical Features

- Newborns and infants may present with lethargy, anorexia, vomiting, and signs of CHF
- ECG may show low voltages, ST-T changes, prolonged QT, and dysrhythmias
- Cardiac x-ray examination may show cardiomegaly
- ↑ ESR ± ↑ SGOT (AST)

Management

- Anti-CHF measures (reduced dosage of digoxin; see p 42)

Follow-Up

- Majority recover completely
- A few develop chronic myocarditis ± CHF

ACUTE PERICARDITIS

Causes

- Viral infection (as in myocarditis)
- Post cardiac surgery (post pericardiotomy syndrome)
- Bacterial infection (*S. aureus, S. pneumoniae, H. influenzae*); TB often chronic
- Kawasaki disease (see p 72)
- Collagen vascular disease
- Acute rheumatic fever (see p 67)

Clinical Features

- Fever
- Precordial pain (sharp, substernal; may radiate to neck)
- Pericardial friction rub
- Cardiomegaly, but quiet and hypodynamic heart
- ± Signs of tamponade: tachycardia, pulsus paradoxus
- Hepatomegaly
- Venous distention

Management

- Investigations
  1. ECG
     - Low voltages
     - Time dependent changes secondary to myocardial involvement: initial ST elevation → return of ST to baseline with T inversion
  2. Chest x-ray: cardiomegaly and effusion, ↑ pulmonary venous marking if tamponade
  3. 2D-ECHO
  4. Pericardiocentesis
- Treatment
  1. Surgical treatment
     - Pericardiocentesis for relief of tamponade

- Surgical drainage of purulent pericarditis
    and 4–6 wk of IV antibiotics
  2. Medical treatment
    - Treatment of underlying condition
    - Digitalis contraindicated in tamponade
      since it blocks tachycardia, the compensa-
      tory response to ↓ venous return

RHEUMATIC FEVER

Clinical Features

TABLE 4–7   Revised Jones Criteria for Guidance in Diagnosis of Rheumatic Fever*

Major manifestations	Minor manifestations

1. Carditis
  a. Murmur
  b. Cardiomegaly
  c. Pericarditis
  d. Congestive heart failure
2. Polyarthritis
3. Chorea
4. Erythema marginatum
5. Subcutaneous nodules
	1. Clinical evidence
	  a. History of rheumatic fever
	  b. Arthralgia
	  c. Fever
	2. Laboratory evidence
	  a. Increased ESR, C reactive protein, WBC count, anemia
	  b. Prolonged P-R and Q-T intervals on ECG
	
	Supportive evidence
	1. Recent scarlet fever
	2. Throat culture positive for group A strep-tococci
	3. Increased ASO or other streptococcal antibodies

* Two major manifestations or one major and two minor manifestations with supportive evidence of recent streptococcal infection
indicate a high probability of rheumatic fever. However, failure to
meet the Jones criteria does not exclude rheumatic fever.
Modified from Rudolph AM, ed. Pediatrics. 17th ed. Norwalk:
Appleton-Century-Crofts, 1982:446.

Management

- Treatment
  1. Benzathine penicillin G, 1.2 million U IM x

one dose (half the dose if <30 kg), *or* penicillin V, 200,000–400,000 U PO, tid–qid × 10 days, *or* erythromycin, 20–40 mg/kg/day (÷ bid or tid) PO × 10 days

2. Then: benzathine penicillin G, 1.2 million U IM monthly, *or* penicillin V, 200,000 U PO bid, *or* sulfadiazine, 1 g PO daily (half the dose if <30 kg) for prophylaxis indefinitely

- Acute treatment
  1. Uncomplicated disease
     - ASA, 70–100 mg/kg/day × 6 wk
     - Bed rest, then gradual ambulation after 2 wk
  2. With carditis
     - Bed rest: duration dependent on severity of carditis
     - Prednisone, 1–2 mg/kg/day, if cardiomegaly present
     - ASA if no cardiomegaly

CORRECTIVE CARDIAC PROCEDURES DEFINED

Procedures

- Blalock-Hanlon: surgical atrial septectomy
- Brock: infundibulectomy or closed pulmonary valvulotomy
- Fontan: connection of right atrium to pulmonary artery either by atrial appendage–PA anastomosis or use of conduit-graft between them
- Mustard: intra-atrial baffle or patch (pericardium) for palliation of simple transposition
- Park: creation of atrial septostomy by use of knife-tipped catheter after passage through foramen ovale
- Rashkind: balloon atrial septostomy with cardiac catheter
- Rastelli
  1. Placement of valved conduit-graft between

right ventricle and pulmonary artery
    2. Repair of CAVSD by resuspension of MV and
       TV upon newly created atrial septum
- Senning: a type of repair of simple TGA by
  intra-atrial baffle using flaps of native atrial sep-
  tum and atrial wall
- Jatene: arterial switch for correction of TGA
- Norwood: two-stage palliation for hypoplastic
  left heart syndrome and other forms of complex
  CHD with systemic outflow obstruction
- Shunts
    1. Blalock-Taussig: subclavian artery to pulmo-
       nary artery
    2. Glenn: superior vena cava to R pulmonary
       artery (e.g., for tricuspid atresia)
    3. Potts: descending aorta to L pulmonary artery
    4. Waterston: ascending aorta to R pulmonary
       artery

DIGOXIN TOXICITY

Clinical Features

- Anorexia, nausea, abdominal pain
- Vomiting, diarrhea
- Restlessness, drowsiness
- Fatigue
- Visual disturbances

Risk Factors

- Renal failure
- Myocardial injury (including myocarditis)
- Hypokalemia, hypercalcemia, acidosis
- Hypoxia
- Hypothyroidism
- Adrenergic or catecholamine stimulation

Management

- Investigations
    1. ECG
       - Early

a. Short QT
b. Scooped ST with T wave inversion
c. Slowing heart rate
- Late
  a. Prolonged PR progressing to heart block
  b. Supraventricular or ventricular arrhyth-
     mias with ectopic beats
  c. Worsening heart failure
2. Digoxin level: normal range, 1–2.5 nmol/L
   (0.8 – 2.0 μg/L)
3. Electrolytes: watch for low K+

- Treatment
1. Stop digoxin
2. Stop diuretics if possible
3. ECG monitoring
4. Individualize:
   - Give KCl if low K+ (0.05 mEq/kg/hr)
   - Tachyarrhythmia
     a. Lidocaine, 1 mg/kg IV bolus → infusion
        10–50 μg/kg/min
     b. Phenytoin, 3–5 mg/kg IV; may repeat x
        1 in 4 hr (maximal total dose = 500 mg)
     c. Propranolol, 0.01 mg/kg slow IV every 2
        min to maximum of 0.1 mg/kg, then 1–4
        mg/kg/day divided 3–4 x/day PO
     d. Cardioversion 0.5–2 joules/kg (only if life
        threatening dysrhythmia resistant to med-
        ical treatment) after sedation
   - Heart block
     a. Atropine 0.01–0.03 mg/kg IV q4–6h
     b. Temporary pacemaker (transvenous or
        transthoracic) if available

CYANOTIC SPELLS IN
TETRALOGY OF FALLOT

General Considerations

- Decreased pulmonary blood flow, therefore ↑ R
  to L shunt

Clinical Features

- Paroxysmal dyspnea with cyanosis; therefore ↑ respiratory rate and ↑ depth of breathing (Kussmaul)
- Quieter and shorter ejection murmur
- Floppy
- Can lead to loss of consciousness, seizures, death

Management

- Investigation
  1. Laboratory studies:
     - ABG–acidosis with hypoxia
     - Chest x-ray: decreased pulmonary blood flow (*rarely* done during episode)
     - ECG: increased P wave
- Treatment
  1. Knee-chest position (↓ venous return, therefore ↓ R → L shunt)
  2. Oxygen by mask or hood (6–8 l/min or 100% oxygen)
  3. Drugs
     - Propranolol, 0.05–0.1 mg/kg slow IV push (over 10 min)
     - Morphine, 0.1 mg/kg IV or SC (may depress respiration)
     - $NaHCO_3$, 1–2 mEq/kg IV, for correction of metabolic acidosis
     - Phenylephrine, 0.10 mg/dose IM (vasoconstrictor: ↑ systemic vascular resistance and therefore ↓ R → L shunt)
  4. Transfuse if anemic (Hb < 150 g/L [15 g/dl])
- At recovery
  1. Color returns
  2. Activity returns
  3. Typical murmur returns
- Consider
  1. Discharge on beta blocker (propranolol, 2–4 mg/kg/day ÷ q6h)

2. Surgical correction of ToF (or palliation with a systemic to PA shunt)

KAWASAKI DISEASE
(Mucocutaneous Lymph Node Syndrome)

General Considerations

- Definition: a syndrome of unknown etiology whose epidemiology suggests an idiosyncratic immunologic response triggered by an infection

Clinical Features

- (Five of six must be present)
  1. Fever persisting for more than 5 days
  2. Conjunctival injection without exudate
  3. Mouth changes
     - Erythema and fissuring of lips
     - Strawberry tongue
     - Diffuse erythema of oral mucosa
  4. Peripheral changes
     - Erythema of palms and soles
     - Indurative edema of hands and feet
     - Membranous desquamation of fingers and toes
  5. Erythematous rash
  6. Swelling of cervical lymph nodes >1.5 cm (70% of cases)
     - Peak frequency 6 mo–5 yr of age
- Stages:
   I. Acute: 0 → 10 days
     - Fever, conjunctivitis, rash, oral changes, cervical adenopathy
     - Usually no obvious cardiac changes (despite generalized microvasculitis)

II.Subacute: 11 → 28 days
  - Irritability, desquamation
  - Cardiac: ± effusion, ± CHF ± AV valve regurgitation, ± coronary artery aneurysms

III.Convalescent: 29 → 45 days
  - Gradual decrease in acute signs and symptoms; persistence of cardiac findings if initially present

Differential Diagnosis

- Viral exanthems
- Stevens-Johnson syndrome

Management

- Investigation
  1. CBC, differential, platelets, ESR
  2. Electrolytes, urea, creatinine, SGOT, alkaline phosphatase, urinalysis
  3. Chest x-ray, ECG, 2D-ECHO
- Treatment
  1. High dosage ASA (100 mg/kg/day divided q6h) until afebrile; then 5 → 10 mg/kg q AM × 2 mo
  2. Dipyridamole, 5 mg/kg/day if coronary artery aneurysm
  3. Low dose ASA/dipyridamole to be continued as long as coronary aneurysms persist
  4. IgG currently under trial

Follow-Up

- Cardiology consultation, ECG, and 2D-ECHO at 3 wk, 2 mo, 6 mo, and 1 yr after onset of fever

CARDIAC CATHETERIZATION VALUES

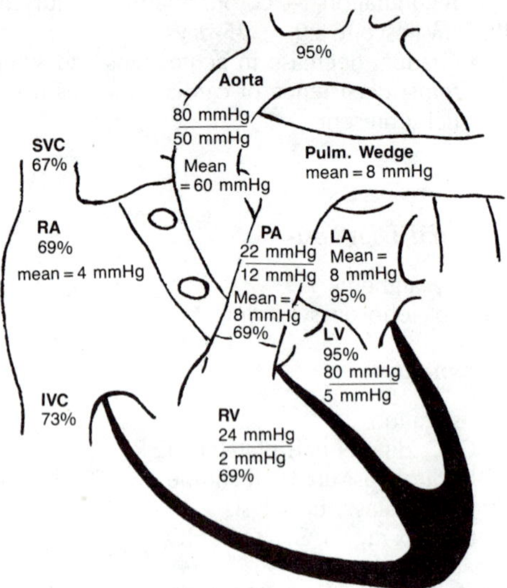

Figure 4–25 Normal cardiac catheterization data in children older than one month of age. Catheterization values: oxygen saturation as % saturation. Pressure as mm Hg.

Suggested Reading

1. Adams FH, Emmanouilides GC, eds. Moss' heart disease in infants, children and adolescents. 3rd ed. Baltimore: Williams & Wilkins, 1983.
2. Garson A Jr. The electrocardiogram in infants and children. Philadelphia: Lea & Febiger, 1983.
3. Park MK. Pediatric cardiology for practitioners. Chicago: Year Book, 1984.
4. Rowe RD, Freedom RM, Mehrizi A. The neonate with congenital heart disease. Philadelphia: W.B. Saunders, 1981.

5 DENTISTRY

DENTAL PAIN

General Considerations and Management

- There are four main causes:
  1. Hyperemia
     - Simple hyperemia due to trauma or large restorations
     - Consult dental service
     - Treatment: removal of source of irritation
  2. Pulpitis due to dental caries
     - Serous pulpitis: tooth sensitive to cold, relieved by heat
     - Suppurative pulpitis
       a. Tooth sensitive to heat; cold may relieve pain
       b. Consult dental service
       c. Treatment: removal of pulp tissue from tooth (pulpectomy)
  3. Pulpal necrosis with abscess
     - May occur without facial swelling or systemic signs
     - Management
       a. Consult dental service
       b. Analgesics for pain
       c. Acetaminophen for fever
       d. Possibly give systemic antibiotics (Pen V)
       e. Removal of offending tooth, if possible
       f. Reassessment by dental service in 24 hr
  4. Periodontal abscess
     - Usually pain (localized or referred) with associated facial swelling and fever
     - Management
       a. Consult dental service
       b. Systemic antibiotic therapy and surgical drainage, if necessary

DENTAL TRAUMA

General Considerations

- Displacement of deciduous teeth interferes with development and eruption of adjacent permanent teeth
- Interference with blood supply may result in pulpal necrosis (indicated by blue-black discoloration of crown) and infection
- After age 20 months, space preservation is unnecessary in anterior segment, but imperative in posterior segments of deciduous dental arch

Management

- Determine
  1. Time of accident
  2. Age of patient
  3. Whether tooth is deciduous or permanent
  4. Whether tooth is loose, out, or fractured, and whether dental pulp is visible
- In all cases consult dental service
- Therapy depends on type of injury and tooth affected
  1. Loosened or displaced anterior teeth
     - Deciduous
       a. Removal of injured tooth
     - Permanent
       a. Consult dental service immediately (the affected tooth will be immobilized with an acrylic splint)
       b. Every 6 wk observe tooth for signs of pulpal necrosis due to interference with neurovascular supply (less likely in younger children and when dental trauma has been treated promptly)
  2. Fractured permanent anterior teeth
     - Most fractures should be assessed by dentist on call, particularly those that are temperature sensitive
     - Even small enamel fractures in teeth may

have associated root fractures, which may require stabilization for a minimum of 6 wk
3. Avulsed teeth
   - Deciduous
     a. No treatment required except roentgenographic search for remnants in the jaw, lips, or lungs, if indicated
     b. *Never* replant an avulsed primary tooth
   - Permanent
     a. Ask patient to bring tooth along ASAP!
     b. *Keep tooth moist in cold milk or ice water*
     c. Call dental service for replanting and immobilization
     d. Prognosis dependent on length of time out of mouth (extraalveolar period < 30 min has ~ 90% chance of longterm retention), contamination of tooth (should avoid handling root surface), and age of patient

DENTAL POSTOPERATIVE HEMORRHAGE

General Considerations (Definition)

- Bleeding longer than 4 hr, or delayed recurrent bleeding

Management

- Consult dental service
- Apply pressure: have patient bite firmly on a folded 2×2 inch gauze pack positioned over the extraction socket
- Recheck in ~ 30 min for hemostasis
- If above unsuccessful:
  1. Local infiltration of 2% Xylocaine with epinephrine 1:100,000
  2. Try topical hemostatic agents (e.g., bovine thrombin)

3. Further therapy (Gelfoam gauze pack or suturing) rarely needed

ACUTE HERPETIC GINGIVOSTOMATITIS

General Considerations and Clinical Features

- Usually affects children ages 1–3 yr, but may occur at any age
- Rapid onset with dramatic pain, profuse salivation, halitosis, fever, and anorexia
- Red to gray-yellow membranous gingivitis with scattered ulcers on tongue and labiobuccal mucosa are commonly seen
- Submandibular lymphadenopathy and tenderness may be present

Management

Mainly supportive
- Topical antiseptics (antiseptic mouthwash, e.g., Dequadin)
- Topical anesthetics (e.g., benzocaine) as oral rinses (N.B.: risk of sensitization)
- Acetaminophen for pain and fever
- Systemic antibiotic *only* for secondary bacterial infection
- Soft bland diet with extra fluids should be encouraged
- Self-limiting disease lasting 10–14 days
- Children occasionally must be hospitalized because of inadequate oral intake. Appropriate isolation guidelines should be followed to prevent nosocomial transmission.

"BABY BOTTLE" SYNDROME ("Nursing" Caries)

General Considerations

- Development of caries as a result of prolonged

use of bottle feeding (delayed weaning) and bedtime bottling with milk or sugar-containing liquids (e.g., fruit juices, pop)
- Prolonged breast feeding also has been implicated
- Teeth affected in the order they erupt—maxillary incisors, maxillary first deciduous molars, maxillary canines, and second deciduous molars. Mandibular teeth are characteristically spared, at least early in development.

Management

- Parent education most important
- Encourage parents to clean child's teeth as soon as they appear (initially with gauze swab and later with soft tooth brush)
- Recommend early weaning from bottle or breast feeding (by age 12 mo)
- Bedtime bottle should be discouraged—or sugar (or milk) content progressively decreased until child receives pure water
- Regular dental visits should be recommended, beginning not later than 36 mo

Suggested Reading

1. Stewart RE, Barber TK, Troutman KC, Wei SHY. Pediatric dentistry. St. Louis: C.V. Mosby, 1982.
2. Worth HM. The principles and practice of oral radiologic interpretation. Chicago: Year Book, 1975.

6 DERMATOLOGY

ACNE

General Considerations and Clinical Features

- Usually self-limited disease of pilosebaceous units in adolescents
- Two types of lesions
  1. Noninflammatory: comedones (open, closed)
  2. Inflammatory: papules, pustules, cysts
- Neonatal acne—due to maternal hormones (usually self-limited)

Management

- General measures
  1. Exclude androgenic causes, if severe
  2. May adjust diet (controversial)
  3. Use drying soaps (benzoyl peroxide)
  4. Do not use moisturizers, steaming, or saunas
  5. Use oil-free make-up
- Topical medication
  1. Benzoyl peroxide (2.5–20%)
     - Apply qhs; start with 2.5%; then increase % prn
     - Oxidizer; therefore inhibits *Propionibacterium acnes*; therefore antibacterial
     - Comedolytic
  2. Vitamin A acid (0.01, 0.025, 0.05%)
     - For noninflammatory acne (particularly comedones)
     - Apply qhs; start at 0.01%
     - Use for a minimum of 6 wk
  3. Antibiotics
     - For inflammatory lesions
     - Staticin (erythromycin) or 2% clindamycin solution bid

- Oral medication (for inflammatory acne)
  1. Antibiotics
     - Bacteriostatic for *P. acnes*; inhibit lipase, which degrades free fatty acids; inhibit polymorphonuclear chemotaxis
     - Tetracycline (not if under 8 yr old or pregnant), 1 g daily × 1 wk and then 500 mg daily, or minocycline, 50–100 mg/day, or erythromycin, 500 mg–1 g/day
     - If taking a specific antibiotic for a prolonged time and it no longer seems to be working, switch to one of the others
  2. Accutane (13–cis retinoic acid)
     - Best used only by a dermatologist or physician familiar with this drug
     - Stop antibiotics while patient is receiving Accutane
     - Anti-inflammatory; decreases sebaceous gland secretion; normalizes keratinization of follicular epithelium
     - For cystic scarring acne that is resistant to oral antibiotics
     - Four month course and regular lab tests (Liver function tests, urinalysis, CBC)
     - MUST AVOID PREGNANCY during and for 3 mo after treatment is finished (do serum β–HCG pregnancy test prior to starting Accutane)
     - Side effects: cheilitis (100%), xerostomia, xerosis, myalgia, facial dermatitis, headache (all reversible when drug is discontinued)

- If necessary, dermatology referral for
  1. Intralesional steroid injections of cysts and scars
  2. Acne surgery (comedone removal)
  3. Treatment of scars
     - Dermabrasion
     - Collagen injections
     - Excise individual scars

ALOPECIA

General Considerations and Differential Diagnosis

- Normal scalp hair growth is 1 cm/mo
- There are many causes of alopecia, and only the more common types are mentioned here. In approaching the differential diagnosis, consider whether the alopecia is:
  1. Scarring vs nonscarring
  2. Congenital vs acquired
  3. Patchy vs diffuse
  4. Inflammatory vs noninflammatory
- The presence or absence of scarring is the best way of generally categorizing the alopecias (Table 6–1)

TABLE 6–1 Causes of Alopecia

Nonscarring	Scarring (Cicatricial)
Alopecia areata	Physical trauma (radiation, thermal or chemical burns)
Trichotillomania or traction alopecia (if prolonged may lead to scarring)	Scarring dermatoses (discoid lupus erythematosus, lichen planopilaris, morphea)
Tinea capitis (note that some types cause scarring)	Developmental defects (aplasia cutis, epidermal nevi)
Telogen effluvium (diffuse hair loss following stress, such as infection, pregnancy, or surgery, as well as drugs, such as beta blockers, vitamin A, retinoids, heparin, Coumadin, propylthiouracil)	Infections (some types of fungi, bacteria, viruses, protozoa)
Anagen effluvium (associated with chemotherapeutic agents or other severe insults to body)	Neoplasms (benign or malignant)
Androgenic alopecia (hereditary male pattern baldness)	
Endocrine related alopecia and deficiency disorders (thyroid disease, severe iron deficiency)	
Hereditary disorders of hair shaft	

Management

- The three most common causes of patchy non-scarring alopecia in children are alopecia areata (see below), trichotillomania, and tinea (see p 100)
- Examine entire skin, mucosal surfaces, nails, and teeth
- Depending on the situation, fungal or other microbiologic studies, Wood's lamp examination, light microscopic examination of hair, or scalp biopsy, may be indicated

Alopecia Areata

- Billiard ball, smooth areas; exclamation mark hairs
- Prognosis unpredictable
- Rarely associated with autoimmune disease
- Potent topical steroids, e.g., fluocinonide, 0.05% tid (Lidex or Topsyn Gel), or intralesional steroids if patient can tolerate injections

ATOPIC DERMATITIS (AD)

- See Fig. 5–1

General Considerations

- Pruritic dermatitis of childhood
- Belongs to IgE atopy triad (AD, asthma, hay fever)
- 60% have family history of AD, asthma, or hay fever
- Usually begins after 3 mo of age (majority present before 1 yr of age)
- Usually improves by age 3–4 yr (75% of patients grow out of disease)

Clinical Features

- Erythema, scaling ± crusting, dry skin (xerosis)
- Lichenification is pathognomonic
- Infants: face, extensor surfaces

- Older children: flexor surfaces
- Dennie-Morgan folds (extra crease of lower eyelid)
- Differential includes contact dermatitis (allergic and irritant) and scabies

Associated Features

- Cutaneous features
  1. Pityriasis alba—hypopigmented, poorly demarcated patches on cheeks and upper outer arms
  2. Keratosis pilaris—keratotic asymptomatic papules on upper outer arms, occasionally cheeks, thighs; treatment not necessary
  3. Juvenile plantar dermatosis—erythema, scaling, fissuring of plantar aspect of toes and anterior third of soles; worse in winter; lasts until puberty; treat with emollients or topical steroids; advise patient to wear cotton socks (washed without bleach) and leather shoes
  4. Dyshidrotic eczema—deep seated tiny vesicles on palms and soles and in interdigital spaces
- Infections
  1. Viral—herpes simplex (Kaposi's varicelliform eruption)
  2. Bacterial—impetigo

Management

- Diet is controversial (some authors suggest avoiding fish, eggs, milk, and nuts before age 2)
- Environment
  1. Prevent overheating—wear cotton clothes, ensure adequate control of ambient temperature (air conditioning if necessary)
  2. Humidification—humidifier, daily bath (add oilated Aveeno, Alpha Keri, or baby oil to bath); pat dry
  3. Chemical—use mild soaps (e.g., Dove or baby soap), make sure clothes are rinsed well

when washed
- Topical agents
  1. Steroids (see p 102)—start with hydrocorti-
     sone, 1% tid to qid; if necessary, use more
     potent steroid to body (NOT on face or
     groin)
  2. Emollients (see p 103)
- Antihistamines: Benadryl, Atarax, or Seldane
  may help (especially if child cannot sleep
  because of itchiness)
- Antibiotics: erythromycin or cloxacillin PO for
  impetigo
- Systemic steroids: avoid if at all possible

BACTERIAL INFECTIONS

Cellulitis: see p 318
Erysipelas: see p 318

Furunculosis

Clinical Features

- A furuncle is an acute infection (usually
  staphylococcal) arising in a hair follicle
- Erythematous, tender, with surrounding cellulitis
- Often "points" then spontaneously drains
- Usually in a hairy area or area of friction
  (posterior neck, axillae, thighs, perineum)
- A carbuncle is a deeper infection of several
  adjacent hair follicles, with multiple draining
  sites

Management

- Hot compresses
- Incise and drain (when "pointing")
- Oral cloxacillin

Impetigo

- See Fig. 5–2

Clinical Features

- Contagious infection by beta hemolytic streptococcus or *S. aureus*
- Child not systemically ill
- Usually occurs on face and limbs
- Strep. impetigo
  1. Honey colored crusts ("classic" impetigo)
  2. Poststrep. glomerulonephritis can occur after
     impetigo or pharyngitis; poststrep. rheumatic
     fever occurs after pharyngitis, not after
     impetigo
- Staph. impetigo
  1. Bullous; often begins in folds (neck, groin)
  2. Staph. reservoir: upper respiratory tract

Management

- Cool compresses in order to dry lesions
- Penicillin or erythromycin PO for 10 days
- If staph. impetigo, use cloxacillin or erythro-
  mycin PO
- Treat underlying eczema if present once infec-
  tion has cleared

POISON IVY CONTACT DERMATITIS

- See Fig. 5–3

General Considerations

- An allergic (not irritant) contact dermatitis
- Vesiculobullous, papular, pruritic
- Usually linear distribution, with scattered
  lesions

Management

- Dry it (Burow's compress, 1:40 tid × 15 min)
- Potent steroid cream (e.g., Synalar Cream,
  0.025%) or lotion if weeping lesions

- Use prednisone (start at 1 mg/kg/day PO and taper over 1–2 wk period) if extensive

DIAPER DERMATITIS

- See Fig. 5–4 and 5–5

Clinical Features and Differential Diagnosis

- Contact (irritant) dermatitis: due to urine, feces, and maceration. Creases may be spared. If severe, it may lead to Jacquet's erosive diaper dermatitis (one or a few red papules with central erosion). More common with cloth diapers that are washed at home.
- Seborrheic dermatitis: greasy, scaly, and erythematous. Other areas may be involved, e.g., cradle cap, ears, and axillae. Creases are involved. If seborrheic dermatitis fails to respond to treatment, consider the possibility of histiocytosis X.
- Candida: very erythematous, satellite pustules or red papules, scaly border. There may be associated oral thrush. Creases are involved.

Management

- Avoid irritants on diapers and rinse out detergents and fabric softeners thoroughly
- Change diaper frequently
- Avoid plastic or rubber pants
- Burow's 1:40 compresses for 10–15 min tid if macerated
- 1% hydrocortisone ointment for contact dermatitis, seborrheic dermatitis
- If Candida primarily or superimposed: 1% hydrocortisone in Canesten cream
- Apply barrier ointment (zinc oxide)

ERYTHEMA MULTIFORME

General Considerations and Etiology

- Infection: herpes simplex, mycoplasma

- Drug: sulfa, phenytoin, and phenobarbital are most common
- Idiopathic, cancer

Clinical Features

- Classic (erythema multiforme [EM] minor)
  1. Asymptomatic, symmetrical, fixed, often acral
  2. Multiforme lesions (i.e., pleomorphic): target lesions (pathognomonic); urticaria; papules; macules; mucosal crusting; vesicles
- Erythema multiforme major
  1. Stevens-Johnson syndrome (see Fig. 5–6)
     - Painful skin lesions; higher morbidity and mortality; most frequently caused by drugs; mucosal lesions
     - Systemically ill; febrile
     - Mouth and genital erosions; lips crusted; ocular lesions (conjunctivitis, keratitis); can have classic EM skin lesions
  2. Toxic epidermal necrolysis (TEN, Lyell syndrome)
     - TEN now considered a severe form of EM
     - Usually a drug etiology
     - Painful sloughing of large areas of epidermis and sometimes of mucous membranes, upper respiratory, and GI tract
     - High mortality rate
     - Differential diagnosis is staphylococcal scalded skin syndrome (in SSSS, the cleavage in the epidermis is much higher)

Management

- Treat cause (e.g., discontinue any possible offending medications)
- In recurrent EM minor with herpes, can often abort episode by prednisone for 2 wk as soon as herpetic prodrome begins
- Ophthalmology consult mandatory for Stevens-Johnson syndrome
- Prednisone for Stevens-Johnson (or TEN) is controversial

- Treat TEN like a burn (depending on severity and extent of sloughing)

ERYTHEMA TOXICUM

General Considerations and Clinical Features

- Usually occurs within first week of life
- Erythematous patches and small pustules (filled with eosinophils)
- Needs no treatment and usually resolves within 1–2 wk

HEMANGIOMAS

- See Fig. 5–7 and 5–8

General Considerations

- Capillary (strawberry) hemangioma
  1. Immature capillaries—may be present at birth; usually appear within first 2 mo; ↑ in size for several months; usually start to involute by end of first year; 90% gone by age 10 yr
- Cavernous hemangioma
  1. Deeper and larger vessels than capillary type; may be present at birth
  2. Fade but less than capillary type
- Nevus flammeus
  1. Dilated mature vessels; present at birth; do not fade

Complications and Associated Syndromes

- Hemangiomas
  1. May enlarge very quickly (bleeding into hemangioma)
  2. May develop Kasabach-Merritt syndrome (see next page)
  3. May be located where it is frequently injured
  4. May affect important organs, especially eyes (amblyopia, glaucoma, strabismus)

- Sturge-Weber syndrome
  1. Definition
     - Congenital nevus flammeus of cranial nerve V_1 (may also involve V_2, V_3)
     - Ipsilateral leptomeningeal vascular anomaly
     - Ocular (choroidal) vascular anomaly
  2. Complications
     - CNS—seizures (80%, often initial symptom), retardation (60%), hemiplegia (30%)
     - Ocular glaucoma
     - Cutaneous—cosmetic importance only
- Rare syndromes
  1. Kasabach-Merritt syndrome—platelet sequestration by large hemangioma
  2. Klippel-Trenaunay syndrome—nevus flammeus with underlying soft tissue or bone hypertrophy of limb
  3. Neonatal hemangiomatosis—multiple cutaneous and visceral hemangiomas, which may lead to cardiac failure and gastrointestinal hemorrhage

Management of Capillary and Cavernous Hemangiomas

- Generally no treatment is necessary
- Prednisone, 1–3 mg/kg/day (may require several months of treatment with careful follow-up), if:
  1. Enlarges very quickly
  2. Affects vital structures
  3. Patient develops Kasabach-Merritt syndrome
- Cosmetic treatment: coverup makeup (Lydia O'Leary Covermark, Dermablend) or argon laser (once child is older)

LICE

General Considerations

- Pediculosis capitis (head louse)
  Adult louse is 3–4 mm long; eggs (nits) are 1

mm, usually white, and firmly adherent to the
hair shafts; usually <10 adults on an individual;
postauricular and occipital regions are most
common sites
- Pediculosis corporis (body louse)
  Slightly larger than the head louse; less common; insect lives in seams of clothing and goes
  onto the body to feed; lesions usually around
  shoulders and waist: papules, urticarial wheals,
  and excoriations
- Pediculosis pubis (crab louse)
  Smaller than head and body louse, with crab-
  like claws anteriorly; they remain in one place
  for days, feeding intermittently; transmitted by
  sexual contact or rarely by shared clothing

Management of Pediculosis Capitis and Pediculosis Pubis

- Lindane (gamma benzene hexachloride) shampoo to affected hair-bearing site. Lather for 10
  min and rinse. Repeat in 7 days
- Pyrethrins (e.g., A-200 Pyrinate) can be used as
  above instead of lindane
- Eyelashes may be involved with pediculosis
  pubis; apply petrolatum to eyelashes bid or tid
  for 10 days
- Remaining nits can be removed with vinegar
  (5% acetic acid) and a fine toothed comb
- Soak comb, brushes, barrettes in lindane shampoo for 10 min
- Clothing and bed linen should be washed in
  hot water or dry cleaned; pillows and mattres-
  ses should be vacuumed

Management of Pediculosis Corporis

- Clothing and bed linen should be washed in
  very hot water or ironed to kill parasites

MOLLUSCUM CONTAGIOSUM

- See Fig. 5–9

General Considerations

- Viral infection, most common in children
- Umbilicated, flesh colored papules
- Occurs anywhere in children; mostly genital in adults
- Is contagious and autoinoculable
- Usually asymptomatic; some develop a surrounding pruritic dermatitis, leading to scratching and further autoinoculation
- Lesions last from a few weeks to 2 yr

Management

- Children: topical cantharidin (0.7%) applied by the physician to lesions (avoid surrounding skin); warn patients to expect blistering
- Older children: can use cantharidin (0.7%), liquid nitrogen, or curettage
- Repeated treatment (every 2–3 wk) often necessary as new crops of lesions arise

PITYRIASIS ROSEA

- See Fig. 5–10

Clinical Features and Management

- Occurs at all ages
- Erythematous scaly patches classically in a "christmas tree" pattern on back; preceded by "herald patch" by days or weeks
- Usually on the upper trunk
- Lasts 6–8 wk and resolves spontaneously
- If pruritic, use warm oilated baths and topical steroids

SCABIES

Clinical Features

- Incubation period: 3–6 wk; primary lesion is a

burrow 2–10 mm in length with the female mite
at the end
- Very pruritic
- Papules, pustules, eczematous patches
- Sites of predilection: finger webs, axillae,
  genitalia, periumbilical area; palms, soles, nape
  of neck, and axillae in infants; face usually not
  involved except in infants and Norwegian
  (extensive) scabies
- If chronic, nodular lesions may develop

Management

- Under age 2 yr: 5% precipitated sulfur in white
  petrolatum bid × 2 wk (entire body)
- Over age 2 yr: Lindane (gamma benzene hexachloride) lotion. Apply from neck down; wash
  off after 12 hr. If done correctly, one application
  is sufficient, but it may be repeated next day.
  Do not use Lindane in children under 2 yr or
  in pregnancy.
- Advise to wash all bedclothing and personal
  clothing used recently
- Treat all household contacts as above, whether
  itchy or not
- Advise that pruritis and rash may persist for
  several weeks after mite eradicated
- Nodular lesions may persist for months after
  active infection is controlled (topical steroids
  may be beneficial)

SEBORRHEIC DERMATITIS

Clinical Features

- Infants
  1. Greasy scales on erythematous skin present
     on scalp (cradle cap), ears, eyebrows,
     nasolabial folds, axillae, diaper area; can also
     be more generalized
  2. Can start in neonatal period; usually lasts
     6–8 wk

3. Children are "fat, and happy" that is, unlike
   everybody who looks at them, they are not
   usually bothered by the skin condition
   (unlike children with atopic dermatitis)
- Adolescents, adults
  1. Erythema and fine scaling on scalp, eye-
     brows, nasolabial folds, eyelid margins, chest

Management

- Scalp: daily tar shampoo; baby oil to remove
  thick scale in infants (1–2 hr before shampoo-
  ing); 1% hydrocortisone lotion qhs
- Body: 1% hydrocortisone cream or ointment bid
  prn

STAPHYLOCOCCAL SCALDED SKIN SYNDROME (SSSS)

- See Fig. 5–11

Clinical Features
- Young children (under 8 yr)
- Due to exfoliative toxin made by certain types
  of *S. aureus* (phage group II)
- Source of staph.—usually nose, pharynx, eyes;
  cannot culture from skin bullae
- Sick, febrile
- Tender erythematous skin, peeling (flaccid bul-
  lae break easily)
- Positive Nikolsky sign
- Can be differentiated from toxic epidermal
  necrolysis by skin biopsy

Management

- Cloxacillin for 7–10 days, IV initially because of
  possibility of bacteremia
- Usually lasts 5–10 days

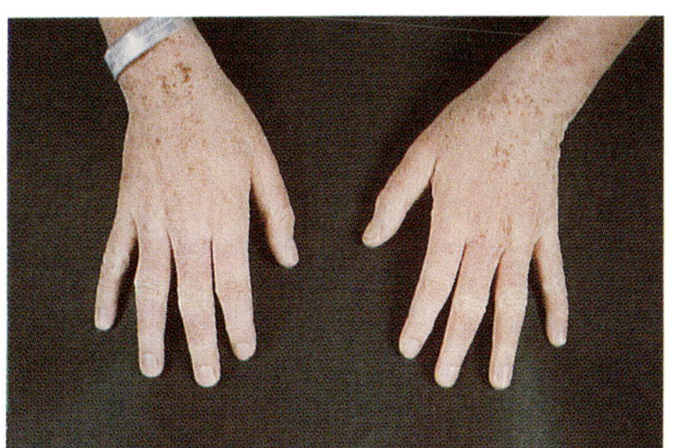

Figure 5–1 Atopic dermatitis.

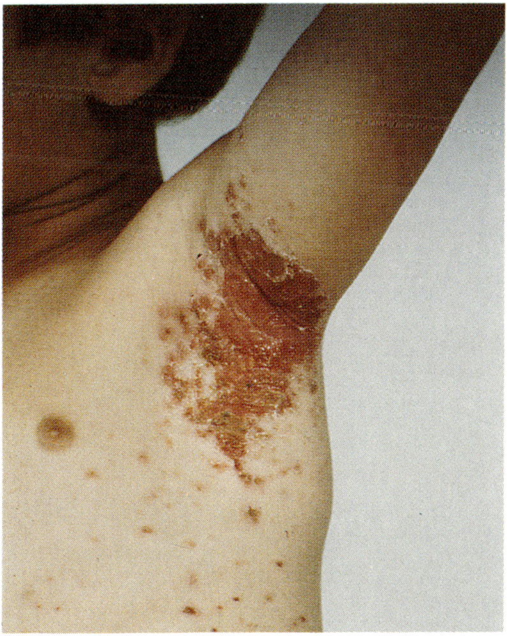

Figure 5–2 Impetigo.

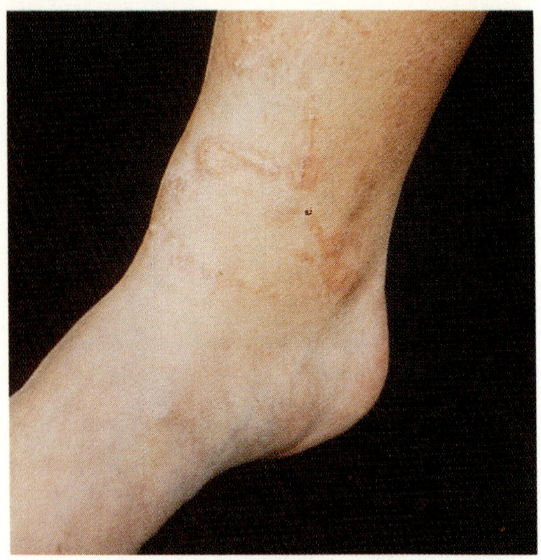

Figure 5-3 Poison ivy dermatitis.

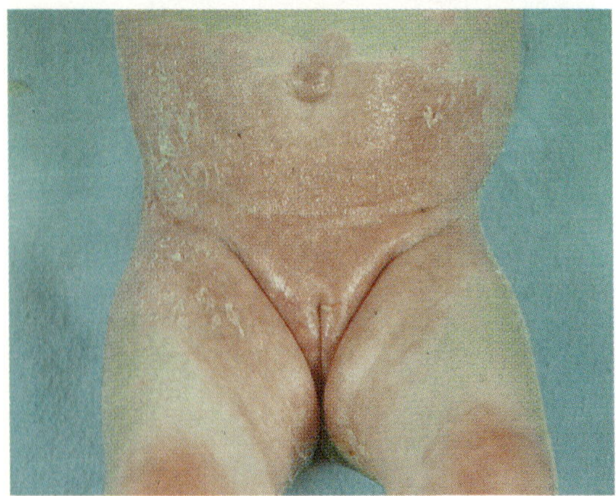

Figure 5-4 Seborrheic diaper dermatitis.

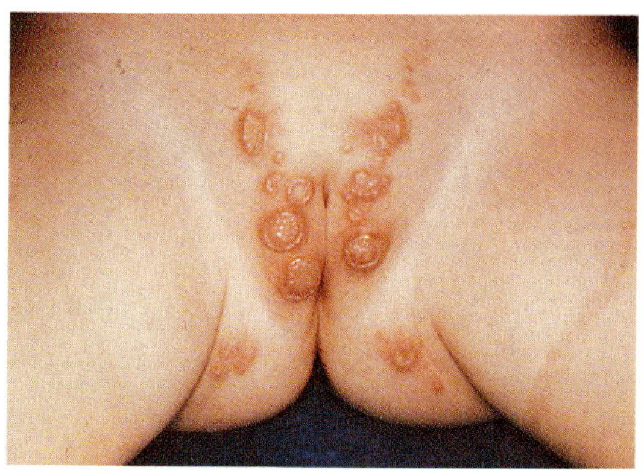

Figure 5-5 Jacquet's diaper dermatitis.

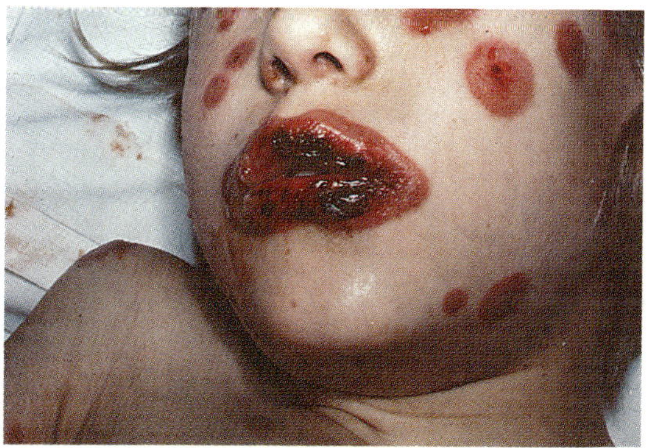

Figure 5-6 Stevens—Johnson syndrome.

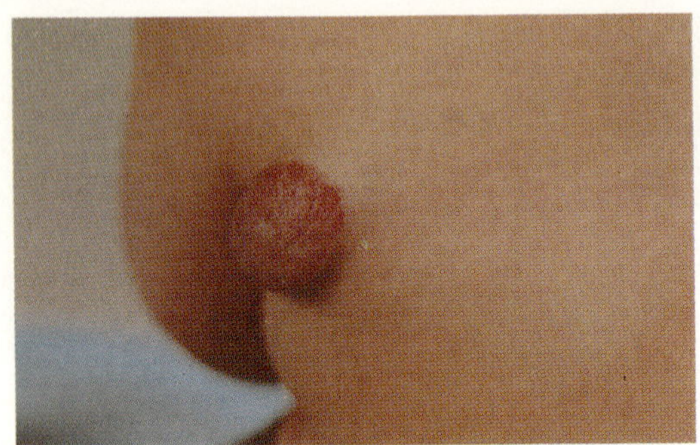

Figure 5–7   Capillary hemangioma.

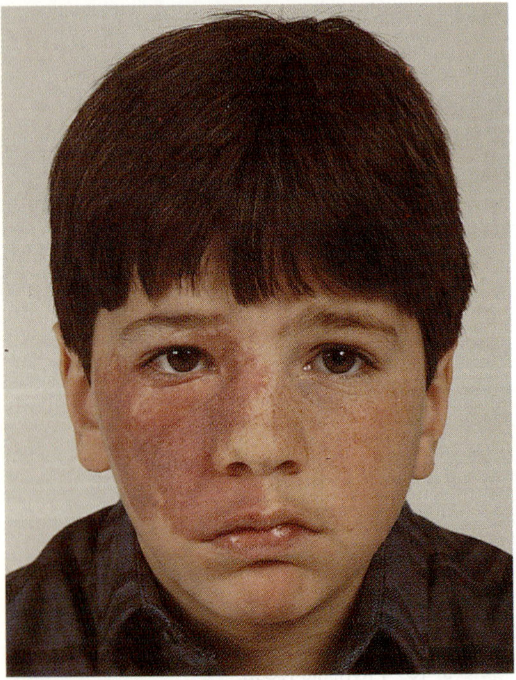

Figure 5–8   Nevus flammeus.

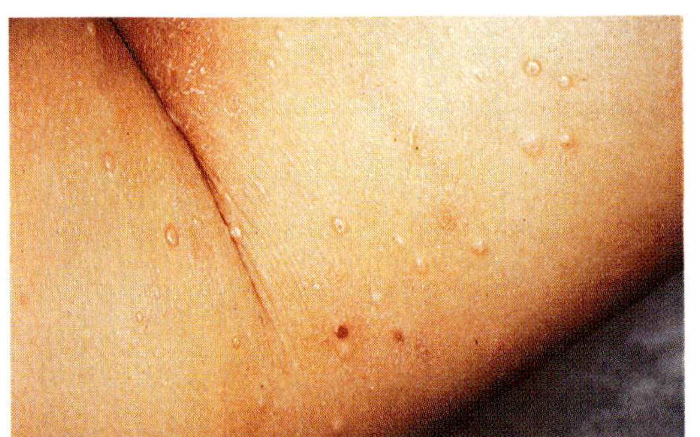

Figure 5–9 Molluscum contagiosum.

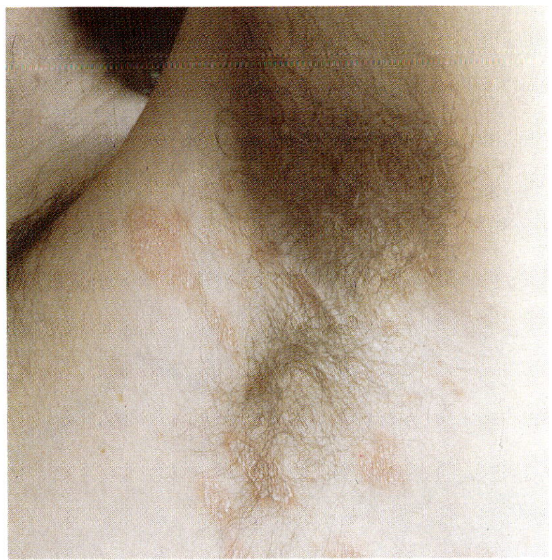

Figure 5–10 Pityriasis rosea.

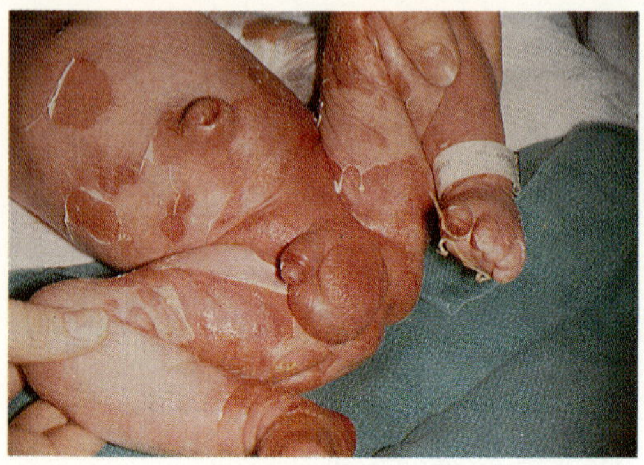

Figure 5–11   Staphylococcal scalded skin syndrome.

TINEA CAPITIS

General Considerations and Clinical Features

- Most frequent organisms: anthropophilic (*Microsporum audouinii, Trichophyton tonsurans*) and zoophilic (*Microsporum canis*)
- Nonscarring alopecia, scaly scalp
- "Black dot alopecia" (hairs very short because they break at scalp level)
- Kerion (often causes scarring)

Management

- Wood's lamp fluorescence (green) if *Microsporum audouinii* or *canis*
- Potassium hydroxide (KOH) prep. of scale and hair (see p 725)
- Fungal culture
- Griseofulvin (microsize preparation), 15 mg/kg/day once daily for 3 mo, or Griseofulvin (ultramicrosize preparation, e.g., Fulvicin P/G) give half the above dose, i.e., 5–10 mg/kg/day once daily for 3 mo

TOXIC EPIDERMAL NECROLYSIS (TEN)

- See p 88

URTICARIA

General Considerations

- Urticaria (hives) consists of transient (lasting less than 24 hr) erythematous pruritic wheals
- May involve eyelids, lips, tongue, pharynx, larynx
- The two serious complications are pharyngolaryngeal edema and anaphylaxis
- Many etiologies (mnemonic: IMPS)
  - I: idiopathic; inherited; inhalants; ingestants (food allergy, drugs); infections (hepatitis); infestations (especially gastrointestinal parasites, insect bites)
  - M: mastocytosis; malignant disease, metabolic
  - P: physical urticarias (cold, hot, cholinergic, solar, aquagenic, vibratory, pressure); psychogenic
  - S: systemic lupus erythematosus (and other connective tissue diseases); Still's disease
- Acute urticaria: lasts 6 wk or less, usually idiopathic or food or drug related
- Chronic urticaria: lasts longer than 6 wk, usually idiopathic

Management

- Find and treat cause if possible (CBC + differential + ESR, urinalysis, and stool for ova and parasites are reasonable initial investigations if nothing is suspected on basis of history or physical examination)
- Symptomatic treatment: antihistamines (oral, not topical)
- For pharyngolaryngeal edema: epinephrine and diphenhydramine parenterally (see p 662)

VERRUCAE

Management

- Verruca vulgaris
  1. Apply 75% salicylic acid in petrolatum and leave on for 1 wk; then debride in office
  2. Repeat until all warty tissue is removed
  3. Liquid nitrogen (if child over 5 yr old)
- Verruca plantaris
  1. Single warts: treat as above
  2. Multiple warts (mosaic): soak feet in 10% glutaraldehyde solution 15 min daily; then apply Duoplant to warts qhs and cover with Bandaid
- Verruca plana
  1. Peeling agent once daily or bid (vitamin A acid, 0.01 or 0.05%; benzoyl peroxide, 5–20%)
- Condyloma accuminata
  1. Apply (in office only) 25% podophyllin and leave on 6 hr (avoid contact with normal surrounding skin)
  2. Patient washes it off at home with soap and water
  3. Repeat weekly

TOPICAL STEROIDS

General Considerations

- Use a lotion on the scalp
- Ointments are used more in the winter (to prevent drying)
- Creams are used more during the summer
- Use creams in flexural areas
- Avoid using fluorinated steroids on face and in flexural areas
- Rule of thumb: 30 g (1 oz) of medication will cover an entire adult body once
- Side effects of topical steroids include degeneration of dermal collagen (atrophy, striae, purpura,

telangiectasia), infection, hypertrichosis, and
decreased pigmentation

TABLE 6–2 Examples of Topical Steroids

Potency	Brand Name	Generic Name
Nonfluorinated, lowest potency		Hydrocortisone (0.5%, 1%)
Nonfluorinated, low potency	Tridesilon	Desonide (0.05%)
	Westcort	Hydrocortisone valerate (0.2%)
Intermediate potency	Betnovate (0.05%, 0.1%)	Betamethasone valerate (0.05%, 0.1%)
	Valisone scalp lotion	Betamethasone valerate (0.1%)
	Kenalog, Aristo-cort (0.1%)	Triamcinolone acetonide (0.1%)
	Synalar (0.025%)	Fluocinolone acetonide (0.025%)
High potency	Cyclocort	Amcinonide (0.1%)
	Halog (0.1%)	Halcinonide (0.1%)
	Lidex (0.05%)	Fluocinonide (0.05%)
	Diprolene	Betamethasone dipro-pionate (0.05%)
Highest potency	Dermovate	Clobetasol propionate (0.05%)

EMOLLIENTS

General Considerations

- Use after bath and prn for dry skin
- Some examples include: 10% urea in hydrous eucerin and proprietary preparations such as Complex 15 cream, Nutraplus, Lachydrin, Aquatain

Suggested Reading

1. Fitzpatrick T, Eisen A, Wolff K, Freedberg I, Austen K, eds. Dermatology in general medicine. New York: McGraw-Hill, 1979.
2. Hurwitz S. Clinical pediatric dermatology. Philadelphia: W.B. Saunders, 1981.

7 ENDOCRINOLOGY

DIABETES MELLITUS

General Considerations

- Diabetes can occur in infants as well as older children
- This outline concentrates on management. For details of incidence, etiology, and so forth, the reader is referred to textbooks of pediatrics, endocrinology, or diabetes (see suggested reading).

Clinical Features

- Polyuria, polydipsia, weight loss, fatigue, monilial vaginal or diaper infections

Management

- Investigations
  1. The diagnosis is based on symptoms of polyuria, polydipsia, and weight loss plus a random blood glucose >11 mmol/L (200 mg/dl) (with or without ketonuria)
  2. If the child does not have ketonuria, electrolyte and acid-base measurements are not necessary. Ketonuria may be present without acidosis.
  3. If there is ketoacidosis, vomiting, abdominal pain, rapid breathing, or unconsciousness may be present. pH, Pco_2, bicarbonate, sodium, potassium, chloride, urea nitrogen, as well as blood glucose determinations are required. Calculate the anion gap: sodium − (chloride + bicarbonate).
     - Mild ketoacidosis: pH 7.2–7.3
     - Moderate ketoacidosis: pH 7.0–7.2
     - Severe ketoacidosis: pH less than 7.0

- Treatment
  1. The child requires hospital admission when a diagnosis of diabetes mellitus is made
  2. The parents are usually quite upset. Do not discuss too many details about diabetes. A positive, optimistic outlook is important.
A. Child without diabetic ketoacidosis. If the child is not vomiting, an intravenous line is not necessary. In this circumstance:
  - Give crystalline insulin, ~ 0.25 U/kg body weight SC, to relieve symptoms
  - Begin lente or NPH insulin the next day, approximately 1 unit per year of age. Human insulin is now being used for newly diagnosed children, but animal insulins are also satisfactory.
  - Increase the dosage 10–20%/day until target values of blood glucose are achieved (see below)
  - Nursing protocols are established in the hospital for the frequency of blood glucose and urine glucose and ketone determinations
  - The dietitian assesses dietary needs and adjusts the diet every 1–2 days
  - A diabetes nurse educator arranges teaching for the parents; usually takes ~ 2 wk
B. Child with diabetic ketoacidosis
  - Start an infusion of 0.9% saline or Ringer's lactate at 15–20 ml/kg body weight/hr for the first 2 hr; then 10–15 ml/kg body weight/hr until acidosis is corrected. A good rule for any child >6 yr is to give 1 liter of fluid in the first hour, 1 liter in the next 2 hr, and 1 liter in the following 3 hr.
  - Add 25 units of regular insulin to 250 ml of saline and infuse using Y tubing or a second infusion line. Do not delay in beginning insulin once the diagnosis is established. Start IV insulin infusion at 0.1 U/kg body weight per hour (1 ml/kg/hr of the diluted insulin solution).

- If serum K >5 mmol/L (mEq/L), wait until patient voids to add KCl; dose 3–5 mmol (mEq)/kg/24 hr. If serum K <4.0 mmol/L (mEq/L), add KCl immediately.
- Evaluate patient's condition frequently: calculate the fluid balance, i.e., the input and output. Use this as a guide to calculating fluid and electrolyte replacement after the first few hours.
- If pH <7.2 and plasma bicarbonate <12, give sodium bicarbonate to correct to those levels using formula [(12 − observed bicarbonate) × body weight in kg × 0.6 = millimoles of bicarbonate necessary to raise the plasma bicarbonate to 12]. Give half the dose stat IV over 10–20 min; then the remainder over ~1–2 hr. Reassess acid-base status q4h.
- Chemstrips bG/blood glucose at least q2h
- Repeat biochemical determinations q4h
- When blood glucose <15 mmol/L (<270 mg/dl), add glucose to IV solution and reduce rate of insulin infusion to 0.02 U/kg body weight/hr. Switch to 5% glucose in 0.2% saline (or 3.33% dextrose and 0.3% saline).
- NPO until child is out of severe acidosis; then begin with fluids and work up to a full diet
- General measures
    1. Establish diabetes coma chart
    2. Accurate intake and output
    3. Vital signs and level of consciousness every hour
    4. Continue insulin infusion until the following morning when intermediate acting insulin can be started if pH >7.3 and bicarbonate >20 mmol/L (mEq/L)
- Complications of diabetic ketoacidosis (DKA)
    1. Hypoglycemia—blood glucose <3 mmol/L (48 mg/dL)

2. Hypokalemia—serum K <3 mmol/L (mEq/L)
3. Slipping back into acidosis when partially corrected
4. Cerebral edema: most children fall
   asleep during treatment of DKA but can be
   easily roused. Any failure to rouse the child
   should raise concern of hypoglycemia or
   cerebral edema. The blood glucose level
   should be determined immediately. If in
   doubt, a bolus of 50% glucose should be administered.
- General comments on the management of diabetes at the Hospital for Sick Children (may
  vary elsewhere)
  1. The education of the child and the family is
     carried out by the diabetes team
  2. Children with diabetes should be seen regu-
     larly for follow-up—more frequently at first
     and then about every 3 mo
  3. All children should monitor their own blood
     glucose using one of the several methods
     available. The target values for blood glucose
     are 4-10 mmol/L (75-180 mg/dl) before main
     meals 70–80% of the time
  4. Urine should be tested for ketones if
     blood glucose levels are over 13 mmol/L
     (235 mg/dl) or an illness is present
  5. The glycosylated hemoglobin value is the
     best index of long-term control and should
     be determined at each clinic visit every 3
     mo. Glycosylated hemoglobin levels for non-
     diabetics are 0.04 to 0.06. The average for
     most children with diabetes is 0.09. Values
     under 0.09 indicate acceptable control.
     Values over 0.12 require action to improve
     control.
  6. Many children can maintain good metabolic
     control with one injection of insulin per day
     until they stop producing their own insulin,
     i.e., until they come out of their "honey-
     moon" phase; then two injections of insulin

are usually necessary. Some children, particularly infants, require two injections initially.
- Surgery in a child with diabetes mellitus
  1. Children with diabetes mellitus tolerate sur-
     gery as well as children without diabetes
  2. Blood glucose control should be reasonable
     and the urine must be free of ketones
  3. For a child in good control, admission to the
     hospital the day before is sufficient
  4. If control is poor, several days in the hospital
     to achieve target values of blood glucose
     (4–10 mmol/L [75–180 mg/dl] before break-
     fast and before supper) is required
- Elective surgery
  1. Minor procedure (less than 1 hr duration,
     with the ability to take fluids shortly after
     surgery is completed, e.g., hernia, T&A)
     - Preferable to book surgery at 0800–0900
       hr. This is not mandatory, since children
       can be managed even when surgery is
       booked for later in the day.
     - The child is kept NPO and an IV of 3.33%
       dextrose and 0.3% saline (⅔:⅓) plus KCl
       at maintenance rates is established at ap-
       proximately 0730–0800
     - SC intermediate acting insulin (Lente or
       NPH) only is given; usually two-thirds the
       total daily dose is administered. No regular
       insulin should be given.
     - Blood sugar values at 0700 to 0730 and
       immediately postoperatively are required
     - Extra crystalline insulin is given to main-
       tain blood glucose between 5 and 15
       mmol/L (90–270 mg/dl) postoperatively
     - Resume usual insulin when the child is
       able to take fluids and solids orally, usually
       the next day
  2. Major procedures (longer than 1 hr in length,
     less likely to drink and eat immediately after
     surgery, e.g., acute appendicitis, wisdom
     teeth)

- Same general principles as for minor surgery
  - No SC insulin on day of surgery
  - An insulin infusion of 0.02 U of regular insulin/kg body weight/hr is a reasonable starting rate. Adjust rate of infusion to maintain blood glucose between 5–15 mmol/L (90–270 mg/dl.
  - Surgery can be booked any time of day
  - Blood glucose every hour, while in the OR, by the laboratory and chemstrips bG
  - Postoperative glucose values are obtained q4h to maintain blood glucose at 5–15 mmol/L (90–270 mg/dl)
  - Check urine for ketones twice a day
  - Discontinue insulin infusion when child can tolerate fluids by mouth
  - Restart SC insulin at half to two-thirds the usual dose and increase as indicated to obtain target values of blood glucose
- Emergency surgery
  1. Determine acid-base and electrolyte status
  2. Correct dehydration and acidosis if present; usually requires only a few hours
  3. Give extra insulin as required either SC or by IV infusion, depending on the time from previous insulin dose and the type of procedure anticipated

Hypoglycemia in a Child with Diabetes Mellitus

- Most children with reasonable metabolic control usually have symptoms of *mild hypoglycemia* with extra activity; they should not occur with the usual activities of daily living
- Most children or their parents can recognize and treat these symptoms themselves with oral glucose, milk, juice, regular pop, corn syrup, honey, or Dextrosol

- Repeated episodes of mild hypoglycemia should be reported and adjustments in diet and insulin made

Severe Hypoglycemia

- Severe hypoglycemia is associated with alteration or loss of consciousness requiring the assistance of another person and should be reported immediately
- The parents should have glucagon for SC injection made available. They may need to be reminded to give it; 1 mg (one vial) should be given SC.
- If a convulsion has occurred, the child should be seen in the nearest emergency department
- If a seizure or unconsciousness has occurred, a bolus of 50% glucose, 0.5 g/kg body weight up to 25 g, should be administered, regardless of the level of consciousness at that time. Do not rely on oral glucose because many children vomit.
- It is recommended that after the bolus of 50% glucose, an IV infusion containing glucose, e.g., D5 with 0.2% saline, be given for several hours to make sure the child has completely recovered
- Most severe reactions have an explanation and steps should be taken to avoid a repetition. If there is no readily apparent explanation for the reaction, changes in insulin or diet are required.

Illness in Child with Diabetes Mellitus

- Should an intercurrent illness occur in the child with diabetes mellitus, the following guidelines are helpful:

1. Measure blood glucose and urine ketones immediately and q4h around the clock. Refer to Table 7–1 for appropriate action.
2. If the child cannot eat, offer sugar-containing fluids such as regular soda pop or juice
3. Give an antipyretic if indicated
4. Should vomiting develop twice in 4–6 h, the child should be seen in the emergency department. If the child has been vomiting clear fluids and is nauseated, do not give oral fluids but establish an intravenous line and keep NPO for a few hours.

AMBIGUOUS GENITALIA

General Considerations

- Requires immediate and urgent action to avoid serious problems for the child and the family
- If masses are present in the scrotum or the groins, a Y chromosome is usually present
- Hypospadias with descended and easily palpable testes and a well developed penis is not as urgent as a small, poorly developed phallus with inpalpable testes and a single opening in the perineum

Management

- Tell the parents the genitalia are "incomplete" or "unfinished" and that you are not sure whether the infant is a boy or a girl
- Blood for 17-hydroxyprogesterone (17-OHP) and chromosome karyotyping are the initial investigations
- If 17-OHP is increased, the diagnosis is congenital adrenal hyperplasia (see p 758 for normal 17-OHP levels)
- If 17-OHP is normal, await chromosome analysis. If chromosomes are 46 XY with a normal 17-OHP, the child is a male pseudohermaphro-

TABLE 7–1   Guidelines for Insulin Adjustment During Intercurrent Illness

Sickness Profile	A	B	C	D	E
Is sickness present?	Yes	Yes (usually more severe)	Yes	Yes	Yes
Blood glucose in mmol/L(mg/dl)	≥ 4.4 and <13.3 (≥ 80 and <240)	≥ 13.3 and <22.2 (≥ 240 and <400)	≥ 22.2 (≥ 400)	≥ 13.3 (≥ 240)	<4.4 (<80)
Urine ketones	Negative or positive	Negative	Negative	Positive	Negative or positive
Action	Wait; continue to monitor carefully	Wait; if the condition persists, increase insulin next day by 10–20%/day until achieve aims	Give extra soluble insulin q4h, equal to approximately 20% of total daily dose until acetone clears and/or blood sugar <13.3 mmol/L (<240 mg/dL); then proceed as for regimen in columns A/B		Decrease daily insulin by 20%/day until blood glucose is between 4.4 mmol/L (80 mg/dl) and 13.3 mmol/L (240 mg/dl)

dite and needs more extensive investigation,
which may include:
1. Gonadotrophins and testosterone level
2. Examination under anesthesia with cysto-
   scopy and a urethrogram
3. Pelvic ultrasound may be helpful, but can
   give false positive and negative results

- Sex of rearing
  1. The sex of rearing depends on a number of
     factors including anatomic configuration of
     the genitalia, possibility of surgical correc-
     tion, and underlying condition, e.g., andro-
     gen sensitivity
  2. In order to make a rational decision concern-
     ing sex of rearing, it is best to have all the in-
     formation necessary. In addition to the above,
     a trial of testosterone to see whether the
     phallus will enlarge, and a laparotomy, in-
     cluding gonadal biopsy, before assigning or
     changing the sex of rearing may be required.
  3. Management involves pediatricians, endo-
     crinologists, urologists, and gynecologists

ADRENAL INSUFFICIENCY

General Considerations

- A rare cause of shock, vascular collapse,
  hypoglycemia, and hyponatremia in infancy and
  childhood
- Usual cause in the newborn is congenital
  adrenal hyperplasia with chronic adrenal insufficiency. Addison's disease is extremely rare in
  childhood. Iatrogenic adrenal suppression is
  common in children taking pharmacologic
  doses of adrenal steroids. Children with diseases of the hypothalamic-pituitary area are
  also at risk for adrenal insufficiency during an
  intercurrent illness.

Clinical Features

- Shock with dehydration, a low sodium (<130 mmol/L [mEq/L]), a high potassium (>5 mmol/L [mEq/L]) with or without hypoglycemia

Management

- Investigation
  1. Plasma cortisol, renin, aldosterone levels plus electrolyte levels at the time of presentation *before treatment*
  2. If ambiguous genitalia are present, a 17-OHP level should be obtained; renin and aldosterone levels are not as important
- Treatment
  1. Glucose and saline to correct the hypoglycemia and hyponatremia. Hyponatremia can be corrected by saline intravenously, but can be maintained only with the addition of a mineralocorticoid. Correction of the hyponatremia usually allows the child to take oral 9-α-fludro cortisone acetate (Florinef); the dose is 0.05 to 0.2 mg/day.
  2. Treat the underlying condition, e.g., meningitis
  3. Solucortef, 100 mg/m^2, stat and q4h intravenously. Larger doses can be given safely in older infants and children.
  4. Initiate appropriate diagnostic tests to determine the underlying cause of the adrenal insufficiency, e.g., chromosomes, adrenal antibodies, 17-OH-progesterone, ultrasound, or CT scan of the abdomen or head

CONGENITAL ADRENAL HYPERPLASIA

- See also section on ambiguous genitalia

Management

- Hydrocortisone, 20–25 mg/m²/day in divided doses orally
- 9-α-fludro cortisone acetate, 0.05 to 0.2 mg/day in divided doses, in most children who are salt losers
- The child's growth in length, weight, and 17-OHP, androstenedione, testosterone, and renin levels (if salt loser) are required at regular intervals
- The dose of hydrocortisone must be tripled if an intercurrent illness develops. Should the child develop persistent vomiting, he must be seen in the emergency department and be given IV fluids.
- The management of chronic adrenal insufficiency, i.e., Addison's disease is similar to that of congenital adrenal hyperplasia

HYPOCALCEMIA

General Considerations

- Definition
  1. Term infant: plasma calcium <1.9 mmol/L (7.5 mg/dl)
  2. Preterm infant: plasma calcium <1.75 mmol/L (7 mg/dl)
  3. Older child: plasma calcium <2.0 mmol/L (8 mg/dl)
  4. Symptoms may or may not be present. Most older children complain of muscle cramps or tingling. The Trousseau and Chvostek signs are often present. In infancy, symptomatic hypocalcemia may lead to cerebral damage or sudden death
  5. See also neonatology section (p 398)
- Causes
  1. Transient neonatal hypoparathyroidism, permanent hypoparathyroidism, vitamin D defi-

ciency, the DiGeorge syndrome, steatorrhea, acute and chronic renal insufficiency

Management

- Calcium gluconate intravenously; dose is 0.1 mmol of elemental calcium/kg body weight/hr. Dilute 10% calcium gluconate to a 2% solution with 5% glucose and water. This dilution provides 0.05 mmol/ml. Therefore, the dose of calcium equals 2 ml/kg body weight/hr, e.g., for 10 kg child equals 20 ml/hr of the 2% calcium gluconate solution. Adjust infusion rate q4h on basis of plasma calcium level. Aim for a plasma calcium of 2 mmol/L (8 mg/dl). Once desired level is reached, reduce infusion rate slowly. If plasma calcium drops, increase rate of infusion.
- Oral calcium, 100 mg/kg (of elemental calcium) per day; usually calcium lactate is used
- Dose of calcitriol (1,25-dihydroxy vitamin D_3)
  1. Newborns: 0.10–0.15 μg/kg body weight/day; reduce to 0.025–0.05 μg/kg body weight/day after 3–4 days
  2. Older children: 0.025–0.05 μg/kg body weight/day
  3. Monitor serum calcium daily

Points to Note

- Symptomatic hypocalcemia is an emergency, particularly in infancy. Oral calcium supplements are insufficient to relieve symptoms.
- Be sure intravenous needle is definitely and securely in a vein
- Watch for evidence of the infusion going interstitial or venous thrombosis developing. The addition of 0.1 ml of 1,000 U/ml heparin to each 100 ml of calcium gluconate reduces the risk of thrombosis.
- Do not administer calcium gluconate and sodium bicarbonate in the same intravenous tubing
- Never give calcium intramuscularly or subcutaneously

HYPERCALCEMIA

Definition and Management

- Serum calcium >3 mmol/L (12 mg/dl). If vitamin D compounds are being given, they should be stopped immediately.
- Treatment consists of a low calcium diet, a high fluid intake, IV fluids to expand the extracellular volume (usually normal saline administered at two and one-half times the maintenance rate), corticosteroids (e.g., hydrocortisone), and furosemide (Lasix), 0.5 to 1.0 mg/kg intravenously q4–6h

THYROID DISORDERS

- Table 7–2 groups thyroid function tests into categories that are considered clinically useful and Table 7–3 interprets the results
- The indications for the tests vary depending on the condition being investigated. Investigation of the commoner thyroid conditions is as follows:
  1. Goiter: T_4, TSH, T_3RU, TT_3, thyroid antibodies
  2. Suspected hypothyroidism: T_4, TSH, T_3RU, thyroid antibodies
  3. Suspected hyperthyroidism: T_4, T_3RU, TSH, TT_3, thyroid antibodies
  4. Thyroid nodule: T_4, TSH, TT_3, thyroid antibodies, nuclear scan, ultrasound, possible needle biopsy

ANTIDIURETIC HORMONE DEFICIENCY

General Considerations and Clinical Features

- ADH deficiency is a cause of diabetes insipidus and can result from a tumor, trauma, or histiocytosis X or can be idiopathic
- There is usually severe polyuria and polydipsia

TABLE 7–2 Thyroid Function Tests

Tests to Determine Thyroid Status	Tests to Determine the Cause of Thyroid Disease	Special Tests
Thyroxine (T_4)	Thyroid antibodies	Radioactive iodine uptake
Thyroid stimulating hormone (TSH)	Ultrasound of thyroid gland	Thyroglobulin
Tri-iodothyronine resin uptake (T_3RU)	Nuclear scan of thyroid	Thyroid stimulating immunoglobulin
Tri-iodothyronine (TT_3)	Thyrotrophin releasing hormone stimulation test (TRH test)	Needle biopsy of thyroid

TABLE 7–3 Interpretation of Results

	T_4	TSH	TT_3	Thyroid Antibodies
Euthyroid	Normal	Normal	Normal	±
Hypothyroid				
Primary	Low	High	Low or normal	±
Secondary	Low	Normal	Low or normal	Negative
Tertiary	Low	Usually normal	Low or normal	Negative
Hyperthyroid	High	Normal	High	±

with a dilute urine that does not contain glucose

Management

- Investigation
  1. Accurate intake and output
  2. Daily weights
  3. Electrolytes, urea nitrogen, creatinine
  4. Water deprivation test (see an endocrinology textbook)
  5. Skull film, CT scan as indicated

- Treatment
  - Treat underlying condition if present
  1. DDAVP (Minirin), 0.05 to 0.1 ml intranasally q12–24h, usually controls symptoms

HYPOGLYCEMIA

Neonatal Hypoglycemia

- See p 395

See p 395

Older Infants and Children

General Considerations

- Hypoglycemia is an uncommon cause of convulsions. Always check blood sugar level in a child with first-time seizures.
- Hyperinsulinism can present after the neonatal period
- Ketotic hypoglycemia is the commonest cause in children 1–4 yr of age

Management

- Critical sample consists of blood glucose, acid-base values, electrolytes, insulin, growth hormone, cortisol, lactate, and 3-hydroxybutyric acid
- If hypoglycemia is detected, take critical sample (about 2 ml of heparinized blood) *before* any treatment, and send to laboratory. Plasma can be frozen for special tests.
- Treat hypoglycemia with 50% glucose (0.5 g/kg IV bolus) plus continuous glucose infusion to maintain normal level of blood glucose
- Recurrent hypoglycemia may require glucagon infusion
- To investigate recurrent hypoglycemia, monitored starvation is carried out by either the endocrine or metabolic service
- Procedure for monitored starvation
  1. Child is not fed after supper for 24 hr

2. Blood glucose level is obtained at 0800, 1200, and 1500 hr the next day *or* if symptoms of hypoglycemia develop. If hypoglycemia occurs—blood glucose <2.2 mmol/L (40 mg/dl)—take blood for acid-base values, insulin, growth hormone, cortisol, lactate, and 3-hydroxybutyric acid.
3. See Table 7–4 for interpretation of results in major differential diagnoses of hypoglycemia

TABLE 7–4 Major Differential Diagnoses of Hypoglycemia*

	Hyper-insulinism	Substrate Deficiency	Ketotic Hypoglycemia	Normal
Glucose	Low	Low	Low	Normal
Insulin	High	Low	Low	Low
Lactic acid	Nor/low	High	Normal	Normal
3-Hydroxybutyric acid	Low	High	Very high	Normal

* From Aynsley-Green A. Hypoglycemia in infancy and childhood. Clin Endocrinol Metab 1982; 11:159.

Suggested Reading

1. Daneman D, Ehrlich R. Management of insulin dependent diabetes mellitus in childhood. Medicine NA 1984; 15:1852.
2. Daneman D, Kooh SW, Fraser D. Hypoparathyroidism and pseudohypoparathyroidism in childhood. Clin Endocrinol Metab 1982; 11:211.
3. Ehrlich RM. Diabetes mellitus in childhood. Clin Endocrinol Metab 1982; 11:195.
4. Hughes IA. Congenital and acquired disorders of the adrenal cortex. Clin Endocrinol Metab 1982; 11:89.
5. National Diabetes Data Group: Classification and diagnosis of diabetes mellitus and other categories of glucose intolerance. Diabetes 1974; 28:1039.
6. Saenger P. Abnormal sex differentiation. J Pediatr 1984; 104:1–14.

8   EPIDEMIOLOGY

DIAGNOSTIC TESTS

Sensitivity, Specificity, and Predictive Values

Disease

		Present	Absent	
Test	Positive	a	b	a + b
	Negative	c	d	c + d
		a + c	b + d	a + b + c + d

a = True positive (TP)
b = False positive (FP)

c = False negative (FN)
d = True negative (TN)

Figure 8–1   2 × 2 table of test results.

- Prevalence of disease (pretest probability of having the disease) =

$$\frac{a+c}{a+b+c+d}$$

- Sensitivity of test (proportion of those with the disease who have a positive test) =

$$\frac{a}{a+c} = \frac{TP}{TP+FN}$$

- Specificity of test (proportion of those without the disease who have a negative test) =

$$\frac{d}{b+d} = \frac{TN}{FP+TN}$$

- Positive predictive value (PV +'ve, post-test probability of having the disease if the test is positive) =

$$\frac{a}{a+b} = \frac{TP}{TP+FP}$$

- Negative predictive value (PV −'ve, post-test probability of *not* having the disease if the test is negative) =

$$\frac{d}{c+d} = \frac{TN}{FN+TN}$$

Likelihood Ratio

- Sensitivity and specificity are usually independent of the prevalence of a disease
- Predictive values (+'ve and −'ve) vary with the prevalence of a disease, which may differ according to the population studied (e.g., hospitalized patients vs patients seen in a private practice)
- Likelihood ratios provide another estimate of the post-test probability of disease that is usually independent of prevalence
- Likelihood ratio for a +'ve test =

$$\frac{a}{a+c} \div \frac{b}{b+d} = \frac{Sensitivity}{1-Specificity}$$

- Likelihood ratio for a −'ve test =

$$\frac{c}{a+c} \div \frac{d}{b+d} = \frac{1-Sensitivity}{Specificity}$$

- To use likelihood ratios, it is useful to express the likelihood of having disease as an odds (ratio of those who have the disease to those who do not) rather than a probability (fraction of the entire population that have the disease). Figure 8–2 demonstrates the difference between probability and odds using an example of a population of 100, of whom 20 have the disease (▥) and 80 do not (▤).

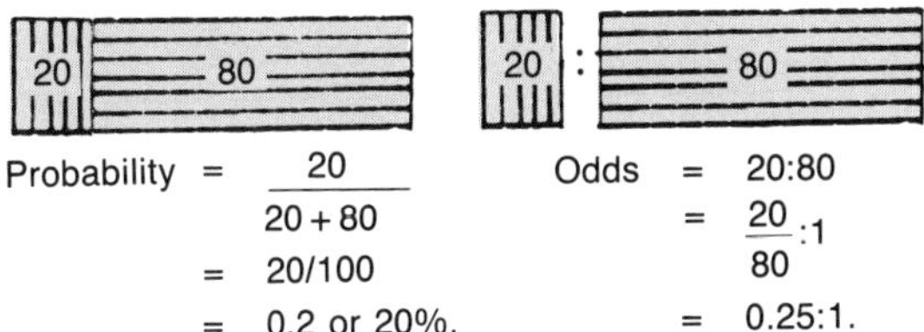

Probability $= \dfrac{20}{20+80}$

$= 20/100$

$= 0.2$ or 20%.

Odds $= 20{:}80$

$= \dfrac{20}{80}{:}1$

$= 0.25{:}1.$

Figure 8–2 Probability vs odds.

To convert from one to other:

$$\text{Odds} = \frac{\text{Probability}}{1-\text{Probability}}$$

$$\text{Probability} = \frac{\text{Odds}}{\text{Odds}+1}$$

- Post-test odds of having the disease (if the test is +'ve) = pretest odds × likelihood ratio (for a +'ve test)
- Post-test odds of having the disease (if the test is −'ve) = pretest odds × likelihood ratio (for a −'ve test)
- Alternatively one can "ignore" the term odds and use the nomogram in Figure 8–3 to determine the post-test probability directly from the pretest probability (prevalence of disease) and the likelihood ratio. (When using the nomogram, note that the pre- and post-test probabilities are expressed in percentages rather than in fractions.)

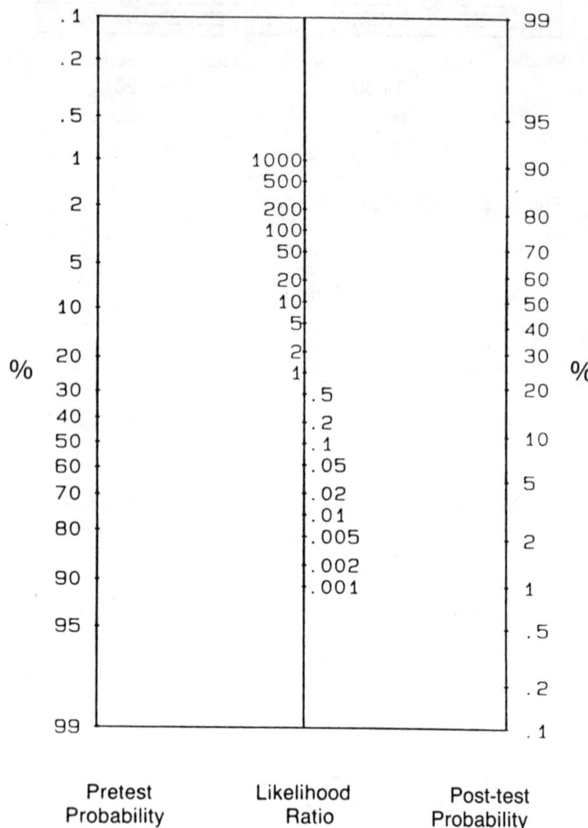

Figure 8–3 Nomogram for applying likelihood ratios. (Adapted from Fagan TJ. Nomogram for Bayes' theorem. N Engl J Med [letter] 1975; 293:257. In: Sackett DL, Haynes RB, Tugwell P. Clinical epidemiology: a basic science for clinical medicine. Boston: Little, Brown, 1985:112.)

Applying a Diagnostic Test[*]

[*] Data from Teele DW, Pelton SI, Grant MJA, et al. Bacteremia in febrile children under 2 years of age: results of cultures of blood of 600 consecutive febrile children seen in a "walk-in" clinic. J Pediatr 1975; 87:227.

<table>
<tr><td rowspan="2"></td><td rowspan="2"></td><td colspan="2" align="center">Bacteremia[†]</td><td></td><td></td></tr>
<tr><td align="center">Present</td><td align="center">Absent</td><td></td><td></td></tr>
<tr><td rowspan="2">WBC</td><td>$\geq 15 \times 10^9$/L</td><td align="center">15</td><td align="center">194</td><td align="center">209</td><td>PV +'ve = 15/209 = 0.07</td></tr>
<tr><td>$< 15 \times 10^9$/L</td><td align="center">4</td><td align="center">387</td><td align="center">391</td><td>PV −'ve = 387/391 = 0.99</td></tr>
<tr><td></td><td></td><td align="center">19</td><td align="center">581</td><td align="center">600</td><td></td></tr>
</table>

Sensitivity = 15/19 = 0.79. Specificity = 387/581 = 0.67. Prevalence of bacteremia (pretest probability of bacteremia) = 19/600 = 0.03.

[†] As determined by the "gold standard," i.e., blood culture

Figure 8–4 The use of the WBC in the diagnosis of bacteremia.

- Pretest odds $= \dfrac{\text{Pretest prob.}}{1 - \text{Pretest prob.}}$

$$= \frac{0.03}{0.97} = 0.03{:}1$$

  (i.e., odds of having bacteremia are 0.03:1) In this case the pretest odds and pretest probability happen to be equal when rounded off to two decimals because the pretest probability is very low
- Likelihood ratio for a WBC $\geq 15 \times 10^9$/L $= \dfrac{\text{Sensitivity}}{1 - \text{Specificity}} = \dfrac{15/19}{194/581} = 2.36$

1. Post-test odds of bacteremia (if WBC $\geq 15 \times 10^9$/L) $=$
$$\frac{0.03}{0.97} \times 2.36 = 0.07{:}1$$

2. Post-test probability of bacteremia (if WBC $\geq 15 \times 10^9$/L) $=$
$$\frac{\text{Post-test odds}}{\text{Post-test odds}+1} = \frac{0.07}{1.07} = 0.065$$
(i.e., if WBC $\geq 15 \times 10^9$/L, the probability of bacteremia is 0.065; in this population the positive test increased the probability of disease from 3% to 6.5%).

- Likelihood ratio for a WBC $< 15 \times 10^9$/L $=$
$$\frac{1-\text{Sensitivity}}{\text{Specificity}} = \frac{4/19}{387/581} = 0.32$$
  1. Post-test odds of bacteremia (if WBC $< 15 \times 10^9$/L) $=$
$$\frac{0.03}{0.97} \times 0.32 = 0.01{:}1$$
  2. Post-test probability of bacteremia (if WBC $< 15 \times 10^9$/L) $=$
$$\frac{0.01}{1.01} = 0.01$$
  (i.e., if WBC $< 15 \times 10^9$/L, the probability of bacteremia is 0.01; a negative test reduced the probability of disease from 3% to 1%)
- Note that the post-test probability of bacteremia if WBC $\geq 15 \times 10^9$/L calculated using the likelihood ratio is identical to the positive predictive value (except for rounding errors in the calculations)

  However, if we have a population that has an extremely high prevalence of bacteremia, say 20%, we can still use the likelihood ratio to calculate post-test probability, as follows:
  1. Pretest odds of bacteremia $= \dfrac{0.2}{0.8} = 0.25{:}1$

2. Post-test odds of bacteremia (if WBC $\geq 15 \times 10^9$/L) = 0.25×2.36 (likelihood ratio, from above) = 0.59:1
3. Post-test probability of bacteremia (if WBC $\geq 15 \times 10^9$/L) =
$$\frac{0.59}{1.59} = 0.37$$
   (i.e., in this population if a patient has a WBC $\geq 15 \times 10^9$/L, there is a 37% chance of his being bacteremic)

- These data were used to demonstrate the use of the equations and *not* to suggest that a WBC is sufficient to differentiate a bacteremic child from a nonbacteremic child. If anything, these data show that a WBC by itself is not a very useful test.

Suggested Reading

1. Feinstein AR. Clinical epidemiology: the architecture of clinical research. Philadelphia: W.B. Saunders, 1985.
2. Fletcher RH, Fletcher SW, Wagner EH. Clinical epidemiology—the essentials. Baltimore: Williams & Wilkins, 1982.
3. Sackett DL, Haynes RB, Tugwell P. Clinical epidemiology: a basic science for clinical medicine. Boston: Little, Brown, 1985.

9 FLUIDS AND ELECTROLYTES

GENERAL INFORMATION

TABLE 9–1 Atomic Weight and Valence of Common Elements

Element	Value	Element	Value
Aluminum (Al)	26.9/3	Lead (Pb)	207.21/2,4
Barium (Ba)	137.4/2	Lithium (Li)	7/1
Calcium (Ca)	40.0/2	Magnesium (Mg)	24.3/2
Carbon (C)	12.0/2,4	Mercury (Hg)	200.6/1,2
Chlorine (Cl)	35.5/1	Nitrogen (N)	14.0/3
Copper (Cu)	63.6/1,2	Oxygen (O)	16.0/2
Fluorine (F)	19.0/1	Phosphorus (P)	31.0/3,5
Gold (Au)	197.0/1,3	Potassium (K)	39.1/1
Helium (He)	4.0/0	Silver (Ag)	107.9/1
Hydrogen (H)	1.0/1	Sodium (Na)	23.0/1
Iodine (I)	126.9/1	Sulfur (S)	32.1/2,4,6
Iron (Fe)	55.9/2,3	Zinc (Zn)	65.4/2

Conversions (mmol, mg, mEq, mOsm)

- Millimole (mmol) to mg. To calculate weight of a substance (mg), multiply number of mmol by molecular weight: e.g., 1 mmol of NaCl = 23 + 35.5 = 58.5 mg; e.g., 2.2 mmol/L of Ca^{++} = 2.2 (40) mg/L = 88 mg/L = 8.8 mg/dl
- Milliequivalent (mEq), measurement of the electrical charge contributed by an ion. To calculate number of mEq from number of mmol, multiply number of mmol by valence: e.g., 1 mmol of Na^+ = 1 mEq; e.g., 1 mmol of Ca^{++} = 2 mEq
- Milliosmoles (mOsm) = mmol × number of particles produced by dissociation, e.g., 1 mmol of $CaCl_2$ = 3 mOsm [1 from Ca^{++}, 2 from Cl^-]

- Osmolality (mOsm/kg) = number of mOsm/kg solvent, e.g., plasma = 275–295 mOsm/kg

Fluid Requirements

- Fluid requirements per 24 hr: 100 ml/kg for the first 10 kg + 50 ml/kg for next 10 kg (e.g., 10–20 kg) + 20 ml/kg for >20 kg; *or* 1500 ml/m². (N.B. These values assume a healthy child with normal renal function and frequently need to be modified. For requirements in the neonatal period, see neonatology section, chapter 17, p 388.)

TABLE 9–2 Conditions Requiring Modification to Daily Fluid Requirements

↑ Requirements	↓ Requirements
Fever: add 12% per rise of 1° C (↑caloric expenditure)	Congestive heart failure
	Meningitis (SIADH)
	Mechanical ventilation
Vomiting, diarrhea	Postoperative
High output renal failure, diabetes insipidus	Oliguric renal failure
Tachypnea	

- Fluid and electrolyte requirements are related to metabolic rate and calculated according to caloric expenditure (basically, normal maintenance H_2O requirements = 100 ml/100 kcal metabolized)

Electrolyte Requirements

- 2–3 mmol(mEq)/kg for Na^+ and K^+
- Maintenance solutions should contain approximately 25–35 mmol(mEq) Na^+/L and 20 mmol (mEq) K^+/L, and dextrose (e.g., D5:0.2% saline with 20 mmol/L (mEq/L) of KCl)

TABLE 9–3   Average Normal Values for Various Body Compartments (L/kg)

	Newborn	Child	Adult Male	Adult Female
TBW*	0.75	0.65	0.60	0.55
ICF*	0.40	0.40	0.40	0.40
ECF*	0.35	0.25	0.20	0.15
Blood volume	0.07–0.09	0.07–0.08	0.07–0.08	0.07–0.08

* TBW = total body water; ICF = intracellular fluid; ECF = extracellular fluid.

DEHYDRATION

General Considerations

- Most common cause in childhood is gastroenteritis

Clinical Features

- See Table 9–5

Management (General Principles)

- Investigation
  1. Determine "type" of dehydration: Measure Na^+ and osmolality. Estimated osmolality = 2[Na] (mmol/L) + glucose (mmol/L) + urea (mmol/L) (or 2[Na] + [BUN/2.8] + [glucose/18] where BUN and glucose are expressed in mg/dl and Na^+ in mEq/L).
  2. Assess biochemical status
     - Acid-base status: Acidosis may occur (diarrhea, diabetic ketoacidosis). Alkalosis may occur with high intestinal obstruction (especially pyloric stenosis).
     - Serum K^+: Usually have total body deficit. May be as high as 12 mmol/kg (mEq/kg), especially with prolonged diarrhea and vomiting.

TABLE 9–4 Approximate Electrolyte Composition of Gastrointestinal Fluids

Fluid	mmol(mEq)/L				
	H^+	Na^+	K^+	Cl^-	HCO_3^-
Gastric	80	40 (20–80)	20 (5–20)	150 (100–150)	0
Small intestinal	0	130 (100–140)	20 (5–25)	120 (100–130)	30
Pancreatic	0	135 (120–140)	15 (5–15)	100 (90–120)	50
Diarrheal	0	40	40	40	40

TABLE 9–5 Clinical Features of Dehydration*

Severity	Age <1 Yr		Age >1 Yr		Clinical Signs
	% Water Loss	Water Loss	% Water Loss	Water Loss	
Minimal	<5%		<3%		Thirst, mild oliguria
Mild	5%	50 ml/kg	3%	30 ml/kg	Dry mucous membranes, axilla, groin
Moderate	10%	100 ml/kg	6%	60 ml/kg	Loss of skin turgor, severe thirst, sunken eyeballs and fontanelle
Severe	15%	150 ml/kg	9%	90 ml/kg	Low BP, poor circulation, CNS changes, fever

* In hypernatremic dehydration, neurologic features predominate early, whereas ECF is preserved.

TABLE 9–6 Classification of Dehydration

	Na mmol/L(mEq/L)	Osmolality mmol/kg(mOsm/kg)
Isotonic	130–150	280–300
Hypertonic	>150	↑
Hypotonic	<130	↓

- Serum Ca^{2+}: May be low in neonates, hypernatremia, alkalemia, and high phosphate states.
- Blood glucose: Hyperglycemia occurs frequently with hypernatremia!
- Treatment
  1. Emergency phase (do not wait for laboratory results)
     - Take blood for electrolytes, urea (BUN), creatinine, glucose, calcium, acid-base status, CBC, Hct
     - Rapid treatment of shock (if present), using:

       Plasma
       Blood (if anemic) } give 20 ml/kg
       5% Albumin } within 1 hr, IV

       Normal saline } 20–40 ml/kg
       Ringer's lactate* } over 20–40 min IV
     - If still in shock, further immediate volume is needed
     - Omit this phase if patient is hemodynamically stable
     - Subtract the volume given from the calculated 24 hour fluid requirement (e.g., maintenance, *plus* deficit [see Table 9–5] *plus* estimated continuing losses)
     - If serum pH ≤ 7.1 (severe metabolic acidosis), give bicarbonate over 1–2 hr, after bolus (p 142)
  2. Repletion phase: Replacement of extracellular deficits (first 8 hr)

* Ringer's lactate has limitation of ↓ metabolism in shocked patient.

- Maintenance fluids...
  - + 50% of calculated fluid *deficit*, to be given over 8 hr (not valid for hyper-natremia)...
  - + Continue to replace ongoing losses...
  - + Correct sodium deficit (if applicable)
3. Recovery phase: Replacement of intracellular deficits (next 16 hr)
   - Maintenance fluids (continue)...
   - + Replace balance of deficit over 16 hr (replacement over 48 hr with hyper-natremia)
   - + Replace ongoing losses...
   - + Replacement of intracellular ions especially K^+. (Note: K^+ replacement starts as soon as patient has voided and continues for up to 4 days).
4. N.B. These are merely guidelines. *Management is based on continuing clinical and biochemical evaluation.*

Specific Forms of Dehydration

Isotonic Dehydration

Management

- Principles of therapy as previously outlined
- The solution used should contain dextrose and 35–50 mmol (mEq)/liter of sodium (e.g., "⅔:⅓" or D5W 0.2% NaCl)
- Potassium should be added only when urine output is adequate

Hypotonic Dehydration

General Considerations

- Be suspicious when a child has been given an electrolyte-free solution for management of gastroenteritis

TABLE 9–7   Composition of Some Common Parenteral Solutions (mmol or mEq/L)

Solution	Na^+	K^+	Cl^-	HCO_3^- *	Comments
Isotonic (0.9%) NaCl (normal saline)	154		154		
Hypertonic (3%) NaCl	513		513		
3.33% Dextrose and 0.33% NaCl ("2/3:1/3")	52		52		Contains 33.3 g/L dextrose; useful maintenance fluid and replacement fluid for Na^+
5% Dextrose + 0.2% NaCl (D5:0.2 normal saline)	34		34		Contains 50 g/L dextrose; useful Na^+ maintenance fluid
8.4% NaHCO$_3$ (1 mmol(mEq)/ml)	1000			1000	1 mmol of Na^+ and bicarbonate/ml
Lactated Ringer's	130	4	109	28	Ca^{2+} 3 mg/dl
0.5 normal saline (0.45%),	77		77		
5% Dextrose (D5W)					50 g/L dextrose

* Bicarbonate or potential bicarbonate.

- Any serum Na^+ <130 mmol (mEq)/L can cause symptomatic hyponatremia if it occurs acutely

Management

- Principles of therapy as outlined above
- In addition, correct the hyponatremia to an isotonic state using the formula:

$$Na^+_{deficit} = (Na^+_{desired} - Na^+_{observed}) \times BW(kg) \times TBW(L/kg)$$

> Note: Na >105 mmol/L (mEq/L): correct to 125–130
>
> : Na <105 mmol/L (mEq/L): correct by no more than 20 mmol/L (mEq/L)
> - ½ correct initially, then reassess
> - Do not correct by more than 2–5 mmol(mEq)/L/hr

- If patient symptomatic (seizures usually), use hypertonic saline (3–5%):
  1. 3% saline = 0.5 mmol (mEq) Na^+/ml
  2. 5% saline = 0.855 mmol (mEq) Na^+/ml
  Give 3% NaCl at a rate such that the $[Na^+]$ is corrected to ~ 125 mmol (mEq)/L in ~ 30–240 min depending on initial $[Na^+]$ and clinical status of patient
- Hyponatremia not associated with dehydration should be treated appropriately with fluid restriction, ± NaCl supplementation, ± diuretic therapy and treatment of underlying disease (see p 138 and 139)

Hypertonic (Hypernatremic) Dehydration

General Considerations

- ECF relatively well preserved, at expense of ICF
- Be suspicious when:
  1. Minimal signs of depleted intravascular volume with CNS disturbances: lethargy

when not stimulated, excessive irritability
with any stimulus, may have nuchal rigidity
and hypertonia
   2. Warm, "doughy," or more commonly
      "velvety" skin
- Predisposing causes: fever or high ambient temperature, low humidity, feeding of boiled
  skimmed milk, extremes of age, mental or
  physical retardation
- Warnings:
   1. Danger of rapid rehydration causing move-
      ment of water across blood-brain barrier into
      cerebral cells $\rightarrow$ cerebral edema and con-
      vulsions
   2. Frequent association with hyperglycemia
      (early) and hypocalcemia (late)
   3. $\uparrow$ ADH

Management

- Emergency phase: rapid plasma expansion, as
  outlined on p 133, if shock present
- Give 75% maintenance fluids because of risk of
  $\uparrow$ ADH with water retention
- Slow correction of fluid deficit over 48 hours
- Use following formula to calculate water load
  required to produce a predictable fall in
  serum Na^+: $LH_2O =$
  $$\frac{(Na_1^+ - Na_2^+) \times TBW}{Na_2^+} \text{ (where}$$
  LH_2O = water load in L/kg;
  Na_1^+ = observed Na^+;
  Na_2^+ = desired Na^+
  [140 mmol(mEq)/L];
  TBW in L/kg)
- Choice of fluid:
  Use fluid containing 30–35 mmol(mEq)/L Na^+
  and 40 mmol(mEq)/L K^+ (if not anuric)
- Check serum Na^+ frequently. If it falls too
  rapidly (>10–15 mmol(mEq)/L/day), either slow
  rate of correction, or change to a solution with
  a higher Na^+ content.

Complications

- Jitteriness: Check Na^+ (? fall too fast). Check Ca^{2+} (may need calcium gluconate). ? Head ultrasound (U/S) or CT scan—intracranial bleed (seizures) or cerebral edema.
- Hyperglycemia: Avoid use of insulin, which $\rightarrow$ rapid reduction in extracellular osmolality by $\downarrow$ glucose $\rightarrow \uparrow$ cerebral edema

SALT POISONING

General Considerations

- Serum Na >200 mmol (mEq)/L may occur
- Both serum and total body Na^+ are increased, thus impairing kidney's ability to excrete excess solute

Management

- Maintenance fluids as above by IV fluids
- Peritoneal dialysis using 7–8% glucose electrolyte-free may be required in severe cases ($Na^+ >180$), or when renal function is poor. This produces hyperglycemia, which offsets Na^+ drop and prevents water intoxication.
- Furosemide, 1 mg/kg, while replacing urine output with D10W, can be used when renal function is good, provided frequent monitoring of electrolytes is instituted

HYPONATREMIA (DILUTIONAL)

General Considerations

- Without edema (see Fig. 9–1)
- Causes
    1. $\uparrow$ Intake (compulsive drinking, excessive electrolyte-free IV fluids)

2. SIADH (CNS trauma, neoplasm, inflammation, asphyxia, drugs, lung disease)

Management

- Fluid restriction ($\pm$ hypertonic saline $\pm$ diuretics if symptomatic)

HYPONATREMIA (WITH EDEMA)

General Considerations

- Causes include congestive heart failure,
  nephrotic syndrome, cirrhosis, and protein-
  losing enteropathies (see Fig. 9–1)

Management

- Fluid and Na^+ restriction
- Diuretics

Pseudohyponatremia

- Associated with $\uparrow$ lipids (depending on technique used to measure Na^+) or $\uparrow$ glucose
- N.B. $[Na^+]$ $\downarrow$ ~1.6 mmol(mEq)/L for each $\uparrow$ in
  glucose of 5.5 mmol/L (100 mg/dl)

HYPOKALEMIA

General Considerations

- Causes include
  1. $\downarrow$ Intake (usually iatrogenic, e.g., parenteral
     fluids not supplemented with KCl)
  2. $\uparrow$ Losses (renal and GI, e.g., vomiting, diar-
     rhea, nasogastric suction, metabolic alkalosis,
     steroids, Na^+ loading, diuretics, renal tubular
     acidosis)

Clinical Features

- Neuromuscular: weakness, $\downarrow$ reflexes, paresthe-

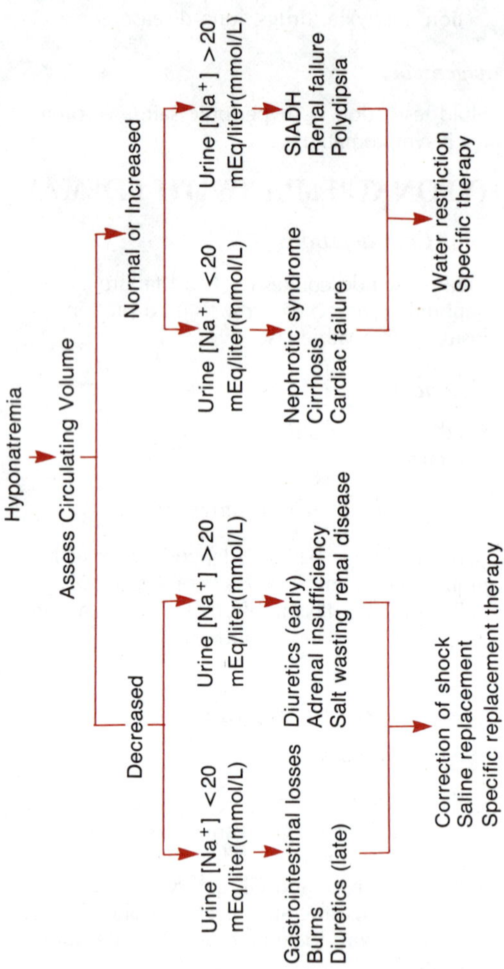

Figure 9–1 Differential diagnosis of hyponatremia and approach to therapy. (From Perkin RM, Levin DL. Common fluid and electrolyte problems in the pediatric intensive care unit. Pediatr Clin North Am 1980; 27:573.)

140

sias, ileus
- Renal: polyuria, polydipsia
- Cardiac (ECG): low amplitude T waves, "u"
  waves, S-T depression, dysrhythmias (atrial and
  ventricular premature beats)

Management

- Investigations
  1. ECG, electrolytes, urinalysis (including uri-
     nary pH, ± electrolytes). Continuous ECG
     monitoring for IV repletion therapy.
- Treatment
  1. Ensure intake of maintenance K^+, e.g., oral
     prophylactic supplementation with diuretic
     therapy
  2. Can go up to 40–60 mmol(mEq)/L by
     peripheral IV infusion. Higher concentrations
     (60–80 mmol(mEq)/L) should be administered
     through a central line. Usually infusion rates
     of <.03 mmol(mEq) K^+/kg/hr are adequate
     for replacement. *Correct with caution, and
     monitor K^+ levels frequently, as rapid infu-
     sion, even in severely depleted patients, may
     → fatal dysrhythmias.*
  3. As most K^+ is intracellular, it is difficult to
     calculate the amount needed to correct
     hypokalemia

HYPERKALEMIA

- See p 429, nephrology section

ACID-BASE DISORDERS

General Considerations and Investigations

- Check that blood gases make sense (Fig. 9–2
  and Tables 9–8 and 9–9)
- Normal pH: 7.38–7.42
- Acid-base disturbances cause vital organ dys-

function when pH <7.1 or >7.6
- Acid-base assessment

TABLE 9–8   pH and Corresponding Hydrogen Ion Concentration*

pH	$[H^+]$ nanomolar
6.9	126
7.0	100
7.1	79
7.2	63
7.3	50
7.4	40
7.5	32
7.6	25
7.7	20
7.8	16

$$* [H^+] = \frac{24\ P_{CO_2}}{[HCO_3^-]}$$

1. Measure serum pH, HCO_3^-, P_{CO_2}, and electrolytes
2. Calculate unmeasured anion gap: $[Na^+]$ − $([Cl^-]+[HCO_3^-])$. Normal value $= 12 \pm 4$.

Management of Metabolic Acidosis

- Treat underlying cause (Fig. 9–3)
- Calculate amount of bicarbonate required
    1. Use formula $(HCO_3^-\ _{desired} - HCO_3^-\ _{recorded}) \times$ BW (kg) $\times$ 0.6 [for desired HCO_3^- use 12 mmol(mEq)/L]
    2. Give half the amount required over 10–15 min IV and the remainder over the next 2 hr
    3. Acidosis needs to be corrected if pH <7.2 and HCO_3^- <12.0 mmol(mEq)/L
- Reassess acid-base status after treatment

TABLE 9–9 Common Patterns of Blood Gas Abnormality*

Respiratory acidosis (acute): pH ($\downarrow$), PCO_2 ($\uparrow$), HCO_3^- (N) or slightly $\uparrow$

Respiratory acidosis (chronic): pH ($\downarrow$ slightly), PCO_2 ($\uparrow$), HCO_3^- ($\uparrow$)

Respiratory alkalosis (acute): pH ($\uparrow$), PCO_2 ($\downarrow$), HCO_3^- (N) or slightly $\downarrow$

Respiratory alkalosis (chronic): pH (N or $\uparrow$), PCO_2 ($\downarrow$), HCO_3^- ($\downarrow$)

Metabolic acidosis: pH ($\downarrow$), PCO_2 ($\downarrow$), HCO_3^- ($\downarrow$)

Metabolic alkalosis: pH ($\uparrow$), PCO_2 (N or $\uparrow$), HCO_3^- ($\uparrow$)

* Rule of thumb:
1. For every 3 mm Hg $\uparrow$ in PCO_2 in chronic respiratory acidosis (CRA), bicarbonate will $\uparrow$ by $\sim$1 mmol/L; e.g., 3:1 ratio.
2. For metabolic acidosis, every 1 mmol/L $\downarrow$ in bicarbonate (HCO_3^-) $\rightarrow$ PCO_2 $\downarrow$ by 1 mm Hg; e.g., 1:1 ratio.

Suggested Reading

1. Hochman HI, Grodin MA, Crone RK. Dehydration, diabetic ketoacidosis and shock in the pediatric patient. Pediatr Clin North Am 1979; 26:803–826.
2. Perkin RM, Levin DL. Common fluid and electrolyte problems in the pediatric intensive care unit. Pediatr Clin North Am 1980; 27:567–585.
3. Winters RW, ed. The body fluids in pediatrics. Boston: Little, Brown, 1973.

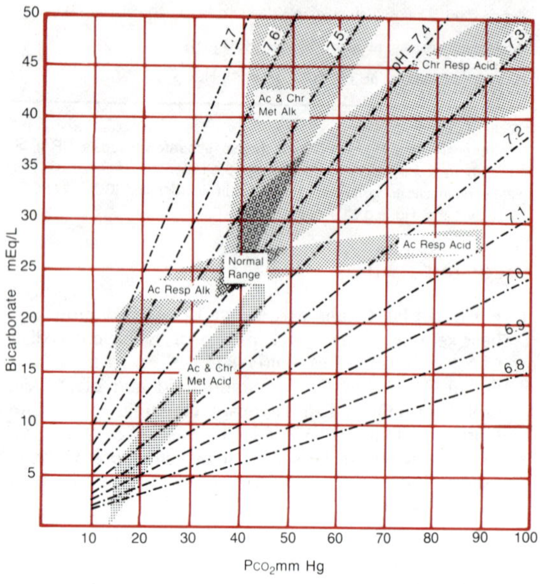

Figure 9–2   An in vivo acid-base nomogram for clinical use. Usually acid-base values falling *within* a shaded band indicate a single disturbance. Occasionally they may indicate a mixed disturbance. Acid-base values falling *outside* shaded bands indicate there are at least two acid-base disturbances. (From Arbus GS. An in vivo acid-base nomogram for clinical use. Can Med Assoc J 1973; 109:291.)

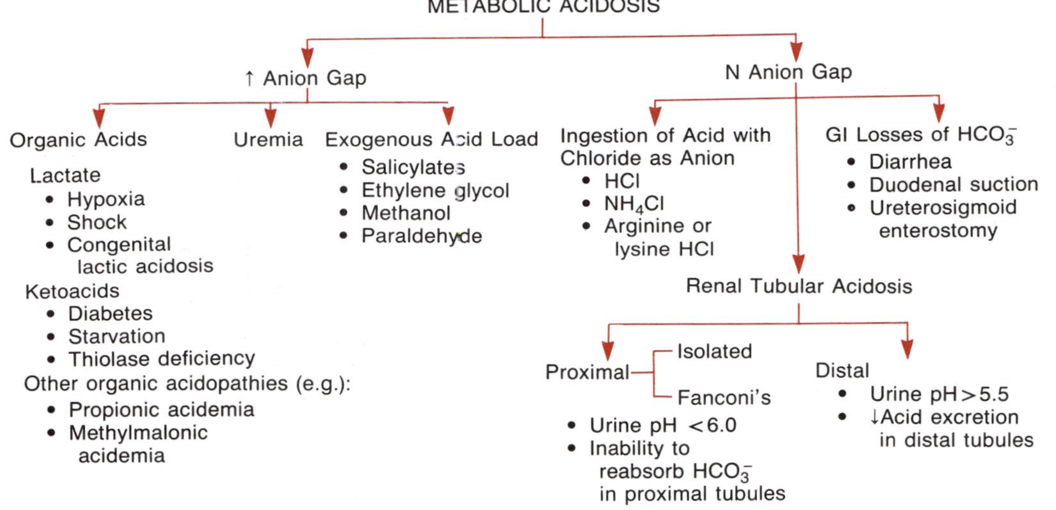

Figure 9–3 Differential diagnosis of metabolic acidosis.

10 GASTROINTESTINAL AND LIVER DISORDERS

GASTROINTESTINAL DISORDERS

Diarrhea

- Definition: excessive loss of fluid and electrolytes in stool

Acute Diarrhea

General Considerations

- Most commonly due to enteric infection (Table 10–1).
- Beware: in infants increased stool frequency and decreased consistency may reflect serious systemic infection (e.g., septicemia, meningitis, urinary tract infection) needing specific investigation and treatment

Principles of Management of Acute Diarrhea

- Prevention and treatment of dehydration and electrolyte imbalance most important
- Early refeeding vital
- Antidiarrheal medications not indicated
- Specific antimicrobial treatment not usually required

Exceptions	Recommended Antibiotic
Clostridium difficile	Vancomycin or metronidazole
Campylobacter (*if* very ill)	Erythromycin
Shigella (if severe)	According to sensitivities
Giardia (if symptomatic)	Metronidazole

TABLE 10–1   Enteric Pathogens Causing Acute Diarrhea in North America

Viral
  Rotavirus
  Norwalk agent
  Other suspect viruses—enteric adenovirus, calcivirus,
    astrovirus, coronavirus, small round viruses

Bacterial
  Campylobacter jejuni
  Salmonella species
  Yersinia enterocolitica
  Shigella species
  Clostridium difficile
  E. coli—enterotoxigenic, enteroinvasive, enteroadherent
  Aeromonas species

Parasites
  Giardia lamblia
  Entamoeba histolytica
  Cryptosporidia

- Fluids and electrolytes
  1. Assess hydration and plan necessary correction of deficits as outlined in the chapter *Fluids and Electrolytes*
  2. Rectal examination to assess stool consistency essential in recognizing potential water loss
  3. Severely dehydrated children need immediate resuscitation with intravenous fluids
  4. Others can be managed with oral rehydration therapy (ORT), which in viral and other invasive diarrheas makes best use of remaining absorptive function (Table 10–2)
  5. Vomiting is not a contraindication to ORT. It is usually transient and overcome by giving small volumes frequently (e.g., 15–30 ml per ½ hr).

TABLE 10–2 Composition of Oral Rehydration Fluids

	Glucose (g %)	Na (mmol/L)	K (mmol/L)	Cl (mmol/L)	Base (mmol/L)
WHO Solution	2.0	90	20	80	30
HSC Toronto Solution	2.0	50	20	40	30
Pedialyte	2.5	45	20	35	30
Gastrolyte	2.0	50	20	52	18

6. Pedialyte (Ross Laboratories) is best available solution for rehydration (composition approximates fecal losses found in rotavirus gastroenteritis)
7. Remember that rehydration involves replacement of fluid deficit, ongoing maintenance requirements, and continuing losses (diarrhea, vomitus)
8. Patients 5–10% dehydrated must be managed in a supervised setting (i.e., hospital or observation ward if possible)
9. Patients < 5% dehydrated may be managed with ORT at home after initial period of surveillance. Careful instructions regarding possible need to return are essential. Rotavirus gastroenteritis, particularly, can still kill through rapid dehydration.
- Nutrition
  1. Essential for repair process in the gut
  2. Breast feeding should be continued during acute phase with supplementary ORT if needed
  3. For weaned babies start half strength formula after 24–48 hr and increase to full strength by third to fourth day
  4. Restart solids when infant or child is receptive
  5. Avoid excessively sweet foods early in convalescence
  6. Transient lactose and other disaccharide intolerance may occur secondary to infectious enteritis, but not sufficiently often to justify routine avoidance of cow's milk formula

Specific Enteritides

- Rotavirus gastroenteritis
  1. The major cause of viral diarrhea in infants and children
  2. More likely to cause dehydration than other North American pathogens

3. Children 6 mo to 3 yr most commonly
   affected (peak 9–12 mo)
4. Prevalence in winter months
5. Typical clinical course 4–7 day illness; fever
   and vomiting followed by watery diarrhea,
   usually nonbloody
6. Pathogenesis: model of enteroinvasive disease
7. Virus invades the mature villous epithelium
   of small intestine, leading to its shedding and
   replacement by rapidly proliferating, relatively
   undifferentiated crypt cells incapable of normal solute transport, and hence to diarrhea
- *Campylobacter jejuni*
  1. Commonest bacterial isolate in diarrheal ill-
     ness at HSC
  2. Typical illness: fever, abdominal pain, diar-
     rhea which becomes bloody
  3. Pathology: an invasive colitis
  4. Most patients do not require an antibiotic
  5. Usually sensitive to erythromycin if patient is
     ill and not improving on his own

Chronic Diarrhea

- Diarrhea lasting >14 days
- Common complaint, especially in toddler age
  group
- Often what is described is simply increased
  stool frequency or decreased consistency rather
  than a truly excessive loss of fluids, electrolytes,
  and nutrients
- Avoid overinvestigation; distinguish chronic diarrhea with failure to thrive (suggests malabsorption) from chronic diarrhea in a well thriving
  child

Malabsorption

- Causes of malabsorption in childhood are listed
  in Table 10–3
- Suspect if child is gaining weight poorly or falling off growth curves

- But remember to assess dietary intake. If unnecessarily limited in response to diarrhea,
  child will fail to thrive in spite of normal
  absorptive capacity.
- Investigations (suggested workup)
  1. Screening tests
     - Stool microscopy for fat globules, fatty acid
       crystals (see p 726, procedures section)
     - Test stools for pH, reducing substances if
       watery (to detect disaccharide intolerance;
       see p 726, procedures section)
     - No reliable screening blood test (CBC,
       albumin probably best)
  2. Biochemical assessment of nutritional status
     (e.g., albumin, Ca^{2+}, phosphate, alkaline
     phosphate, Mg^{2+}, Zn^{2+}, Fe studies, folate,
     vitamins E and A, PT/PTT)
  3. Quantitative immunoglobulins
  4. Best available test for documentation of
     malabsorption is quantitative 3 day fecal fat
     estimation
  5. Further investigation as clinically indicated—
     small bowel biopsy, sweat chloride, pancreat-
     ic stimulation test
- Specific malabsorptive conditions
  1. Cystic fibrosis
     - Most common lethal genetic defect of
       white populations
     - Autosomal recessive inheritance
     - Multiple exocrine gland involvement with
       obstructive lesions, disordered mucus, and
       electrolyte secretion
     - 90% have exocrine pancreatic insufficiency
     - GI presentations include
       a. Intrauterine intestinal perforation with
          meconium peritonitis
       b. Meconium ileus as a newborn
       c. Failure to thrive with steatorrhea (charac-
          teristically hungry infants with voracious
          appetites)
       d. Rectal prolapse

  e. Syndrome in infancy (usually <6 mo) of
     edema, hypoalbuminemia, anemia (often
     due to vitamin E deficiency), and bruis-
     ing (vitamin K deficiency)
  f. Meconium ileus equivalent in older
     children and teenagers
  g. Rarely intussusception or volvulus
  h. Prolonged self-limited cholestasis in new-
     born period
  i. Biliary cirrhosis—presenting usually in
     late childhood or teenage years with por-
     tal hypertension
  j. Gallstones, cholecystitis
  k. Recurrent acute pancreatitis in patients
     with residual pancreatic function
- Prognosis improved significantly with nutritional support, pancreatic enzyme replacement, and intensive respiratory
  management
- Diagnosis
  a. Compatible clinical presentation plus
     sweat chloride (by pilocarpine ionto-
     phoresis method) >60 mEq/L (mmol/L)
  b. Exocrine pancreatic function assessed by
     measuring 3 day fecal fat excretion
- Treatment of exocrine pancreatic
  insufficiency—enzyme replacement titrated
  to patients' needs
  a. 1 capsule of uncoated enzyme per 3–4
     oz of formula in infancy (mixed with
     some vehicle, e.g., rice cereal immedi-
     ately before feeding)
  b. 2–3 capsules of enteric coated enzymes
     per meal, 1 per snack given once able
     to swallow capsules; dosage increased
     with age to 5–6 per meal, 2–3 per
     snack
- Caloric requirements 120–150% RDA for
  age
- Fat soluble vitamin supplements

2. Shwachman's syndrome
   - Second most common cause of exocrine pancreatic insufficiency in childhood, but far less common than CF
   - Other features
     a. Neutropenia often intermittent ± anemia ± thrombocytopenia
     b. Short stature (out of proportion to steatorrhea)
     c. Skeletal abnormalities
     d. Developmental delay
     e. Increased susceptibility to infections
   - Steatorrhea often disappears with age
   - Pancreatic enzyme replacement may not be necessary
   - Screening tests: chest x-ray (for rib flaring), long bone x-rays, serial CBCs, fecal fat estimation, serum trypsinogen
3. Celiac disease
   - Disease of proximal small intestine characterized by abnormal small intestinal structure with a permanent intolerance to dietary gluten (wheat, rye, barley, ± oats)
   - Latent period between introduction of gluten into diet and onset of symptoms
   - Most common childhood presentation
     a. Infant 9–18 mo
     b. Gradual failure to gain weight or weight loss
     c. Irritability, anorexia, apathy
     d. Abdominal distention
     e. Large foul, pale stools
     f. May be vomiting
     g. Finger clubbing, edema
   - Sometimes presents in later childhood with short stature and only subtle signs of specific malabsorption (e.g., anemia)
   - Diagnosis: may screen as for malabsorption, but definitive diagnosis based on typical "flat" jejunal biopsy (villous atrophy,

crypt hypertrophy, inflammatory cell
infiltrate)
- Treatment: gluten-free diet for life
- Gluten challenge, with re-biopsy usually
withheld until growth is completed unless
original diagnosis is doubtful

TABLE 10–3   Malabsorption in Childhood

Intestinal causes
CELIAC DISEASE
POSTINFECTIOUS ENTEROPATHY
CHRONIC INFECTION (especially if immune deficient)
SHORT GUT (congenital or ACQUIRED)
Abetalipoproteinemia
Bacterial overgrowth—blind loop syndrome, malrotation,
  motility disorder
Lymphangiectasia
Acrodermatitis enteropathica
Congenital villous atrophy
Autoimmune villous atrophy
Allergic (e.g., cow's milk protein) enteropathy

Pancreatic causes
CYSTIC FIBROSIS
SHWACHMAN'S SYNDROME

Hepatic causes
BILIARY ATRESIA
OTHER CIRRHOTIC OR CHOLESTATIC CONDITIONS

Miscellaneous
Neoplasm—neural crest tumor (neuroblastoma,
  ganglioneuroma)

Commoner conditions in CAPITAL LETTERS.

Chronic Diarrhea Without Failure to Thrive

- Consider
  1. Chronic enteric infection (especially Giardia)
  2. Chronic parenteral infection (urinary tract, ears)
  3. Disaccharidase deficiency (primary or secondary)
  4. "Toddler's diarrhea"
     - Label given to loose stools in an otherwise well toddler
     - At times starts with an infection
     - Pathophysiologic mechanism unknown (? maturational lag, lack of bowel control,? increased colonic bile acids)
     - Treatment
       a. Reassurance
       b. Full normal diet (avoid hyperosmolar, full strength fruit juices; stools said to be more formed when normal amount of fat given in diet)
       c. Elimination diets *to be avoided*
     - Stools will form up by age 3 yr or when toilet trained

Protein Losing Enteropathy

- Excessive exudation of protein into gastrointestinal tract
- Suspect in a child who presents with edema, hypoproteinemia, but no proteinuria
- Confirmation by fecal α_1-antitrypsin clearance
- May be associated with many diseases of gastrointestinal tract via altered mucosal permeability or stasis of lymph flow
- Consider (commoner causes in CAPITALS)
  1. Esophagitis
  2. Menetrier's disease
  3. CELIAC DISEASE
  4. ALLERGIC GASTROENTEROPATHIES (especially COW'S MILK PROTEIN INTOLERANCE in infants)

5. CROHN'S DISEASE
6. ULCERATIVE COLITIS
7. Henoch-Schönlein purpura
8. INFECTIONS
9. HIRSCHSPRUNG'S ENTEROCOLITIS
10. Intestinal lymphangiectasia
11. Congestive heart failure, constrictive pericarditis

- Cow's milk protein intolerance. Two major gastrointestinal syndromes are recognized:
  1. Proctitis, colitis
     - Usually young infant (first few months)
     - Loose stools with blood
     - Eosinophils in stool smear (Wright's stain)
     - Resolution off cow's milk protein unless also reactive to soy protein (50%)
  2. Edema, hypoproteinemia
     - Usually somewhat older infants (3–4 mo to as late as 18 mo)
     - Improvement off cow's milk protein with same (50%) chance of reacting to soy
     - Site of intestinal lesion often not identified, although small bowel biopsy and rectal biopsy results variably abnormal
     - May have peripheral eosinophilia
     - IgE and RAST testing usually normal
  3. In both syndromes milk tolerated by 2 yr of age or sooner
  4. Role of milk and other food antigens in other less well documented gastrointestinal complaints (e.g., diarrhea without evidence of colitis) more controversial, harder to document objectively
  5. Cow's milk protein intolerance not to be confused with lactose intolerance, which is simply the result of a primary or secondary mucosal lactase deficiency
- Inflammatory bowel disease
  1. Chronic inflammation in the gastrointestinal tract in the absence of a detectable pathogenic agent

2. Two major types—Crohn's disease and ulcerative colitis

General Considerations

- Incidence of ulcerative colitis stable in past 30 yr; incidence of Crohn's disease has been rising
- More common in Jewish populations than other races
- Genetic predisposition exists; about 20% of patients have a positive family history
- Symptoms begin before 20 yr of age in about 15% of patients with ulcerative colitis and 18–30% with Crohn's disease

Clinical Features

- Crohn's disease
  1. Mean age of onset in pediatric population is 12 yr
  2. Rarely manifest before age 5 yr
  3. Major presenting features may be
     - Recurrent abdominal pain, with anorexia, some diarrhea
     - Weight loss
     - Perianal disease
     - Extraintestinal manifestations—arthritis, mouth ulcers, erythema nodosum, liver disease, episcleritis
     - Anemia
     - Recurrent fever
     - Growth retardation and pubertal delay
- Ulcerative colitis
  1. More uniform clinical presentation
     - Bloody diarrhea ± urgency, tenesmus, abdominal pain, weight loss
     - May have extraintestinal manifestations similar to those of Crohn's disease
  2. Mean age of onset 10 years; does occur in very young children and infants

Investigations

- Aimed at
  1. Excluding other identifiable causes of inflammatory bowel disease
  2. Differentiating Crohn's disease from ulcerative colitis and defining disease extent and localization

Differential Diagnosis

- Infections (Self-limited but enter differential in first 4–6 wk)
  1. *Campylobacter jejuni*
  2. *Yersinia enterocolitica*
  3. *Entamoeba histolytica*
  4. *Salmonella, Shigella*
  5. Antibiotic associated colitis
- Henoch-Schönlein purpura
- Hemolytic uremic syndrome
- Eosinophilic gastroenteritis
- In infants consider allergic colitis, necrotizing enterocolitis, Hirschsprung's enterocolitis
- Behçet's disease

Pathologic Distinctions

Crohn's Disease	vs	*Ulcerative Colitis*
Any part of gastrointestinal tract		Colon only
Segmental disease with "skip lesions"		Continuous disease, usually worse distally
Transmural inflammation—granulomas may be present		Mucosal inflammation Crypt abscesses common

Usual Diagnostic Work-Up

- CBC, ESR, iron studies, albumin, stool cultures, Yersinia, Widal and amebic titers
- Small bowel follow-through
- Double contrast barium enema or colonoscopy
- Rectal (or colonic) biopsy

- Both diseases have relapsing course with exacerbations and remissions
- In more severe forms, disease activity is continuous and chronic
- Colectomy is curative for ulcerative colitis, whereas resection for Crohn's disease, while often necessary, is never curative

Management

- Ulcerative colitis
  1. Mild attack
     - Salazopyrin (50–75 mg/kg/day) or Asacol (30–60 mg/kg/day) + Cortenemas/Cortifoam (if very distal disease)
     - 5-ASA enemas an alternative
  2. Moderate attack
     - As above
     - Early recourse to oral steroids if not responding (1 mg/kg/day prednisone)
  3. Severe attack
     - Hospitalization
     - NPO
     - NG suction
     - IV steroids
     - Steroid/5-ASA enemas if able to retain
     - Consider broad spectrum IV antibiotics
     - Blood transfusion as needed
     - Avoid barium studies
     - Monitor electrolyte and Hct levels
     - Monitor flat plates of abdomen—BEWARE TOXIC MEGACOLON
     - Colectomy if not settling on full medical therapy in 5–7 days

     N.B. The prognosis in severe pancolitis is poor; at least 50% do not respond to medical treatment
  4. Maintenance therapy
     - Salazopyrin (and presumably Asacol) of

value in preventing exacerbations of ulcerative colitis
  - Continue until asymptomatic at least 2 yr
- Crohn's disease
  1. Prednisone 1 mg/kg/day (maximum 40–60 mg/day) for 6 wk, then tapering
  2. 5-ASA preparations may be of value in mild-moderate disease, depending on location
     - Salazopyrine: colonic disease only
     - Asacol: ? ileum + colon
     - Pentasa: ? small bowel
  3. Metronidazole useful in perianal disease, possibly in colonic disease
  4. Elemental feeds an alternate to prednisone; also useful when child is malnourished or growth retarded
  5. TPN: as per elemental feeds, but with greater risks
  6. Immunosuppressants (6MP, azathioprine)
     - Useful in control of inflammation
     - Probably justified in severe extensive disease that is running a chronic course
  7. Resection: never curative, but often necessary. Most indications are relative rather than absolute.
  8. Maintenance therapy—no drug of proven value in prophylaxis of attacks

Recurrent Abdominal Pain

General Considerations

- Common complaint in children aged 5–15 yr
- Most often (>90%) no organic cause found; labeled RAP or psychophysiologic pain
- Features suggesting organic cause
  1. Age <5 yr—BEWARE!
  2. Location other than periumbilical
  3. Night-time pain
  4. Associated symptoms—protracted vomiting (suggests intestinal obstruction, which must

be excluded by normal location of cecum
and placement of D–J flexure on lower and
upper barium studies), significant diarrhea,
weight loss (think IBD)
- Features suggesting psychophysiologic pain
    1. Often vaguely, variably, imprecisely described
    2. Often other somatic complaints (headaches, limb pain)
    3. General appearance of good health maintained
    4. Often supportive evidence of psychopathologic disorder in home or school
- All patients deserve full history with attention to above organic and psychophysiologic features, thorough physical examination, and screening tests (CBC, ESR, urinalysis, stool for occult blood)
- Should proceed to explanations, reassurance, advice if comfortable with diagnosis of RAP on these grounds; i.e., more invasive investigation not warranted
- GI causes to consider if pain does not "ring" of RAP
    1. Inflammatory bowel disease
    2. Intestinal obstruction (most commonly malrotation or malfixation of gut with intermittent volvulus)—BEWARE!
    3. Recurrent acute pancreatitis
    4. Peptic ulcer disease
    5. Lactose intolerance
    6. Constipation

Peptic Ulcer Disease

General Considerations and Investigations

- Not a common pediatric problem

Primary	*Secondary*
That is, without other systemic illness or drug ingestion	That is, in association with major underlying systemic illness (e.g.,

	shock, sepsis, burns) or drug ingestion (e.g., aspirin, nonsteroidal anti-inflammatory agents—more often cause erosive gastritis)
Extremely rare under age 10 yr	Seen in all age groups
Spectrum of symptomatology as in adults; in general, more benign presentation than secondary	Often presents with severe hemorrhage or perforation
Great tendency to recurrent relapsing course for duodenal ulcer	*Not* recurrent
Duodenal more common than gastric	Same
Role of *Campylobacter pyloridis* in pathogenesis under intense investigation	? This organism not associated with secondary PUD

- Diagnosis best made by fiberoptic endoscopy (single contrast barium study notoriously unreliable)

Management

- Acute
  1. Intravenous access, blood replacement as needed
  2. Antacids—30 cc q2h via NG tube
  3. H_2 blocker—cimetidine 20 mg/kg/day PO/IV divided qid, or ranitidine 5 mg/kg/day PO divided bid or 4 mg/kg/day IV divided bid
- Chronic
  1. Continue oral H_2 blocker for 6 wk in primary PUD; then 1 mo as a nightly dose
  2. Alternates—sucralfate 1 g qid, or bismuth subcitrate and antibiotics if *Campylobacter* is found

Constipation

General Considerations

- Infrequent passage of hard stools with difficulty
- In children
    1. Usually functional
    2. Voluntary fecal retention (e.g., resistance to toilet training, painful anal fissure, preoccupation with play, repression of urge to defecate); initiates cycle of stool accumulation; dulled defecation reflexes due to rectal dilation; further stool retention
- If onset in early infancy still likely functional, consider
    1. Hypothyroidism
    2. Neurogenic bowel (e.g., spinal dysraphism)
    3. Abnormal motility (e.g., Hirschsprung's disease, chronic intestinal pseudo-obstruction)
    4. Polyuric states with chronic dehydration
- Few investigations required unless clinical examination suggests underlying organic cause. Urine should be checked to exclude urinary tract infection, which can complicate chronic constipation.

Management

- Dietary advice regarding fiber intake
- Habit training: regular attempts at defecation—after a meal, waiting 5–10 min, hips flexed, feet pressing on flat surface
- These measures should suffice in early, mild stages, but in longstanding chronic cases, particularly if encopretic, a stool softener is required
    1. >1 yr
        - Mineral oil nightly
        - In older child begin with 15–30 cc qhs; increase until passing oil; then decrease slightly
        - Long-term therapy required (e.g., 3–6 mo) with cautious weaning

- Enemas—either saline (300 cc + 20 cc/kg) or hypertonic phosphate—may be required at start, especially if encopretic
2. <1 yr
  - Avoid mineral oil (risk of aspiration)
  - Alternate: Lactulose 5–10 ml/day starting dose, to be increased until stool is soft
- Follow-up conversations or visits required to prevent slipping back into old habits

Encopresis

General Considerations

- Usually the result of longstanding chronic constipation
- Assessment and management as above

Gastroesophageal Reflux

General Considerations and Investigations

- Chalasia
  1. Regurgitation after feeding in infants up to 15 mo of age
  2. Common: 40% of infants
  3. "Spitting up" often worse in recumbent position or with inadvertent pressure on stomach
  4. Infant healthy, growing well
  5. No investigations required; no treatment other than attention to positioning unless complications ensue
- Pathologic reflux
  1. Gastroesophageal reflux with suspected complications (make sure no other cause of "vomiting," e.g., CNS lesions, renal disease)
     - Failure to thrive
     - Respiratory—aspiration pneumonia, wheezing, apnea
     - Esophageal—hematemesis, melena, stricture, Barrett's esophagus, Sandifer's syndrome

2. Investigate
   - Upper GI series for anatomy, assess gastric outlet, *not* to document reflux (50% false negative)
   - Esophageal biopsy (blind suction biopsy or via esophagoscopy) if esophagitis queried
   - Milk scintiscan may be attempted to document association with pulmonary symptoms
   - 24 hr pH probe—not always necessary but may help document reflux in doubtful cases

Treatment

- Medical
  1. Positioning—45 degrees prone
  2. Thickened feeds (1 tbsp infant cereal per 1 oz formula)
  3. Drugs
     - Metoclopramide (0.125 mg/kg/dose given qid) or domperidone (0.03–0.06 mg/kg/dose given qid) to facilitate gastric emptying, increase lower esophageal tone
     - H_2 blockers if esophagitis
- Surgical: antireflux procedure, such as Nissen fundoplication, if medical treatment fails or if complications of reflux deemed too severe to justify trial of medical therapy

LIVER DISORDERS

General Features

- Jaundice
- Hepatomegaly—a palpable liver does not necessarily mean that the liver is enlarged, as thoracic deformities or chronic lung disease may make the liver palpable. Therefore, include liver span by percussion; also texture, firmness and presence of bruits (Fig. 10–1).

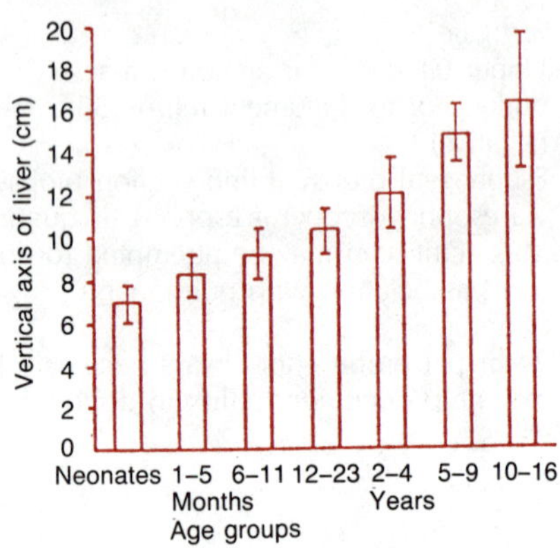

Figure 10-1 Normal (average) values for liver spans in various age groups. (Adapted from Deligeorgis D, et al. Normal size of liver in infancy and childhood. Arch Dis Child 1973; 48:792.)

- Splenomegaly—tip may be palpable in normal children < 4 yr old
- Pain or vague ache in right upper abdominal quadrant
- Fatigue, anorexia, nausea or vomiting, diarrhea, failure to thrive
- Spider angiomas, palmar erythema, collateral abdominal circulation, clubbing
- Pruritus, xanthomas (with cholestasis)

Investigations

- CBC and reticulocyte count. Anemia may be present—normochromic normocytic anemia of chronic disease, hypochromic microcytic anemia related to blood loss, or hemolysis.
- Blood smear—may show changes as above, or target cells or burr cells or evidence of hemolysis as in crisis of Wilson's disease

- Stool and urine—for bilirubin. No bilirubin
  should be detectable in urine; if it is detectable,
  conjugated hyperbilirubinemia is present.
- Bilirubin—total and direct (or conjugated)
- Hepatic enzymes: aminotransferases—aspartate
  aminotransferase or AST (SGOT), alanine
  aminotransferase or ALT (SGPT)—both elevated
  in hepatocellular disease; AST released from
  liver and muscle; ALT predominantly from liver.
  Alkaline phosphatase (ALP)—elevated in
  cholestasis, diffuse hepatic infiltration (e.g.,
  granulomatosis), biliary obstruction; also elevated in bone disease and during pubertal growth
  spurt. To differentiate liver ALP from bone or
  other ALP, measure 5′-nucleotidase (5′NT) or
  gamma-glutamyl transpeptidase (GGT): either
  will be elevated if hepatic ALP is elevated.
  Ethanol and inducers of hepatic microsomal enzymes can also elevate GGT.
- Bile acids—elevated levels may be found in
  both acute and chronic liver disease. Usefulness
  as liver function test in children still being investigated.
- Serum proteins—hypoalbuminemia may reflect
  chronic liver disease. Protein electrophoretic
  patterns may suggest specific disease states: absent α_1-globulin in α_1-Antitrypsin deficiency and
  elevated gamma globulin in chronic active
  hepatitis.
- Serum ammonia (specimen must be transported
  to laboratory and measured promptly)
- PT, PTT
- Vitamin E, 25-hydroxy-vitamin D, and
  carotene—deficiencies with prolonged cholestasis may lead to neurologic abnormalities, rickets, and night blindness, respectively
- Viral studies
  1. Hepatitis B surface antigen (HBsAg), anti-
     hepatitis B surface antibody (anti-HBs), anti-
     hepatitis B core antibody (anti-HBc)—see
     Infectious Disease section (p 358)

2. Anti-HAV antibody (specify IgM for acute disease)
3. EBV, CMV, HSV titers; CMV growth from urine
4. Adeno-, ECHO-, Coxsackie B virus titers

Radiologic studies
1. Ultrasound of liver $\pm$ Doppler flow studies
2. CT scan of abdomen
3. Liver scan—sulfur colloid (RE cell uptake—image liver and spleen), HIDA/DISIDA/PIPIDA (uptake by hepatocytes—image liver cells and biliary system)
4. Angiography (to define vascular anatomy, tumors)
5. Percutaneous transhepatic cholangiogram (PTC) and endoscopic retrograde cholangiopancreatogram (ERCP) to visualize the biliary system when extrahepatic obstruction or sclerosing cholangitis is suspected. PTC likely to succeed when intrahepatic bile ducts shown dilated on ultrasound examination of liver.

Liver biopsy
1. Prebiopsy investigations—CBC and platelet count, PT, PTT, bleeding time (BT) if thrombasthenia suspected
2. Type and crossmatch (10 ml/kg blood on hold)
3. Rethink indication if Hb <100, platelet count $<60,000$, PT or PTT or BT prolonged
4. Frequent pulse and blood pressure measurements afterward

Other studies
1. Slit lamp eye examination: Kayser-Fleischer ring in Wilson's disease, posterior embryotoxon in Alagille's syndrome
2. PI typing: α_1-antitrypsin deficiency
3. Lipoprotein electrophoresis: cholesterol ester storage disease
4. Serum copper, ceruloplasmin

Hepatomegaly ± Splenomegaly ± Jaundice

General Considerations

- Etiology in infants (essentially the differential diagnosis of neonatal cholestatic jaundice)
  1. Infections
     - TORCHS
     - Hepatitis A, B, non-A/non-B
     - Adenovirus, ECHOvirus, Coxsackie virus, varicella
     - Bacterial (liver or elsewhere), TB, listeriosis
  2. Structural
     - Extrahepatic biliary atresia
     - Choledochal cyst
     - Hepatic fibropolycystic disease with renal cystic disease
     - Extrahepatic bile duct (EHBD) stenosis, hypoplasia
     - EHBD obstruction by gallstone, tumor, thick bile
     - Spontaneous perforation of bile duct
     - Paucity of interlobular bile ducts (e.g., Alagille's syndrome)
  3. Metabolic
     - α_1-Antitrypsin deficiency
     - Cystic fibrosis
     - Galactosemia
     - Fructosemia
     - Tyrosinemia
     - Glycogen storage disease, type IV
     - Lipidoses (e.g., Wolman's, Gaucher's, Niemann-Pick disease)
     - Zellweger's syndrome (and other peroxisomal disorders)
     - Primary cholestatic syndromes (e.g., Byler's, Aagenaes' syndrome)
     - Perinatal hemochromatosis
     - Endocrinopathies (e.g., idiopathic hypopituitarism)

4. Genetic (e.g., trisomy E)
5. Toxic
   - Total parenteral nutrition
   - Drugs (administered to infant or absorbed from breast milk)
   - Severe or prolonged unconjugated hyper- bilirubinemia usually secondary to hemoly- sis ("inspissated bile syndrome")
6. Tumor (e.g., hepatoblastoma, metastatic neu- roblastoma, histiocytosis X)
7. Vascular
   - Congestive heart failure
   - Budd-Chiari syndrome
   - Shock
8. Idiopathic ("giant cell hepatitis")
- Etiology in childhood and adolescence (differential diagnosis includes diseases that may present with hepatomegaly but no jaundice)
  1. Infectious
     - Hepatitis A, B, non-A/non-B
     - Mononucleosis syndrome (EBV, CMV, tox- oplasmosis)
  2. Structural
     - Congenital hepatic fibrosis ⎫
     - Caroli's syndrome ⎬ "Hepatic fibropolycystic disease"
     - Choledochal cyst ⎭
     - Cholecystitis, choledocholithiasis
     - Alagille's syndrome
  3. Metabolic
     - Glycogen storage disease (notably types III, VI, IX)
     - Fatty liver (various etiologies)
     - Wilson's disease
     - α_1-Antitrypsin deficiency
     - Cholesterol ester storage disease
  4. Toxic
     - Reye's syndrome (still common in adolescents)
     - Drug induced (e.g., acetaminophen, valpro- ate, phenytoin, erythromycin)
  5. Tumor

6. Vascular
  • Portal vein thrombosis (typically presents as
    variceal bleeding or splenomegaly-
    hypersplenism; hepatomegaly uncommon)
  • Budd-Chiari syndrome (oral contraceptive
    pill may predispose)
  • Veno-occlusive disease (some antineoplastic
    treatments may predispose)
7. Others
  • Autoimmune chronic active hepatitis
  • Sclerosing cholangitis
  • Cirrhosis (secondary to metabolic disease,
    biliary tract disease, chronic viral infection)

Jaundice Without Hepatosplenomegaly

General Considerations

- Congenital defects in bilirubin metabolism
  1. Unconjugated hyperbilirubinemia—Crigler-
     Najjar syndrome, types I and II, Gilbert's
     syndrome
  2. Conjugated hyperbilirubinemia—Dubin-
     Johnson syndrome, Rotor's syndrome
- Hemolysis (splenomegaly may occur)
- Neonatal hypothyroidism
- Breast milk jaundice
- Other (e.g., sepsis in infants)

Acute or "Fulminant" Hepatic Failure

General Considerations

- Defined as liver failure occurring within 8 wk
  after the acute liver disease
- Most commonly follows acute viral hepatitis or
  drug and/or toxin ingestion or may be first sign
  of Wilson's disease (typically with severe intravascular hemolysis). In infants, metabolic disease (e.g., galactosemia) may present in this
  way.

Clinical Features

- Deepening jaundice
- Profound anorexia
- Vomiting (often after a period of apparent clinical improvement)
- Marked lethargy, unsteady gait, confusion, stupor, asterixis
- Fetor hepaticus
- Hypoalbuminemia, azotemia, bleeding disorder

Investigation

- As previously discussed (liver biopsy rarely possible because of severe coagulopathy) plus drug screen

Complications Associated with Hepatic Failure

- Cerebral edema
- Renal failure
- Respiratory failure
- Circulatory failure
- Pancreatitis
- Bleeding
- Sepsis

Management

- This involves no specific therapy but intensive, supportive, symptomatic care
- Isolation procedures for patient and body products, e.g., secretions, blood
- Monitor vital signs, including neurologic vital signs (for increased ICP)
- Daily weights with strict monitoring of fluid balance
- Monitor electrolytes (with specific attention to K^+, phosphate, ionized calcium concentrations), amylase, renal function, albumin
- Frequent measurement of blood glucose. Give 10% glucose solutions with appropriate electrolyte replacement.

- Monitor CBC and coagulation tests daily. Give FFP if active bleeding or risk of severe bleeding (e.g., intracranial); avoid saline overload secondary to FFP.
- Medical measures to reduce intracranial pressure
- High dose steroids of no proven benefit
- Neomycin and/or lactulose for encephalopathy; these may be given as enemas. No sedatives or analgesics.
- Antacids or histamine H_2 receptor blockers (e.g., ranitidine)
- Daily blood culture

Chronic Persistent (CPH) and Chronic Active Hepatitis (CAH)

General Considerations and Management

- These are defined by histopathology. Definition of chronicity in adults (>6 mo) cannot be applied to children; these diagnoses should be considered after 1–2 mo of illness in children. Autoimmune CAH and Wilson's disease should be considered in any child presenting with acute hepatitis.
  1. CPH
     - Syndrome related to viral hepatitis
     - Patients are mostly asymptomatic; if symptoms do occur, they are usually mild
     - Aminotransferase levels are usually mildly elevated and the prognosis is good. Progression to CAH is rare.
  2. CAH
     - Majority on an autoimmune basis. Approximately 20% are HBsAg positive; non-A/non-B hepatitis, Wilson's disease, drug toxicity, and α_1-antitrypsin deficiency are other possible causes of chronic active hepatitis.

- Patients with autoimmune CAH are unwell, with anorexia, fatigue, and abdominal discomfort. Joint pains, rashes, and polyserositis may occur. Serum bilirubin is elevated, although clinical jaundice may not be present. Presentation may mimic acute hepatitis.
- Strong association with other autoimmune diseases
- Biochemical features include
  a. Elevated aminotransferases (AST, ALT)
  b. Hypergammaglobulinemia
  c. Positive (a) smooth muscle antibody (SMA)—commonly, (b) antinuclear antibody (ANA)—usually, (c) antimitochondrial antibody (AMA)—sometimes
- Therapy involves immunosuppression with prednisone; azathioprine may be added to permit prednisone dose reduction if steroid side effects severe

Suggested Reading

1. Clin Gastroenterol 1986; 15(1):entire issue.
2. Sem Liver Dis 1982; 2(4):entire issue.
3. Sherlock S. Diseases of the liver and biliary system. Oxford: Blackwell, 1985.
4. Walker-Smith JA, Hamilton JR, Walker WA. Practical pediatric gastroenterology. London: Butterworths, 1983.

11 GENETICS

APPROACH TO THE CHILD WITH MULTIPLE ANOMALIES

General Considerations

- The practical approach to a dysmorphic child in terms of management and to prevention in other family members depends on the cause and pathogenesis of the defects present.
- Definitions of abnormal morphogenesis
    1. Malformation: a morphologic defect of an organ, part of an organ, or a larger region of the body resulting from an *intrinsically* abnormal developmental process, e.g., malformations present in Down syndrome
    2. Disruption: a morphologic defect of an organ, part of an organ, or a larger region of the body resulting from the *extrinsic* breakdown or interference with an originally normal developmental process, e.g., a teratogen or amniotic bands
    3. Deformation: an abnormality of form, shape, or position of a part of the body caused by mechanical forces, as in deformation secondary to breech presentation (e.g., abnormal head shape, asymmetry of ears and shoulders, and hip dislocation resulting from constrained position in utero)
    4. Dysplasia: an abnormal organization of cells into tissue(s) and its morphologic result(s)

Management

- Investigations
    1. Physical examination
        - Particular attention to unusual physical features, including measurements of hands, in-

ner canthal distance, position of eyes and ears
- All major and minor anomalies should be noted
- Photographs and x-ray views are useful documentation

2. Clinical investigations. To delineate underlying anomalies, the following may be useful: ophthalmologic assessment, cardiac assessment, skeletal survey, renal ultrasound, and other tests as indicated by clinical status.
3. Biochemical or molecular investigations. Indicated when a particular diagnosis is to be established or ruled out, e.g., urinary mucopolysaccharides in Hurler syndrome.
4. Chromosome analysis
   - Frequently indicated in diagnosis of dysmorphic children, except when the syndrome present is known not to be chromosomal
   - When the disorder is known to be chromosomal, chromosome analysis should be done for confirmation
   a. Blood
      - Anticoagulated (usually heparinized) blood is required
      - Full karyotype to rule out rearrangement (4 wk)
      - Rapid count to rule out aneuploidy can be done in less time (about 5 days)
      - The laboratory should be notified if the fragile X syndrome or a chromosome breakage syndrome is suspected
   b. Bone marrow
      - Rapid analysis of marrow cells to rule out aneuploidy
      - Test results ready within hours
      - Indicated if urgent decisions (e.g., use of life support) depend on chromosome results

c. Skin biopsy for fibroblast culture
- Indicated if blood results are ambiguous or in the event of mosaicism
- Can culture skin or other tissues post mortem

d. Buccal smear
- Most labs prefer full karyotypes

5. When stillbirth or perinatal death occurs:
- A complete autopsy should be done unless the cause of demise is obvious
- If malformations or dysmorphic features are present, chromosome analysis and photographs should be done
- A post mortem x-ray examination can be very helpful

- Treatment
1. Supportive care for the child (e.g., investigation and treatment of heart failure in a child with Down syndrome)
2. Supportive care for the parents
3. It may not be possible to reach a definitive diagnosis. DO NOT LABEL A CHILD WITH A DIAGNOSIS UNLESS YOU ARE SURE.

GENETIC COUNSELING

General Considerations

- When the child's disorder may be hereditary, the parents are advised of the consequences of the disorder, both immediate and long term, the probability of developing or transmitting it, and the possible ways to prevent recurrence or reduce the risk
- A family history should include at least the patient's parents, sibs, and second degree relatives (grandparents, uncles and aunts, nieces and nephews). Age (or age at death), clinical conditions in relatives, stillbirths or miscarriages in the child's sibship, ethnic background, parental consanguinity, and so forth should be recorded.

- Physical examination of family members may be important
- The risk of recurrence of a disorder in family members depends chiefly on its genetic mechanism, although other factors (e.g., penetrance, variable expressivity, age of onset) must also be assessed. Genetic disorders are classified broadly as:

1. Single gene (Mendelian) disorders: autosomal dominant, autosomal recessive, X-linked
2. Chromosomal disorders
   - Aneuploidy (abnormal chromosome number)
   - Structural rearrangement—may be balanced (with all the chromosome material present) or unbalanced (with extra or missing chromosome segments)
   - Other chromosome abnormalities, resulting from single gene disorders, e.g., fragile site on X chromosome (fragile X syndrome), chromosome breakage syndromes (e.g., Fanconi anemia)
3. Multifactorial disorders
   - Usually single, common, morphologic defects, e.g., neural tube defects, many cases of cleft lip and cleft palate
   - Before counseling as multifactorial, must rule out any underlying syndrome
   - Recurrence risk is usually low, 3 to 5% in first degree relatives
4. Teratogens
   - A teratogen is defined as any agent that causes or increases the risk of defects
   - Teratogens are environmental, not genetic, causes of multiple anomalies
   - There are only a few proven teratogens in man. Examples include some congenital infections (rubella, cytomegalovirus, toxoplasmosis, syphilis), some drugs (thalidomide, warfarin, alcohol, aminopterin, methotrexate, retinoic acid, and proba-

bly some anticonvulsant drugs), and some
maternal factors (e.g., mental retardation
and microcephaly occur in offspring of
mothers with phenylketonuria, as a result
of the mother's abnormally high serum
phenylalanine levels).
- It is often hard to prove or disprove a tera-
togenic effect because of lack of population experience. Up to date information
about teratogens can be obtained through
clinical pharmacologists or geneticists.

CHROMOSOME DISORDERS

- See Table 11–1 (p 180)

Suggested Reading

1. Emery AEH, Rimoin DL. Principles and practice of medical genetics. New York: Churchill Livingstone, 1983.
2. Harper PS. Practical genetic counselling. 2nd ed. Bristol:
   John Wright, 1984.
3. McKusick VA. Mendelian inheritance in man. 7th ed. Baltimore: Johns Hopkins University Press, 1986.
4. Smith DW. Recognizable patterns of human malformation.
   3rd ed. Philadelphia: W.B. Saunders, 1982.
5. Thompson JS, Thompson MW. Genetics in medicine. 4th
   ed. Philadelphia: W.B. Saunders, 1986.

TABLE 11–1 Common Disorders of Chromosomes

Chromosome Finding	Maternal Age	Newborn Incidence	Distinguishing Features
Trisomy 13 (Patau syndrome)		1/20,000	Holoprosencephaly, cleft lip-palate, cutis aplasia, polydactyly, eye and heart abnormalities; usually incompatible with life
Trisomy 18 (Edwards syndrome)		1/8,000	SGA, fine features, abnormal ears, hypertonia, hypoplastic nails, overlapping fingers, short sternum, cardiac defects; usually incompatible with life
Trisomy 21 (Down syndrome)	Overall	1/800	Epicanthal folds, upslanting eyes, Brushfield spots on iris, flat occiput, excess skin at back of neck, hypotonia, simian crease, in-curving of fifth fingers, characteristic dermatoglyphics; mental retardation; increased risk of leukemia (1%); increased risk of respiratory infections in childhood; increased risk of antithyroid antibodies and hypothyroidism
	20–24	1/1,550	
	25–29	1/1,050	
	30–34	1/700	
	35	1/350	
	40	1/100	
	>45	1/25	
47,XXY (Klinefelter syndrome)		1/1,000 males	Hypogonadism, infertility, long limbs
45,X (Turner syndrome)		1/10,000 females 1/5,000 females (including mosaics)	Short stature, webbed neck, low posterior hairline, increased carrying angle, lymphedema in newborn period, gonadal dysgenesis; normal intelligence but may have visual-spacial problems; increased risk of cardiac defects, renal abnormalities, and hearing loss
Fragile X syndrome		1/1,100 males;less frequent in females	Mental retardation, prominent jaw, large ears, macro-orchidism (most obvious after puberty); caused by X-linked gene

180

12 Growth and Development

In a developmental assessment, one attempts to examine the degree of maturation of the child's central nervous system in relation to his age. This can lead to identification of motor, sensory, and mental handicaps.

As Illingworth notes, it is difficult to draw a dividing line between normal and abnormal development. However, the further away from average the child is in anything, the more likely this is to be abnormal.

One should note the importance in developmental assessment and predictive value of what Gesell termed "insurance factors," such as the child's alertness, responsiveness, interest in surroundings, determination, and concentration. These factors are often of greater relevance than the more easily scored specific milestones from psychologic tests or other developmental screening inventories.

It will always be difficult to make accurate predictions of future intelligence and achievements routinely from developmental assessments early in childhood. This is because of the profound effect of environment and familial milieu on development, and the unforeseen effects of possible future neurologic disease or impairment.

As with any other kind of diagnosis (but of particular importance in developmental assessment), the pediatrician must base his evaluation on a full history (medical, psychosocial, and developmental), a full physical examination (including detailed "classic" neurologic and developmental examinations), ancillary data collected from other professionals (e.g., psychologists, occupational therapists, speech pathologists), and a full knowledge of the child's family situation and interpersonal dynamics.

Figure 12–1 and Tables 12–1 to 12–4 outline the various aspects of child development from birth through school age; in addition to a summary of developmental milestones, a guide for pediatricians on psychologic testing is included.

INTRODUCTION TO GROWTH CHARTS

The following pages contain comprehensive height, weight, height velocity, and head circumference charts for boys and girls from birth through 19 years of age. Please note carefully when plotting whether the age on the growth chart is calculated using decimal years (Table 12–5 is included to allow easy calculation of decimal age) or months. We have included the traditional British Tanner charts as well as the Serono Laboratory version of Tanner's recently published longitudinal standards for height of North American children. For fast approximations of height and weight for age, one can use the formulas listed in Table 12–6.

The following is a list of the growth charts and illustrations found in this section:

Boys:
Birth–5 years: height and weight, p 206 and 207.
Girls:
Birth–5 years: height and weight, p 208 and 209.
Boys:
Birth–19 years: height and weight, p 210 and 211.
Girls:
Birth–19 years: height and weight, p 212 and 213.
Boys:
Birth–19 years: height velocity, p 214.
Girls:
Birth–19 years: height velocity, p 215.

Boys:

Birth–19 years: height (North American standards), p 216.

Girls:

Birth–19 years: height (North American standards), p 217.

Boys:

Birth–18 years: head circumference, p 218.

Girls:

Birth–18 years: head circumference, p 219.

Fraction of adult height attained at each bone age, p 220, 221, and 222.

Male genital and pubic hair development, p 223.

Female breast development, p 224.

Female pubic hair development, p 225.

Chronological order of appearance of osseous centers, p 226, 227, 228, and 229.

Stretched penile length, p 230.

Chronology of human dentition, p 231 and 232.

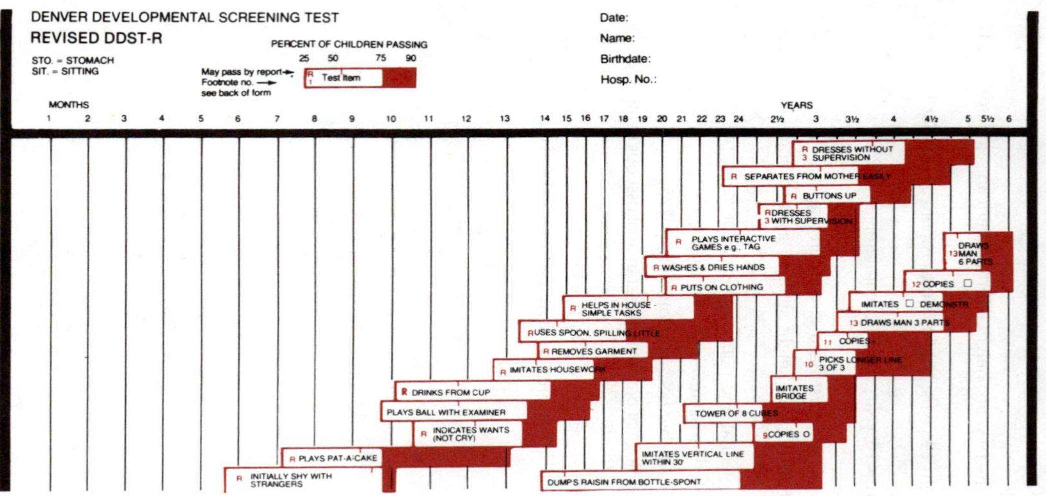

Figure 12–1 Denver developmental screening test. (From Frankenburg WK, Dodds JB. Denver: University of Colorado Medical Center, 1978.)

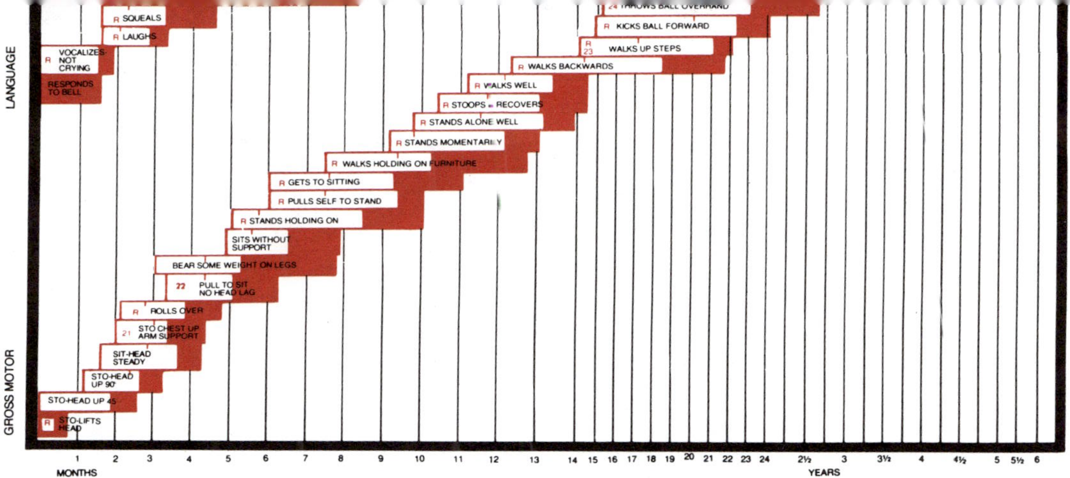
LANGUAGE
GROSS MOTOR
RESPONDS TO BELL
VOCALIZES - NOT CRYING
R SQUEALS
R LAUGHS
R STO-LIFTS HEAD
STO-HEAD UP 45
STO-HEAD UP 90
SIT-HEAD STEADY
21 STO CHEST UP ARM SUPPORT
R ROLLS OVER
22 PULL TO SIT NO HEAD LAG
BEAR SOME WEIGHT ON LEGS
SITS WITHOUT SUPPORT
R STANDS HOLDING ON
R PULLS SELF TO STAND
R GETS TO SITTING
R WALKS HOLDING ON FURNITURE
R STANDS MOMENTARILY
R STANDS ALONE WELL
R STOOPS - RECOVERS
R WALKS WELL
R WALKS BACKWARDS
R 23 WALKS UP STEPS
R KICKS BALL FORWARD
24 THROWS BALL OVERHAND
MONTHS
1 2 3 4 5 6 7 8 9 10 11 12 13 14 15 16 17 18 19 20 21 22 23 24
YEARS
2½ 3 3½ 4 4½ 5 5½ 6

PERSONAL-SOCIAL
FINE MOTOR-ADAPTIVE
LANGUAGE
GROSS MOTOR
185
2 RESISTS TOY PULL
50% PLAYS PEEK-A-BOO
WORKS FOR TOY OUT OF REACH
R FEEDS SELF CRACKERS
R SMILES SPONTANEOUSLY
F SMILES 1 RESPONSIVELY
REGARDS FACE
TOWER OF 4 CUBES
R SCRIBBLES SPONTANEOUSLY
DUMPS RAISIN FROM BOTTLE-DEMONSTR
TOWER OF 2 CUBES
8 NEAT PINCER GRASP OF RAISIN
R BANGS 2 CUBES HELD IN HANDS
7 THUMB-FINGER GRASP
RAKES RAISIN ATTAINS
SIT. TAKES 2 CUBES
6 SIT. LOOKS FOR YARN
R PASSES CUBE HAND TO HAND
R REACHES FOR OBJECT
REGARDS RAISIN
5 GRASPS RATTLE
4 FOLLOWS 180°
R HANDS TOGETHER
4 FOLLOWS PAST MIDLINE
EQUAL MOVEMENTS
100% pass at birth
FOLLOWS TO
R IMITATES SPEECH SOUNDS
R DADA OR MAMA NONSPECIFIC
R DADA OR MAMA SPECIFIC
R 3 WORDS OTHER THAN MAMA, DADA
R POINTS TO 1 NAMED BODY PART
R COMBINES 2 DIFFERENT WORDS
14 NAMES 1 PICTURE
15 FOLLOWS DIRECTIONS/2 OF 3
R USES PLURALS
R GIVES 1ST & LAST NAME
16 COMPREHENDS COLD, TIRED HUNGRY/2 OF 3
17 COMPREHENDS PREPOSITIONS/3 OF 4
R RECOGNIZES COLORS/3 OF 4
18 OPPOSITE ANALOGIES 2 OF 3
19 DEFINES WORD/6 OF 9
20 COMPOSITION OF/3 OF 3
87%
87%
JUMPS IN PLACE
R PEDALS TRICYCLE
BALANCE ON 1 FOOT 1 SECOND/2 OF 3
25 BROAD JUMP
BALANCE ON 1 FOOT 5 SECONDS/2 OF 3
HOPS ON 1 FOOT
26 HEEL TO TOE WALK/2 OF 3
27 CATCHES BOUNCED BALL/2 OF 3
BALANCE ON 1 FOOT 10 SECONDS/2 OF 3
28 BACKWARD HEEL-TOE/2 OF 3

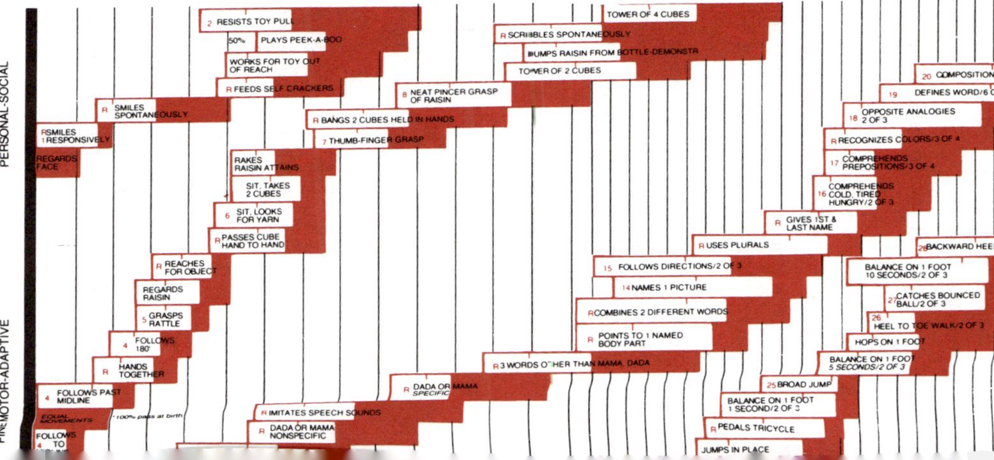

185

1. Try to get child to smile by smiling, talking, or waving to him. Do not touch him.
2. When child is playing with toy, pull it away from him. Pass if he resists.
3. Child does not have to be able to tie shoes or button in the back.
4. Move yarn slowly in an arc from one side to the other, about 6″ above child's face. Pass if eyes follow 90 degrees to midline. (Past midline; 180 degrees)
5. Pass if child grasps rattle when it is touched to the backs or tips of fingers.
6. Pass if child continues to look where yarn disappeared or tries to see where it went. Yarn should be dropped quickly from sight from tester's hand without arm movement.
7. Pass if child picks up raisin with any part of thumb and a finger.
8. Pass if child picks up raisin with the ends of thumb and index finger using an over hand approach.
9. Pass any enclosed form. Fail continuous round motions.
10. Which line is longer? (Not bigger.) Turn paper upside down and repeat. (3/3 or 5/6)
11. Pass any crossing lines.
12. Have child copy first. If failed, demonstrate.

When giving items 9, 11, and 12, do not name the forms. Do not demonstrate 9 and 11.

13. When scoring, each pair (2 arms, 2 legs, etc.) counts as one part.
14. Point to picture and have child name it. (No credit is given for sounds only.)

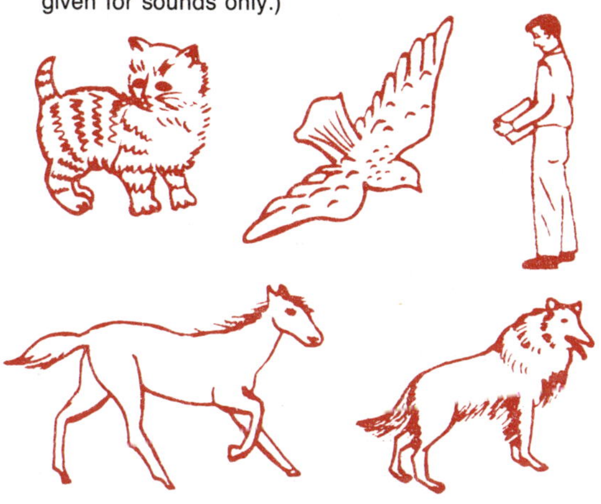

15. Tell child to: Give block to Mommie; put block on table; put block on floor. Pass 2 of 3. (Do not help child by pointing, moving head or eyes.)
16. Ask child: What do you do when you are cold? ..hungry? ..tired? Pass 2 of 3.
17. Tell child to: Put block *on* table; *under* table; in front of chair, *behind* chair. Pass 3 of 4. (Do not help child by pointing, moving head or eyes.)
18. Ask child: If fire is hot, ice is ?; Mother is a woman, Dad is a ?; a horse is big, a mouse is ?. Pass 2 of 3.
19. Ask child: What is a ball? ..lake? ..desk? ..house? ..banana? ..curtain? ..ceiling? ..hedge? ..pavement? Pass if defined in terms of use, shape, what it is made

of or general category (such as banana is fruit, not just yellow). Pass 6 of 9.

20. Ask child: What is a spoon made of? ..a shoe made of? ..a door made of? (No other objects may be substituted.) Pass 3 of 3.

21. When placed on stomach, child lifts chest off table with support of forearms and/or hands.

22. When child is on back, grasp his hands and pull him to sitting. Pass if head does not hang back.

23. Child may use wall or rail only, not person. May not crawl.

24. Child must throw ball overhand 3 feet to within arm's reach of tester.

25. Child must perform standing broad jump over width of test sheet. (8½ inches)

26. Tell child to walk forward, heel within 1 inch of toe. Tester may demonstrate Child must walk 4 consecutive steps, 2 out of 3 trials.

27. Bounce ball to child who should stand 3 feet away from tester. Child must catch ball with hands, not arms, 2 out of 3 trials.

28. Tell child to walk backward, toe within 1 inch of heel. Tester may demonstrate. Child must walk 4 consecutive steps, 2 out of 3 trials.

DATE AND BEHAVIORAL OBSERVATIONS (how child feels at time of test, relation to tester, attention span, verbal behavior, self-confidence, etc).

TABLE 12–1 Emerging Patterns of Behavior from Birth Through Five Years*†

Neonatal Period (First 4 Weeks)
Prone: Lies in flexed attitude; turns head from side to side; head sags on ventral suspension
Supine: Generally flexed and a little stiff
Visual: May fixate face or light in line of vision; "doll's-eye" movement of eyes on turning of the body
Reflex: Moro response active; stepping and placing reflexes; grasp reflex active
Social: Visual preference for human face

At 4 Weeks
Prone: Legs more extended; holds chin up; turns head; head lifted momentarily to plane of body on ventral suspension
Supine: Tonic neck posture predominates; supple and relaxed; head lags on pull to sitting position
Visual: Watches person; follows moving object
Social: Body movements in cadence with voice of other in social contact; beginning to smile

At 8 Weeks
Prone: Raises head slightly farther; head sustained in plane of body on ventral suspension
Supine: Tonic neck posture predominates; head lags on pull to sitting position
Visual: Follows moving object 180 degrees
Social: Smiles on social contact; listens to voice and coos

TABLE 12–1   Emerging Patterns of Behavior from Birth Through Five Years[*][†] (Continued)

At 12 Weeks

Prone:	Lifts head and chest, arms extended; head above plane of body on ventral suspension
Supine:	Tonic neck posture predominates; reaches toward and misses objects; waves at toy
Sitting:	Head lag partially compensated on pull to sitting position; early head control with bobbing motion; back rounded
Reflex:	Typical Moro response has not persisted; makes defense movements or selective withdrawal reactions
Social:	Sustained social contact; listens to music; says "aah, ngah"

At 16 Weeks

Prone:	Lifts head and chest, head in approximately vertical axis; legs extended
Supine:	Symmetrical posture predominates, hands in midline; reaches and grasps objects and brings them to mouth
Sitting:	No head lag on pull to sitting position; head steady, held forward; enjoys sitting with full truncal support
Standing:	When held erect, pushes with feet
Adaptive:	Sees pellet, but makes no move to it
Social:	Laughs out loud; may show displeasure if social contact is broken; excited at sight of food

At 28 Weeks

Prone:	Rolls over; may pivot
Supine:	Lifts head; rolls over; squirming movements
Sitting:	Sits briefly, with support of pelvis; leans forward on hands; back rounded
Standing:	May support most of weight; bounces actively
Adaptive:	Reaches out for and grasps large object; *transfers* objects from hand to hand; grasp uses radial palm; rakes at pellet
Language:	Polysyllabic vowel sounds formed
Social:	Prefers mother; babbles; enjoys mirror; responds to changes in emotional content of social contact

At 40 Weeks

Sitting:	Sits up alone and indefinitely without support, back straight
Standing:	Pulls to standing position
Motor:	Creeps or crawls
Adaptive:	Grasps objects with *thumb and forefinger*; pokes at things with forefinger; picks up pellet with assisted pincer movement; uncovers hidden toy; attempts to retrieve dropped object; releases object grasped by other person
Language:	Repetitive consonant sounds (mamma, dada)
Social:	Responds to sound of name; plays peek-a-boo or pat-a-cake; waves bye-bye

At 52 Weeks (1 Year)

Motor:	Walks with one hand held; "cruises" or walks holding on to furniture
Adaptive:	Picks up pellet with unassisted pincer movement of forefinger and thumb; releases object to other person on request or gesture
Language:	A few words besides mama, dada
Social:	Plays simple ball game; makes postural adjustment to dressing

15 Months

Motor:	Walks alone; crawls up stairs
Adaptive:	Makes tower of 2 cubes; makes a line with crayon; inserts pellet in bottle
Language:	Jargon; follows simple commands; may name a familiar object (ball)
Social:	Indicates some desires or needs by pointing; hugs parents

TABLE 12–1   Emerging Patterns of Behavior from Birth Through Five Years*[†] (Continued)

18 Months

Motor:	Runs stiffly; sits on small chair; walks up stairs with one hand held; explores drawers and waste baskets
Adaptive:	Piles 3 cubes; imitates scribbling; imitates vertical stroke; dumps pellet from bottle
Language:	10 words (average); names pictures; identifies one or more parts of body
Social:	Feeds self; seeks help when in trouble; may complain when wet or soiled; kisses parent with pucker

24 Months

Motor:	Runs well; walks up and down stairs, one step at a time; opens doors; climbs on furniture
Adaptive:	Tower of 6 cubes; circular scribbling; imitates horizontal stroke; folds paper once imitatively
Language:	Puts 3 words together (subject, verb, object)
Social:	Handles spoon well; often tells immediate experiences; helps to undress; listens to stories with pictures

30 Months

Motor:	Jumps
Adaptive:	Tower of 8 cubes; makes vertical and horizontal strokes, but generally will not join them to make a cross; imitates circular stroke, forming closed figure
Language:	Refers to self by pronoun "I"; knows full name
Social:	Helps put things away; pretends in play

36 Months

Motor:	Goes up stairs alternating feet; rides tricycle; stands momentarily on one foot
Adaptive:	Tower of 9 cubes; imitates construction of "bridge" of 3 cubes; copies a circle; imitates a cross
Language:	Knows age and sex; counts 3 objects correctly; repeats 3 numbers or a sentence of 6 syllables
Social:	Plays simple games (in "parallel" with other children); helps in dressing (unbuttons clothing and puts on shoes); washes hands

48 Months

Motor:	Hops on one foot; throws ball overhand; uses scissors to cut out pictures; climbs well
Adaptive:	Copies bridge from model; imitates construction of "gate" of 5 cubes; copies cross and square; draws a man with 2 to 4 parts besides head; names longer of 2 lines
Language:	Counts 4 pennies accurately; tells a story
Social:	Plays with several children with beginning of social interaction and role-playing; goes to toilet alone

60 Months

Motor:	Skips
Acaptive:	Draws triangle from copy; names heavier of 2 weights
Language:	Names 4 colors; repeats sentence of 10 syllables; counts 10 pennies correctly
Social:	Dresses and undresses; asks questions about meaning of words; domestic role-playing

* From Behrman RE, Vaughan VC, eds. Nelson textbook of pediatrics 12th ed. Philadelphia: WB Saunders, 1983.

† Data are derived from those of Gesell, Shirley, Provence, Wolf, Bailey, and others. After 5 years the Stanford-Binet, Wechsler-Bellevue, and other scales offer the most precise estimates of developmental level. In order to have their greatest value, they should be administered only by an experienced and qualified person.

TABLE 12–2   Physician's Speech and Language Checklist: Birth to Five Years

Birth to 6 Months
Startles to loud, sudden noises
Sometimes stirs or awakens when sleeping quietly and someone makes a loud noise
(3 to 6 months) stops moving when called

6 to 12 Months
Turns toward a sound or when his name is called
Babbles, laughs, or makes sounds like "ga-ga," "ma-ma," or "ba-ba"

12 to 15 Months
Repeats sounds
Understands some simple phrases like "Come here," "Don't touch"
Recognizes telephone or doorbell ringing

15 to 18 Months
Says four to six words
Tells what he wants by pointing and saying a word
Understands phrases like "Give me that" when gestures are used
Recognizes names of common objects like ball, table, bed, car
Uses names of familiar things like water, cup, cookie, clock

18 to 24 Months
Uses two word combinations
Says about 20 or more words
Uses words to express physical needs
Follows simple directions like "Sit down," "Give me that ball"
Points to appropriate picture when you say "Show me the dog (hat, man, etc.)"

2 to 3 Years
Uses three word sentences
Tells a story or expresses his feelings in words
Remembers some recent past events
Counts to 3
Tells his first and last names
Is understood in 40 to 50% of what he says by people outside the family

3 to 4 Years
    Uses four to five word sentences
    Tells a story
    Asks a lot of questions
    Repeats a sentence of eight to nine syllables, e.g.,
    "We are going to buy some candy"
    Names three colors
    Uses plurals like "toys," "balls"
    Can repeat three or four numbers

4 to 5 Years
    Can define four or more common words or tell how the
    objects are used (e.g., hat, dish, apples)
    Can name a penny, a nickel, and a dime
    Is understood in 80 to 90% of what he says by people
    outside the family
    Likes to look at books and have someone read to him
    Uses I, me, you, he, and him properly

Adapted from Speech and hearing checklist for the family physician. Toronto, Ontario: The Ontario Association Speech-Language Pathologists and Audiologists.

TABLE 12–3   Clinical Guide to Commonly Encountered Psychodiagnostic Tests*

Type of Test	Age Range	Uses	Limitations
Tests to Evaluate General Intelligence			
Stanford-Binet Intelligence Scale	2 yr–adult	Yields mental age and IQ Used frequently for preschool age children and preferred by some professionals over the WISC-R up to 8 yr Can be used with children considered to be mentally retarded	Provides one global score No differentiation of strengths and weaknesses through test construction Is heavily weighted with verbal items Requires normal sensory and motor skills
Wechsler Intelligence Scale for Children—Revised (WISC-R) and	6–16 yr	Yields a verbal IQ, performance IQ, and full scale IQ Tests constructed according to skill areas permitting delineation of child's strengths and weaknesses	Caution indicated in interpretation of individual subtest scores at certain ages owing to lower reliability
Wechsler Preschool and Primary Scale of Intelligence (WPPSI)	4–6½ yr	May use one of the verbal or performance scales alone to estimate overall level of intelligence if administration of the full scale is precluded by child's handicap	

McCarthy Scales of Children's Abilities	2½–8½ yr	Multiple subtests tap different areas of function Verbal, perceptual-performance, and quantitative scales make up a general cognitive index comparable to an IQ Motor abilities recorded separately	Administration of full scale often too lengthy for some handicapped children in this age range
Peabody-Picture Vocabulary Test	2–18 yr	Effective test of receptive language Particularly useful for testing children with severe speech or motor impairment, since the test requires only a pointing response	Measures only one area of functioning (listening vocabulary) Can be misleading to generalize from this to other areas of intellectual or language ability
Leiter International Performance	2–18 yr	Designed for use with deaf children and is useful in assessment of speech-language handicapped children Measures nonverbal intelligence Test administration allows observation of learning ability	Limited range of abilities are sampled Manipulation of materials can be difficult for motor handicapped children
Hiskey-Nebraska Test of Learning Aptitudes	4–12 yr	Designed and standardized for deaf children	Does not evaluate language skills

TABLE 12–3   Clinical Guide to Commonly Encountered Psychodiagnostic Tests* (Continued)

Tests to Evaluate Perception			
Bender Visual-Motor Gestalt	5 yr–adult	Assesses visual-motor functioning in relation to maturation Nonthreatening, easy to administer, well researched	Open to overinterpretation in terms of IQ estimate and emotional status Requires functional graphomotor skills to provide useful information See limitation below (Beery)
Beery and Buktenica Developmental Test of Visual-Motor Integration	2–16 yr	Assesses visual motor performance Useful in evaluation of younger children compared to Bender Gestalt Not used to gauge IQ or emotional status	Like the Bender, measures visual motor copying of shapes and designs, which may or may not correlate with ability to copy (print or write) letters or words
Wepman Auditory Discrimination	5–8 yr	Examines ability to detect likeness and difference between sounds in pairs of words presented aurally	Requires mastery of concepts of "same" vs "different" to respond to test items
Tests to Evaluate Academic Achievement			
Wide Range Achievement Test (WRAT)	Kindergarten to 12th grade	Used to assess quickly the level of academic skills and improvement from one evaluation to the next	Has been normed several times with different inaccuracies associated with each set of norms Reading subtest taps only word identification, not comprehension Math subtest taps limited concepts and problem solving ability

Peabody Individual Achievement Test (PIAT)	Kindergarten to high school	Provides overview of mathematics, reading, spelling, and general information Requirement for only a pointing response and use of large, clear response choices make it useful in evaluation of handicapped children	Considered by authors to be a screening instrument Manual suggests use of alternate instruments when more intensive study is required
Social/Adaptive Scales			
Vineland Social Maturity †	Infant to adult	Questionnaire type instrument for measurement of general social competences as reflected in eight different areas Constructed as age scale and yields social age equivalent and social quotient comparable to a mental age and IQ	Tends to have some cultural and socioeconomic bias Data obtained through interview with an informant who may not provide reliable information
Emotional and Projective Assessment Tests			
Children's Apperception Test (CAT) and Thematic Apperception Test (TAT)	3–10 yr >10 yr	Assesses child's adjustment patterns and social relationships	Marked controversy exists concerning reliability and validity data
Rorschach Ink Blot Test	3 yr to adult	Evaluates personality structure, including ego strengths, reality testing, and defense mechanisms	Same as CAT Requires freedom from significant perceptual problems

TABLE 12–3 Clinical Guide to Commonly Encountered Psychodiagnostic Tests* (Continued)

Figure Drawings (e.g., draw a person, house-tree-person, kinetic family drawing)	4 yr to adult	Reveals self-image and perception of interpersonal relationships in addition to providing estimate of level of development or intelligence Appealing task for most children	Requires good graphomotor ability in order to interpret for emotional factors
Self-Report Inventories	Varied	Assesses perception of individual regarding his own functioning level	Subject to intentional distortion
Test for Infants Gesell Development Schedules	4 wk–6 yr	Forerunner in systematic observation of infant development Useful standardized procedure for evaluating and observing behavior in four major areas of functioning, including adaptive, gross and fine motor, language, and personal-social skills	Note: For all infant tests, scales are most useful for providing an indication of current developmental levels and not for prediction. They can be weighted with motor items, which limit predictive accuracy for physically handicapped children; in children with language delays, their true cognitive potential may be masked by their verbal inadequacy
Bayley Scales of Infant Development	2–30 mo	Provides separate mental and motor scales and an index for reporting quality of infant's behavior during evaluation	

| Cattell Infant Intelligence Scale | 2–30 mo | Yields mental age
For 18–30 mo age children pro-vides transition from infant scale to preschool Stanford-Binet
Assesses level of sensorimotor and problem solving skills and taps emerging language abilities |

* Adapted from Molnar GE, ed. Pediatric rehabilitation. Baltimore: Williams & Wilkins, 1985:ch.3.
† N.B. There exists a revised edition (1984), which involves conducting a semistructured interview with the caregiver and provides data regarding adaptive skills in such areas as communication, daily living, socialization, and motor behavior as well as the assessment of maladaptive behavior. Covers birth to 18 years.

TABLE 12–4 Levels of Mental Retardation and Associated Features

Borderline (IQ 68–83)	Children with IQ's above 69 are not retarded, strictly speaking, but are vulnerable to educational problems. They are usually able to function adequately in slow sections of regular classes. Most achieve independent social and vocational adjustment.
Mild (IQ 52–67)	This group includes 90% of children formerly classified as retarded. Most need special class placement, and some can achieve 4th–6th grade reading levels. Those who are well adjusted may be able to function independently as adults.
Moderate (IQ 36–51)	Children in this group usually function in classes for the trainable retarded, with emphasis on gaining maximal self-care and perhaps some academic skills. Those who are well adjusted may be able to function semi-independently in supervised living and sheltered workshop settings.
Severe (IQ 20–35)	Children in this group can learn minimal self-care skills and simple conversational skills. They need much supervision and are often institutionalized.
Profound (IQ below 20)	Children in this group need total supervision. Very minimal self-care skills are possible. Some may be toilet trained. Language development will be minimal.

From Behrman RE, Vaughan VC, eds. Nelson textbook of pediatrics. 12th ed. Philadelphia: W.B. Saunders, 1983:124.

TABLE 12–5 Calculation of Decimal Age*†

Table of Decimals of Year

	1 Jan	2 Feb	3 Mar	4 Apr	5 May	6 June	7 July	8 Aug	9 Sept	10 Oct	11 Nov	12 Dec
1	000	085	162	247	329	414	496	581	666	748	833	915
2	003	088	164	249	332	416	499	584	668	751	836	918
3	005	090	167	252	334	419	501	586	671	753	838	921
4	008	093	170	255	337	422	504	589	674	756	841	923
5	011	096	173	258	340	425	507	592	677	759	844	926
6	014	099	175	260	342	427	510	595	679	762	847	929
7	016	101	178	263	345	430	512	597	682	764	849	932
8	019	104	181	266	348	433	515	600	685	767	852	934
9	022	107	184	268	351	436	518	603	688	770	855	937
10	025	110	186	271	353	438	521	605	690	773	858	940
11	027	112	189	274	356	441	523	608	693	775	860	942
12	030	115	192	277	359	444	526	611	696	778	863	945
13	033	118	195	279	362	447	529	614	699	781	866	948
14	036	121	197	282	364	449	532	616	701	784	868	951
15	038	123	200	285	367	452	534	619	704	786	871	953
16	041	126	203	288	370	455	537	622	707	789	874	956

TABLE 12–5 Calculation of Decimal Age*† (Continued)

	Jan 1	Feb 2	Mar 3	Apr 4	May 5	June 6	July 7	Aug 8	Sept 9	Oct 10	Nov 11	Dec 12
17	044	129	205	290	373	458	540	625	710	792	877	959
18	047	132	208	293	375	460	542	627	712	795	879	962
19	049	134	211	296	378	463	545	630	715	797	882	964
20	052	137	214	299	381	466	548	633	718	800	885	967
21	055	140	216	301	384	468	551	636	721	803	888	970
22	058	142	219	304	386	471	553	638	723	805	890	973
23	060	145	222	307	389	474	556	641	726	808	893	975
24	063	148	225	310	392	477	559	644	729	811	896	978
25	066	151	227	312	395	479	562	647	731	814	899	981
26	068	153	230	315	397	482	564	649	734	816	901	984
27	071	156	233	318	400	485	567	652	737	819	904	986
28	074	159	236	321	403	488	570	655	740	822	907	989
29	077		238	323	405	490	573	658	742	825	910	992
30	079		241	326	408	493	575	660	745	827	912	995
31	082		244		411		578	663		830		997

* From Tanner JM, Whitehouse RH. Growth and development records. London: University of London, Institute of Child Health, 1966.
† Decimal age. The year is divided into 10, not 12. Each date in the calendar is marked (from the table) in terms of thousandths of the year. Thus January 7, 1987, is 87.016. The child's birth date is similarly recorded; e.g., a child born on June 23, 1984, has the birth day 84.474. The age at examination is then obtained by simple subtraction; e.g., 87.016 − 84.474 = 2.542, and the last figure is rounded off. This system greatly facilitates the computing of velocities, since the proportion of the year between two examinations is easily calculated.

TABLE 12–6 Formula for Calculating Approximate Average Height and Weight of Normal Infants and Children

Weight	Kilograms	(Pounds)
at birth	3.25	(7)
3–12 mo	$\dfrac{age(mo) + 9}{2}$	(age[mo] + 11)
1–6 yr	age(yr) × 2 + 8	(age[yr] × 5 + 17)
6–12 yr	$\dfrac{age(yr) \times 7 - 5}{2}$	(age[yr] × 7 + 5)
Height	**Centimeters**	**(Inches)**
at birth	50	(20)
at 1 yr	75	(30)
2–12 yr	age(yr) × 6 + 77	(age[yr] × 2½ + 30)

From Behrman RE, Vaughan VC, eds. Nelson textbook of pediatrics. 12th ed. Philadelphia: W.B. Saunders, 1983:19.

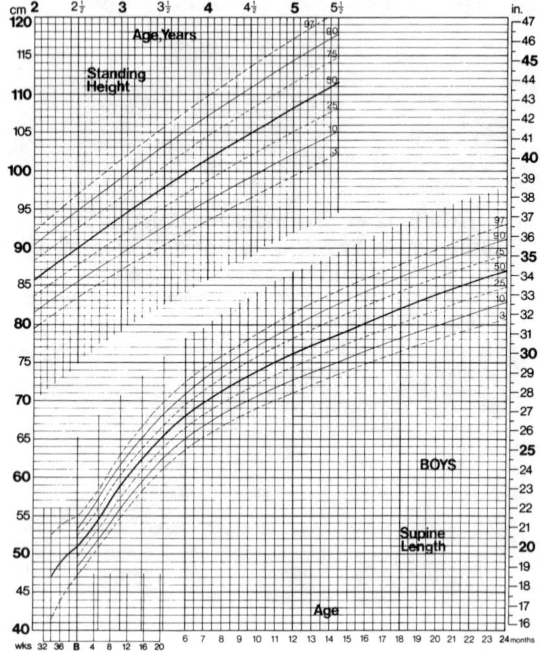

Figure 12–2 Boys: birth–5 years: height. Note: Age scale is divided into months. (From Tanner JM, Whitehouse RH. Growth and development record. Swains Mill, Herts, England: Castlemead Publications, Ward's Publishing Services, 1984.)

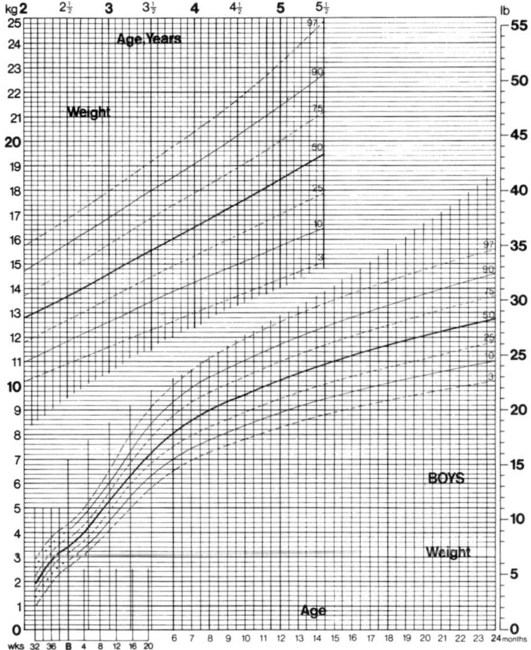

Figure 12–3   Boys: birth–5 years: weight. Note: Age scale is divided into months. (From Tanner JM, Whitehouse RH. Growth and development record. Swains Hill, Herts, England: Castlemead Publications, Ward's Publishing Services, 1984.)

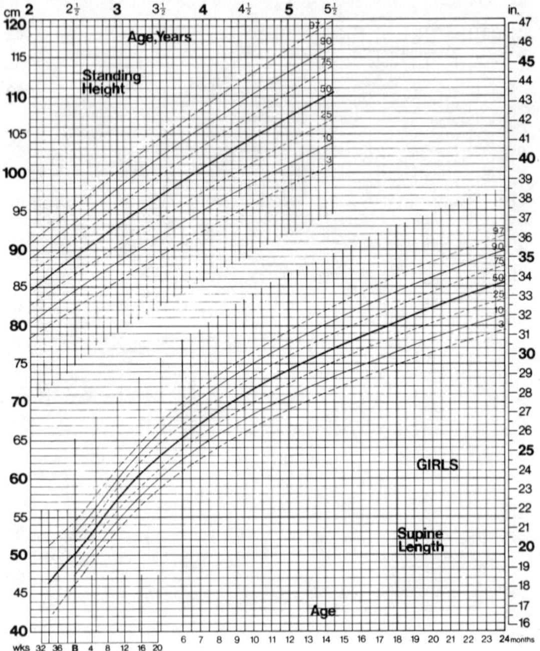

Figure 12–4   Girls: birth–5 years: height. Note: Age scale is divided into months. (From Tanner JM, Whitehouse RH. Growth and development record. Swains Mill, Herts, England: Castlemead Publications, Ward's Publishing Services, 1984.)

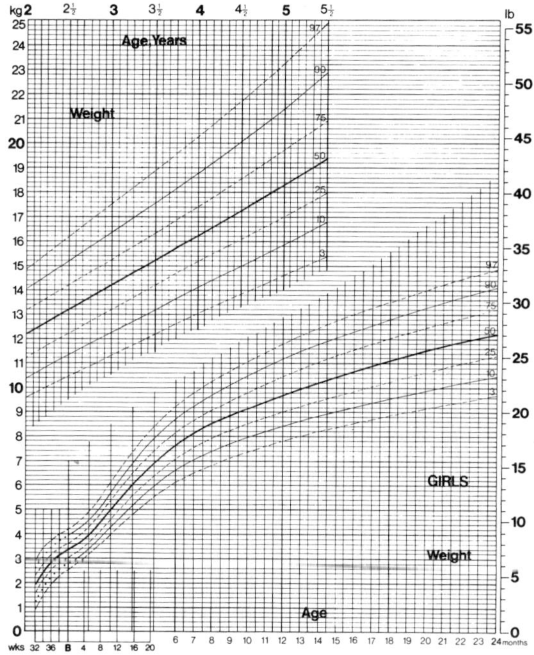

Figure 12–5 Girls: birth–5 years: weight. Note: Age scale is divided into months. (From Tanner JM, Whitehouse RH. Growth and development record. Swains Mill, Herts, England: Castlemead Publications, Ward's Publishing Services, 1984.)

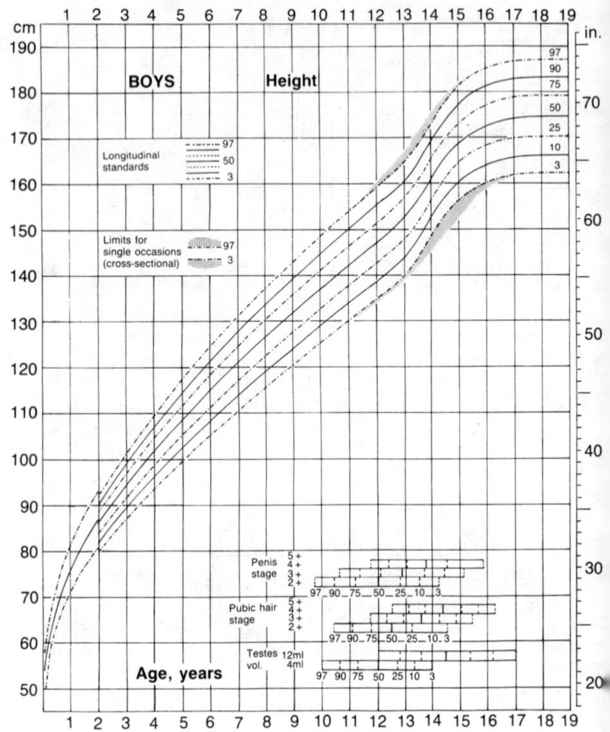

Figure 12–6 Boys: birth–19 years: height. (From Tanner JM, Whitehouse RH. Growth and development record. London: University of London, Institute of Child Health, 1966.)

210

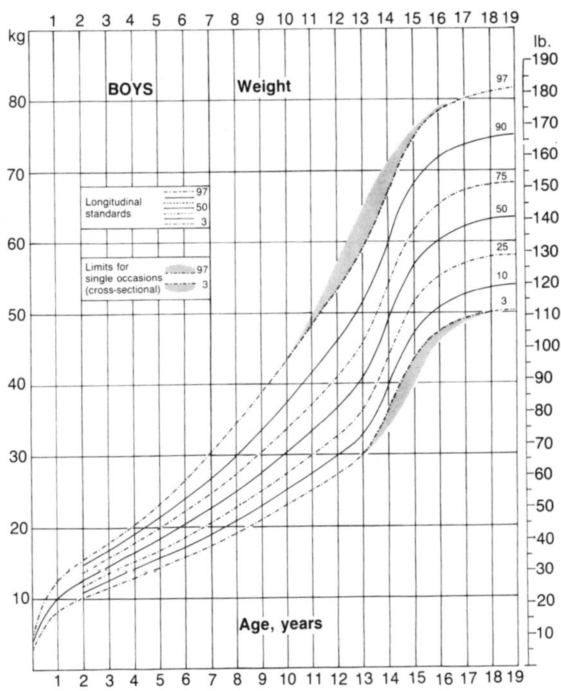

Figure 12–7 Boys: birth–19 years: weight. (From Tanner JM, Whitehouse RH. Growth and development record. London: University of London, Institute of Child Health, 1966.)

211

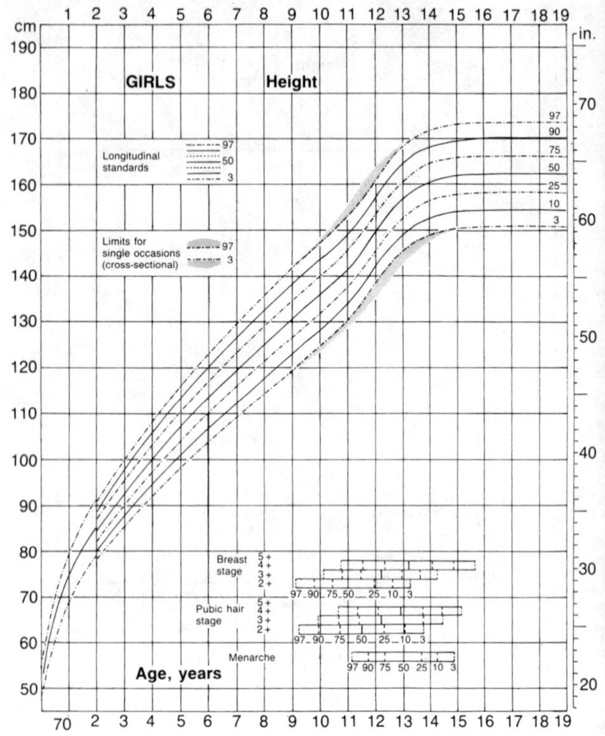

Figure 12–8 Girls: birth–19 years: height. (From Tanner JM, Whitehouse RH. Growth and development record. London: University of London, Institute of Child Health, 1966.)

212

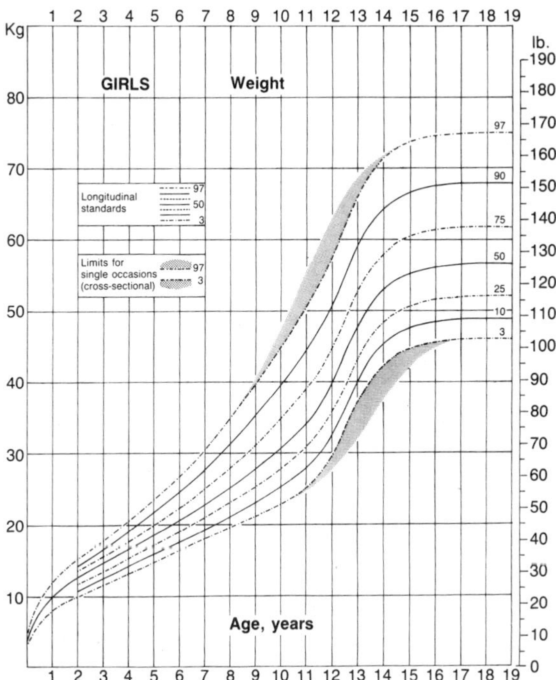

Figure 12–9 Girls: birth–19 years: weight. (From Tanner JM, Whitehouse RH. Growth and development record. London: University of London, Institute of Child Health, 1966.)

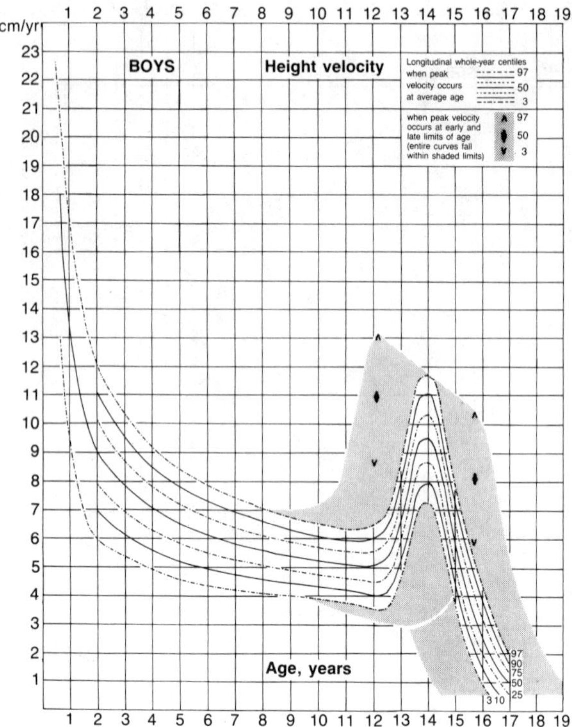

Figure 12–10 Boys: birth–19 years: height velocity. (From Tanner JM, Whitehouse RH. Growth and development record. London: University of London, Institute of Child Health, 1966.)

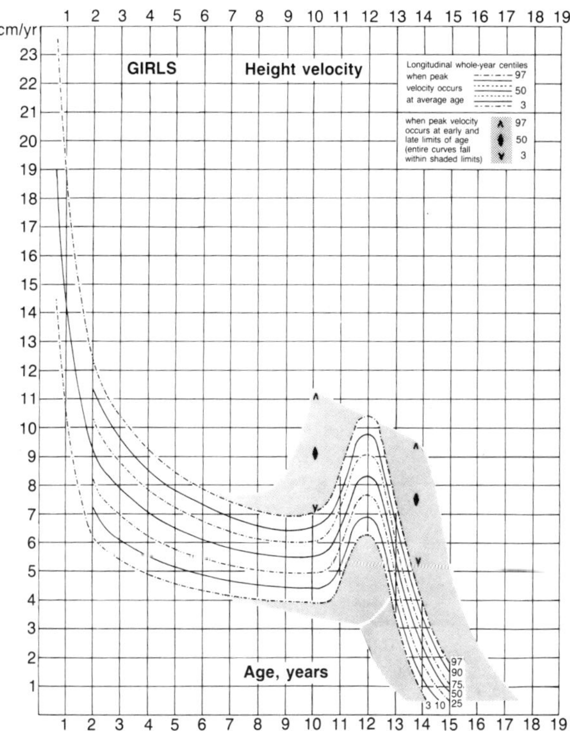

Figure 12–11 Girls: birth–19 years: height velocity. (From Tanner JM, Whitehouse RH. Growth and development record. London: University of London, Institute of Child Health, 1966.)

215

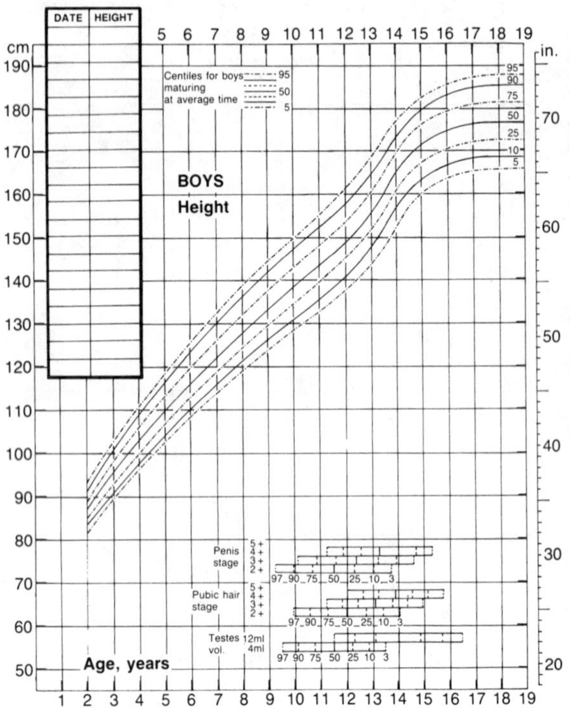

Figure 12–12 Boys: birth–19 years: height (North American standards). (Modified from Tanner JM, Davies PSW. Clinical longitudinal standards for height and height velocity for North American children. J Pediatr 1985; 107:320.)

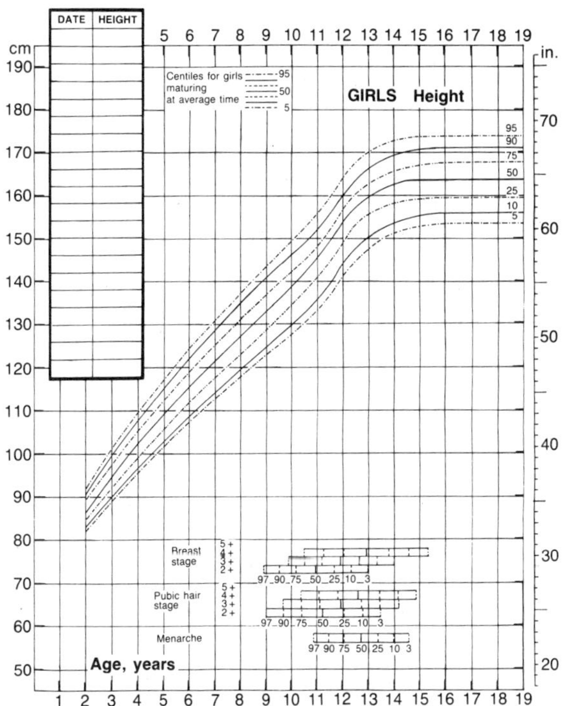

Figure 12–13   Girls: birth–19 years: height (North American standards). (Modified from Tanner JM, Davies PSW. Clinical longitudinal standards for height and height velocity for North American children. J Pediatr 1985; 107:322.)

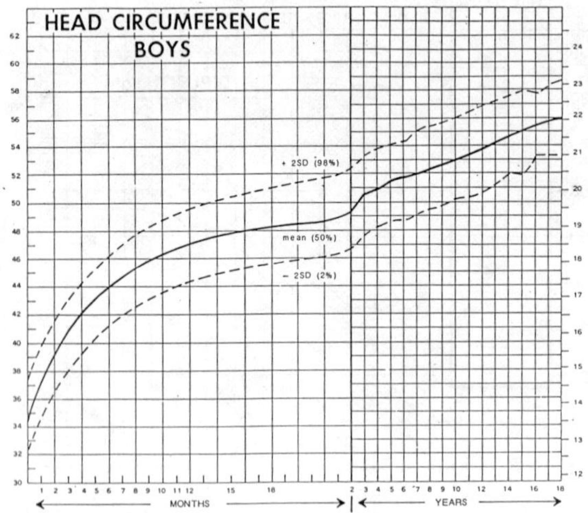

Figure 12–14 Boys: birth–18 years: head circumference. (From Nelhaus. Pediatrics 1968; 41:106.)

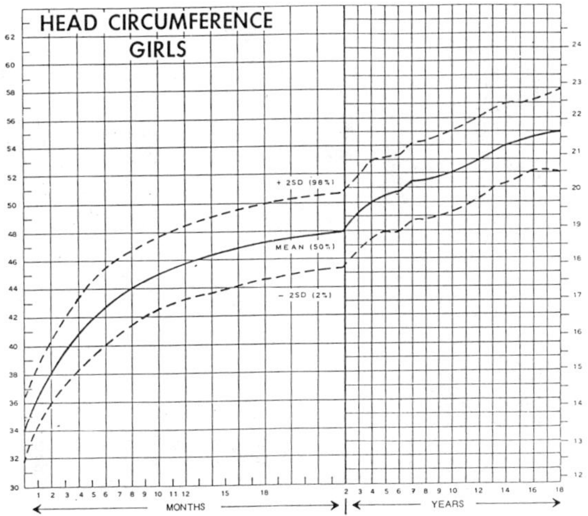

Figure 12–15 Girls: birth–18 years: head circumference. (From Nelhaus. Pediatrics 1968; 41:106.)

TABLE 12–7 Fraction of Adult Height Attained at Each Bone Age[†]

Bone Age	Girls			Boys		
yr–mo	Retarded*	Average**	Advanced***	Retarded*	Average**	Advanced***
6–0	0.733	0.720		0.680		
6–3	0.742	0.729		0.690		
6–6	0.751	0.738		0.700		
6–9	0.763	0.751		0.709		
7–0	0.770	0.757	0.712	0.718	0.695	0.670
7–3	0.779	0.765	0.722	0.728	0.702	0.676
7–6	0.788	0.772	0.732	0.738	0.709	0.683
7–9	0.797	0.782	0.742	0.747	0.716	0.689
8–0	0.804	0.790	0.750	0.756	0.723	0.696
8–3	0.813	0.801	0.760	0.765	0.731	0.703
8–6	0.823	0.810	0.771	0.773	0.739	0.709
8–9	0.836	0.821	0.784	0.779	0.746	0.715
9–0	0.841	0.827	0.790	0.786	0.752	0.720
9–3	0.851	0.836	0.800	0.794	0.761	0.728
9–6	0.858	0.844	0.809	0.800	0.769	0.734
9–9	0.866	0.853	0.819	0.807	0.777	0.741
10–0	0.874	0.862	0.828	0.812	0.784	0.747
10–3	0.884	0.874	0.841	0.816	0.791	0.753
10–6	0.896	0.884	0.856	0.819	0.795	0.758
10–9	0.907	0.896	0.870	0.821	0.800	0.763

11–0	0.918	0.906	0.883	0.823	0.804	0.767
11–3	0.922	0.910	0.887	0.827	0.812	0.776
11–6	0.926	0.914	0.891	0.832	0.818	0.786
11–9	0.929	0.918	0.897	0.839	0.827	0.800
12–0	0.932	0.922	0.901	0.845	0.834	0.809
12–3	0.942	0.932	0.913	0.852	0.843	0.818
12–6	0.949	0.941	0.924	0.860	0.853	0.828
12–9	0.957	0.950	0.935	0.869	0.863	0.839
13–0	0.964	0.958	0.945	0.880	0.876	0.850
13–3	0.971	0.967	0.955		0.890	0.863
13–6	0.977	0.974	0.963		0.902	0.875
13–9	0.981	0.978	0.968		0.914	0.890
14–0	0.983	0.980	0.972		0.927	0.905
14–3	0.986	0.983	0.977		0.938	0.918
14–6	0.989	0.986	0.980		0.948	0.930
14–9	0.992	0.988	0.983		0.958	0.943
15–0	0.994	0.990	0.986		0.968	0.958
15–3	0.995	0.991	0.988		0.973	0.967
15–6	0.996	0.993	0.990		0.976	0.971
15–9	0.997	0.994	0.992		0.980	0.976

TABLE 12–7   Fraction of Adult Height Attained at Each Bone Age[†] (Continued)

Bone Age yr–mo	Girls			Boys		
	Retarded*	Average**	Advanced***	Retarded*	Average**	Advanced***
16–0	0.998	0.996	0.993		0.982	0.980
16–3	0.999	0.996	0.994		0.985	0.983
16–6	0.999	0.997	0.995		0.987	0.985
16–9	0.9995	0.998	0.997		0.989	0.988
17–0	1.00	0.999	0.998		0.991	0.990
17–3					0.993	
17–6		0.9995	0.9995		0.994	
17–9					0.995	
18–0		1.00			0.996	
18–3					0.998	
18–6					1.00	

  * Retarded: Bone age more than 1 year below chronologic age
 ** Average: Bone age within 1 year of chronologic age
*** Advanced: Bone age more than 1 year above chronologic age

Predicted height $= \dfrac{\text{Present height}}{\text{Decimal fraction}}$

[†] From Post EM, Richman RA. A condensed table for predicting adult stature. J Pediatr 1981; 98:441.

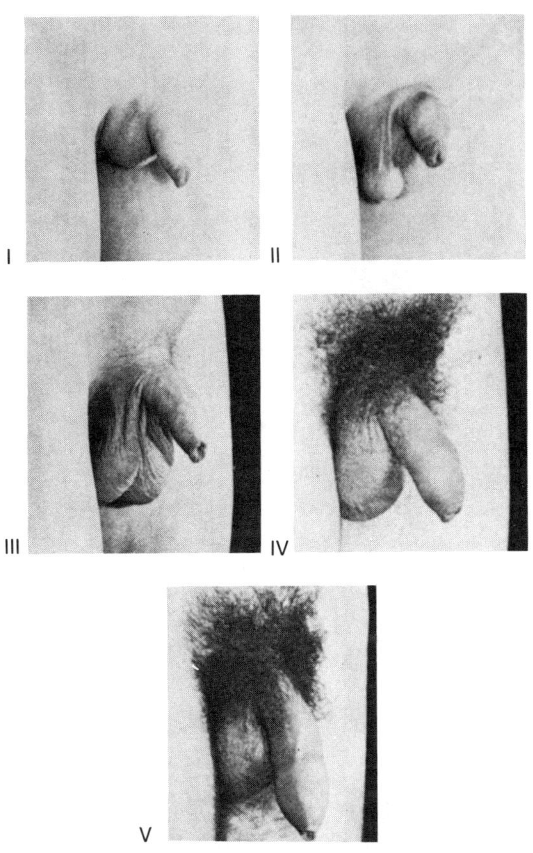

Figure 12–16 Male genital and pubic hair development. Stage I: prepubertal. Stage II: enlargement of testes, appearance of scrotal reddening, and increase in scrotal rugations. Stage III: increase in length and, to a lesser extent, breadth of penis, with further growth of testes. Stage IV: further increase in size of penis and testes and darkening of scrotal skin. Stage V: adult. (Modified from Van Wieringen, et al. Growth diagrams, 1965. Netherlands: Wolters-Noordhoff, 1971.)

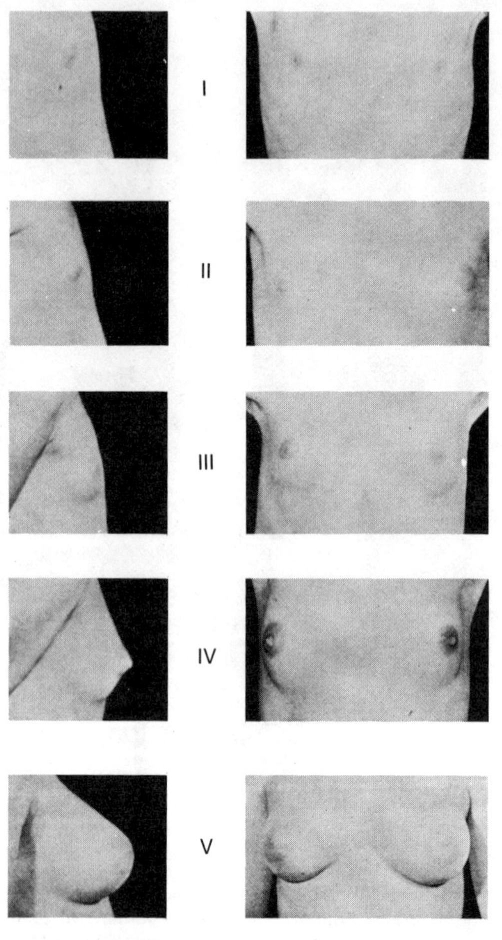

Figure 12–17 Female breast development. Stage I: prepubertal. Stage II: budding. Stage III: appearance of small adult breast. Stage IV: areola and papilla form a secondary mound. Stage V: adult (Modified from Van Wieringen, et al. Growth diagrams, 1965. Netherlands: Wolters-Noordhoff, 1971.)

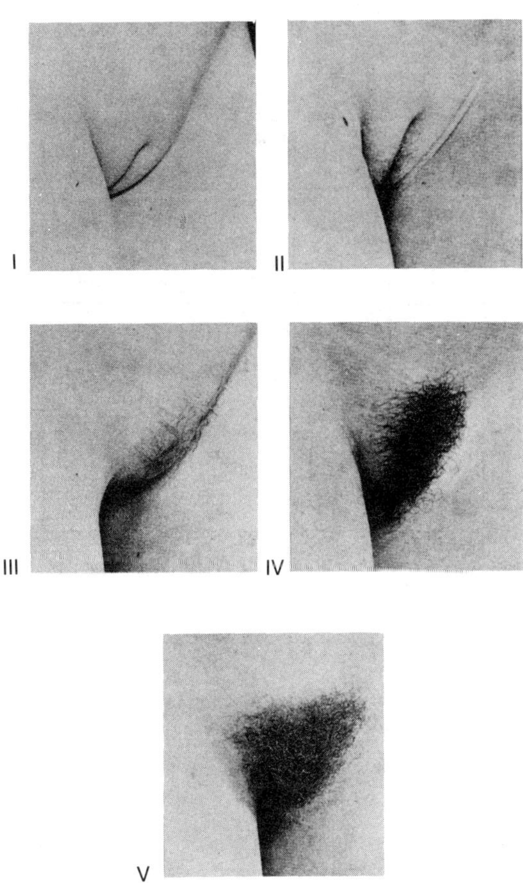

Figure 12–18 Female pubic hair development. Stage I: prepubertal. Stage II: sparse growth of long, slightly pigmented hair. Stage III: hair darker, coarser, and curlier, and beginning to spread over symphysis pubis. Stage IV: hair is adult in character but not distribution, without spread to medial surface of thigh. Stage V: adult (From Van Wieringen, et al. Growth diagrams, 1965. Netherlands: Wolters-Noordhoff, 1971.)

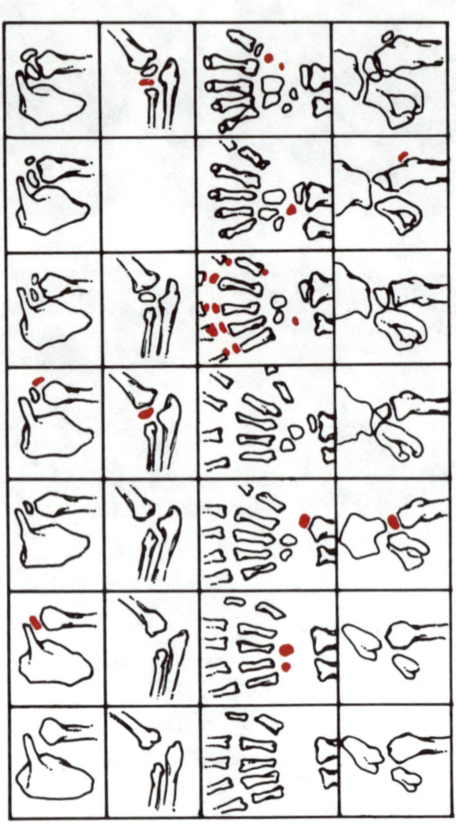

Figure 12–19 Chronological order of appearance of osseous centers. The new centers of ossification that appear at each year are shown in red. (From Wilkins L. The diagnosis and treatment of endocrine disorders in childhood and adolescence. 3rd ed. Springfield, Illinois: Charles C Thomas, 1965:38.)

	BIRTH	1 YR	2	3	4	5
Shoulder	0	Head of humerus (*3 months*)	Great tuberosity			
Elbow	0		Capitellum			Head of radius
Hand	0	Hamate (*4 mos.*) Capitate (*6 mos.*) Ep. radius		Triquetrum Ep. metacarpals Ep. phalanges	Lunatum	Trapezium Scaphoid
Hip	0	Head of femur (*9 mos.*)			Great trochanter	
Knee	Ep. femur & tibia				Head of fibula	Patella
Foot	Cuboid	Ext. cuneiform Ep. tibia	Ep. fibula	Int. cuneiform Ep. metatarsals	Mid cuneiform Navicular	

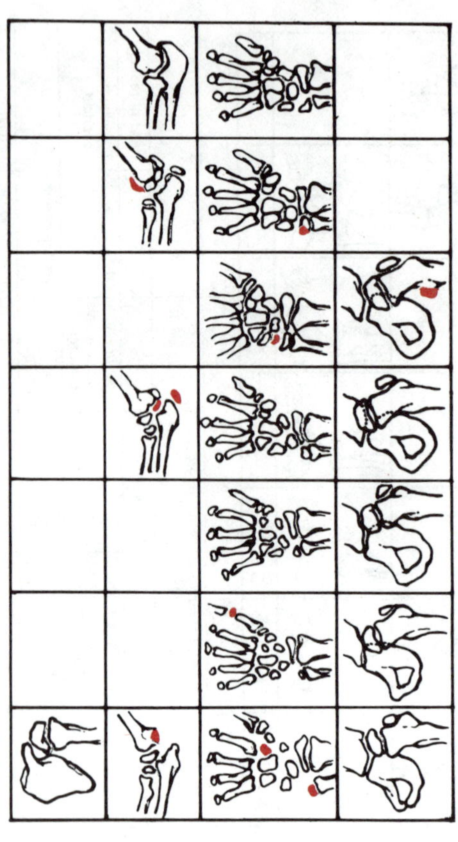

Figure 12–19 Six to thirteen years (Continued)

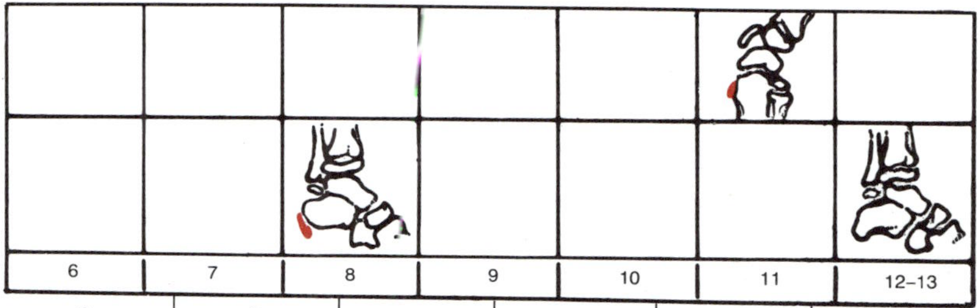

	6	7	8	9	10	11
Shoulder	*Union* head & tuberosity					
Elbow	Int. epicondyle			Trochlea Olecranon		Ext. epicondyle
Hand	Trapezoid Ep. ulna				Pisiform	Styloid ulna
Hip		*Union* ischium & pubis			Ep. lesser trochanter	
Knee						Tibial tubercle
Foot			Ep. os calcis			

TABLE 12–8 Stretched Penile Length

Stretched penile Length (cm) in Normal Males		
	Mean ± S.D.	Mean – 2½ S.D.
Newborn: 30 wk	2.5 ± 0.4	1.5
34 wk	3.0 ± 0.4	2.0
term	3.5 ± 0.4	2.5 – 2.4
0–5 mo	3.9 ± 0.8	1.9
6–12 mo	4.3 ± 0.8	2.3
1–2 yr	4.7 ± 0.8	2.6
2–3 yr	5.1 ± 0.9	2.9
3–4 yr	5.5 ± 0.9	3.3
4–5 yr	5.7 ± 0.9	3.5
5–6 yr	6.0 ± 0.9	3.8
6–7 yr	6.1 ± 0.9	3.9
7–8 yr	6.2 ± 1.0	3.7
8–9 yr	6.3 ± 1.0	3.8
9–10 yr	6.3 ± 1.0	3.8
10–11	6.4 ± 1.1	3.7
Adult	13.3 ± 1.6	9.3

Adapted from Lee PA, Mazur T, Danish R, et al. Micropenis I. Criteria, etiologies and classification. Johns Hopkins Med J 1980; 146:158.

TABLE 12–9 Chronology of Human Dentition

	Calcification		Eruption		Shedding	
	Begins At	Complete At	Maxillary	Mandibular	Maxillary	Mandibular
Primary or Deciduous Teeth						
Central incisors	5th fetal mo	18–24 mo	6–8 mo	5–7 mo	7–8 yr	6–7 yr
Lateral incisors	5th fetal mo	18–24 mo	8–11 mo	7–10 mo	8–9 yr	7–8 yr
Cuspids (canines)	6th fetal mo	30–36 mo	16–20 mo	16–20 mo	11–12 yr	9–11 yr
First molars	5th fetal mo	24–30 mo	10–16 mo	10–16 mo	10–11 yr	10–12 yr
Second molars	6th fetal mo	36 mo	20–30 mo	20–30 mo	10–12 yr	11–13 yr

TABLE 12–9 Chronology of Human Dentition (Continued)

	Calcification		Eruption	
	Begins At	Complete At	Maxillary	Mandibular
Secondary or Permanent Teeth				
Central incisors	3–4 mo	9–10 yr	7–8 yr	6–7 yr
Lateral incisors	Max., 10–12 mo Mand., 3–4 mo	10–11 yr	8–9 yr	7–8 yr
Cuspids (canines)	4–5 mo	12–15 yr	11–12 yr	9–11 yr
First premolars (bicuspids)	18–21 mo	12–13 yr	10–11 yr	10–12 yr
Second premolars (bicuspids)	24–30 mo	12–14 yr	10–12 yr	11–13 yr
First molars	Birth	9–10 yr	6–7 yr	6–7 yr
Second molars	30–36 mo	14–16 yr	12–13 yr	12–13 yr
Third molars	Max., 7–9 yr Mand., 8–10 yr	18–25 yr	17–22 yr	17–22 yr

From Behrman RE, Vaughan VC, eds. Nelson textbook of pediatrics. 12 ed. Philadelphia: W.B. Saunders, 1983:25.

Suggested Reading

1. Illingworth RS. The development of the infant and young child. London: Churchill Livingstone.
2. Knobloch H, et al. Manual of developmental diagnosis. Philadelphia: Harper and Rowe, 1980.
3. Levine M, et al, eds. Developmental-behavioral pediatrics. Philadelphia: W.B. Saunders, 1983.
4. Lowrey GH. Growth and development of children. 8th ed. Chicago: Year Book, 1986.

VAGINAL BLEEDING

General Considerations

- Definition: any bloody vaginal discharge other than normal menstrual flow
- Always do a complete history and physical
- Consider first the age and maturity of the patient when determining likely etiology
  1. Premenarchal: neonatal 0–8 wk, early and late childhood (8 wk–10 yr)
  2. Perimenarchal (10–13 yr)
  3. Postmenarchal (13+yr)

Neonatal

Clinical Features

- Usually occurs between 5–10 days of age
- Difficult to distinguish from hematuria
- May be accompanied by other signs of a bleeding diathesis
  1. Bruising and petechiae
  2. Bloody umbilical stump
  3. GI bleeding and hematuria

Differential Diagnosis

- Maternal estrogen effects
- Gynecologic disease (infection; tumor)
- Bleeding diathesis

Management

- Investigations
  1. CBC, PT, PTT and bleeding time, platelets
  2. Swab for C+S
  3. Urinalysis and C+S

- Treatment
  1. If physical and lab data normal, diagnosis is likely maternal estrogen effects and withdrawal bleeding. Follow-up in 6–8 wk.
  2. All other causes need a gynecologic referral and assessment
  3. Bleeding disorder—refer to hematology and gynecology

Premenarchal: Early and Late Childhood

Clinical Features

- Pertinent points in history
  1. Trauma or sexual abuse
  2. Foreign body
  3. Pubertal changes
  4. Bleeding diathesis
  5. Hormone ingestion or vaginal cream
- Pertinent points in physical
  1. Signs of pubertal changes
  2. Patient's behavior (re: abuse)
  3. Other signs of systemic illness
  4. Perineal examination for trauma or discharge

Differential Diagnosis

- Trauma
- Foreign body
- Sexual abuse
- Precocious puberty
- Hormone withdrawal
- Vaginitis (group A beta strep, Shigella; uncommon)
- Bleeding disorder (rare)
- Uterine, vaginal, urethral disease (uncommon)

- Investigations
  1. CBC
  2. Vaginal C+S
  3. Maturation index
- Treatment: Refer to gynecology for vaginoscopy and therapy unless only superficial trauma, foreign body easily removed, or vaginitis with positive culture

Perimenarchal

Clinical Features

- Similar in pattern to those of premenarchal group
- Always consider pregnancy, as it is possible to become pregnant prior to first menses

Differential Diagnosis

- Menarche
- Trauma
- Sexual abuse
- Bleeding disorder (would present as heavy flow at menarche)
- Uterine, vaginal disease (uncommon)
- Pregnancy complication

Management

- Investigations
  1. CBC
  2. Platelets, PT, PTT, and bleeding time (if bleeding considered excessive for normal menarche)
  3. Pregnancy test (serum β-HCG)

- Treatment
  1. Refer to gynecology if bleeding disorder (and hematology), sexual abuse, trauma requiring examination under anesthesia (EUA) or stitches, pregnancy complication, or uterine and vaginal disease suspected
  2. Otherwise reassure

Postmenarchal

Clinical Features

- Always consider this female sexually active until proven otherwise
- Pregnancy is a strong possibility
- Dysfunctional uterine bleeding is a diagnosis of exclusion
- A complete menstrual and sexual history is mandatory, but remember that it may not be completely reliable
- Determine contraceptive use and compliance
- Examine with other systemic illnesses in mind
- Do as complete a pelvic examination as possible

Differential Diagnosis

- Pregnancy and its complications
  1. Ectopic pregnancy
  2. Threatened and incomplete abortions. NB: Urine pregnancy test positive at 42 days (from date of last normal menstrual period [DLNMP]); serum β-HCG positive at 29 days (from DLNMP).
- Dysfunctional uterine bleeding (DUB)
  1. Approximately three fourths of the cases
  2. Anovulatory cycles
  3. Common in first 2 yr post menarche
- Coagulation disorders: approximately 20%

- Gynecologic disease:
  1. Infections: PID and endometritis
  2. IUD problems
  3. Oral contraceptive misuse

Management

- Investigations
  1. CBC, differential, platelets
  2. PT, PTT, bleeding time
  3. Thyroid function (T_4, T_3RU, TSH), prolactin
  4. Cervical swabs for gonorrhea and Chlamydia
  5. Pap smear
  6. Pregnancy test—serum β-HCG
  7. Urinalysis
  8. Blood sugar
- Treatment
  1. Principles of management depend on clinical diagnosis and patient's status
  2. Obtain a gynecologic consult if in doubt or concerned
  3. Mild bleeding (DUB)
     - Chronic bleeding with normal hemoglobin
     - Erratic menses only
     - Reassure patient and arrange close follow-up after two cycles (8 wk)
  4. Moderate bleeding (DUB)
     - Hemoglobin $\geq$100 g/L ($\geq$10 g/dL) and is stable
     - Birth control pill (BCP)
       a. Ovral: Two tabs initially and then one tab qid until bleeding stops (5 days maximum)
       b. When bleeding stops, continue one to two tabs PO daily for a total of 21 days; then withdraw for 7 days
       c. Pre-empt next two cycles with BCP
     - Alternatively: Provera chemical curettage with 5 mg bid PO $\times$ 7 days every 40–60 days

5. Grossly irregular menses with profuse or
   prolonged bleeding (DUB)
   • Gynecologic consult
   • Possible admission for observation
   • BCP therapy as in moderate bleeding
6. Severe acute bleeding (DUB +/− coagulation
   disorder)
   • Hemoglobin <100 g/L (<10 g/dL)
   • Admit to hospital; always consult gyne-
     cology
   • IV fluid resuscitation and blood transfusion
     as necessary
   • Premarin, IV 25 mg q4h PRN, for a maxi-
     mum of 24 hr to stop bleeding
   • Simultaneously Ovral, 2 tabs initially and
     then 1 tab qid and continue as for "moder-
     ate bleeding"
   • Replace clotting factors as needed (fresh
     frozen plasma, cryoprecipitate, or platelet
     concentrations)
   • Give antinauseants with the IV Premarin
   • Hematology referral for bleeding problems

VULVOVAGINITIS

General Considerations

- The approach to the diagnosis of vulvovaginitis
  depends on whether the patient is prepubertal
  or postpubertal
- Infection with gonorrhea, herpes, Chlamydia,
  condylomata, and Trichomonas generally means
  venereal transmission. Although nonvenereal
  transmission of any of these is possible, it is
  rare, and sexual assault must always be ruled
  out. Consultation should be sought.

Prepubertal

General Considerations

- Nonbloody discharge and pruritus are common in children because of poor hygiene, proximity to anus, and susceptibility of thin vaginal mucosa to infection

Differential Diagnosis

- Noninfectious
  1. Poor hygiene
  2. Trauma or sexual assault
  3. Chemical irritant
  4. Generalized skin disease
  5. Foreign body
- Infectious
  1. Nonspecific bacterial (usually coliforms from bowel, *not* Gardnerella as in adults)
  2. Pinworms
  3. Group A beta-hemolytic streptococcus
  4. Sexually transmitted disease (STD) (gonorrhea [GC], Trichomonas)
  5. Monilia is very uncommon before hormonal changes of perimenarchal stage
  6. Prepubertal girls do not develop cervicitis

Management

- Investigations
  1. Perineal examination
  2. Culture vagina (use soft plastic eyedropper to collect specimen if needed) for GC and beta-hemolytic strep if discharge present
  3. Wet prep for Trichomonas (only if profuse purulent discharge or sexual assault possible)
  4. Referral to gynecology for vaginoscopy if
     - Bloody discharge
     - Foreign body suspected and unable to remove with gentle irrigation with normal saline with Foley catheter (one attempt)
     - Symptoms recurrent or not resolving

- Treatment
  1. The most helpful management is symptomatic
     - Hygiene education
     - Sitz baths tid
     - Avoid soaps
     - Burow's solution, 1:20–1:50, or calamine lotion, or 15% zinc oxide + 15% talc + 10% glycerine + H_2O qhs to vulva
  2. Remove foreign bodies (see above)
  3. Pinworms: give mebendazole, 100 mg PO once and repeat in 2 wk for children >2 yr
  4. Streptococcus: give Amoxil or penicillin V
  5. Gonorrhea (see p 341)

Postpubertal

- The infections in this age group are the same as those in an adult.

Differential Diagnosis

- Physiologic leukorrhea
- Noninfectious—generalized dermatitis, poor hygiene, retained tampon
- Infectious
  1. Nonspecific vaginitis ("Gardnerella vaginitis")
     - Synergistic infection caused by Gardnerella and anaerobes together
     - Gardnerella may be normal vaginal flora
     - Grey malodorous discharge with "clue cells"
  2. Moniliasis ("yeast")—cheesy white discharge, pruritic; common after antibiotics, in diabetics, pregnancy
  3. Trichomonas—green frothy foul discharge, often pruritic
  4. Gonorrhea—often asymptomatic; may be purulent cervical discharge
  5. Chlamydia—often asymptomatic; may be cervicitis; may be concomittant with GC or present after treatment of GC

6. Herpes—usually painful, vesicles ulcerate, inguinal adenopathy
7. Condylomata accuminata—nonplanar perineal warts
8. Parasites—scabies, pediculosis pubis
9. Mycoplasma—role controversial

Management

- Investigation
  1. Perineal examination
  2. Vaginal swab—KOH prep for Candida; wet prep for Trichomonas + "clue cells" (organisms on epithelial cell surface)
  3. Cervical swabs for GC and Chlamydia if sexually active
  4. Herpes—electron microscopy → viral particles; viral culture of lesion; scrapings with Wright stain → multinucleated giant cells
  5. Bimanual pelvic examination necessary in all sexually active girls
- Treatment
  1. No treatment for physiologic leukorrhea
  2. Hygiene education
  3. Treat specific infection
     - (Nonspecific vaginitis)—Metronidazole, 500 mg bid × 7 days
     - Trichomonas—Metronidazole as above or 2 g PO × one dose (adult); treat partner
     - Monilia—Monistat-3 cream intravaginally × three nights
     - Gonorrhea (see p 341)
     - Chlamydia (see p 341)
     - Herpes—symptomatic
     - Condylomata—gynecology consult for podophyllin (see p 102), freezing, or cautery
     - Scabies (see p 92)
     - Pediculosis (see p 90)

LABIAL FUSION

General Considerations and Management

- Generally an asymptomatic condition, which presents because of maternal concern about appearance of vulva
- Benign condition that resolves when endogenous estrogen is produced. It may be corrected by application of exogenous estrogen (Premarin, bid × 14 days to vulva) if
  1. Urethral meatus is obstructed
  2. Strong parental anxiety
  3. Confusion with other diagnoses (i.e., congenital absence of vagina)
- Do not force labia apart or allow surgical revision

PELVIC INFLAMMATORY DISEASE

General Considerations

- Should always be included in differential diagnosis of abdominal pain and vaginal discharge in adolescent
- Definition: upper genital tract infection often associated with pain and systemic symptoms of infection; commonly sexually transmitted
- Causative organisms—gonococcus; Chlamydia; mixed bacterial including anaerobes, particularly Bacteroides; mycoplasma (controversial)
- Remember the risks of sterility and ectopic pregnancies after pelvic inflammatory disease (PID)

Clinical Features

- Symptoms
  1. Fever and abdominal pain
  2. Vaginal discharge or bleeding
  3. Usually occurs following a period

4. Anorexia and diarrhea
5. Pain increasing with walking and intercourse
6. Both acute and subacute clinical courses
- Signs
    1. Bilateral lower quadrant tenderness or guarding
    2. Cervical excitation pain and adnexal tenderness
    3. Perihepatic pain with Fitz-Hugh–Curtis syndrome
    4. Vaginal discharge
    5. May have ↑ WBC with left shift and ↑ ESR

Differential Diagnosis

- Ectopic pregnancy with bleeding
- Appendicitis
- Ovarian cyst or torsion
- Peritonitis (primary or secondary)

Management

- Gynecology assessment essential
- Inpatient treatment
    1. Parenteral antibiotics (for at least 4 days)
        - Cefoxitin: 2 g initially and then 2 g q6h
        - Alternatives: erythromycin, tetracycline, or penicillin
        - If tetracycline is not given as the parenteral antibiotic, it should be given concurrently PO (because of risk of Chlamydia)
    2. Oral therapy (to follow)
        - Doxycycline, 100 mg bid × 10–14 days
        - Metronidazole, 1 g bid × 10–14 days

BIRTH CONTROL METHODS

General Considerations

- There are many problems with contraception in the adolescent patient
- 90% or more of all adolescents seeking birth control information are sexually active
- Often adolescents are poorly compliant with any method prescribed
- Often they are unlikely to properly use or regularly employ mechanical and barrier methods
- IUDs are not recommended in nulliparous women but may be the method of choice in individual patients
- Tables 1 through 4 deal with contraceptives

TABLE 13–1 Methods of Birth Control Available and Efficacy with Full Compliance

Method	Efficacy* per 100 ♀ years
Oral contraceptives	98 +
Intrauterine devices	96–98
Diaphragm and spermicide[†]	82–85
Condom and spermicide[†]	85–95
Condom alone[†]	85–95
Spermicide alone[†]	70–75
Rhythm[†]	65–70
Withdrawal[†]	<65–70
Postcoital interception (Ovral, 2 tabs q12h × 2 doses)	98
Abstinence[†]	100

* Efficacy may be less in adolescents

† NB: These methods are notoriously poorly used in adolescents. From Special Advisory Committee on Reproductive Physiology to the Health Protection Branch, Health and Welfare, Canada. Report on oral contraceptives, 1985:12–13.

TABLE 13–2 Oral Contraceptives Available in Canada[1]

Product	Manufacturer	Estrogen	μg/Tablet	Progestogen	μg/Tablet
20, 30, & 35 μg Estrogen				(days in parentheses for biphasics & triphasics)	
Minestrin 1/20	Parke-Davis	Ethinyl Estradiol	20	Norethindrone Acetate	1000
Min-Ovral	Wyeth	Ethinyl Estradiol	30	d-Norgestrel[2]	150
Loestrin 1.5/30	Parke-Davis	Ethinyl Estradiol	30	Norethindrone Acetate	1500
Demulen 30	Searle	Ethinyl Estradiol	30	Ethynodiol Diacetate	2000
Ortho 1/35	Ortho	Ethinyl Estradiol	35	Norethindrone	1000
Ortho 0.5/35	Ortho	Ethinyl Estradiol	35	Norethindrone	500
Brevicon 0.5/35	Syntex	Ethinyl Estradiol	35	Norethindrone	500
Brevicon 1/35	Syntex	Ethinyl Estradiol	35	Norethindrone	1000
Ortho 10/11[3,5]	Ortho	Ethinyl Estradiol	35 (21)	Norethindrone	500 (10) 1000 (11)
Ortho 7/7/7[4,5]	Ortho	Ethinyl Estradiol	35 (21)	Norethindrone	500 (7) 750 (7) 1000 (7)

Triphasil[4,5]	Wyeth	Ethinyl Estradiol	30 (6) 40 (5) 30 (10)	d-Norgestrel[2]	50 (6) 75 (5) 125 (10)

50 μg Estrogen—For conception control only when lower dosage estrogen formulations prove to be unsatisfactory.[6]

Ovral	Wyeth	Ethinyl Estradiol	50	d-Norgestrel[2]	250
Norlestrin 1/50	Parke-Davis	Ethinyl Estradiol	50	Norethindrone Acetate	1000
Norlestrin 2.5/50	Parke-Davis	Ethinyl Estradiol	50	Norethindrone Acetate	2500
Demulen 50	Searle	Ethinyl Estradiol	50	Ethynodiol Diacetate	1000
Ortho-Novum 1/50	Ortho	Mestranol	50	Norethindrone	1000
Norinyl 1/50	Syntex	Mestranol	50	Norethindrone	1000

1. Most of the estrogen-progestogen combination products listed in this table are also available with inert tablets that permit uninterrupted 28-day cycles of therapy.
2. Supplied as the dl--racemate in double the amount shown.
3. Biphasic product.
4. Triphasic product.
5. The number of days each dosage of estrogen and progestogen is to be taken is shown in brackets in the dosage columns.
6. Prolonged use of products with ≥50 μg of estrogen should only be used under the supervision of a gynecologist.

Modified from Special Advisory Committee on Reproductive Physiology to the Health Protection Branch, Health and Welfare, Canada. Report on oral contraceptives, 1985:16–17.

TABLE 13–3 Contraindications to Birth Control Pill Use

Absolute contraindications
  Thromboembolic disorders
  Cerebrovascular accident
  Coronary artery disease
  Hepatic adenoma
  Breast or gynecologic estrogen dependent
    malignant disease
  Pregnancy
  Undiagnosed vaginal bleeding

Relative contraindications
  Hypertension
  Diabetes mellitus
  Acute phase mononucleosis
  Sickle cell disease
  Impaired liver function within last year
  Cardiac or renal disease
  Depression
  Epilepsy (pill may not be as effective if patient is
    taking anticonvulsants concurrently)
  Lipid disorders
  Migraine
  Smoking

TABLE 13–4 Side Effects of Oral Contraceptives

Problems related to estrogen excess
  Nausea
  Vomiting
  Diarrhea
  Edema
  Chloasma
  Hypertension
  Breast tenderness

Problems related to progesterone excess
  Acne
  Hirsutism
  Alopecia
  Depression
  Increased appetite
  Amenorrhea

Use of BCP

- Workup prior to birth control pills
  1. Complete history including menstrual and sexual history and physical with blood pressure and pelvic examination if sexually active
  2. Smoking history
  3. Pap smear and cultures for GC and Chlamydia
  4. Pregnancy test
  5. Urinalysis
  6. Blood smear
  7. VDRL and rubella titer
- NB: In the healthy adolescent the risks to health from pregnancy outweigh those of the low dose birth control pills
- Begin with low dose estrogen pill, i.e., <50 μg/pill (e.g., Ortho 1/35, Min-Ovral)
- Follow up more frequently than adults for problems and compliance

SEXUAL ASSAULT

General Considerations

- If the assault occurred within 24 hr, a complete examination should be done immediately; otherwise examination can wait and be done at the physician's and patient's convenience
- Contact Children's Aid Society and the police (if patient <16 yr)

Management

- Obtain a brief history from the parents or guardians and then a full history from the patient. Record specific data and use the patient's own words.
- Obtain written consent prior to the examination from patient or guardian

- Use the sexual assault kit to collect appropriate specimens, and label them carefully. Follow enclosed guidelines (i.e., label slides with a diamond pencil; put clothing into paper bags), and give the evidence directly to the police officer. Have a signed receipt for the evidence.
- Perform a full physical and record all pertinent data carefully
  1. Illustrate with diagrams
  2. Obtain medical photographs whenever possible
- Assess and record the patient's emotional state
- Examine the following specimens immediately
  a. Urine for Hgb, RBCs, and sperm
  b. Wet mount of vaginal swab for motile sperm
- Take appropriate samples for STDs
  1. GC swabs—endocervix, vaginal, urethral, rectal, and oral
  2. Chlamydia—endocervix, oral, rectal
  3. VDRL and follow-up in 8 wk with repeat VDRL
- Consult gynecology if a surgical problem is found—e.g., cervical or vaginal tear
- Prevent pregnancy ("morning-after" pill)
  1. Treatment for all peri- and postmenarchal women regardless of the timing in the cycle
  2. Treatment within 72 hr after coitus
  3. Ovral, two tabs PO q12h $\times$ 2 doses
  4. NB: serum β-HCG is positive at 29 days post DLNMP
- Give STD prophylaxis: ampicillin or amoxicillin, 50 mg/kg (max 3.5 g for ampicillin; 3.0 g for amoxicillin), and probenecid, 25 mg/kg (max 1.0 g) $\times$ 1 dose PO (if not allergic to penicillin) and treat for Chlamydia as well (see p 341)
- Arrange good follow-up
  1. Psychological-emotional counseling
  2. Medical—STD follow-up

- Refer to a rape crisis center if desired by patient or family
- Consider hepatitis B prophylaxis (see p 302)

Suggested Reading

1. Cowell CA, ed. Pediatric and adolescent gynecology. Pediatr Clin North Am 1981; 28(2).
2. Emans SJ, Goldstein PG. Pediatric and adolescent gynecology. 2nd ed. Boston: Little, Brown, 1981.

14 HEMATOLOGY AND ONCOLOGY

HEMATOLOGY

Anemia

General Considerations

- Definition: hemoglobin or hematocrit less than the age appropriate values (see laboratory values section, p 731)
- Certain conditions decrease hemoglobin determination thereby leading to an incorrect diagnosis of anemia (e.g., volume overload), while others cause higher hematocrit, causing a diagnosis of anemia to be missed (e.g., dehydration, heel prick in newborns)

Clinical Features

- In history, inquire about diet (e.g., vegetarianism, milk and meat intake), drugs, bleeding episodes, foreign travel (e.g., parasitic infestations), family history, pica, neonatal history (e.g., exchange transfusions), diarrhea, weight loss, jaundice
- On examination carefully assess following systems:
  1. Mucocutaneous—pallor, jaundice, petechiae
  2. Cardiovascular—tachycardia, cardiac murmur, cardiac failure
  3. Reticuloendothelial—lymphadenopathy, hepatosplenomegaly
  4. Central nervous system—irritability, lethargy, poor concentration, retinal hemorrhage

5. Gastrointestinal—bleeding mucous membranes, smooth tongue, cheilosis, blood in stools (melena, hematochezia)

Management

- Basic investigations (Table 14–1)
  1. Hb, Hct, RBC number, MCV
  2. Reticulocyte count
  3. Blood smear.
     N.B. Examination of blood smear is most important investigation.
  4. WBC, differential, platelet count (Fig. 14–1)
- Other investigations as indicated
  1. Iron studies—Fe, TIBC, ferritin
  2. HB electrophoresis
  3. Haptoglobin
  4. Bilirubin T and D
  5. Antibody studies—Coombs' test, cold agglutinins, and Donath-Landsteiner test
  6. Heinz body prep.
  7. Red cell enzymes (e.g., G6PD, pyruvate kinase)
  8. Unstable Hb
  9. Hb H prep.
  10. Bone marrow aspiration and biopsy
  11. Osmotic fragility
  12. Vitamin studies: vitamin B_{12}, folate on serum and whole blood
     * N.B. If patient *must* be transfused before diagnosis is made, obtain blood for Hb electrophoresis, Hb H prep., unstable Hb, Heinz body prep., red cell enzymes, vitamin B_{12} and folate

TABLE 14–1 Hematologic Parameters in Various Types of Anemia

Test	Aplastic Anemia	Thalassemia Major	Thalassemia Minor	Iron Deficiency	Anemia of Chronic Disease
Hemoglobin	↓*	↓	↓	↓	↓
MCV	↑*	↓	↓	↓	N or ↓
MCHC	N*	↓	↓	↓	N
Iron	N	↑	N or ↑	↓	N or ↓
TIBC	N	↓	N	↑	↓
Ferritin	N	↑	N or ↑	↓	↑
Transferrin	N	↓	N	↑	↓
Bone marrow iron store	N	↑	↑	Absent	N or ↑
Reticulocyte count	↓	N	N	↓	N

* N, normal. ↑, increased. ↓, decreased.

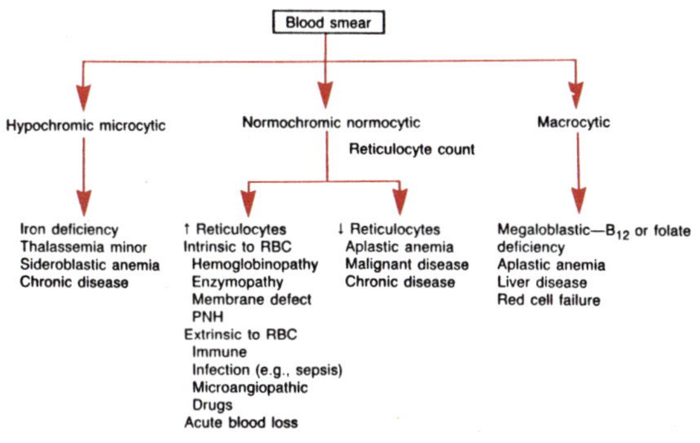

Figure 14–1 Morphologic approach to anemia.

Iron Deficiency Anemia

General Considerations

- Commonest cause of anemia in children
- Commonest nutritional deficiency in children
- Iron depletion from bone marrow before development of anemia
- Causes are age dependent
  1. <6 mo—perinatal blood loss, prematurity
  2. 6–24 mo—nutritional
  3. >24 mo—blood loss, especially from GI tract

Pathogenesis of Nutritional Iron Deficiency

- Decreased total body iron at birth
- Prematurity
- Rapidly expanding blood volume during first yr
- Decreased iron intake, excessive milk drinking, blood loss

- Cow's milk sensitivity
- Because a premature starts with decreased total body iron and the blood volume expands extremely rapidly in the first few months, he becomes iron deficient earlier (e.g., 2–4 mo) than a full term infant
- All premature infants should therefore receive prophylactic iron supplementation starting at age 2 mo or before

Investigations

- Serum Fe ↓, TIBC ↑, ferritin ↓
- Free erythrocyte protoporphyrin ↑
- Marrow iron stores ↓ (usually unnecessary)
- To differentiate thalassemia minor, family studies and Hb electrophoresis can be done. (Note: Hb electrophoresis will be normal in α-thal. minor.)

Treatment

- Treat underlying cause, e.g., diet, source of blood loss
- 6 mg elemental iron/kg/day divided in 3 doses on empty stomach ½ hr before meals (ferrous sulfate, ferrous fumarate, ferrous glutamate are equivalent)
- Expect reticulocyte response at 7–10 days
- After Hb becomes normal, treat for 2–3 mo to replenish iron stores
- Therapeutic trial of iron: In an infant 6–24 mo old with hypochromic microcytic anemia, a therapeutic trial of iron can be given for 4 wk without further investigation. If the anemia responds, continue iron therapy. If the anemia fails to respond, further investigation is required.

Thalassemia Syndromes

General Considerations

- Caused by decreased or absent globin chain synthesis
- Autosomal recessive inheritance
- Most important are α- and β-thalassemias
  1. α-Thalassemia
     - Decreased production of α-chains
     - Relative excess of β-chains
     - Degree of anemia depends on number of deleted α-chain genes
     - α-Thalassemia trait
       a. Asymptomatic
       b. Peripheral smear: hypochromic microcytic red cells
       c. Hb H prep. positive
       d. *No* treatment required
  2. β-Thalassemia
     - Decreased production of β-chains
     - Relative excess of α-chains
     - Autosomal recessive
     - Geographic distribution: Mediterranean region, Africa, Middle East, Pakistan, India, China
     - β-Thalassemia trait
       a. Heterozygous state
       b. Usually asymptomatic
         - Peripheral smear $\rightarrow$ microcytic hypochromic red cells
         - Electrophoresis $\rightarrow$ $\uparrow$ HbA_2
         - No therapy required
  3. β-Thalassemia major
     - Homozygous state
     - Usually diagnosed in first yr of life: pallor, fatigue, failure to thrive, hepatosplenomegaly

- Management (of β-Thal. Major):
  1. Investigations (Table 14–1)
     - CBC (↓ Hb, severe hypochromia, microcytosis, bizarre aniso- and poikilocytosis)
     - Hb electrophoresis → ↓ or absent HbA, ↑ HbF
  2. Treatment
     - Mainstay is *blood transfusion*, either high transfusion regimen (maintain Hb >100 g/L) or supertransfusion (Hb >120 g/L)
     - Chelation therapy—deferoxamine (desferrioxamine) infused subcutaneously overnight (12 hr)
     - Vitamin C—enhances chelation, but may cause cardiac toxicity; maximum daily dosage 100 mg
     - Splenectomy when transfusion requirements excessive

Hemolytic Anemia

General Considerations

- Anemia, unconjugated hyperbilirubinemia, reticulocytosis, and suggestive red cell changes in smear indicate hemolysis
- Degree of anemia depends on balance between hemolysis and marrow compensation (manifested by reticulocytosis)

Management

- Investigations
  1. See Figure 14–2
- Treatment
  1. Depends on cause

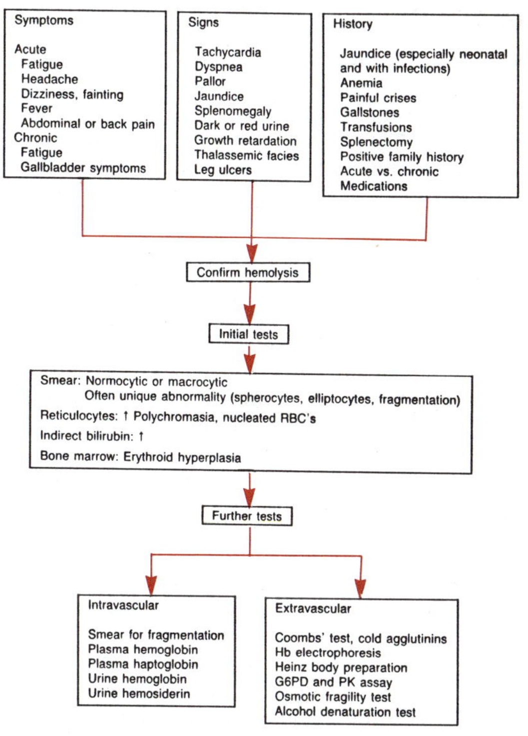

Figure 14–2 Diagnostic approach to hemolytic anemias.

Sickle Cell Disease

General Considerations

- Those disorders in which one or both of the major hemoglobins are sickle hemoglobin. These include sickle cell trait (SA), sickle cell anemia (SS), sickle-C disease (SC), sickle-beta° thalassemia ($S\beta°$), and sickle-beta$^+$ thalassemia ($S\beta^+$).

Management

- Diagnosis: see Tables 14–2, 14–3, 14–4
- Therapy
  1. Vaso-occlusive crises
     - Pulmonary crisis—"acute chest syndrome"
       a. Difficult to distinguish from pulmonary infection; often appears during painful crises; may be severe and fatal
       b. See Table 14–5
       c. Treatment consists of supplemental oxygen, antibiotic coverage, transfusion with packed RBCs
     - Musculoskeletal (painful bony) crises
       a. Difficult to distinguish from osteomyelitis
       b. Appears as dactylitis (hand-foot syndrome) in infants between 3–20 mo; rare after 48 mo
       c. In older children, common sites include humerus, tibia, femur; may present as acute monoarticular or polyarticular arthritis
       d. See Table 14–6

TABLE 14–2　Diagnosis of the Sickling Disorders

	Sickle		Erythrocyte Shape			Major Hemoglobins				
	Prep.	Anemia	Sickle	Target	Micro	S	A	F	C	A_2
SA	+	0	0	0	0	30–40%	60%	<2%	0	2–4%
SS	+	+ + +	+ + +	+	0	80–90%	0	2–20%	0	2–4%
SC	+	+	+	+ + +	±	50%	0	2%	<50%	*
SB⁺thal.	+	+	±	+ + +	+	55–75%	10–30%	1–13%	0	3–6%
SB°thal.	+	+ +	+	+ + +	+ +	80–95%	0	1–15%	0	3–6%

* Not available because of difficulty in determining HbA_2 in presence of HbC.

TABLE 14–3 Clinical Features of Sickle Cell Disorders

	SA (Trait)	SS	SC	$S\beta + Thal.$	$S\beta°Thal.$
Chronic anemia	0	+ + +	+	+	+ +
Impaired growth and development	0	+ + +	0	±	±
Painful ("vaso-occlusive") Crises	0	+ + +	+ +	+	+ +
Pulmonary					
Musculoskeletal					
Abdominal					
Neurologic—stroke					
Priapism					
Anemic crises	0	+ + +	+ + +	+	+ +
Splenic sequestration					
Aplastic					
Infections	0	+ + +	+ + +	+	+ +
Chronic organ damage					
Eye—proliferative retinopathy	0	+ +	+ + +	+	+ +
MSK—aseptic necrosis, femoral head	0	+ +	+ + +	+	+ +
Renal—medullary infarction with hematuria	+	+ +	+ + +	+	+ +
Tubular dysfunction with hyposthenuria	+	+ +	+ +	+	+ +
Hepatobiliary system—cholelithiasis	0	+ +	+	+	+ +

TABLE 14–4   Approximate Hematologic Values in Sickle Cell Disease (Mean ± SD)

	Hb (g/L)	HbF (%)	HbA$_2$ (%)	Retics ($\times 10^9$/L)	MCV (f1)
SS disease					
Birth	210 ± 30	75 ± 10	<2.0	150–450	103 ± 8
6 mo	87 ± 15	24 ± 8	<2.0	100–450	75 ± 7
1 yr	79 ± 15	16 ± 6	<2.0	100–500	77 ± 9
3 yr	80 ± 14	11 ± 6	<2.5	150–550	82 ± 9
5 yr	79 ± 12	8 ± 6	<3.0	150–550	85 ± 7
Adult	78 ± 12	6 ± 4	<3.5	150–550	94 ± 10
SC disease					
Birth	210 ± 30	75 ± 10	*	150–450	105 ± 7
6 mo	90 ± 10	12 ± 7	–	<200	67 ± 8
1 yr	90 ± 10	7 ± 4	–	<200	66 ± 8
3 yr	100 ± 10	3 ± 1	–	<200	70 ± 8
5 yr	105 ± 10	<2	–	<200	74 ± 8
Adult	115 ± 15	<2	–	<200	74 ± 8

TABLE 14–4 (Continued)

S thalassemia (Sβ^+ contains HbA 18–30%; S$\beta°$ contains no HbA)					
Birth	210±30	75±10	<2.0	150–450	103±6
1 yr: β^+	100±20	14±5	3.5±1.0	100–200	67±8
$\beta°$	85±15		3.8±1.0	150–400	65±8
3 yr: β^+	105±10	11±4	4.0±1.0	100–200	67±8
$\beta°$	90±10		4.0±1.0	150–400	65±8
5 yr: β^+	105±10	9±4	4.2±1.0	100–200	67±8
$\beta°$	90±10		4.5±1.0	150–400	65±8
Adult: β^+	105±15	5±5	4.8±1.0	100–200	67±8
$\beta°$	85±15		5.0±1.0	150–400	65±8

* Information not available because of difficulty in determining HbA$_2$ in the presence of HbC.

TABLE 14–5 Differentiation Between Pneumonia and Pulmonary Infarction

Common features

Chest pain
Cough
Fever
CXR infiltrates
Leukocytosis
Hypoxemia
Pleural effusion

Features favoring pneumonia

Age $\leq$ 5 yr
Shaking chills
Upper lobe disease
Bands >1000 cells/mm^3
Sputum Gram stain ⎫
Cultures ⎬ Positive
Cold agglutinins ⎭

Features favoring infarction

Associated painful bone crisis
Clear radiograph at onset
Lower lobe disease

Modified from Platt OS, Nathan DG. Sickle cell disease. In: Nathan DG, Oski FA, eds. Hematology of infancy and childhood. 2nd ed. Philadelphia: W.B. Saunders, 1981:703.

TABLE 14–6   Differentiation Between Bone Infarction and Osteomyelitis

Common features

Local pain, tenderness, swelling, and erythema
Fever
Leukocytosis

Features favoring infarction

Multiple sites
Patient description of "crisis"
History of predisposing factor
Negative cultures
Response without antibiotics

Features favoring osteomyelitis

Single site
Bands >1000 cells/mm^3
Positive cultures

Modified from Platt OS, Nathan DG. Sickle cell disease. In: Nathan DG, Oski FA, eds. Hematology of infancy and childhood. 2nd ed. Philadelphia: W.B. Saunders, 1981:702.

- Abdominal crisis
  a. Must be differentiated from acute surgical abdomen
  b. Common features include abdominal pain and classic rebound tenderness; other sites of pain, patient's previous experience, and presence of bowel sounds favor crisis
  c. Two types of crises: transient intrahepatic obstruction (10%)—self-limited, mild LFT abnormalities; and the rarer intrahepatic cholestasis—bilirubin grossly elevated, fulminant hepatic failure
  d. High incidence of cholelithiasis (30% of children older than 10 yr)
  e. Treatment consists of supportive care ± transfusion, surgical consultation (elective cholecystectomy for recurrent episodes of pain and gallstones)

- Central nervous system
  a. Two-thirds of strokes occur in children; mean age of 8 yr; 5% of sicklers sustain a cerebral infarction and two-thirds will have a second
  b. Predisposing factors—previous bacterial meningitis, acute precipitating events (e.g., shock, severe anemia, hypoxia)
  c. Treatment consists of exchange transfusion, and for long-term management—hypertransfusion to maintain hemoglobin >100 g/L
- Priapism
  a. Occurs in 40% of SS male patients; 25% develop impotence, particularly after a severe prolonged episode
  b. Treatment consists of early surgical consultation, sedation, analgesia, fluids, possibly exchange transfusion

- General treatment of painful crisis
  1. First 24 hr
     - Demerol 1.0–1.5 mg/kg IV q2-4h or morphine on a regular basis
     - Acetaminophen PO q6h for additive effect
     - Fluids at 1.5 × maintenance
     - Reassess frequently
  2. Subsequently
     - Taper narcotics (10–20% decrements in dose, maintain frequency); change to oral medication when dose is decreased by 50%; adjust oral dose but avoid returning to parenteral administration
     - Early discharge
     - Small quantities of oral narcotic plus an alternative analgesic for use at home
- Anemic crises
  1. Aplastic anemia
     - Usually associated with acute infection (parvovirus)
     - Rapid and pronounced fall in hemoglobin with a reduced reticulocyte count

- Treatment consists of supportive care and transfusion
  2. Acute splenic sequestration
     - Rapid fall in hemoglobin, elevation of reticulocyte count, and enlarging spleen; may occur very rapidly → shock
     - Occurs in infants and young children
     - Treatment consists of urgent transfusion, and supportive care; predictive of subsequent episodes; consider splenectomy
- Infections
  1. Bacterial sepsis (*S. pneumoniae*, *H. influenzae*) is a leading cause of death in SS patients (secondary to RES blockade and impaired splenic function as a result of auto-infarction of spleen)
  2. May follow a rapidly fulminant course with shock and death within a few hours
  3. Other pathogens include *E. coli*, *Salmonella*, *Shigella*, and *Mycoplasma*
  4. Prevention
     - Pneumococcal vaccination (initially at 2 yr and give booster 5 yr later)
     - *H. influenzae* vaccine—give at 2 yr of age
     - Influenza vaccination—for those >6 mo old, given each fall
     - Antibiotic prophylaxis
       <35 mo—Pen-VK 125 mg PO bid
       >35 mo—Pen-VK 250 mg PO bid
  5. Acute management (compliance with prophylaxis and response to vaccination cannot be assumed)
     - Temp. <38.5° C orally: assess, culture. If not admitted, reassess within 24 hr
     - Temp. >38.5° C orally: culture, admit, and cover with IV Cefuroxime until culture results available

- Surgery
    1. In black children a sickle cell prep., and if positive a hemoglobin electrophoresis, should be done on an elective basis prior to any surgery
    2. SA disease (trait): require no specific preparation
    3. SS, SC, S thal.: routine quantitation of HbS unnecessary; transfuse to a Hb > 100 g/L for routine or emergency surgery or radiologic procedures using contrast materials. Under high risk conditions (cardiovascular, neurosurgical, tourniquets in orthopaedic procedures, eye surgery patients with previous stroke), it is appropriate to reduce HbS to <30% preoperatively.
    4. Unknown status: elective procedures should be postponed. Emergency procedures may be done following consultation with a hematologist.

Thrombocytopenia

General Considerations

- Definition: platelet count <150,000
- Inquire about drug history, recent viral illness, skin rashes, bruises, bleeding episodes, family history
- Look for petechiae, bruising, mucous membrane bleeding, jaundice, hepatosplenomegaly, skeletal abnormalities (e.g., TAR syndrome, cardiac murmur)

Management

- Investigations
    1. Sepsis work-up (exclude LP if platelet count <50,000), to be considered
    2. Autoimmune work-up
    3. Platelet antibody studies (especially in newborn)

4. Hb, platelet count, white cell count, and differential
5. Peripheral blood smear
6. Coagulation screen (bleeding time must not be done)
7. Bone marrow examination

Idiopathic Thrombocytopenia Purpura (ITP), Acute

General Considerations and Clinical Features

- Usually a history of preceding viral illness followed by petechiae, bruising, and mucous membrane bleeding
- Physical examination—well looking child with petechiae and bruising

Management

- Investigations
  1. CBC, platelet count, peripheral smear
  2. Coombs' test
  3. Platelet antibody
  4. Rheumatoid factor
  5. ANF (antinuclear factor)
  6. Immunoglobulin electrophoresis
  7. Bone marrow examination
- Treatment
  1. High dose steroids—4 mg/kg/day prednisone with rapid taper
  2. High dose IV gamma globulin—1 gm/kg/day × 2 doses
  3. Splenectomy (see below)
  4. In cases of *life-threatening* bleeding, IV gamma globulin or emergency splenectomy is the treatment of choice
  5. May observe if platelet count >20,000

Neonatal Thrombocytopenia

General Considerations

- If maternal history of ITP, SLE, or previously affected infant
  1. Monitor maternal platelet count during pregnancy
  2. At time of delivery, measure fetal platelet count by fetal scalp sampling
  3. If fetal platelet count >50,000, proceed to deliver normally, but if <50,000, perform cesarean section
- Measure infant and maternal PL^{A1} antigen and antibody

Management

- Investigations
  1. Measure platelet count in cord blood at birth
  2. If normal, monitor for 1 mo as it may fall
- Treatment
  1. Platelet count normal—no therapy
  2. Maternal PL^{A1} negative—infuse maternal platelets into baby if thrombocytopenic. If mother's platelets not available, use random donor.
  3. Mother PL^{A1} positive, give IV gamma globulin or use steroids. (Platelet infusion may be effective.)

Coagulation Disorders

General Considerations

- Adequate hemostasis depends on vascular integrity, normally functioning platelets, coagulation factors, and clot stability
- Disorders are either inherited (e.g., deficiencies of factors VIII, IX, vWF) or acquired (DIC, vitamin K deficiency, liver disease, and others). In the inherited disorders the key to diagnosis is a

careful patient and family history of a bleeding tendency. In the acquired disorders the nature of the problem and the presence or absence of clinical bleeding are most important.

- See Figure 14–3

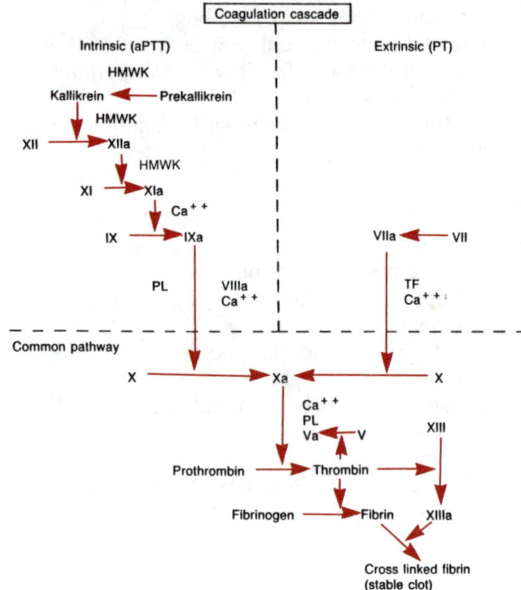

Figure 14–3 Coagulation cascade. Defects in either intrinsic or extrinsic pathways lead to prolongation of indicated tests. Defects in common pathway prolong both tests. Deficiency of XIII does not prolong either aPTT or PT. TT measures conversion of fibrinogen to fibrin. HMWK, high molecular weight kininogen. PL, phospholipid. TF, tissue factor.

Management

- Investigations: see Table 14–7, 14–8, 14–9
- Treatment
  1. Factor VIII deficiency (classic hemophilia or hemophilia A)
     - Supportive measures (physiotherapy, patient education, home care programs)
     - Early treatment of bleeds with either cryoprecipitate or factor VIII concentrates (1 U/kg increases VIIIc activity by 2%, with a half-life of 8–12 hr)
     - See Table 14–10

TABLE 14–7 Abbreviations in Use for Coagulation Disorders

aPTT	Activated thromboplastin time
PT	Prothrombin time
BT	Bleeding time
TT	Thrombin time
vWD	von Willebrand's disease
VIII:C	Factor VIII coagulant activity
vWf	von Willebrand factor (sometimes designated VIII related antigen)
VIIIR:RCo	Factor VIII related ristocetin cofactor
FDP	Fibrin degradation product

TABLE 14–8 Investigation of Inherited Coagulation Disorders

Inherited Deficiency	VIII	vWD*	IX
Type of bleeding	Muscle, joint	Skin bruising, mucosal (e.g., epistaxis, menorrhagia)	Muscle, joint
Inheritance	Sex linked	Autosomal (dominant and recessive)	Sex linked
Lab:			
PT	N	N	N
PTT	I	N or I	I
BT	N	I	N
IX	N	N	D
VIII:C	D	D	N
vWf	N	D	N
VIIIR:RCo	N	D	N

* Subtypes of vWD can be differentiated by multimer analysis and ristocetin induced platelet aggregation (RIPA). N, I, D, = normal, increased, decreased.

TABLE 14–9   Investigation of Acquired Coagulation Disorders

Acquired Disorder	DIC		Liver Dysfunction	Vitamin K Deficiency
History	Shock	Sepsis	Jaundice	Diet, diarrhea, anti-biotics, malabsorption, obstructive jaundice
Bleeding	Generalized*		Generalized	Generalized
Lab:				
PT	I	I	I	I
PTT	I	I	N or I	I
Platelets	N or D	D	N or D	N
Fibrinogen	D	N or D	N or D	N
FDP	I	N or I	N or I	N
Factors				
V	D	N or D	D	N
VII	N	N	D	D
VIII	D	N or D	I	N
IX	N or D	N or D	D	D
X	D	N or D	D	D

* Particularly in the newborn infant, clinical bleeding is much more severe in the infant with DIC secondary to shock. N, I, D = normal, increased, decreased.

TABLE 14–10   Initial Doses of Factor Replacement in Hemophilia

Indication for Replacement	Amount of VIII Required	Amount of IX Required
Hemarthrosis	15–20 U/kg once daily	15 U/kg once daily
Mucous membrane*	40 U/kg once	30 U/kg once
Hematuria[†]	40 U/kg daily or bid × 3–5 days	40 U/kg daily × 3–5 days
Major bleeding (CNS, surgery, retroperitoneal)	40 U/kg q12h as long as indicated	40 U/kg q12h as long as indicated

* Epsilon aminocaproic acid 100 mg/kg q6h × 3–5 days may also be of value.
[†] Prednisone 2 mg/kg/day (maximum 60 mg) may also be considered.

2. von Willebrand disease (vWD)
   - Minor bleeding may require only suppor-
     tive measures
   - 1-Desamino-8-D-arginine-vasopressin
     (DDAVP 0.1–0.3 μg/kg intravenously in
     normal saline at a concentration of
     0.5 μg/ml to a maximum of 24 μg over 20
     min) may be used in selected cases—
     should not be used in type IIb vWD, as
     may cause thrombocytopenia
   - Replace with cryoprecipitate (20–40 U/kg
     daily; 1 bag of cryoprecipitate contains
     80–100 U of factor VIII activity), as factor
     VIII concentrate of no value in this disorder
3. Factor IX deficiency (Christmas disease or
   hemophilia B)
   - Supportive measures as per factor VIII defi-
     ciency
   - Bleeds can be treated with factor IX con-
     centrates (1 U/kg increases activity by
     0.8–1.2%) with a half-life of 18–24 hr—
     usual dose is 15–40 U/kg daily (see Table
     14–10)

4. Disseminated intravascular coagulation (DIC)
   - Supportive care; treat underlying cause
   - Blood product support, e.g., packed RBC's
     and platelets as needed, fresh frozen
     plasma 10 ml/kg every 8 hr, and
     cryoprecipitate (approx. 1 bag/5 kg) for
     hypofibrinogenemia
5. Hepatic failure
   - Supportive care; treatment of underlying
     liver disease
   - Blood product support as needed (see DIC
     for guidelines)
   - Vitamin K_1 1 mg subcutaneously or by
     slow intravenous injection should also be
     given

6. Vitamin K deficiency
   - Look for possible absorptive problem
   - Treat with vitamin K_1 1 mg subcutaneously or slow intravenous administration
   - For oral supplementation, vitamin K_3 is better absorbed
   - To reverse therapeutic anticoagulation, larger doses of vitamin K_1 may be required (2.5–5 mg)
   - For urgent reversal, FFP 10 ml/kg as well as vitamin K_1 should be used

Transfusion Reactions

General Considerations

- There are inherent risks associated with transfusion of blood and blood products. Thus it is important to exercise sound clinical judgment in ensuring that the expected benefits of the transfusion outweigh the risks.
- Clinical manifestations of a transfusion reaction may occur immediately or several days to months after the transfusion
- Immediate reactions include
   1. Fever
   2. Allergic manifestations—urticaria, anaphylaxis
   3. Bacteremia from infected blood
   4. Hemolysis
   5. Hemorrhagic state
   6. Circulatory overload
- Delayed reactions include
   1. Hemolysis
   2. Sensitization to red cell antigens
   3. Infectious diseases, e.g., CMV, hepatitis, AIDS
- See Table 14–11, 14–12

TABLE 14–11   Recipient-Donor Blood Group Compatibility

Recipient's Blood Group	Compatible Donor Red Cells	Compatible Donor Plasma
O	O	O,A,B,AB
A	A,O	A,AB
B	B,O	B,AB
AB	A,B,AB,O	AB

Management of Transfusion Reaction

- Fever due to leukocyte antibodies, especially in multitransfused patients, is the commonest adverse reaction. This is treated by acetaminophen/antihistamines. Depending on the severity of the reaction, it may be possible to continue the transfusion. Such reactions can be prevented by the administration of leukocyte poor red cells in patients requiring red cell transfusions.
- The hemolytic transfusion reaction due to incompatible blood is much less common, but when it occurs it is a medical emergency because of the possible complications of renal failure and acute disseminated intravascular coagulation. Symptoms include fever, dyspnea, pain in chest, flank, and site of infusion, shock, and bleeding. The following measures must be instituted as soon as a hemolytic transfusion reaction is suspected:
  1. Discontinue the transfusion, but keep the vein open with intravenous fluids using a new administration set

TABLE 14–12 Clinical Use of Blood Products

Blood Component	Indications for Use	Dose
Platelet concentrate (30–50 ml/unit)	Bleeding due to thrombocytopenia	1 unit platelets/5 kg ↑ platelet count by 50,000#100,000
Fresh frozen plasma (200–250 ml/unit)	Treatment of coagulation disorders	10 ml/kg
Stored plasma (200–250 ml/unit)	Expansion of blood volume and replacement of all coagulation factors except V and VII	5–10 ml/kg
Cryoprecipitate (an average of 80 units of factor VIII activity per 5–10 ml bag)	Hemophilia A, von Willebrand's disease, and fibrinogen deficiency	1 bag/10 kg (1 U/kg ↑ factor VIII activity in plasma by ~ 2%)
Pooled factor VIII concentrate (~ 300 units/10–30 ml [varies from ~ 250–1000 units])	Hemophilia A	10–40 units/kg; t½ 8–12 hr; (1 U/kg ↑ activity by 2%)
Factor IX complex	Hemophilia B	15–40 units/kg; t½ 18–24 hr; (1 U/kg ↑ activity by 0.8–1.2%)
Packed RBC's (250–300 ml/unit)	Severe anemia	10 ml/kg ↑ Hb by 20–30 g/L

2. Monitor blood pressure and urine output
3. If in shock, treat appropriately (see emergency section, p 659)
4. Notify and return to the blood bank the offending blood product, together with a 5 ml sample of the patient's blood carefully taken without anticoagulant and the first post-transfusion urine specimen

ONCOLOGY

Side Effects of Common Chemotherapy Agents

- See Table 14-13

TABLE 14–13   Side Effects of Some Common Chemotherapy Agents*

Drug	Nausea and Vomiting	Myelosuppression	Alopecia	Mucositis	Neuropathy	Pulmonary	Cardiac	Renal	Tissue Necrosis	Skin	Liver	Diarrhea	Other
Actinomycin D	+ +	+ +	+ +	+ +					+ +	+ +		+ +	Radiation reaction, abdo. pain
Adriamycin	+ +	+ +	+ +	+			+ +	±	+ +	+			Radiation react, red urine, fever, pigmentation
BCNU	+ +	+ +[1]	+	±		+ +		±	+	+	+		Pigmentation, dizziness, ataxia
Bleomycin	+	±	+	+ +		+ +		+		+ +			Fever, hypotension, systemic sclerosis
Busulphan	+	+ +[1]				+ +							Pigmentation, cataracts, gynecomastia
CCNU/methyl CCNU	+ +	+ +[1]	±	±		+		+			+		CNS dysfunction
Chlorambucil	+	+ +[1]				±					±		
Cyclophosphamide	+ +	+ +	+ +	+			±						Hemorrhagic cystitis, H$_2$O retention
Cytosine arabinoside	+ +	+ +	+	+						+	±	+	Fever
Daunorubicin	+ +	+ +	+ +	+			+ +			+			Fever
DTIC	+ +	+ +	+				±	+	+ +		+	+	Flu-like illness, Facial paresthesia

Agent											Comments
3-Fluorouracil	+	+ +	+	+ +		±			+		+	Conjunctivitis, ataxia and drowsiness
Melphalan	+	+ +[1]				±						
Methotrexate	+	+ +	+	+ +	+		+	+		+ +		Conjunctivitis
Mithramycin	+ +	+ +					+	+				Bleeding, fever, hypocalcemia, CNS dysfunction
Mitomycin C	+	+ +[1]	+	+	±	±	+	+ +	±	+		Hemolytic anemia
6MP	+	+ +		±				+	+ +			Fever
Nitrogen mustard	+ +	+ +	+				+	+ +				Encephalopathy
Cis-platinum	+ +	+			±		+ +					Ototoxic, hypersensitivity
Procarbazine	+ +	+ +		+	±			+		+		CNS dysfunction, MAOI, Antabuse, allergy
Streptozotocin	+ +	+			±		+ +		+	+		Hyperglycemia, ataxia, dizziness
Thioguanine	+	+ +		+				+				
Vinblastine	+	+ +	+	+	±		+ + +			+		Abdo. pain
Vincristine	±	+	+		+ +		+	+				Constipation, ataxia, inappropriate ADH, abdo. pain
Vindesine	±	+	+		+ +		+	±		+		Abdo. pain, constipation, fever
VP16–213	+	+ +	+		±							Fever, hypotension
M-AMSA	+	+ +	+	+ +	±		+	±	±	+		Phlebitis, correct serum electrolyte imbalances prior to administration to avoid enhanced cardiotoxicity
Mitoxantrone	+	+ +	±	±	±				±	±		Phlebitis, blue/green urine discoloration, blue streaking of vein

*   From Acronyms in cancer chemotherapy, Eli Lilly Canada, Inc., 1985 revised edition pamphlet, pp 54–55.

+ +   Major toxicity

+   Less frequent or less severe

±   Infrequent, mild or uncertain

1   Delayed myelosuppression

Tumor Lysis Syndrome

General Considerations

- Occurs as a result of release into the blood of breakdown products of tumor cells in leukemia and lymphoma. Often peaks with institution of therapy but may precede it.
- May cause sudden death

Clinical Features

- Hyperkalemia from rapid cell turnover, accentuated by chemotherapy. May cause cardiac dysrhythmia and arrest. May occur and progress rapidly.
- Hyperphosphatemia and hypocalcemia, which may cause tetany and cardiac dysrhythmia
- Metabolic acidosis
- Increased urea from protein catabolism
- Anuria and renal failure secondary to precipitation of urate or phosphate in tubules

Management

- Prevention
  1. Must have large bore central venous line inserted
  2. Monitor electrolytes, calcium, urea, creatinine, phosphate, uric acid q3–4h
  3. Accurate fluid balance and daily weight; assess urine output q2h
  4. Hydrate with fluids at 3–4 L/m²/day as long as urine output is maintained. If urine output drops to less than 60% of input, give intravenous furosemide.
  5. Withhold potassium supplementation during initiation of chemotherapy
  6. Allopurinol 400 mg/m²/day in 3–4 divided doses (10–12.5 mg/kg/day)

7. Alkalinize the urine to maintain a urine of pH 6.5–7.5. This usually requires 100 mEq (mmol) sodium bicarbonate/m²/day. Do not allow pH to exceed 7.5, as phosphates precipitate in alkaline urine. Reassess bicarbonate dose after each void.
8. Requires continuous cardiac monitoring
9. Monitor BP q2h
10. Hemodialysis may be required prior to institution of chemotherapy if good diuresis is not achieved

- Treatment
  1. Dialysis is required for deteriorating renal function, rising potassium, and symptomatic hypocalcemia despite adequate preventive management
  2. For management of rising potassium (see nephrology section, p 429)
  3. For management of hyperphosphatemia, discontinue alkalinization and treat as per nephrology section, (p 435)
  4. Do *not* treat hypocalcemia unless symptomatic because of risk of precipitating calcium phosphate crystals. If necessary, give intravenous calcium gluconate *slowly and carefully* after discontinuing sodium bicarbonate infusion.

Airway Compression

General Considerations

- Extrinsic compression of trachea or major bronchi usually due to a mediastinal or hilar mass (most commonly Hodgkin or non-Hodgkin lymphoma; occasionally neuroblastoma or teratoma in an infant)

Clinical Features

- Respiratory system—stridor, wheezing, indrawing, worse when supine
- May be associated with features of superior vena caval obstruction

Management

- Investigations
  1. Chest x-ray shows mediastinal mass with widening of the superior mediastinum
  2. CT scan of chest shows compression of vena cava, trachea, and bronchi
- Treatment
  1. Urgent attention to airway status is mandatory. Alert anesthetist, radiotherapist, and surgeon, since intubation beyond the block may be necessary. *DO NOT ATTEMPT INTUBATION YOURSELF!*
  2. Steroids: IV dexamethasone 10 mg/m²/day in three divided doses
  3. Do not delay making a specific diagnosis (e.g., lymph node biopsy, bone marrow aspiration, pleural tap), as not all masses will shrink dramatically with steroid therapy
  4. In acute impending respiratory failure, radiotherapy to the mediastinum may have to be considered
  5. No sedation or spinal taps until airway is secure

Spinal Cord Compression

General Considerations

- Compression of spinal cord by tumor or vertebral collapse

Clinical Features

- Motor weakness, early loss of reflexes, overt paraplegia
- Pain due to root compression, aggravated by coughing, straight leg raising
- Absence of pain does not exclude the diagnosis
- Local pain or backache
- Sensory loss and paresthesia in affected dermatomes
- Loss of autonomic function (urinary retention, dribbling, fecal incontinence)

Management

- Requires immediate investigation and treatment
  1. Investigations
     - X-ray of chest, abdomen, and relevant spine
     - CT scan of relevant area and urgent CT myelogram (the latter after neurosurgical consultation)
     - Lumbar puncture may precipitate or worsen paralysis
     - Establish tissue diagnosis (lymph node biopsy, bone marrow aspirate-biopsy, or laminectomy specimen)
- Treatment
  1. Dexamethasone to reduce edema (see formulary)
  2. Urgent neurosurgical consult for consideration of decompression laminectomy
  3. Radiation or chemotherapy

Fever and Neutropenia

General Considerations

- Common side effects of aggressive chemotherapy

- Major risk is overwhelming sepsis
- A nadir in neutrophil count occurs 7–10 days following initiation of a chemotherapy cycle
- Risk of developing a life-threatening infection escalates sharply when the absolute neutrophil count is $< 0.5 \times 10^9$/L (500/mm³)
- Patients with indwelling central lines are more likely to have gram positive infections
- Suggested advice to parents: Seek medical help without delay for fever $>38.5°$ C (orally or equivalent) on one measurement or $>38°$ C on two measurements 4 hr apart, OR if child appears unwell

Management

- Investigations
  1. CBC with differential and platelet count
  2. Full sepsis work-up, including peripheral site and central venous line (if present). LP should only be done if indicated (requires platelet transfusion if count $<50,000$/mm³)
  3. Chest x-ray
  4. Stools for virology
  5. Skin lesions—send vesicular fluid or aspirate from lesion for electron microscopy, Gram stain, and culture
- Treatment
  1. For persistent neutropenia and fever, *ADMIT*
  2. Start antibiotics as soon as blood cultures are drawn
  3. Use broad spectrum coverage, e.g., tobramycin and piperacillin or ticarcillin. If penicillin allergy exists, use ceftazidime and tobramycin.
  4. Broad spectrum coverage should continue despite a positive culture and the initiation of more specific antibiotic coverage
  5. If fever persists >5 days, consider fungal infection, e.g., *Candida, Aspergillus*

6. If blood culture negative, antibiotics may be discontinued when patient is afebrile and absolute neutrophil count is $>0.5 \times 10^9/L$
7. If blood culture is positive, antibiotics should be continued for 14 days in the presence of a central line, 10 days otherwise

Interstitial Pneumonitis

General Considerations

- Patients immunocompromised by chemotherapy are at risk for interstitial pneumonitis caused by nosocomial agents, e.g., *Pneumocystis carinii*
- Can occur when the neutrophil count is normal

Clinical Features

- Fever, tachypnea, shortness of breath, indrawing in the absence of auscultatory findings; late in the course, cyanosis and crepitations may be present
- Chest x-ray usually shows bilateral interstitial infiltrates

Management

- Investigations
  1. Chest x-ray
  2. Blood culture, throat swab, or sputum culture if available
  3. Mycoplasma and CMV titers, cold agglutinins, and urine for CMV
  4. Baseline arterial blood gas levels; repeat as necessary
- Treatment
  1. High dose trimethoprim-sulfamethoxazole (20 mg TMP component/kg/day in three divided doses)
  2. In the absence of biopsy confirmation and when neutropenia coexists, broad spectrum antibiotics should be started

3. In nonresponsive patients a lung biopsy should be done
4. No further chemotherapy until patient is better
5. Oxygen supplementation as indicated

Varicella-Zoster Infections

General Considerations

- Varicella-Zoster is potentially lethal in immuno-compromised patient
- Parents should be instructed to call immediately if child is exposed

Management

- Prophylaxis
    1. (Varicella) zoster immune globulin for direct contacts (1 vial/10 kg IM) will suppress or modify disease
    2. More effective the earlier after exposure it is given
    3. Of doubtful value if given >72 hr after exposure
- Treatment
    1. Acyclovir is drug of choice—1500 mg/m²/day, divided q8h for 7–10 days
    2. Acyclovir topical applications may be used for local (dermatomal) shingles

Recommendations for Platelet Transfusions in Children with Cancer

General Considerations

- Any patient who
    1. Has active clinical bleeding (mucosal, orbital, intramuscular) with significant thrombocytopenia
    2. Is being given chemotherapy with a platelet count of <10,000

3. Has count <100,000 and requires a surgical
   procedure
4. Has count <50,000 and is hypertensive, or
   has significant headache

Treatment

- Dose of platelets—standard dose 1 unit of random donor platelets/5 kg will raise platelet count approximately 50,000/mm³

Hypercalcemia in Malignant Diseases

General Considerations

- Hypercalcemia in patients with malignant disease may occur because of
   1. Bone involvement with malignant disease
   2. Ectopic parathyroid hormone, androgen and estrogen production
   3. Osteoclast activating factor released by tumor
- Hypercalcemia may be exacerbated by
   1. Dehydration
   2. Immobilization
   3. Thiazide diuretics
- May be accompanied by
   1. Hypokalemia
   2. Hypophosphatemia
   3. Hyper-Mg^{2+}

Clinical Features

- Early signs and symptoms include nocturia, polyuria, polydipsia
- Late signs and symptoms include
   1. Neurologic—drowsiness, lethargy, confusion, muscular weakness, coma
   2. Gastrointestinal—anorexia, nausea, vomiting, constipation
   3. Renal—as in acute renal failure
   4. Cardiac—(see cardiology section, p 50 and 62)
   5. Metabolic—alkalosis, hypokalemia

Treatment

- Must be prompt!
- If serum calcium
  1. 2.8–3.5 mmol/L (12–13 mg/dl)
     - Hydrate rapidly with saline at 3 L/m²/day
     - Follow with furosemide 1 mg/kg IV
  2. >3.5 mmol/L (14 mg/dl)
     - Vigorous hydration until brisk urine flow
     - IV furosemide 1 mg/kg—repeat q2h if necessary to maintain urine output
     - Cardiac monitor
     - Serial measurements of serum K^+, Na^+, Ca^{2+}
     - In patients who fail to respond to above measures, may try mithramycin 25 μg/kg IV over 4 hr × 1 dose only (potentially toxic if used more often)
  3. To maintain normocalcemia
     - Encourage ↑ ambulation
     - Low calcium diet
     - Avoid dehydration
     - Steroids (require days or weeks to work; hence not useful for *acute* hypercalcemia)

Suggested Reading

1. Altman AJ, ed. Symposium on pediatric oncology. Pediatr Clin North Am 1985; 32:541–857.
2. Dacie JV, Lewis SM. Practical haematology. New York: Churchill Livingstone, 1984.
3. Lampkin BC, Gruppo RA, et al. Pediatric hematologic and oncologic emergencies. Emerg Med Clin North Am 1983; 1:63–86.
4. Nathan DG, Oski FA. Hematology of infancy and childhood. Philadelphia: W.B. Saunders, 1981.
5. Pochedly C, ed. Symposium on supportive care and late effects of cancer treatment. Pediatr Ann 1983; 10:428–460.

15 INFECTIOUS DISEASES

IMMUNIZATION AND PROPHYLAXIS

General Precautions

- In febrile illness, immunizations should be deferred. Minor infections (e.g., colds) are not considered a reason to withhold immunizations.
- A history of anaphylactic or urticarial reactions after eating eggs is a contraindication to vaccination against measles, mumps, influenza, and yellow fever
- Live attenuated virus vaccines should not be given in the following cases:
  1. Pregnant women
  2. Immunodeficient and immunosuppressed patients
  3. People with HIV infection
  4. Oral polio vaccine should not be given to household contacts of immunodeficient patients
- Pertussis vaccination should be avoided in patients with progressive neurologic disorders
- Live vaccine administration should be postponed if immune globulin was given in the previous 3 mo

Administration

- For dosages and mode of administrations, consult manufacturer's package insert
- Inactivated vaccines can be administered simultaneously with live attenuated virus vaccines, bacterial polysaccharide vaccines, or other inactivated vaccines

Prophylaxis in Special Situations

- Premature infants: Begin immunizations at the usual chronologic age. If patient is still in the nursery when immunization is due to start, give DPT. Defer OPV or give IPV.
- Hemodialysis patients: Give hepatitis B vaccine if HBsAg negative
- Immigrants and refugees: Update routine immunizations
- Pregnancy:
  1. Bacterial and killed virus vaccines and immune globulins may be given
  2. Live virus vaccines are contraindicated— except yellow fever if travel to an endemic area cannot be avoided
- Anatomic or functional asplenia: Patient should receive
  1. The following vaccinations at 2 yr of age or older (if possible give prior to splenectomy): (i) pneumococcal, (ii) Haemophilus type b, (iii) meningococcal
  2. Continuous antibiotic prophylaxis (compliance is important):
     - <5 yr: TMP-SMX—5 mg of TMP/kg PO once daily, or amoxicillin—20 mg/kg/day PO ÷ bid
     - >5 yr: penicillin V 250 mg PO bid
  3. Medic-Alert bracelet
- Hemophilia-thalassemia patients: hepatitis B vaccine
- Cancer patients:
  1. Vaccination
     - Live virus vaccines are contraindicated
     - Inactivated vaccines can be given, but antibody responses will be lower than those in healthy recipients
  2. TMP-SMX may be used for *Pneumocystis carinii* prophylaxis

Routine Immunizations

TABLE 15–1A Schedule of Routine Immunizations for Infants and Children

Age	Immunization Against			
2 mo	Diphtheria	Pertussis	Tetanus	Poliomyelitis
4 mo	Diphtheria	Pertussis	Tetanus	Poliomyelitis
6 mo	Diphtheria	Pertussis	Tetanus	Poliomyelitis*
12–15 mo[‡]	Measles	Mumps	Rubella[†]	
18 mo	Diphtheria	Pertussis	Tetanus	Poliomyelitis
24 mo	Haemophilus influenzae type b			
4–6 yr	Diphtheria	Pertussis	Tetanus	Poliomyelitis
14–16 yr	Diphtheria[§]		Tetanus[§]	Poliomyelitis*

TABLE 15–1B Immunization Schedule for Children Not Immunized in Early Infancy

Timing	Immunization Against			
For children 1 through 6 yr of age				
First visit[#]	Diphtheria	Pertussis	Tetanus	Poliomyelitis
Interval after first visit:				
1 mo	Measles	Mumps	Rubella[†]	
2 mo	Diphtheria	Pertussis	Tetanus	Poliomyelitis
4 mo	Diphtheria	Pertussis	Tetanus	Poliomyelitis*
16 mo	Diphtheria	Pertussis	Tetanus	Poliomyelitis
Preschool: see Note**				
At age:				
2–5 yr	Haemophilus influenzae type b			
14–16 yr	Diphtheria[§]		Tetanus[§]	Poliomyelitis*
For children 7 yr of age and over				
First visit#	Diphtheria[§]		Tetanus[§]	Poliomyelitis
Interval after first visit:				
1 mo	Measles	Mumps	Rubella[†]	Poliomyelitis*
2 mo	Diphtheria		Tetanus	Poliomyelitis
14 mo	Diphtheria		Tetanus	Poliomyelitis
10 yr	Diphtheria		Tetanus	Poliomyelitis*

* This dose may be omitted if live (oral) polio vaccine is being used.

† Rubella vaccine is also indicated for all girls and women of child bearing age who lack proof of immunity. At all medical visits the opportunity should be taken to check whether such a patient has received rubella vaccine.

‡ MMR vaccine is recommended to be given at 12 mo in Canada and at 15 mo in the United States.

§ Diphtheria and tetanus toxoid (Td), a combined adsorbed "adult type" preparation for use in persons 7 yr of age or more, contains less diphtheria toxoid than preparations given to younger children and is less likely to cause reactions in older persons.

\# Measles, mumps, and rubella vaccines may also be given at the first visit if it is considered likely that a child will not return for further immunization. It has not been shown, however, that a full response to all antigens will occur.

** When the last of the above doses are given before the fourth birthday, consideration should be given to the administration of an additional dose at the time of school entry.

Modified from Canadian Medical Association. CMA policy summary: Immunization. Can Med Assoc J Dec. 15, 1985; 133:1248B.

Diphtheria, Pertussis, Tetanus, and Poliomyelitis

Preparations

- For use under 7 yr: combined DPT-polio (inactivated polio virus, IPV), or DPT and OPV (oral live polio virus) separately. If pertussis vaccine is contraindicated, give DT and IPV separately, or DT and OPV separately.
- For use above 7 yr: combined Td-polio (IPV). Td, OPV, and IPV are also available as individual products.

Administration

- See Table 15–1
- A booster dose of Td should be given every 10 yr following primary immunization
- If a child recovers from culture proven pertussis, no further doses of the pertussis vaccine are required
- OPV may rarely produce paralytic illness in the recipient (~1 in 8 million doses); there is a greater risk in adults
- If giving OPV, ask parents whether they were immunized against poliomyelitis, since OPV may rarely produce paralytic illness in unimmunized household contacts (~1 in 5 million doses)

- Contraindications against pertussis vaccine
  1. Any serious reactions developing within 72 hr following vaccination
     - Fever >40.5° C
     - Persistent inconsolable crying (>3 hr)
     - Collapse episodes (hypotonia, lethargy, pallor)
     - Convulsions
     - Acute encephalopathy (within 7 days after vaccination)
  2. Progressive neurologic disorders (e.g., progressive encephalopathy, uncontrolled epilepsy) but not contraindicated in static lesions (e.g., cerebral palsy) or children with a family history of convulsions or nonprogressive CNS disorders. In a child with a history of seizures there may be an increased risk of a seizure following vaccination.
  3. Children 7 yr of age or older
- Contraindications against diphtheria and tetanus toxoids
  1. Hypersensitivity or anaphylactic reactions following a previous dose
  2. Giving Td doses frequently may produce a local arthus-like reaction
- Contraindications against polio vaccine
  1. OPV: pregnancy, immunodeficient children, or families with immunodeficient members
  2. IPV: hypersensitivity reactions in children who are sensitive to streptomycin or neomycin

Measles, Mumps, and Rubella

Indications

- Primary immunization (MMR)
- Measles revaccination if
  1. Measles immunization before 12 mo of age
  2. Previous immunization with killed measles vaccine

   3. Patient has received the present measles
      vaccine simultaneously with, or within 3 mo
      after receiving immune globulin
- Rubella vaccination of susceptible prepubertal
  and nonpregnant female adolescents

Side Effects

- General: fever (day 6 or later), rash, hypersensitivity reactions in children allergic to eggs
- Measles and mumps:
  1. Encephalitis (rare)
  2. TB skin test reactivity may be suppressed if
     administered 1–6 wk following measles vacci-
     nation
- Rubella: arthralgia, arthritis

Contraindications

- Febrile illness
- Pregnancy. Rubella vaccine is contraindicated 3
  mo prior to and during pregnancy. However, if
  vaccine is inadvertently given to a pregnant
  woman, termination of pregnancy is *not* recommended (congenital rubella syndrome has not
  occurred in >500 infants born to rubella susceptible mothers vaccinated during the first
  trimester).
- Hypersensitivity or anaphylactic reactions to
  eggs or neomycin
- Administration of immune globulin or blood in
  preceding 3 mo
- Cell mediated immune deficiency, malignant
  disease, and immunosuppression

Postmeasles Exposure Prophylaxis

- Immune globulin to
  1. Infants under 1 yr: Give 0.25 ml/kg IM within
     6 days after exposure
  2. Susceptible persons in whom the vaccine
     is contraindicated (e.g., leukemics): Give

0.5 ml/kg (maximum 15 ml) IM within 6 days
after exposure
- Measles vaccine: Might be protective if given to susceptible persons (in whom the vaccine is *not* contraindicated) up to 3 days following exposure

Postrubella Exposure Prophylaxis in Pregnant Women

- Serology immediately following exposure
  1. If rubella immune, there is no risk of congenital infection. Reassure mother.
  2. If rubella susceptible, repeat serology in 4 wk
     - If repeat serology is negative, no infection has occurred. Reassure mother. Arrange for vaccination following delivery.
     - If seroconversion, rubella infection has occurred
- If exposure occurs early in pregnancy in a susceptible woman and termination of pregnancy is not an option, immune globulin may be given (0.55 ml/kg; maximum 20 ml)

Prophylaxis for Specific Diseases

Diphtheria Prophylaxis

- All close contacts should
  1. Have nose and throat cultures
  2. Be observed for clinical evidence of diphtheria
- If asymptomatic and previously fully immunized
  1. If no booster given within last 5 yr, give booster dose of diphtheria toxoid preparation—DPT, DT, or Td (if >7 yr)
  2. If cultures are positive
     - Start antibiotic therapy with erythromycin—40 mg/kg/day PO÷q6h (maximum 2 g/day)×7 days
     - If compliance is not assured, give

benzathine penicillin G
a. >30 kg=1.2 million units IM once only
b. <30 kg=600,000 units IM once only
- Reculture following treatment. If still positive, retreat with erythromycin for 10 days.
- If asymptomatic and unimmunized or of doubtful status
1. Start antibiotic therapy immediately (as above) following cultures
2. Initiate immunization with toxoid—DPT, DT, or Td (if >7 yr)

Haemophilus Influenzae Type b Prophylaxis

- Active immunization (Haemophilus type b polysaccharide vaccine)
1. Indications
- All children at 2 yr of age
- Unimmunized children between 2 and 5 yr of age
- Unimmunized high risk children older than 5 yr (e.g., asplenia, sickle cell disease, or immunosuppression)
2. Precautions and contraindications
- Not recommended under 2 yr of age
- Revaccination not recommended at present time (unless patient received the vaccine prior to 2 yr of age)
- Not protective against nontypable strains of *H. influenzae*; therefore not recommended for recurrent otitis media or sinusitis
3. Side effects: local pain and erythema, mild fever
- Post-exposure prophylaxis with rifampin
1. In cases of invasive *H. influenzae* type b disease (e.g., meningitis, arthritis, pneumonia), rifampin is given to
- The index case
- All household contacts if there is a child (other than index case) less than 4 yr of age at home

- Day care center attendees, if two or more cases are detected within 60 days
2. Do *not* give rifampin to pregnant women
3. Dosage: 20 mg/kg/day (maximum 600 mg) PO once daily × 4 days

Hepatitis A Prophylaxis

Preparations: passive—immune globulin (IG)

Indications

- Pre-exposure: travelers to developing countries where hepatitis A may be prevalent
- Post-exposure
  1. Household contacts
  2. Sexual contacts
  3. In day care centers where all children are toilet trained—attendees and staff who are in the same room as the index case
  4. In day care centers where some children are not toilet trained—all attendees and staff if one or more cases occur among the children or employees, or if there are cases in two or more households of attendees. Give IG to all new employees and attendees for 6 wk following diagnosis of last case. If cases occur in three or more households, consider giving IG to household contacts of all attendees <3 yr.
  5. Residents and staff having close contact with patients in custodial institutions
  6. In food or water-borne hepatitis A epidemics, if source is identified within 2 wk
  7. If an infected food handler has hepatitis A, IG is recommended for other food handlers in same establishment
  8. School, hospital, or place of work contacts are generally not immunized unless an outbreak has originated in these areas
  9. Newborns born to infected mothers who

are jaundiced at delivery

Administration

- Pre-exposure
  1. Travel less than 3 mo—0.02 ml/kg IM once only
  2. Prolonged travel—0.06 ml/kg IM every 5 mo
- Post-exposure—0.02 ml/kg IM within 2 wk after exposure

Hepatitis B Prophylaxis

Indications

- Pre-exposure
  1. Household and sexual contacts of HBsAg carriers
  2. Health care workers frequently exposed to blood or blood products
  3. Residents and staff of institutions for mentally retarded
  4. Hemodialysis patients, hemophiliacs, and other recipients of blood products
  5. Active homosexuals
  6. Users of illicit injectable drugs
  7. Heterosexually active persons with multiple partners
- Post-exposure
  1. Infant born to an HBsAg positive mother
  2. Sexual exposure to and household contacts of an HBsAg positive person
  3. Percutaneous or mucosal exposure to blood that may contain HBsAg

Administration

- Pre-exposure
  1. Three doses of hepatitis B vaccine (suspension of purified surface antigen protein), the second and third doses given 1 and 6 mo, respectively, after the first

TABLE 15–2   Post-exposure Recommendations for Hepatitis B

Type of Exposure	HBIG*	Vaccine[†]
Perinatal[‡]	Within 12 hr after birth (repeat at 3 mo if vaccine was not given)	Within 7 days after birth; repeat at 1 and 6 mo
Sexual	Single dose within 14 days after sexual contact (repeat at 3 mo if contact is still HBsAg positive and vaccine was not given)	Recommended for sexual contacts of HBsAg carriers and active homo-sexual men
Percutaneous[§]		
HBsAg positive blood	Within 24 hr; repeat in 1 mo if vaccine was not given	Initiate vaccine series (or give booster if previously immunized)
Unknown status of blood		
High risk source e.g., acute hepatitis	Within 24 hr. Test source: if positive, repeat in 1 mo if vaccine was not given	Test source: if positive, as above
Intermediate risk source[#]	IG within 24 hr. Test source: if positive, give HBIG. Repeat HBIG in 1 mo if vaccine was not given	Test source: if positive, as above
Low risk or un-known source	Depends on cir-cumstances. Treat-ment is optional. If decide to treat, give IG	Test source: if positive, as above

* Use HBIG unless IG specifically mentioned. Doses of HBIG (or immune globulin [IG]): Perinatal = 0.5 ml IM. Sexual or percutaneous exposure = 0.06 ml/kg IM.

† Give vaccine at a different site than HBIG or IG.

‡ Check infant's serology at 9 mo: If HBsAg and anti-HBs are

negative, repeat dose of vaccine. If HBsAg is positive:
prophylaxis has failed, follow as a carrier. If anti-HBs is
positive, vaccination was successful.
§ If contact has been vaccinated and has a recently
documented protective antibody level, no treatment is
necessary.
Blood of immigrants from HBV endemic areas, residents of
custodial institutions, hemodialysis patients, users of illicit
drugs, homosexuals.
  2. Doses
      • HEPTAVAX-B
         1. <10 years: 10 μg (0.5 ml)
         2. ≥10 years: 20 μg (1.0 ml)
      • RECOMBIVAX-HB
         1. <10 years: 5 μg (0.5 ml)
         2. ≥10 years: 10 μg (1.0 ml)
      • Hemodialysis and immunosuppressed patients: 2 ×
        usual dose for age
  3. Should be given IM in deltoid (older children and
     adults) or anterolateral thigh (infants). (Suboptimal an-
     tibody responses have been seen when vaccine is
     given in the buttocks).
• Post-exposure: vaccine as above and HBIG if
  appropriate. For details see Table 15–2

Influenza Prophylaxis

• Influenza vaccine
  1. Preparations
      • The vaccine contains polyvalent killed flu
        strains (A and B); strains vary by location
        and year. It is available in two preparations:
        "whole virus" and "split virus."
      • Use "split virus" for children less than 12
        yr of age
      • It is usually given annually around October
  2. Indications
      • Children with severe chronic disease, e.g.,
        heart disease associated with cardiac failure
        or pulmonary congestion, chronic pulmo-
        nary disease (e.g., cystic fibrosis, severe
        asthma), chronic renal disease, diabetes
        mellitus, sickle cell anemia and other
        hemoglobinopathies, and immunosup-
        pressed children
      • Children taking long-term aspirin therapy

3. Contraindications
   - Children under 6 mo
   - Hypersensitivity reactions to egg ingestion
- Amantadine (post-exposure prophylaxis against influenza A virus only)
   1. Indications
      - During outbreaks in custodial institutions
      - High risk groups, during influenza A epidemics, for those in whom the vaccine is contraindicated or those not expected to have a good antibody response
   2. Administration
      - Dosage
         a. <9 yr: 4 mg/kg/day (maximum 100 mg/day) PO÷bid
         b. ≥9 yr: 200 mg/day PO÷bid
      - For treatment: Start as soon as possible after symptoms begin and continue for 5 days or until asymptomatic × 48 hr
      - For prophylaxis: Give × 10–14 days (may be given throughout an epidemic up to 90 days)
   3. Precautions
      - Not recommended for infants under 1 yr
      - Children with impaired renal function
      - Children with active seizure disorder
   4. Side effects: 5–10% insomnia, lightheadedness, irritability

Measles Prophylaxis

See p 298

Meningococcal Prophylaxis

- Active immunization
   1. Preparations: monovalent (A or C), bivalent (A and C), quadrivalent (A, C, Y, and W–135)
   2. Indications
      - Control of outbreaks (due to serogroups represented in the vaccine) in a closed population

- As adjunct to chemoprophylaxis in household contacts during epidemics
- Travel to endemic or epidemic areas
- May be helpful in children with complement deficiencies or asplenia
3. Efficacy: Adequate antibody levels are achieved with group A vaccine in children 3 mo or older and with other vaccine groups in children 2 yr or older
4. Side effects: Local erythema and discomfort (rare), transient fever (2%)

- Post-exposure prophylaxis with rifampin
1. Indications
  - The index case
  - Household contacts
  - Day care contacts
  - Intimate contact, e.g., mouth to mouth resuscitation
2. Do *not* give rifampin to pregnant women
3. Dose: 20 mg/kg/day (maximum 1200 mg/day) PO÷q12h×2 days
4. If organism is known to be sensitive to sulfonamides, use sulfisoxazole instead of rifampin
  - Dose of sulfisoxazole
    a. <1 yr: 500 mg PO once daily × 2 days
    b. 1–12 yr: 500 mg PO q12h × 2 days
    c. >12 yr: 1 g PO q12h × 2 days

Pertussis Prophylaxis

See p 338

Pneumococcal Vaccination

Preparation

- Purified capsular polysaccharides of 23 serotypes of *S. pneumoniae*

Indications

- Children 2 yr of age or older with
  1. Anatomic or functional asplenia
  2. Sickle cell disease
  3. Nephrotic syndrome
  4. Immunosuppression

Administration

- 0.5 ml IM/SC single dose; if possible give 2 wk prior to splenectomy or immunosuppression. Revaccination is not recommended at present time (in children who were previously vaccinated at age 2, the need for revaccination is currently being re-evaluated).
- 70–80% of recipients achieve adequate antibody levels to the antigens in the vaccine (a partial response is seen in Hodgkin's disease and renal transplant patients)

Precautions and Contraindications

- Febrile illness
- Reimmunization not recommended for those who received the previous vaccine (14-valent)
- Avoid in pregnancy unless there is a high risk of pneumococcal infection
- N.B. This vaccine does not represent all the pneumococcal serotypes. Therefore antimicrobial coverage in certain patients, e.g., splenectomized children, is still advised (see p 294).

Side Effects

- Soreness, erythema, fever, myalgias, anaphylactic reactions (rare)

Rabies Prevention

- See also p 315 for general treatment of animal bites

Preparations

- Active: human diploid cell vaccine (HDCV)
- Passive: human rabies immune globulin (RIG)

Indications for Active and Passive Immunization Following a Bite

- See Table 15–3

Administration Following a Bite

- Not previously immunized:
  1. HDCV: 1 ml IM—days 0, 3, 7, 14, and 28 (5 doses)
  2. RIG: 20 IU/kg—half IM and half infiltrated around the bite site
  3. Always give HDCV and RIG with different syringes at different sites
- Previously immunized (with HDCV or other type of vaccine with documented positive antibody response), HDCV: 1 ml IM—days 0 and 3 (no RIG)
- N.B. Follow-up serology recommended only in immunocompromised patients

Precautions

- Immunosuppression: can interfere with development of active immunity
- Allergies (including anaphylaxis) can occur
- Pregnancy: may be given if substantial risk of rabies exists

Side Effects

- HDCV (common): pain, erythema and swelling, headache, nausea, abdominal pain, myalgias, dizziness, serum sickness-like reactions following boosters
- RIG: local pain and low grade fever

TABLE 15–3 Rabies Post-exposure Prophylaxis Guide*

Animal Species	Condition of Animal at Time of Attack	Treatment of Exposed Person[†]
Domestic dogs and cats	Healthy and available for 10 days of observation	None, unless animal develops rabies[‡]
	Rabid or suspected rabid	RIG[§] and HDCV
	Unknown (escaped)	Consult public health officials. If treatment is indicated, give RIG[§] and HDCV
Wild Skunk, bat, fox, coyote, racoon, bobcat, and other carnivores	Regard as rabid unless proven negative by laboratory tests[**]	RIG[§] and HDCV
Other Livestock, rodents, and lagomorphs (rabbits and hares)	Consider individually. Local and state public health officials should be consulted on questions about the need for rabies prophylaxis. Bites of squirrels, hamsters, guinea pigs, gerbils, chipmunks, rats, mice, other rodents, rabbits, and hares almost never call for antirabies prophylaxis.	

* These recommendations are only a guide. In applying them, take into account the animal species involved, the circumstances of the bite or other exposure, the vaccination status of the animal, and presence of rabies in the region. Local or state public health officials should be consulted if questions arise about the need for rabies prophylaxis.

† *All bites and wounds should immediately be thoroughly cleansed with soap and water.* If antirabies treatment is indicated, both rabies immune globulin (RIG) and human diploid cell rabies vaccine (HDCV) should be given as soon as possible, *regardless* of the interval from exposure. Local reactions to vaccines are common and do not contraindicate continuing treatment.

Discontinue vaccine if fluorescent-antibody tests of the animal are negative.

‡ During the usual holding period of 10 days, begin treatment with RIG and HDCV at first sign of rabies in a dog or cat that has bitten someone. The symptomatic animal should be killed immediately and tested.

§ If RIG is not available, use antirabies serum, equine (ARS). Do not use more than the recommended dosage.

** The animal should be killed and tested as soon as possible. Holding for observation is not recommended.

From Centers for Disease Control. Rabies prevention. MMWR 1984; 33:393–402.

Rubella Prophylaxis

- See p 299

Tetanus Prophylaxis (in Wound Management)

- Attention to wound cleaning and debridement when indicated
- Proceed as in Table 15–4

Tuberculosis Prophylaxis

- BCG vaccine
  1. Indications
     - High risk groups with high rates of new infections
     - Health workers at increased risk of repeated exposure to groups of people with high prevalence rates of TB
     - Infants and other individuals who are tuberculin skin test negative and who are repeatedly exposed to household members with active untreated TB
  2. Precautions and contraindications
     - Should be given to PPD or 5TU skin test negative persons only (not necessary to test infants <6 wk old)
     - Contraindicated in persons with impaired cell mediated immune response, e.g., malignant disease, steroids, HIV infection
     - Contraindicated during pregnancy
  3. Side effects
     - Local: skin ulceration, keloid formation, axillary adenitis
     - Systemic (rare): osteomyelitis, anaphylaxis, generalized BCG infection (in immunodeficient children)
- Chemoprophylaxis for TB contacts
  1. See page 349

TABLE 15–4   Guide to Tetanus Prophylaxis in Wound Management

Type of Wound	Patient not Immunized or Partially Immunized (<3 doses or unknown)	Patient Completely Immunized Time Since Last Booster‡ 5–10 yr	>10 yr
Clean, minor (<6 hr; no debris)	Td* Complete the immunization series	None	Td*
All other wounds	Td* TIG† 250–500 U IM Complete the immunization series	Td*	Td*

* For children less than 7 yr, use DPT (DT if pertussis is contraindicated).
† Tetanus immune globulin—use separate syringes and deliver at a site other than that used for toxoid.
‡ If patient completely immunized and last booster was within 5 yr, no prophylaxis is necessary.
Modified from Giagrasso et al. Misuse of tetanus immunoprophylaxis. Ann Emerg Med 1985; 14:573–579.

- Varicella vaccine: still investigational
- Varicella-zoster immune globulin (VZIG): prepared from plasma of outdated blood with high
  V–Z antibody titers
  1. Indications
     - Immunocompromised susceptible patients
       exposed to V–Z infection (exposure to
       household contact, indoor playmate con-
       tact >1 hr, or hospital contact—same room
       or prolonged face to face contact)
     - Neonates whose mothers have developed
       varicella $\leq$5 days prior to or within 4 days
       after delivery
     - Exposed premature infants <28 wk gesta-
       tion or $\leq$1 kg
     - Exposed premature infant $\geq$28 wk gesta-
       tion whose mother lacks a history of
       chickenpox
  2. Dose: to be given within 96 hr after
     exposure (preferably sooner)
     - <10 kg = 125 U (one vial)
     - >10 kg = 125 U/10 kg; maximum
       625 U (5 vials)
  3. Precautions: Strict isolation of exposed pa-
     tient is necessary between days 10 and 21
     following exposure. If VZIG was given,
     isolate until 35 days following exposure.

DISEASES AND SYNDROMES

Arthritis, Septic

Clinical Features

- May have history of trauma
- Systemic symptoms: e.g., fever, skin rashes
- Local symptoms: erythema, swelling, pain, and
  limitation of motion
- Neonates: may have irritability and refusal to
  feed in addition to the preceding

TABLE 15–5 Etiologic Organisms and Empiric Therapy of Septic Arthritis*

Age	Potential Organisms	Empiric Antibiotic Therapy
Neonates	Group B strep., *S. aureus*, *N. gonorrhoeae*, coliforms	Cloxacillin + ampicillin + aminoglycoside or Cloxacillin + cefotaxime
Infants and children <5 yr	*H. influenzae, S. aureus, S. pneumoniae*	Cloxacillin + chloramphenicol or Cefuroxime
Children >5 yr	*S. aureus, S. pneumoniae*	Cloxacillin
Immunocompromised	*S. aureus, S. pneumoniae*, gram negative organisms	Cloxacillin + aminoglycoside or Cloxacillin + cefotaxime

* In children with hemoglobinopathies consider Salmonella and *H. influenzae* in addition to usual pathogens. In sexually active adolescents consider *N. gonorrhoeae* in addition to usual pathogens.

Differential Diagnosis

- Noninfectious (see p 621)
- Nonbacterial infections
  1. Viral (rubella, viral hepatitis, EBV, influenza, mumps)
  2. Mycobacterial
  3. Fungal

Management

- Investigation
  1. Joint aspiration for WBC and differential, glucose, Gram stain, latex agglutination, culture (see p 624)
  2. CBC and differential, ESR
  3. Blood cultures
  4. X-ray examination
  5. Bone and gallium radionuclide scans may be useful if adjacent osteomyelitis is suspected
- Treatment
  1. *Rapid joint drainage (consult orthopaedics) and institution of IV antibiotic treatment are crucial* (it is not necessary to wait for results of x-ray examination or scans before treating)
  2. Continuous passive movement reduces stiffness and speeds healing; avoid weight bearing during the acute illness
  3. Analgesics for pain control
  4. Antibiotic therapy
     - For empiric therapy, see Table 15-5 (adjust therapy to results of Gram stain and culture)
     - Antibiotics should be given by IV route initially. Once the signs of acute inflammation have resolved, one can switch to an *equivalent oral dose* of antibiotics if the following conditions are met:
       a. Patient can tolerate oral medications and strict compliance is ensured
       b. Serum bactericidal titers (SBT) can be determined; postlevels should be $\geq 1:8$

    c. Follow-up can be maintained with weekly monitoring of clinical condition, ESR, and SBT. Follow-up x-ray examination should be done if osteomyelitis is suspected.
- Duration
    1. Antibiotics should be given for a minimum of 2 wk
    2. Shorter courses (1 wk) can be given for gonococcal arthritis
    3. Longer courses (3–4 wk) are advised for underlying osteomyelitis, *S. aureus* arthritis of hip joint, neonates, immunocompromised patients, gram negative arthritis
- N.B. Intra-articular instillation of antibiotics is unnecessary and frequently causes chemical arthritis

Bites

Animal Bites

General Considerations and Clinical Features

- Organisms: anaerobes, aerobes including streptococci, *S. aureus, Pasteurella multocida*
- Document the type and health status of the animal; also the circumstances surrounding delivery of the bite
- Note the location and severity of the wound and any signs of infection

Management and Follow-Up

- High pressure irrigation with copious amounts of sterile saline using a syringe
- Debridement of dead tissues
- Leave unsutured if wound involves the hand or if more than 6–8 hr have elapsed since injury
- Prophylactic antibiotics (controversial)—use in major or hand injuries
    1. Penicillin or amoxicillin-clavulanic

acid × 5 days
  2. Penicillin allergic patients: tetracycline (if over
     8 yr) or erythromycin (but 50% of *P. multo-
     cida* are resistant)
- Tetanus prophylaxis (see p 310)
- Rabies prophylaxis (see p 308)
- If presenting late (>12 hr)
  1. Irrigation and debridement as above, drain
     pus, obtain cultures
  2. Leave unsutured (consult plastic surgery)
  3. Start antibiotics × 10 days
  4. Elevate and immobilize affected part
- Instruct parents to return if fever develops,
  wound becomes infected, or infection is
  spreading

Human Bites

General Considerations and Clinical Features

- Organisms: *S. aureus*, streptococci, anaerobes
- Document: location, severity of wound
  (involvement of deep structures), and any signs
  of infection

Management

- If there is a question of joint involvement, consult plastic surgery immediately; this is a surgical emergency and requires *urgent* surgical
  exploration, debridement, and irrigation
- Consult plastic surgery
- Irrigation, debridement (see animal bites)
- Leave unsutured
- Elevate limb (if involved)
- Tetanus prophylaxis (see p 310)
- Prophylactic antibiotics
  1. Penicillin ± cloxacillin
  2. Amoxicillin-clavulanic acid
  3. In penicillin allergic patient, use clindamycin
- If there is evidence of infection, admit. Consult
  plastic surgery immediately (surgical exploration

and debridement will likely be needed). Gram
stain and culture wound. Elevate and immobilize affected part. Administer antibiotics IV.
- Baseline x-ray views may be needed
- Observe for complications, e.g., tenosynovitis,
septic arthritis, or osteomyelitis

Brain Abscess

General Considerations

- Organisms: aerobic and anaerobic streptococci,
Bacteroides, *S. aureus*, gram negative bacilli;
polymicrobial in 30%

Clinical Features

- Maintain a high level of suspicion
- Suspect an abscess if a child develops signs
and symptoms of increased ICP, focal neurologic signs, or seizures, in the presence of the following predisposing conditions: otitis media,
sinusitis, dental infections or surgery, cyanotic
heart disease, immunocompromised host, or
following trauma or neurosurgery

Management

- WBC and differential, ESR
- CT scan (with contrast)
- Brain scan (if CT not available or CT negative
and still a high index of suspicion)
- LP is contraindicated
- Suggested antibiotics
  1. Penicillin (meningitic doses) and
     chloramphenicol (or metronidazole)
  2. In chronic otitis media or immunocom-
     promised patients, use ceftazidime and
     metronidazole
  3. In post-trauma or postneurosurgery cases, use

cloxacillin (or vancomycin) and ceftazidime
- Duration of therapy: 4–6 wk; monitor with
  serial CT scans
- Surgical drainage (aspiration or excision);
  consult with neurosurgery

Cellulitis

General Considerations and Clinical Features

- Etiologic organisms: group A streptococci, *S.
  aureus, H. influenzae* (if < 5 yr), group B streptococci (in neonates)
- Erythema, swelling, heat, tenderness
- If patient is toxic and lesion is spreading very
  quickly and is extremely tender or anesthetic,
  consider necrotizing fasciitis. Although rare, this
  requires immediate surgical debridement and IV
  antibiotics (to cover streptococci, staphylococci,
  gram negative organisms, and anaerobes).

Management

- CBC, blood culture
- Needle aspiration of advancing edge for culture
- If unsure of etiology, can use amoxicillin-
  clavulanic acid PO or cefaclor PO × 10 days
  for minor infections
- For more severe infections, can use IV
  cloxacillin and chloramphenicol in combination
  or IV cefuroxime by itself

Erysipelas

- Caused by group A streptococci
- Elevated and distinct margins, bright red,
  tender; child often toxic
- Obtain CBC, blood culture, needle aspirate for
  culture and sensitivity
- Treat with penicillin

Periorbital and Orbital Cellulitis

General Considerations and Clinical Features

- Etiologic organisms: *H. influenzae, S. aureus, S. pneumoniae*
- Often associated with sinusitis
- Periorbital cellulitis should be differentiated from orbital cellulitis by absence of proptosis, and presence of full ocular movement, and normal vision

Management

- CBC, blood culture
- Sinus x-ray views
- CT scan if orbital cellulitis is a possibility
- Orbital cellulitis requires urgent surgical drainage in addition to IV antibiotics (in addition to orbital damage, untreated orbital cellulitis can lead to cavernous sinus thrombosis)
- Treat with IV cloxacillin and chloramphenicol in combination or cefuroxime by itself

Cervical Adenitis

General Considerations

- Organisms
  1. Acute
     - Common: group A streptococci, *S. aureus*, group B streptococci (neonates)
     - Less common: anaerobes, adenovirus, enterovirus, EBV
  2. Subacute and chronic (1–3 wk): cat scratch fever, anaerobes, EBV, CMV, atypical mycobacteria, *M. tuberculosis*, toxoplasmosis, histoplasmosis

Clinical Features

- History
  1. Preceding illness: URI, sore throat, skin or dental infections

2. Exposure to TB, cat scratch, insect bites
3. Travel history
4. Systemic findings: fever, malaise, myalgia
- Physical examination
  1. Fever
  2. Skin, dental, pharyngeal findings
  3. Nodes: size, distribution, character
  4. Other lymphatic involvement, liver and spleen size

Differential Diagnosis

- Malignant disease
- Drugs (e.g., Dilantin, INH)
- Kawasaki disease
- Neck anomalies (e.g., cystic hygroma, branchial cleft cyst, thyroglossal cyst)

Management

- CBC and differential, ESR
- Cultures (skin, throat, $\pm$ blood culture)
- If node is fluctuant, consider incision and drainage (send sample for Gram stain and culture)
- In mild infection, cloxacillin or erythromycin PO $\times$ 10 days
- If a dental source is suspected, use penicillin V or clindamycin PO
- Neonatal infections and more severe infections may need IV therapy and surgical drainage
- If no improvement or chronic infection, investigate for mycobacterial (atypical or TB), viral, cat scratch, or malignant disease

Clostridium Difficile Infections

General Considerations and Clinical Features

- Gram positive anaerobic bacillus; some strains produce A and B toxins

- Spectrum of disease may range from asymptomatic carriage or mild diarrhea to severe pseudomembranous colitis (PMC)
- Usually associated with or occurs after receiving antibiotics
- Children under 2 yr are most prone to asymptomatic carriage

Management

- Investigations
  1. Stool for
     - Anaerobic culture on a selective media
     - Filtration and detection of cytotoxin B
  2. Sigmoidoscopy-colonoscopy if PMC suspected
- Treatment
  1. Supportive care: Institute fluid and electrolyte replacement. Avoid antidiarrheal drugs.
  2. If symptomatic
     - Enteric isolation
     - Discontinue antibiotics if feasible (mildly symptomatic patients may benefit by stopping antibiotics alone and may not require metronidazole or vancomycin)
     - Metronidazole 20–30 mg/kg/day (maximum 1 g/day) PO ÷ q6h × 7 days (less expensive and better tolerated than vancomycin) or vancomycin 50 mg/kg/day (maximum 500 mg/day) PO ÷ q6h × 7 days
     - If patient cannot tolerate PO antibiotics, can use metronidazole IV (same dose as given for PO)
     - Relapses are common; may require an additional course of treatment
  3. N.B. Asymptomatic patients do not require treatment. It is suggested, however, that neutropenic patients be treated even if asymptomatic, since they may be at higher risk for severe infections.

Congenital Infections

General Considerations

- These infections are also known as the TORCH infections (TO=toxoplasmosis, R=rubella, C=cytomegalovirus [CMV], H=herpes simplex)
- HIV, syphilis, and enteroviruses can also cause congenital infection
- They are acquired in utero (by transplacental transmission) or perinatally (by passage through birth canal)

Clinical Features (see also Table 15–6)

- Congenital infections are suspected if the child presents with some of the following:
  1. Small for gestational age
  2. Prematurity
  3. Congenital defects, e.g., CNS, eye, CVS abnormalities
  4. Hepatosplenomegaly
  5. Rash (may be petechial or purpuric)
  6. Multisystem involvement, e.g., encephalitis, pneumonitis, myocarditis, hepatitis
  7. Lab test abnormalities
     - Hemolytic anemia
     - Thrombocytopenia
     - Hyperbilirubinemia
     - CSF pleocytosis

Management

- CBC, platelet count
- ± PT, PTT
- Liver function tests
- Electron microscopy of skin vesicles (herpes)
- Darkfield examination of nasal discharge (syphilis)
- Viral cultures of throat (rubella, herpes, CMV)
- Urine for CMV, rubella
- Maternal and newborn serology for toxoplasmo-

sis, herpes, rubella, CMV; follow titers over time
- Specific IgM for rubella, herpes, toxoplasmosis, CMV
- Maternal and newborn VDRL and FTA-ABS
- LP for CSF serology and viral culture
- X-ray views of long bones (syphilis, rubella), skull for intracranial calcifications (CMV, toxoplasmosis)
- Head ultrasound, cranial CT scan for hydrocephalus, calcifications
- Ophthalmology consult
- Placenta (if available)—histologic examination and culture (routine and viral)

Encephalitis, Herpes Simplex

Clinical Features

- Patient may present with fever, headache, vomiting, personality changes, changes in level of consciousness, seizures, or focal neurologic signs
- Needs to be distinguished from other viral encephalitides, TB or fungal meningitis, brain abscess, tumor, and vascular disease

Management

- Investigations
  1. Brain scan, CT scan: focal (usually temporal) lesions
  2. Lumbar puncture: CSF usually has normal or increased protein, normal glucose, pleocytosis ($\pm$ increased RBC). If focal signs or signs of $\uparrow$ ICP are present on history or physical, lumbar puncture should not be done until a CT scan has been interpreted.
  3. CSF culture
  4. Blood, CSF serology
  5. EEG: often focal findings

TABLE 15–6 Congenital Infections

CMV	Rubella	Herpes Simplex	Syphilis	Toxoplasmosis
Specific clinical features				
Most asymptomatic Microcephaly Periventricular calcifications Mental retardation Hearing loss Chorioretinitis	Microcephaly Mental retardation Chorioretinitis Cataracts, glaucoma, microphthalmia Hearing loss Congenital heart defects Rash, dermal erythropoiesis Bone radiolucencies	Localized or disseminated Mucocutaneous rash Conjunctivitis, keratitis Meningoencephalitis Sepsis/DIC picture	Asymptomatic Rash Rhinitis Osteochondritis Periostitis	Most are asymptomatic Chorioretinitis Intracranial calcifications Hydrocephalus, microcephaly
Therapy				
No specific therapy	No specific therapy	Symptomatic; newborn should be treated with acyclovir Acyclovir treatment of asymptomatic newborn born to mother with active genital herpes lesions is controversial	Penicillin (see p 346)	Treatment regimen with sulfadiazine, pyrimethamine, and folinic acid is complex; suggest infectious diseases consult

Isolation

Avoid contact with pregnant women; an infected newborn may excrete the virus for months and even years	Avoid contact with pregnant women; an infected newborn may excrete the virus for months	Newborns with clinical disease	Barrier until 24 hr after start of antibiotics	None

Pre- and perinatal prevention

Careful hand washing for nonimmune pregnant women in nurseries and day care centers	Females of child bearing age should have serology checked; if not immune, should receive vaccination at least 3 mo prior to any planned pregnancy	If mother has genital herpes at or near time of delivery and membranes are intact or ruptured <6 hr, cesarean section is recommended	Pregnant females should have a VDRL; if confirmatory serology is positive, treat	Avoid ingestion of raw meat No contact with cat litter

6. Brain biopsy: most definitive way of making diagnosis (used for pathology, EM, IF, viral culture)
- Treatment
  1. Supportive care, including treatment of seizures, treatment of ↑ ICP (see p 478), and monitoring for SIADH
  2. IV acyclovir for 10 days

Infectious Mononucleosis

General Considerations

- Agent: Epstein-Barr virus (a herpes group virus)
- Incubation period: 2–7 wk

Clinical Features

- Fever, malaise, headache, fatigue, sore throat
- Enlarged tonsils with patchy exudate, petechiae on palate
- Cervical adenopathy ± hepatosplenomegaly
- Maculopapular rash, especially if patient has been taking ampicillin
- Complications: splenic rupture, upper airway obstruction

Management

- Investigations
  1. WBC and differential (↑atypical lymphocytes)
  2. Presence of heterophile antibodies: Monospot test, Paul-Bunnell
  3. Specific EBV serology (see p 790)
- Treatment
  1. Isolation: none required
  2. Symptomatic: bed rest, encourage fluids, warm saline gargles for sore throat, acetaminophen
  3. Admit if upper airway obstruction or complicated course
  4. Steroids indicated in airway obstruction

(start with equivalent of 1–2 mg/kg/day of prednisone; give PO in divided doses and taper over 1–2 wk)

Follow-Up

- Usually resolves over 2–3 wk period, although fatigue may persist for weeks
- Contact sports should be avoided while spleen is enlarged

Measles

- See p 353

Meningitis, Bacterial

General Considerations

- *This is a medical emergency*
- Organisms
    1. Neonates: group B streptococci, *E. coli*, Listeria, group D streptococci
    2. Infants and children <10 yr: *H. influenzae, S. pneumoniae, N. meningitidis*
    3. Adolescents: *S. pneumoniae, N. meningitidis, H. influenzae* (rare)
    4. Compromised hosts: in addition to the preceding, *S. aureus,* gram negative bacilli, Listeria

Clinical Features

- The younger the patient, the less specific the clinical picture
- Neonates: fever or hypothermia, irritability, poor feeding, apnea, bulging fontanelle, seizures
- Infants: fever; vomiting; change in mental status, behavior, activity, and feeding habits; seizures; rash
- Older children: fever, headache, vomiting, rash,

neck stiffness, positive Kernig and Brudzinski
signs

Management

- Emergency treatment
  1. Vital signs; assess respiratory, cardiovascular,
     and neurologic status
  2. Assess state of hydration
  3. Start IV infusion; NPO depending on level of
     consciousness
  4. Treat shock if present with normal saline or
     plasma (see p 659)
  5. Treat seizures with diazepam followed by
     either phenobarbital or phenytoin (see p
     469)
  6. Treat ↑ ICP if present (see p 478)
- Investigations
  1. CSF examination: A lumbar puncture should
     be done as soon as the possibility of menin-
     gitis is raised (for procedure and precautions,
     see p 715). If the child is comatose, or if
     there are focal neurologic signs or signs of
     increased intracranial pressure, CT should be
     performed and an LP done only if CT shows
     no signs of ↑ ICP. *Antibiotic therapy should
     never be delayed while waiting for CT scan.
     Start appropriate antibiotics (see Table 15–8)
     while waiting for CT scan.* Examine CSF for
     (see Table 15–7 for interpretation):
     - Cell count and differential
     - Gram stain, culture and sensitivity
     - Protein and glucose
     - Antigen detection testing (e.g., latex agglu-
       tination) if patient has been taking an-
       tibiotics
     - Save one tube for other investigations, e.g.,
       virology, TB
  2. CBC, differential, platelet count
  3. Blood glucose, electrolytes, BUN, creatinine
  4. Blood cultures
  5. PT, PTT, fibrin split products (if indicated)

6. Urine: latex agglutination, specific gravity, electrolytes and osmolality (if SIADH is suspected)

- Treatment
  1. Antibiotic therapy (see Table 15–8)
     - Drugs: switch to appropriate antibiotic once organism is identified and sensitivities are known
     - Duration
       a. Neonates = 2 wk (3 wk in gram negative meningitis)
       b. *H. influenzae, S. pneumoniae, N. meningitidis*—7 days in uncomplicated cases
       c. *S. aureus*—minimum 3 wk
       d. Gram negative bacilli—minimum 3 wk
     - In *H. influenzae* and meningococcal meningitis, the patient should also receive rifampin prophylaxis (see p 300 for *H. influenzae* and p 306 for *N. meningitidis*)
  2. Fluid restriction (60% of maintenance fluids) to prevent SIADH. Follow hydration, weight, and serum and urine electrolytes and osmolalities.
  3. Treat fever if present
  4. Monitor closely
     - Vital signs
     - Respiratory status
     - Cardiovascular status: pulse, blood pressure
     - Neurologic status: level of consciousness, pupillary responses, symmetry of movement, deep tendon reflexes (DTR)
  5. Assess daily
     - Head circumference, skull transillumination (infants)
     - CNS examination, including vision and hearing evaluation
     - For metastatic foci
  6. Prophylaxis for family if indicated
     - See p 300 (*H. influenzae*) or p 306 (*N. meningitidis*)

TABLE 15–7 Interpretation of CSF Findings

	Bacterial	Viral	TB	Partially Treated
Cell count*	Usually >1,000	Usually <300	<1,000	>1,000
Predominate cell	Polys	Early polys, then mononuclear	Lymphocytes	Polys or mononuclear
Gram stain	Usually positive	Negative	Negative (acid-fast stain may be positive)	May be negative
Glucose	Low†	Normal	Low† or normal	Low† or normal
Protein	High	Normal or high	Very high	High
Bacterial culture	Usually positive	Negative	Culture for TB may be positive	Often negative

* The WBC count in normal spinal fluid should be at most 5×10^6/L (5/mm^3). Neonates may have higher numbers of WBC. Even though WBC are usually quite high in bacterial meningitis, any count above normal must be viewed suspiciously.
† CSF glucose: <50% of blood glucose.

Neonate	Ampicillin + aminoglycoside
	or
	Ampicillin + cefotaxime
Infant 1–3 mo	Ampicillin + cefotaxime
Children 3 mo to 10 yr	Cefuroxime, cefotaxime or ceftriaxone
	or
	Ampicillin + chloramphenicol
>10 yr	Penicillin
Immunocompromised	Cefotaxime (or ceftazidime) + ampicillin
Shunt related	Vancomycin + cefotaxime

- Prolonged or recurrent pyrexia (more than 5 days) may be due to
  1. Nosocomial illness, e.g., URI, gastroenteritis
  2. Phlebitis
  3. Secondary focus: arthritis, pneumonia, pleural effusion, pericarditis
  4. Subdural effusions (common; in most cases medical intervention not needed; aspirate if increasing head circumference, vomiting, seizures, or focal neurologic findings)
  5. Drug fever
  6. Failure to cure meningitis

Follow-Up

- All patients should routinely have
  1. Hearing testing within 1 mo after discharge
  2. Psychological testing assessment prior to starting school or before that if developmental delay is suspected
  3. Neurologic assessment and follow-up if indicated

Mumps

General Considerations

- Caused by a paramyxovirus
- Incubation period: 16–18 days (range, 12–25 days)

- May be contagious as long as 7 days prior to onset of parotid swelling and up to 9 days after onset. Asymptomatic infections occur and can be communicable.

Clinical Features

- Fever may be present
- Can cause unilateral or bilateral parotitis (pain and swelling)
- May be complicated by meningoencephalitis (including sensorineural deafness), orchitis, oophoritis, or pancreatitis
- Immunity is life-long
- There are many other causes of parotid swelling
    1. Viral (parainfluenza III, Coxsackie, influenza A), bacterial (*Staphylococcus aureus*)
    2. Drugs
    3. Metabolic disorders (e.g., diabetes), malnutrition, parotid tumor, obstruction of Stensen's duct from any cause, chronic recurrent sialectasia of childhood

Management

- For confirmation of diagnosis
    1. Saliva, urine, CSF (if indicated) for viral isolation
    2. Mumps serology
- Treatment
    1. Respiratory isolation
    2. Symptomatic treatment only (acetaminophen for pain; cold or warm packs to areas of swelling)
    3. No post-exposure prophylaxis is available

Osteomyelitis

General Considerations

- Organisms
    1. Neonate: *S. aureus*, gram negative bacilli,

group B streptococci
2. Infants and children: *S. aureus*
   * Rare: *S. pneumoniae, H. influenzae*, group A streptococci
   * Hemoglobinopathy: Salmonella
   * Foot puncture wound: *Pseudomonas aeruginosa*

Clinical Features

* Fever usually present (but may be absent)
* Pain, swelling, point tenderness (usually metaphyseal in long bones)
* Limitation of motion, refusal to move limb

Differential Diagnosis

* Cellulitis, arthritis, fracture, bone cyst, bone infarction (sickle cell disease)

Management

* Investigations
  1. WBC, ESR ($\uparrow$)
  2. Blood cultures
  3. X-ray: soft tissue swelling, subperiosteal elevation (bone changes not evident for first 10 days)
  4. Bone scan $\pm$ gallium scan
  5. CT scan: vertebral, sacroiliac osteomyelitis
  6. Needle aspiration or incision and drainage if point tenderness, focal swelling, or an x-ray or scan suggestive of subperiosteal pus collection
* Treatment
  1. Immobilize limb for comfort
  2. Analgesics for pain control
  3. Antibiotic therapy
     * Neonate: cloxacillin and aminoglycoside or cloxacillin and cefotaxime
     * Child below 5 yr: cefuroxime by itself or cloxacillin and chloramphenicol in combination

- Child above 5 yr: cloxacillin (if penicillin allergic can use clindamycin)
- Sickle cell disease: add ampicillin
- Puncture wound foot: add aminoglycoside
- Once organism and sensitivities are identified, switch to appropriate antibiotic
- Duration of antibiotic treatment
  a. Acute osteomyelitis: minimum 4 wk, until all clinical signs have resolved and ESR is normal
  b. Pseudomonas osteomyelitis secondary to puncture wound of foot: for 2 wk *after* surgical debridement
  c. Chronic osteomyelitis requires long term treatment (minimum 6 mo)
- Route = IV. When switching to oral therapy, observe same guidelines as outlined in section on septic arthritis (see page 314)

4. Surgical therapy
  - Drainage if
    a. Poor response within 72 hr
    b. Subperiosteal pus
    c. Femoral head osteomyelitis with hip joint involvement
    d. Vertebral osteomyelitis with neurologic signs
  - Excision: sequestra
  - Debridement: puncture wound of foot

Parasitic Infections

- See Table 15–9

Pertussis

General Considerations

- Agent: *Bordetella pertussis*
- Incubation period: 7–21 days
- Communicability: early catarrhal to 3 wk after onset of cough

TABLE 15–9 Parasitic Diseases

Disease	Treatment
I. Intestinal nematodes	
Ascariasis[*]	Pyrantel pamoate (see p 844) or mebendazole (see p 829)
Hookworm (*Ancylostoma duodenale, Necator americanus*)	Mebendazole (see p 829) or pyrantel pamoate (see p 844)
Pinworm (Enterobius)	Pyrantel pamoate (see p 844) or mebendazole (see p 829)
Whipworm (*Trichuris trichiura*)	Mebendazole (see p 829)
Strongyloidiasis	Thiabendazole[†,‡] 50 mg/kg/day (maximum 3g/day) PO ÷ q12h × 2 days
II. Tissue nematodes	
Trichinosis	Steroids and thiabendazole[‡,§] 50 mg/kg/day (maximum 3g/day) PO ÷ q12h × 5 days
Visceral larva migrans (Toxocara)	Thiabendazole[‡,§] 50 mg/kg/day (maximum 3g/day) PO ÷ q12h × 5 days
Cutaneous larva migrans	Thiabendazole[‡] (15% cream prepared using crushed tablets) applied topically tid × 5 days
III. Cestodes (Tapeworms)	
Intestinal disease	Niclosamide[#] 30 mg/kg (maximum 2g) PO × 1 dose or Praziquantel[#] 10-20 mg/kg PO × 1 dose
Cysticercosis	Praziquantel[#] 50 mg/kg/day PO ÷ q8h × 14 days

TABLE 15–9 Parasitic Diseases (Continued)

Disease	Treatment
IV. Trematodes Schistosomiasis	Praziquantel[#] 60 mg/kg/day PO ÷ q8h × 1 day
V. Protozoa Amebiasis: Asymptomatic intestinal disease	Iodoquinol (see p 824)
Symptomatic intestinal or invasive disease	Metronidazole and iodoquinol (see p 831, 824)
Giardiasis	Metronidazole (see p 831) or quinacrine 6 mg/kg/day (maximum 300 mg/day) PO ÷ q8h × 7 days or furazolidone 5 mg/kg/day PO ÷ q6h × 10 days
Malaria[**]	
Vivax, ovale, and malariae and chloroquine sensitive falciparum malaria	Chloroquine (see p 808)
Chloroquine resistant falciparum malaria	Quinine (see p 845) + one dose PO of pyrimethamine/ sulfadoxine (Fansidar):[#,††] 2–11 mo: ¼ tablet 1–3 yr: ½ tablet 4–8 yr: 1 tablet 9–14 yr: 2 tablets >14 yr: 3 tablets

| To achieve radical cure for vivax and ovale[‡‡] | In addition to chloroquine, give primaquine 0.3 mg base/kg/day (maximum 15 mg base) PO once daily × 14 days (DO NOT GIVE PRIMAQUINE UNLESS PERSON IS TESTED AND DOES NOT HAVE G-6-PD DEFICIENCY) |

* In mixed infections treat Ascariasis first.

† Treat for 5 days in disseminated infections.

‡ Available in Canada only at designated centers.

§ Mebendazole in high doses may be used as an alternative to thiabendazole. There is no established pediatric dose.

Available in Canada on emergency release only.

** Severe infections may require IV quinine or quinidine; suggest consult infectious disease or tropical medicine specialist.

†† One tablet contains 25 mg of pyrimethamine and 500 mg of sulfadoxine.

‡‡ Not necessary for congenital or transfusion related malaria.

Clinical Features

- Catarrhal: simple cough, rhinitis (lasts 7–10 days)
- Paroxysmal: violent cough ± vomiting, whoop (lasts 2–6 wk)
- Convalescent: 2–6 wk
- Complications: otitis media, bacterial pneumonia, apnea and hypoxia (common in infants), seizures, encephalopathy, major neurologic sequelae

Management

- WBC and differential (lymphocytosis)
- Nasopharyngeal aspirate or swab for culture
- Direct fluorescent antibody (DFA) smears are unreliable because of false positive and false negative reactions
- Admit if severe illness or apnea, or family cannot provide adequate observation and handling of paroxysmal episodes at home
- Supportive care
  1. Clear airway secretions
  2. Oxygen for cyanotic episodes
- Antibiotics
  1. Erythromycin estolate 40 mg/kg/day (maximum 1 g/day) PO ÷ q6h × 14 days (may prevent paroxysmal stage if started in catarrhal stage and may shorten period of communicability)
  2. Treat secondary bacterial infections

Prevention

- Chemoprophylaxis
  1. Indications: household or close contacts if
     - <1 yr regardless of immunization status
     - <7 yr and not fully immunized
     - Some authorities believe that all contacts should receive chemoprophylaxis

2. Give erythromycin estolate 40 mg/kg/day
   (maximum 1 g/day) PO ÷ q6h × 14 days
3. Alternative to erythromycin: TMP-SMX
- Active immunization of contacts. Give DPT if
  <7 yr and either (i) unimmunized or immunizations are not up to date, (ii) partially immunized and third dose was ≥6 mo ago, or
  (iii) no DPT in last 3 yr

Pharyngitis, Streptococcal

Management

- Diagnosis: Throat culture or latex agglutination
  test for rapid detection of group A streptococcal antigen in pharyngeal secretions
- Therapy: Rationale—prevents suppurative complications (e.g., peritonsillar abscess), prevents
  rheumatic fever, and alleviates symptoms
  1. Drugs
     - Penicillin—penicillin V 25 mg/kg/day
       (maximum 1–1.2 g/day) PO ÷ bid–tid
       × 10 days or benzathine penicillin G as a
       single IM dose (<27 kg, 600,000 units;
       >27 kg, 1.2 million units)
     - Penicillin allergic patients—erythromycin
       estolate 25 mg/kg/day (maximum 1 g/day)
       PO ÷ bid–tid × 10 days
  2. Follow-up cultures not necessary unless pa-
     tient or member of family has rheumatic
     fever; then culture and, if positive, retreat
  3. Carriers are not treated unless a family mem-
     ber has rheumatic fever
  4. Clindamycin by itself × 10 days, or rifampin
     × 5 days together with penicillin × 10 days,
     is more effective than oral penicillin therapy
     alone in eradicating carrier state

Rubella

- See p 354

Septic Shock

Management

- For monitoring and the acute management of shock and its complications, see p 659
- Determine underlying risk factors
  1. Infant
  2. Predisposing conditions, e.g., neutropenia, immunosuppression, nephrotic syndrome, sickle cell anemia
  3. Intravascular or prosthetic devices
  4. Medications—steroids, chemotherapy
- Obtain necessary cultures
  1. Blood, urine, $\pm$ CSF
  2. Gram stain and cultures of infected sites
- Remove intravascular catheters; send tip for culture
- Radiologic (e.g., CXR, ECHO, CT scan) or nuclear scan studies if indicated
- Prompt institution of antibiotics
  1. Empiric choice of antibiotics depends on
     - Potential organisms
     - Underlying risk factors
     - Host factors, e.g., renal failure
  2. In normal host >3 mo: cefuroxime; alternative = cloxacillin and cefotaxime
  3. Normal infant (<3 mo): ampicillin and aminoglycoside; alternative = ampicillin and cefotaxime
  4. In neutropenia: extended spectrum penicillin (e.g., piperacillin) and aminoglycoside; alternative = ceftazidime and aminoglycoside or ceftazidime and vancomycin
  5. Line related infections: vancomycin and aminoglycoside
  6. Respiratory tract related; aspiration— clindamycin and aminoglycoside
  7. Intra-abdominal sepsis: clindamycin and aminoglycoside; alternative = metronidazole and aminoglycoside

8. Urinary tract: ampicillin and aminoglycoside
- Steroids: use is controversial (may even be contraindicated)

Sexually Transmitted Diseases

Chlamydia Trachomatis Infections

General Considerations and Clinical Features

- Causes inclusion conjunctivitis (neonates)—see p 517, pneumonia (ages 3 wk–4 mo), trachoma, and LGV infection
- Also causes cervicitis, salpingitis, and PID (see p 243) as well as urethritis, pharyngitis, and proctitis (males and females), and epididymitis
- Asymptomatic carriage can occur at all ages
- Nongonococcal urethritis usually presents 1–2 wk following intercourse (may take up to 5 wk); it also can be caused by organisms other than Chlamydia

Investigations and Treatment of Nongonococcal Cervicitis, Urethritis, and Epididymitis

- Investigate and treat if necessary for gonococcal infection (see p 342)
- Swabs for Chlamydia culture or Chlamydia antigen
- Treat for 7 days (10 days for epididymitis)
    1. If >8 yr old: tetracycline 500 mg PO qid or doxycycline 100 mg PO bid
    2. If ≤8 yr old or pregnant: erythromycin 40 mg/kg/day (maximum 2 g/day) PO ÷ qid
- Treat sexual partners

Gonococcal Infections

General Considerations

- Organism: *Neisseria gonorrhoeae*
- Incubation period: 2–7 days
- If gonococcal infection in prepubertal child,

strongly consider possibility of sexual abuse

Investigations

- Gram stain: eyes (neonates), urethra (males), vagina (prepubertal), endocervix (postpubertal)
- Cultures
  1. Males
     - Heterosexuals: urethral swabs
     - Homosexuals: urethral, pharyngeal, rectal swabs
  2. Females: endocervical, rectal, pharyngeal swabs
  3. Newborns: conjunctival swabs
  4. Children: vaginal swabs
  5. Swabs should be plated promptly onto Thayer-Martin agar plates or placed in transport medium
- Joint aspirate, blood, and CSF for culture and Gram stain if indicated
- VDRL
- Urethral (male), vaginal, and cervical cultures or antigen test for Chlamydia

Treatment

- Newborn
  1. Asymptomatic infant born to mother with gonorrhea
     - Gastric and rectal cultures (for gonorrhea and Chlamydia)
     - Routine eye prophylaxis
     - Penicillin G 100,000 units IM/IV × 1 dose
     - If resistance is suspected, use ceftriaxone 250 mg IM × 1 dose
  2. Gonococcal ophthalmitis (see p 517)
  3. Disseminated infection
     - Penicillin G IV (see p 865)
     - Use cefotaxime or ceftriaxone IV if a resistant organism is suspected
- Older children and adolescents (if evidence of sexual abuse, see also p 249)

1. Uncomplicated gonorrhea
   - Ampicillin or amoxicillin 50 mg/kg (maximum 3.5 g for ampicillin, 3 g for amoxicillin) PO and probenecid 25 mg/kg (maximum 1 g) PO single dose—or procaine penicillin G 100,000 units/kg (maximum 4.8 million units, total dose divided and given IM in two separate sites) and probenecid 25 mg/kg (maximum 1 g, single PO dose)
   - In penicillin allergy or if organism is penicillin resistant, use spectinomycin 40 mg/kg (maximum 2 g) single IM dose
   - Amoxicillin and spectinomycin are not effective for pharyngeal or anorectal gonorrhea. Therefore when treating these, use procaine penicillin G IM, or if the organism is penicillin resistant use ceftriaxone 250 mg single IM dose.
   - N.B. Everyone, *in addition* to foregoing treatment, should receive simultaneous treatment for *Chlamydia trachomatis* with either tetracycline, doxycycline, or erythromycin (see p 341)
   - Treat sexual partners
2. Disseminated infection (sepsis, arthritis)
   - Penicillin G 100,000–200,000 units/kg/day IV ÷ q6h
   - Ceftriaxone IV may be used for penicillin resistant organisms
3. Pelvic inflammatory disease (PID), see p 243
4. Epididymitis
   - Must be differentiated from testicular torsion
   - As well as gonorrhea, can be caused by *Chlamydia trachomatis*, viruses, gram negative organisms (associated with UTI), and TB
   - Treat gonorrheal epididymitis as for uncomplicated gonorrhea (see above). Remember to treat for Chlamydia (with 10 days of tetracycline, doxycycline, or erythromycin) as well.

- Report to public health for contact tracing
- Repeat VDRL in 8 wk
- Follow-up cultures in 7 days

Syphilis

General Considerations

- Agent: *Treponema pallidum*
- Incubation period: 10 days to 10 wk

Management

- Microscopic darkfield examination to identify spirochetes in material obtained from primary chancre, and skin and mucocutaneous lesions
- Serology
  1. Screening test: VDRL—if negative, repeat in 8 wk
  2. Serology may be negative early, i.e., in contacts or in patients with primary lesion
  3. Confirmatory, specific tests: FTA-ABS (fluorescent treponemal antibody absorption), MHA-TP (microhemagglutination test for TP)
  4. Antibiotic therapy (treat contacts of positive cases as if they have the disease); see Table 15–10

Follow-Up

- Report to public health for contact tracing
- Repeat VDRL at 3, 6, and 12 mo to follow response to treatment

Sinusitis

General Considerations

- Acute: *S. pneumoniae, H. influenzae, B. catarrhalis*
- Chronic: Bacteroides, anaerobic and aerobic streptococci, *S. aureus, H. influenzae*, fungus

Management

- Sinus x-rays: complete opacity, thickening of
  mucous membrane (diagnostic specificity in
  children not proven)
- Antimicrobials
    1. Acute: amoxicillin, TMP-SMX, or cefaclor
       × 10 days
    2. If severe and periorbital cellulitis, see p 319
- Antihistamines and decongestants: clinical
  efficacy not proven and also may reduce local
  resistance

Toxic Shock Syndrome

General Considerations

- Caused by toxin producing *S. aureus*
- Epidemiologically linked to use of highly
  absorbent tampons in menstruating women,
  but may occur also in younger children

Clinical Features

- Temperature ≥ 38.9° C
- Rash (diffuse, erythematous, nonpruritic, involv-
  ing soles and palms—desquamation in 1–2 wk)
- Hypotension (< 5th percentile by age for
  children)
- Involvement of three or more of the following:
    1. Gastrointestinal: vomiting, diarrhea at onset
    2. Mucous membranes: conjunctival, pharyn-
       geal, or vaginal hyperemia
    3. Muscular: severe myalgias or CK (CPK)
       ≥ 2× normal
    4. Renal: BUN or creatinine ≥ 2× normal or
       ≥ 5 WBC/HPF, in absence of UTI
    5. Hepatic: total bilirubin, AST (SGOT), or ALT
       (SGPT), ≥ 2× normal
    6. CNS: change in level of consciousness or
       disorientation with no focal neurologic signs
    7. Hematologic: platelets < 100 × 10⁹/L

TABLE 15–10   Antibiotic Therapy for Syphilis

	Without Penicillin Allergy	With Penicillin Allergy
Congenital—proven or suspected (VDRL positive baby with inadequate or unknown history of treatment of mother)		
1. Asymptomatic with normal CSF (some recommend treating all congenital syphilis, including asymptomatic, with 10 days' therapy [see below])	Benzathine penicillin G 50,000 units/kg IM single dose	
2. Symptomatic, or asymptomatic with abnormal CSF	Penicillin G 50,000 units/kg/day IM/IV ÷ q12h for a minimum of 10 days or procaine penicillin G 50,000 units/kg/day IM once daily for a minimum of 10 days	
Acquired		
1. Primary, secondary, or early latent (duration <1 yr)	Benzathine penicillin G 50,000 units/kg IM (maximum 2.4 million units—1.2 million units in each buttock)	Tetracycline (if >8 yr) or erythromycin[†] 40 mg/kg/day PO ÷ q6h (maximum 2 g/day) × 15 days

2. Latent of duration >1 yr*
   a. Normal CSF

   Benzathine penicillin G 50,000 units/kg (maximum 2.4 million units) IM once weekly × 3 wk

   Tetracycline (if >8 yr) or erythromycin[†] 40 mg/kg/day PO ÷ q6h (maximum 2 g/day) × 30 days

   b. Abnormal CSF

   Penicillin G 200,000 units/kg/day (maximum 12–18 million units/day) IV ÷ q4h × 10 days; then benzathine penicillin G 50,000 units/kg (maximum 2.4 million units) IM once weekly × 3 doses

   OR

   Procaine penicillin G 50,000 units/kg (maximum 2.4 million units) IM daily + probenecid 500 mg PO qid × 10 days; then benzathine penicillin G 50,000 units/kg (maximum 2.4 million units) IM once weekly × 3 doses

* CSF should be examined for cells, protein, and VDRL if neurosyphilis is suspected or if the patient is symptomatic. Also, the CSF should be examined in any case of syphilis of >1 year's duration when the patient is not treated with penicillin G.
† Erythromycin has not been proven to be effective; careful follow-up is required.

Differential Diagnosis

- Exclude Rocky Mountain spotted fever, meningococcemia, leptospirosis, scarlet fever, viral exanthems, Kawasaki disease

Management

- Investigation
  1. CBC and differential, platelets, PT, PTT
  2. BUN, creatinine, LFT, muscle enzymes
  3. Urinalysis
  4. Blood, urine, throat, CSF (if indicated), rectal, and vaginal cultures
  5. Serology to exclude other diagnoses (if indicated)
- Treatment
  1. Supportive care: monitoring, and respiratory and cardiovascular support (see p 659 for treatment of shock)
  2. Antibiotics
     - Cloxacillin 200 mg/kg/day IV ÷ q6h × 1–2 wk
     - In penicillin allergic patients: vancomycin

Tuberculosis

General Considerations

- Agent: *Mycobacterium tuberculosis*
- Incubation period: 4–12 wk

Management

- Investigation
  1. History of exposure
  2. Skin testing
     - Mantoux/PPD 5TU
     - Positive $\geq$ 10 mm of induration at 48–72 hr (5–10 mm may be significant in household contacts)
  3. Radiologic evidence: CXR (AP and lateral)
  4. Stains for acid-fast bacilli and TB cultures: sputum, gastric aspirate, urine, CSF (if indicated)

5. Histologic study and TB culture when indicated: lymph nodes, liver, pleura, bone marrow
- Treatment
  1. In all cases
     - Isolate if active pulmonary TB
     - Inform public health
     - Supportive care
     - In adolescents and adults, give pyridoxine when INH is used
  2. Pulmonary TB
     - INH and rifampin once daily × 9 mo (longer if known INH resistance or if cultures remain positive beyond 3 mo)
     - Alternatively: INH and rifampin once daily × 2 mo and then INH 20–40 mg/kg/dose and rifampin 10–20 mg/kg/dose twice weekly
     - If resistance is suspected, use an additional drug (e.g., streptomycin or pyrazinamide) until sensitivities are known; for treatment of drug resistant TB, suggest infectious disease consult
  3. Extrapulmonary TB
     - Meningitis
       a. INH and rifampin × 12 mo
       b. Streptomycin or pyrazinamide for the first 4–8 wk
       c. Prednisone × 4–6 wk (if there is evidence of ↓ level of consciousness, ↑ ICP, or focal signs); start with 1–2 mg/kg/day and start to taper after 1–2 wk
     - Adenitis: INH and rifampin × 9 mo

Prevention

- In all cases, if INH resistance is suspected, use INH and rifampin together instead of INH by itself
  1. Management of close household contacts of a person with active TB: If asymptomatic and

CXR is normal, do a 5TU skin test
- If 5TU is positive, INH × 12 mo
- If 5TU is negative
  a. Give INH to children <6 yr, persons who have impaired immunity, and contacts of highly infectious patients
  b. Retest all contacts in 3 mo
    - If 5TU is still negative and the infection in the index case has been controlled by treatment, stop INH (unless patient is immunosuppressed)
    - If 5TU is positive, continue or start INH as appropriate for a total of 12 mo
2. Management of 5TU skin test positive individuals ≤35 yr who are asymptomatic with normal CXR: give INH for 6–12 mo
3. Management of perinatal exposure
- Mother is 5TU positive, there is no active disease in mother or family members to whom infant will be exposed, and infant is clinically well
  a. Skin test infant at 4–6 wk and, if negative, repeat at 3 and 12 mo
  b. If family members cannot be investigated, give INH to infant until investigations are done
  c. If at any time infant develops clinical or radiologic evidence of disease, treat with INH and rifampin × 9 mo
- Mother has active TB; infant is asymptomatic (and has a normal CXR)
  a. Separate infant and mother unless or until mother is being treated and is no longer infectious
  b. Give INH for 6 mo
  c. Skin test infant at 4–6 wk and, if negative, repeat at 3 and 6 mo
  d. If maternal compliance is not assured or infant is at risk for repeated exposure, consider BCG (see p 310)
  e. Follow infant at monthly intervals

f. If skin test at 6 mo is negative and maternal infection is under control, stop therapy

g. If skin test becomes positive and infant remains asymptomatic, use INH for a total of 12 mo

h. If at any time infant develops clinical or radiologic evidence of disease, treat with INH and rifampin × 9 mo

Follow-Up

- LFT if being treated with INH (in children only if clinically indicated)
- Follow-up cultures and x-ray examinations
- Follow-up by public health

Varicella (Chicken Pox)

General Considerations

- Incubation period: 10–21 days
- Contagious from 48 hr prior to appearance of rash until 6 days after onset (immunosuppressed patients may be contagious for longer periods)

Clinical Features

- Prodrome: fever, malaise
- Rash
  1. Rapid evolution from macules →papules→vesicles
  2. Lesions in different phases are present
  3. Central distribution mainly over trunk; also present over scalp, face, and extremities
- Complications
  1. Secondary infection
  2. Pneumonia
  3. Visceral dissemination in immunocompromised hosts and newborns infected perinatally (encephalitis, pneumonia, hepatitis)

- Differential diagnosis
  1. Herpes simplex infections
  2. Zoster
  3. Impetigo
  4. Insect bites

Management

- Isolation (strict)
- Symptomatic therapy
- If immunosuppressed, IV acyclovir

Viral and Other Common Childhood Exanthems

- See Figure 15–1

Viral Hepatitis

General Considerations

- Caused by hepatitis A virus (HAV); hepatitis B virus (HBV); delta virus (δ); non-A, non-B hepatitis (NANB); CMV; EBV
- Adenovirus, enterovirus, and herpes virus can cause hepatitis in neonates
- Epidemiologic features (Table 15–11)

Clinical Features

- Jaundice may be associated with or preceded by a flulike illness
- HAV infection: usually anicteric in young children; in older children, typically a brief illness with jaundice; rarely, has a prolonged relapsing or a cholestatic course; very rarely, fulminant
- HBV infection: "healthy carriers" frequent; severity ranges from inapparent or brief illness to fulminant hepatitis; may also be associated with serum sickness-like illness (rash, arthralgia), papular acrodermatitis of childhood (Gianotti-Crosti syndrome), and membranous glomerulonephritis

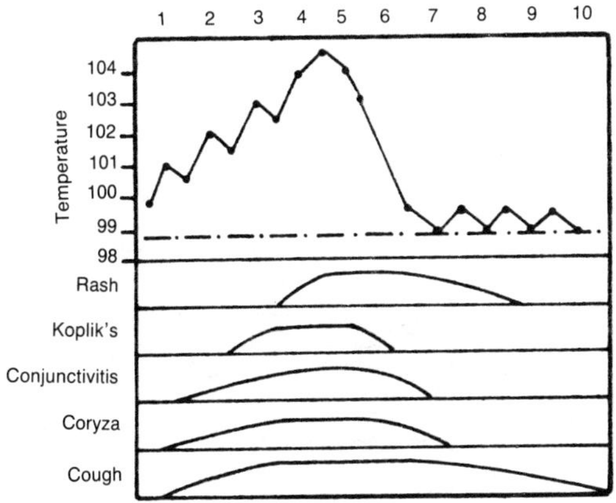

1. Measles

Rash
- Erythematous
- Maculopapular
- Starts at hairline, behind ears and
  upper neck
- Spreads to face and neck and then
  extends to trunk and extremities
- Fades in order of appearance
- Desquamates (except palms, soles)

Incubation period
- 8–13 days

Period of communicability
- 1–2 days before symptoms to
  4 days after rash appears

Therapy
- See p 298 for post-exposure
  prophylaxis

Isolation
- Respiratory

Figure 15-1 Common childhood exanthems. (Diagrams from Krugman S, Katz S, Gershon AA, Wilfert C. Infectious diseases of children, 8th ed. St. Louis: C.V. Mosby, 1985:456.)

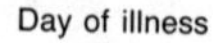

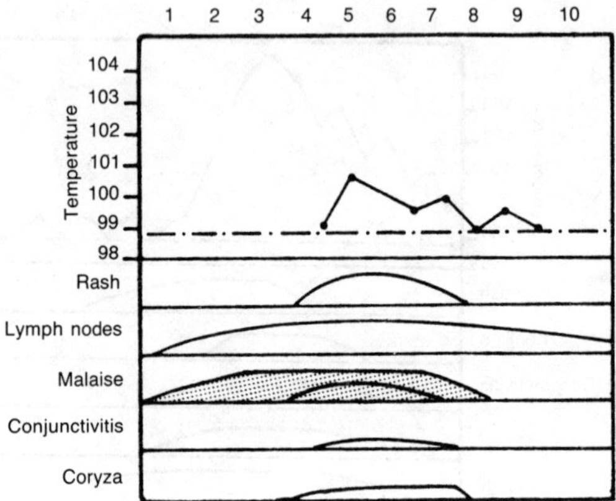

2. Rubella

Rash
- Pink
- Maculopapular
- Lesions on extremities may be
  discrete
- Starts on face, neck→trunk,
  extremities (spreads more quickly
  than measles)

Incubation period
- 14–21 days

Period of communicability
- 7 days pre-rash to 7 days after
  rash appears

Therapy
- None

Isolation
- Respiratory

Figure 15–1 Continued

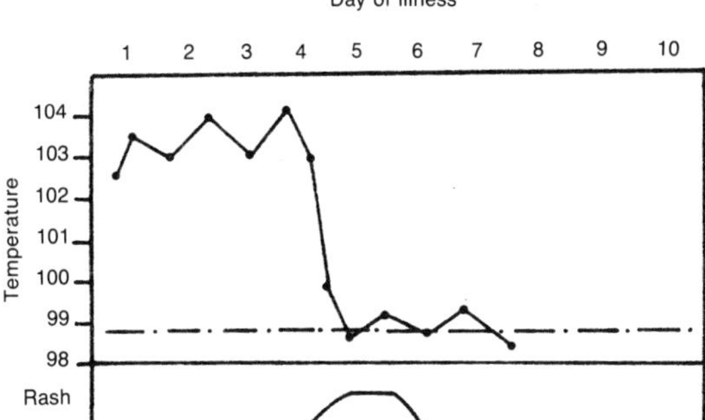

3. Roseola infantum

Rash
- Macular-maculopapular
- Neck-arms-trunk ± face
- Onset of rash accompanies
  disappearance of fever

Incubation period
- 5–15 days

Period of communicability
- Unknown

Therapy
- None

Isolation
- None

Figure 15–1 Continued

**4. Erythema infectiosum
(a parvovirus infection)**

Rash
- Red flushed face, slapped-cheek
  appearance
- Maculopapular rash over trunk and
  extremities with lacelike
  appearance

Incubation period
- 4–14 days

Period of communicability
- Unknown

Therapy
- None

Isolation
- Respiratory (for 7 days following
  onset of illness)

Figure 15–1 Continued

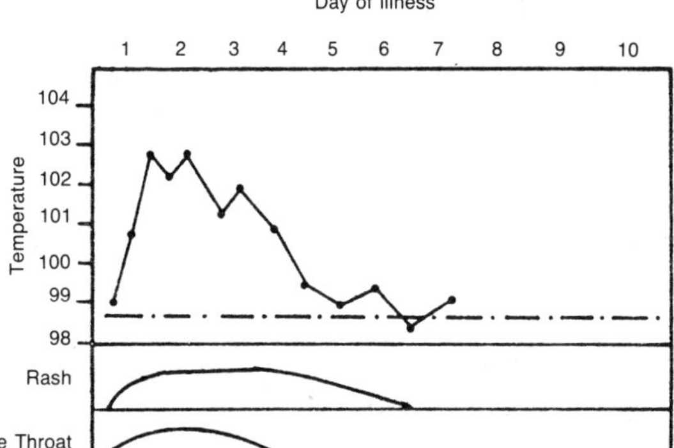

5. Scarlet fever

Rash
- Erythematous
- Blanches on pressure
- Starts in axillae, groin, and neck
  → generalized
- Circumoral pallor
- Desquamates (palms, soles
  involved)

Incubation period
- Occurs 2–5 days following streptococcal pharyngitis or impetigo

Period of communicability
- Maximum during the acute
  infection

Therapy
- Penicillin or erythromycin
  × 10 days

Isolation
- Barrier until on antibiotics for 24 hr

Figure 15–1 Continued

- NANB infection: specific agents not identified; severity ranges from mild (biochemical abnormalities only) to fulminant
- Delta infection: may be severe; causes disease only in persons who have HBV infection (i.e., HBsAg positive)

Management

- Investigation
  1. CBC, bilirubin (total, direct), AST (SGOT), ALT (SGPT), PT, PTT
  2. Hepatitis B serology
     - HBsAg (its presence indicates infectivity)—occurs in either acute infection or chronic infection-carrier state
     - Anti-HBs—indicates either past infection, passive acquisition of antibody (transplacental or parenteral immune globulin), or immune response from HBV vaccination (anti-HBc negative)
     - If HBsAg is positive
       a. IgM anti-HBc—indicates recent infection with HBV (remains positive for 4–6 mo); sometimes may be the only indication of recent infection when HBsAg has been cleared but anti-HBs has not yet appeared
       b. Anti-HBc—indicates previous infection with HBV
       c. HBeAg—serum is highly infective
       d. Anti-HBe—serum has comparatively low infectivity
  3. Delta serology (ordered in severe acute hepatitis B or deterioration of a stable chronic HBsAg carrier)
     - If positive and IgM anti-HBc is positive, assume coinfection with HBV
     - If positive and IgM anti-HBc is negative, assume superimposed infection on HBV carrier

TABLE 15–11 Epidemiology of Viral Hepatitis

	HAV	HBV	NANB	
			Sporadic/Epidemic Form(s)	Post-transfusion Form(s)
Incubation period—usual (range)	25–30 days (15–50 days)	60–90 days (50–180 days)	26–42 days (15–64 days)	42–63 days (14–180 days)
Route of transmission	Fecal-oral	Exposure to infected serum or secretions (transfusion, IV drug abuse, intimate contact)	Probably fecal-oral (e.g., contaminated water)	Exposure to infected serum
Infectivity	2 wk prior to and 1 wk after onset of jaundice	While HBsAg is positive Carrier state exists	Unknown May be similar to HAV Carrier state may exist	Unknown Carrier state exists

    4. Hepatitis A serology: IgM anti-HAV = recent
       infection; positive for 4–6 mo
    5. EBV, toxoplasmosis, CMV titers
    6. Cultures for CMV (urine), adenovirus (stools),
       enterovirus (stools, throat), and herpes virus
       when indicated

- Treatment
  1. Supportive; no diet or exercise restriction necessary
  2. Corticosteroids are not indicated
  3. Admit if confusion, high temperature, dehydration, renal impairment, severe jaundice, prolongation of PT, or social considerations
  4. Fulminant liver failure, see p 171
  5. Post-exposure prophylaxis, see p 301 (hepatitis A) and p 302 (hepatitis B)

Follow-Up

- Advise patient or parents to return in case of increased jaundice, confusion, recurrence of vomiting, or bleeding—i.e., signs of fulminant hepatitis
- Monthly follow-up necessary until clinical resolution to exclude chronic disease
- Apparent acute hepatitis is a possible presentation of either chronic active hepatitis or Wilson's disease (see p 173)

Suggested Reading

1. Benenson AS, ed. Control of communicable diseases in man. 14th ed. Washington, D.C.: American Public Health Association, 1985.
2. Feigin RD, Cherry JD. Textbook of pediatric infectious diseases. 2nd ed. Philadelphia: W.B. Saunders, 1987.
3. Krugman S, Katz S, Gershon AA, Wilfert C. Infectious diseases of children. 8th ed. St. Louis: C.V. Mosby, 1985.
4. National Advisory Committee on Immunization. A guide to immunization for Canadians. 2nd ed. Ottawa: Health Protection Branch, Laboratory Centre for Disease Control (Health & Welfare Canada), 1984.

5. Peter G, Giebink GS, Hall CB, Plotkin SA. Committee on infectious diseases, American academy of pediatrics. Report of the committee on infectious diseases (the "red book"). 20th ed. Elk Grove Village, Illinois: American Academy of Pediatrics, 1986.
6. Remington JS, Klein JO. Infectious diseases of the fetus and newborn infant. 2nd ed. Philadelphia: W.B. Saunders, 1983.

PROTOCOL FOR THE MANAGE-MENT OF THE PATIENT WITH HYPERPHENYLALANINEMIA

General Considerations

- A positive phenylketonuria (PKU) screening test must be followed up immediately, but is not diagnostic of PKU
- It is important to confirm hyperphenylalaninemia and to rule out acquired causes of increased plasma phenylalanine levels, such as transient tyrosinemia of the newborn and parenteral hyperalimentation

Clinical Features

- There may be no clinical abnormalities, especially in early infancy. Older infants with classic PKU usually show marked developmental delay.
- Infants with biopterin defects show microcephaly, intractable seizures, and progressive developmental deterioration in spite of apparently adequate dietary treatment of hyperphenylalaninemia

Management

- Investigations
  1. Urine amino acid screen (thin layer chromatography) to identify infants with neonatal tyrosinemia
  2. Quantitative plasma phenylalanine analysis daily to monitor response to treatment
  3. Random urine for biopterin-neopterin and tetrahydrobiopterin (BH_4) analysis to identify biopterin defects:

Transfer 15–20 ml fresh urine immediately into container with 500 mg ascorbic acid, and store frozen and protected from light until analysis

4. Random urine for urinary catecholamines and metabolites (to rule out BH$_4$ deficiency): Transfer at least 20 ml of urine (pooling specimens if necessary) into acid-washed container obtained from laboratory

5. BH$_4$ loading test (to identify biopterin biosynthesis defects)
   - Must be done while the patient is hyperphenylalaninemic, >600 μmol/L (>10 mg/dl)
   - After urines have been collected for biopterin-neopterin and catecholamine analyses, administer BH$_4$ by nasogastric tube at a dosage of 2 mg/kg or a total of 20 mg, whichever is greater. Flush tubing with water.
   - Take blood samples for quantitative measurement of plasma phenylalanine immediately before and then at 3, 6, and 18–24 hr after the BH$_4$. A sharp drop in the plasma phenylalanine level by 3 hr suggests a defect in biopterin biosynthesis.

6. The most reliable test for dihydropteridine reductase deficiency is direct measurement of the enzyme in blood or cultured skin fibroblasts

7. Electroencephalogram

- Treatment
  1. Begin dietary therapy with phenylalanine-restricted formula with no milk or conventional prepared formula added until plasma phenylalanine level is 365–730 μmol/L (6–12 mg/dl). Then add formula or breast milk to increase phenylalanine intake until plasma level is maintained at 365–730 μmol/L (6–12 mg/dl) on measurements done three times weekly.

2. Treatment should be done in consultation with the therapeutic dietitian
3. Patients with biopterin defects require treatment with the neurotransmitter precursors, L-dopa, carbidopa, and 5-hydroxytryptophan

Follow-Up

- Treatment requires regular measurements of blood phenylalanine levels (e.g., by Guthrie test) initially at intervals of two to three times weekly and then two to four times monthly as the patient becomes older and stabilized
- Close consultation with a therapeutic dietitian is critical to the long term success of management

NEUROLOGIC PRESENTATION OF METABOLIC DISEASE

- See Table 16–1

... gic Presentation of Metabolic Disease

Presentation	Characteristics	Examples
Psychomotor retardation	Progressive, severe, associated with CNS signs	Aminoacidopathies: maple syrup urine disease (MSUD), PKU, infant of maternal PKU, homocystinuria Organic acidopathies: methylmalonic acidemia (MMA), propionic acidemia (PA) CNS storage disease: Tay-Sachs, metachromatic leukodystrophy (MLD) Krabbe, Sanfilippo, neuronal ceroid lipofuscinosis (NCL) Primary lactic acidosis, Lesch-Nyhan, Leigh disease
Seizures	Early onset, multiple types, resistant to conventional anticonvulsants	Nonketotic hyperglycinemia, pyridoxine dependency, NCL, hypoglycemia, hypocalcemia, hypomagnesemia, Menkes
Hypotonia	Peripheral	Glycogen storage disease II, myopathic carnitine deficiency, mitochondrial myopathies
	Central	Zellweger, Ehlers-Danlos, Menkes, nonketotic hyper-glycinemia
Movement disorders	Progressive or intermittent ataxia	Urea cycle enzyme disorders (UCED), MSUD, Hartnup, MLD, MMA, PA, GM2 gangliosidosis, Refsum, abetalipoproteinemia
	Chorea, athetosis, dystonia	Wilson, Lesch-Nyhan
Disorders of conscious-ness	Intermittent lethargy and drowsiness, especially with intercurrent febrile illness	MSUD, systemic carnitine deficiency (recurrent "Reye syndrome"), UCED, MMA, PA

HEPATIC PRESENTATION OF METABOLIC DISEASE IN THE OLDER CHILD

Clinical Features

- Hepatomegaly, hypoglycemia, hyperammonemia
- Hepatic dysfunction—vomiting, irritability, jaundice, abnormal enzymes, coagulation defects
- Table 16–2 lists hepatic disorders

Management

- Investigations
  1. Blood ammonium
  2. Venous blood gases, electrolytes (anion gap), glucose
  3. Lactic acid, 3-hydroxybutyrate
  4. Uric acid
  5. AST (SGOT), alkaline phosphatase, bilirubin—total and direct, albumin, prothrombin time (PT), bleeding time
  6. Galactosemia screen (RBC assay, before transfusion, for galactose-1-phosphate uridyl transferase)
  7. Quantitative plasma amino acids (0.5 ml heparinized blood)
  8. Serum carnitine, α_1-antitrypsin protease inhibitor (PI) typing
  9. Urine—Dextrostix, Clinitest tablets, routine urinalysis, ketones, organic acids
  10. Sweat chloride
- Initial treatment
  1. Discontinue protein
  2. Withhold fructose and lactose containing food
  3. Correct hypoglycemia (see p 119)
  4. Correct acidosis (if $HCO_3^- < 8$) slowly
  5. Vitamin K, fresh frozen plasma.

TABLE 16–2 Hepatic Disorders

Disorder	Special Features	Results of Investigation	Specific Treatment
Galactosemia	See p 402. Older children may present with cirrhosis, mental retardation, recurrent hypoglycemia		
Hereditary fructose intolerance	Symptoms only upon ingestion of fructose, sucrose, sorbitol, variable in severity Seizures, colic, vomiting, diarrhea, jaundice, hepatomegaly May cause acute liver failure or renal Fanconi syndrome	Hypoglycemia, marked metabolic acidosis, ↑ uric acid, ↓ phosphate Urine—negative Clinistix (glucose), positive Clinitest tablets (reducing substances) Chromatography of urine shows generalized aminoaciduria	Elimination of fructose, sucrose, sorbitol from diet
Tyrosinemia, type I	Presents acutely at 8–12 weeks or with acute-on-chronic liver disease, ↑ bleeding, ↑ risk of hepatocellular carcinoma	↑ plasma methionine and tyrosine, ↑ α-fetoprotein, ↑ PT, ↑ PTT, abnormal LFTs, ↑ urinary succinylacetone, renal tubular defects	Diet restricted in tyrosine and phenylalanine Liver transplant
α_1-Antitrypsin deficiency	Pulmonary dysfunction, emphysema Liver disease-cirrhosis, cholestatic jaundice, hepatomegaly, ↑ risk of hepatocellular carcinoma	Abnormal pulmonary function tests, abnormal LFTs, ↓ serum α_1-antitrypsin, missing α_1 globulin peak on protein electrophoresis P typing Characteristic liver biopsy	Supportive therapy

Continued

TABLE 16-2 (continued)

Glycogen storage disease, type IV—brancher glycogenosis	Hepatosplenomegaly, ascites, liver failure, early cirrhosis	Abnormal LFTs, liver biopsy—electron microscopy	Supportive therapy
Glycogen storage disease, type III	Hepatomegaly, may be hypoglycemic, hypotonic, short stature	Glucagon stimulation test Liver biopsy for debrancher enzyme assay	Supportive therapy
Glycogen storage disease, type I—Von Gierke	Characteristic facies, massive hepatomegaly, hypoglycemic seizures, short stature, bleeding diathesis	Hypoglycemia, ↑ lactate, ↑ uric acid, ↑ triglycerides, ↑ urinary ketones, ↑ bleeding time (platelet dysfunction), ↓ response to glucagon	Overnight glucose, uncooked cornstarch before bed
Wilson disease—hepatolenticular degeneration	Possible presentations: hepatitis-like illness, acute liver failure, cirrhosis, hemolytic anemia, neurologic, psychiatric, Kayser-Fleischer rings (slit lamp)	Abnormal LFTs, ↓ serum ceruloplasmin, ↓ total serum copper, ↑ urinary copper after penicillamine loading Peripheral smear may show hemolysis Renal tubular dysfunction, generalized aminoaciduria Liver biopsy—copper deposition	D-penicillamine
Systemic carnitine deficiency	Recurrent attacks resembling Reye syndrome of hypoglycemia, hyperammonemia, and hepatic encephalopathy Skeletal myopathy May have cardiomyopathy	Abnormal LFTs, ↑ NH_4^+, ↓ glucose, may have metabolic acidosis, ↓ carnitine in plasma, muscle (skeletal and cardiac), and liver Dicarboxylic acids in urine	Fat restriction Glucose supplementation L-carnitine administration

STORAGE DISORDERS

Clinical Features

- Somatic dysmorphism—facies, hepatosplenomegaly
- Skeleton—dysostosis multiplex, joint contractures, short stature
- Corneal clouding
- Deafness

Management

- Urinary mucopolysaccharide screen (MPS spot test)
- Urinary oligosaccharide screen (thin layer chromatography)
- X-ray views of hands, chest, and spine—dysostosis multiplex
- Peripheral smear—leukocyte inclusions
- Bone marrow—storage cells
- WBC—↓ lysosomal enzyme activity
- Cultured skin fibroblasts for enzyme assay
- Treatment is supportive only

- See Table 16-3

TABLE 16–3 Storage Disorders

Disorder*	Mental Retardation	Corneal Clouding	Hepatosplenomegaly	Skeletal Abnormalities	Urine Spot Test
MPS IH (Hurler)	+ + +	+ +	+ +	+ + +	MPS + + +
MPS IS (Scheie)	0	+ +	+ +	+ +	MPS + + +
MPS II (Hunter)†	+ → + + +	0	+ +	+ +	MPS + +
MPS III (Sanfilippo)	+ + +	0	±	±	MPS ±
MPS IV (Morquio)	0	+	±	+ + +	MPS ±
MPS VI (Maroteaux-Lamy)	0	+ + +	+	+ +	MPS + + +
MPS VII (Sly)	+ + +	0	+	+ +	MPS + +
GM1 gangliosidosis	+ + +	±	+ + +	±	Oligo + + +
I-Cell disease	0 → + + +	0	0 → + + +	+ +	Oligo ±
Sialidosis	+ + +	±	+ +	±	Oligo ±
Gaucher disease					
Type I (adult)	0	0	+ + +	±	0
Type II (infantile)	+ + +	0	+ + +	0	0
Niemann-Pick disease type A	+ + +	0	+ + +	0	0

* MPS = mucopolysaccharidosis.
† X-linked.

DIFFERENTIATION BETWEEN LARGE AND SMALL MOLECULE DISEASE

- See Table 16–4

Suggested Reading

1. Adams RD, Lyon G. Neurology of hereditary metabolic diseases of children. New York: McGraw-Hill, 1982.
2. Ampola MG. Metabolic diseases in pediatric practice. Boston: Little, Brown, 1982.
3. Cohen RM, Roth KS. Metabolic disease: a guide to early recognition. Philadelphia: W.B. Saunders, 1983.
4. Stanbury JB, Wyngaarden JB. The metabolic basis of inherited disease. 5th ed. New York: McGraw-Hill, 1983.

TABLE 16–4 Differentiation Between Large and Small Molecule Disease

	Large Molecule	Small Molecule
Onset	Gradual	Acute
Course	Relentlessly progressive	Exacerbations and remissions; responsive to treatment
Features	Often with somatic dysmorphism	Normosomatic
Secondary metabolic phenomena	Subtle	Prominent
Histopathology	Often helpful	Rarely helpful
Investigations	Urinary MPS and oligosaccharides, bone marrow and peripheral leukocyte inclusions	Venous blood gases, electrolytes, blood glucose, NH_4^+, serum lactate, serum carnitine, 3-hydroxybutyrate, plasma and urine amino acids, urine organic acids
	X-ray films	
	Tissue biopsy: skin fibroblasts, liver enzyme assay	Urinalysis—reducing substances and ketones
Treatment	Usually no treatment except symptomatic	Specific treatment may be available
Examples	Mucopolysaccharidoses I-VII	Aminoacidopathies: tyrosinemia, homocystinuria, Hartnup disease, MSUD
	Mucolipidoses, e.g., GM1 gangliosidosis, I-cell disease	Organic acidopathies: methylmalonic acidemia, propionic acidemia
	Sphingolipidoses, e.g., Tay-Sachs, MLD, Krabbe	

17 NEONATOLOGY

CLASSIFICATION OF THE NEWBORN

- By gestational age (GA) (in completed weeks from the first day of the last menstrual period)
  1. Preterm: <37 wk
  2. Term: 37–42 wk
  3. Post-term: >42 wk
- By intrauterine growth standards based on intrauterine growth curves of the population between the -2 SD and $+2$ SD (appropriate for GA) and $>+2$ SD (LGA) or <-2 SD (SGA)(where SD = standard deviation); (Fig. 17–1, 17–2)

The SGA Infant

- Associated with
  1. Maternal hypertensive disease, severe toxemia, class D diabetic, disseminated lupus erythematosus. Putative cause: placental insufficiency due to maternal uterine vascular disease.
  2. Congenital infections (TORCH)
  3. Congenital malformations, chromosomal abnormalities
  4. Other causes: smoking, alcohol, multiple pregnancy
- Neonatal risk
  1. Small brown fat reserves: avoid hypothermia
  2. Small glycogen and fat reserves predisposing to hypoglycemia: early feeding and blood sugar monitoring
  3. Polycythemia with hyperviscosity syndrome: measure hematocrit, partial exchange transfusion (see p 423)

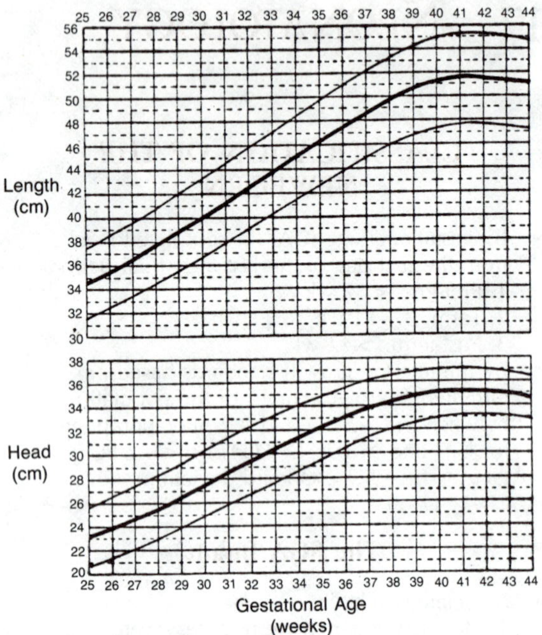

Smoothed curve values for the mean ± 2 standard deviations of crown-heel length and head circumference against gestational age.

Figure 17–1 Length and head circumference in relation to gestational age. (From Usher R, McLean F. Intrauterine growth of live-born Caucasian infants at sea level. J Pediatr 1969; 74:906.)

The LGA Infant

- Associated with
  1. Maternal diabetes or prediabetes, gestational diabetes
  2. Islet cell dysplasia
  3. Rh isoimmunization
  4. Beckwith-Wiedemann syndrome
  5. Racial or familial

374

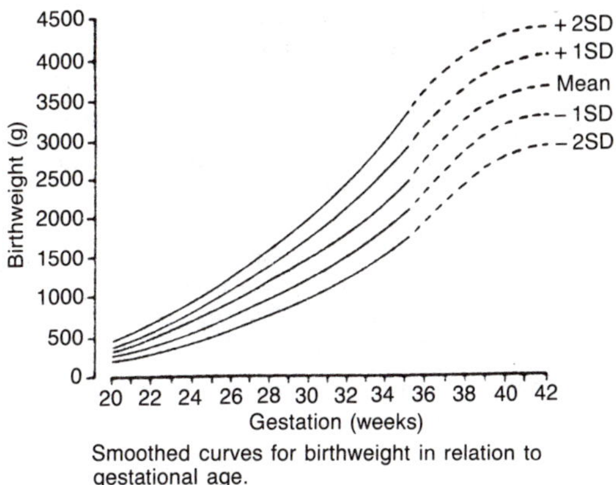

Smoothed curves for birthweight in relation to gestational age.

Figure 17–2 Birthweight in relation to gestational age. (From Keen DV, Pearse RG. Birthweight between 14 and 42 weeks' gestation. Arch Dis Child 1985; 60:443.)

- Neonatal risk
  1. Hyperinsulinism with hypoglycemia: early feeding and blood sugar monitoring

Clinical Assessment of Gestational Age (GA)

- These assessments are accurate ± 1 wk only over about 32 wk GA. Full Dubowitz assessment (see Fig. 17–3) should be delayed in the VLBW infant needing minimal handling. Further, the neurologic component may be quite inaccurate initially in the sick infant.
  1. In all babies admitted, perform a Parkin assessment (Table 17–1)
  2. Measure length and head circumference yourself
  3. Always plot the measurements on charts provided. Note discrepancies between SDs and explain

TABLE 17–1 Parkin Assessment of Gestational Age

Soft Tissue Assessment
  a. Skin texture
     Tested by picking up a fold of abdominal skin between finger and thumb and by inspection
     0: Very thin with gelatinous feel
     1: Thin and smooth
     2: Smooth and of medium thickness; irritation rash, and superficial peeling may be present
     3: Slight thickening and stiff feeling with superficial cracking and peeling, especially evident in the hands and feet
     4: Thick and parchment-like with superficial or deep cracking
  b. Skin color
     Estimated by inspection when the baby is quiet
     0: Dark red
     1: Uniformly pink
     2: Pale, pink, though the color may vary in different parts of the body; some parts may be very pale
     3: Pale, nowhere really pink except on the ears, lips, palms, and soles
  c. Breast size
     Measured by picking up the breast tissue between finger and thumb
     0: No breast tissue palpable
     1: Breast tissue palpable on one or both sides, neither being more than 0.5 cm in diameter
     2: Breast tissue palpable on both sides, one or both being 0.5–1.0 cm in diameter
     3: Breast tissue palpable on both sides, one or both being more than 1.0 cm in diameter
  d. Ear firmness
     Tested by palpation and folding of the upper pinna
     0: Pinna feels soft and is easily folded into bizarre positions without springing back into position spontaneously
     1: Pinna feels soft along the edge and is easily folded but returns in places and the pinna springs back readily after being folded
     2: Cartilage can be felt to the edge of the pinna, though it is thin in places and the pinna springs back readily after being folded
     3: Pinna firm with definite cartilage extending peripherally and springs back immediately into position after being folded

Score	GA in weeks
1	27
2	30
3	33
4	34½
5	36
6	37
7	38½
8	39½
9	40
10	41
11–12	>41

From Parkin M, Hey E, Clowes YS. Rapid assessment of gestational age at birth. Arch Dis Child 1976; 51:529.

NEONATAL EMERGENCIES

Delivery Room Care

Anticipating Problems

- Early identification of "high risk" pregnancies should lead to anticipation and therefore prevention of potential catastrophic events in the delivery suite. The following are examples of conditions that mandate the presence of a skilled neonatal resuscitator at the delivery:
1. Maternal and delivery related problems
   - Severe toxemia
   - Multiple pregnancy ($\geq$ two fetuses)
   - Prolonged rupture of membranes or maternal fever
   - Antepartum hemorrhage (APH), e.g., placenta previa, abruption
   - Medical problem (e.g., diabetes mellitus) in mother
   - Cesarean section or midforceps deliveries, breech extraction
   - Previous perinatal deaths
2. Fetal conditions
   - Evidence of fetal distress
     a. Loss of beat to beat variability

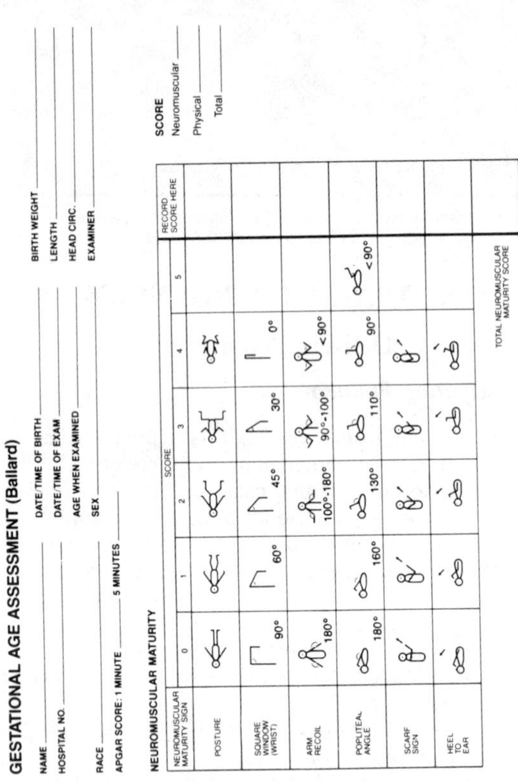

Figure 17–3 Modified Dubowitz assessment. Sample of a form used to estimate gestational age by evaluation of various aspects of maturity. Sl. = slightly (Reproduced with permission of the Mead Johnson Nutritional Group, Evansville, IN 47721)

PHYSICAL MATURITY

PHYSICAL MATURITY SIGN	SCORE						RECORD SCORE HERE
	0	1	2	3	4	5	
SKIN	gelatinous, red, transparent	smooth, pink, visible veins	superficial peeling and or rash, few veins	cracking pale area, rare veins	parchment deep, cracking, no vessels	leathery, cracked, wrinkled	
LANUGO	none	abundant	thinning	bald areas	mostly bald		
PLANTAR CREASES	no crease	faint red marks	anterior transverse crease only	creases anterio 2/3	creases cover entire sole		
BREAST	barely perceptible	flat areola, no bud	stippled areola, 1-2mm bud	raised areola, 3-4mm bud	full areola, 5-10mm bud		
EAR	pinna flat, stays folded	slightly curved pinna; soft with slow recoil	well-curved pinna; soft, but ready recoil	formed & firm with instant recoil	thick cartilage, ear stiff		
GENITALS (Male)	scrotum empty, no rugae		testes descending, few rugae	testes down, good rugae	testes pendulous, deep rugae		
GENITALS (Female)	prominent clitoris & labia minora		majora & minora equally prominent	majora large, minora small	clitoris & minora completely covered		

TOTAL PHYSICAL MATURITY SCORE

Reference
Ballard JL, Novak KK, Driver M. A simplified score for assessment of
fetal maturation of newly born infants. *J Pediatr* 95:769-774, 1979
Reprinted by permission of Dr Ballard and *Journal of Pediatrics*

MATURITY RATING

TOTAL MATURITY SCORE	GESTATIONAL AGE (WEEKS)
5	26
10	28
15	30
20	32
25	34
30	36
35	38
40	40
45	42
50	44

GESTATIONAL AGE (weeks)

By dates _____________

By ultrasound _____________

By score _____________

b. Late decelerations
        c. Decreased fetal movements
        d. Thick meconium stained liquor
  • Prematurity/intrauterine growth retardation
    (IUGR)
  • Antenatally diagnosed life threatening malfor-
    mation or metabolic disorder

Resuscitation

- In the case (delivery) room, ensure that resuscitation equipment is ready
  1. Laryngoscope (with blade sizes 0 and 1)
     functioning
  2. Endotracheal tubes (ETTs) of appropriate sizes
     available (2.5–3.5 mm) and Magill forceps
  3. Radiant heater *on*, and clean warm towels
     available
  4. Anesthesia bag (with O_2 connected) and
     masks of appropriate size (0, 1, 2)
  5. DeLee suction or suction tubes available
     (with suction functioning)
  6. Umbilical catheterization tray with 3.5 and
     5.0 F catheters at hand
  7. EMERGENCY DRUGS
     • Na bicarbonate, 8.4%—diluted to 4.2%
       with D5W or sterile water
     • 10–25% Dextrose
     • 5% albumin
     • Naloxone
     • Epinephrine, 1:10,000
- Following delivery
  1. Note time, and take baby from obstetrician in
     a warm towel
  2. Transfer to radiant heater cot and dry
     thoroughly; 85–90% of newborns require no
     further intervention (N/G suctioning can be
     done after 5 min APGAR)
- The remainder are managed as follows
  1. Gently suction oropharynx and nares, limit-
     ing insertion of catheter via nose and mouth
     to 4 cm (to avoid vagal response)

2. APGAR scores (Table 17–3) calculated at 1 min and infant approached accordingly (Fig. 17–4, Table 17–4)

- *Resuscitation measures should precede the APGAR assessment at 1 min if deemed necessary; the heart rate is the best guide in this situation.*

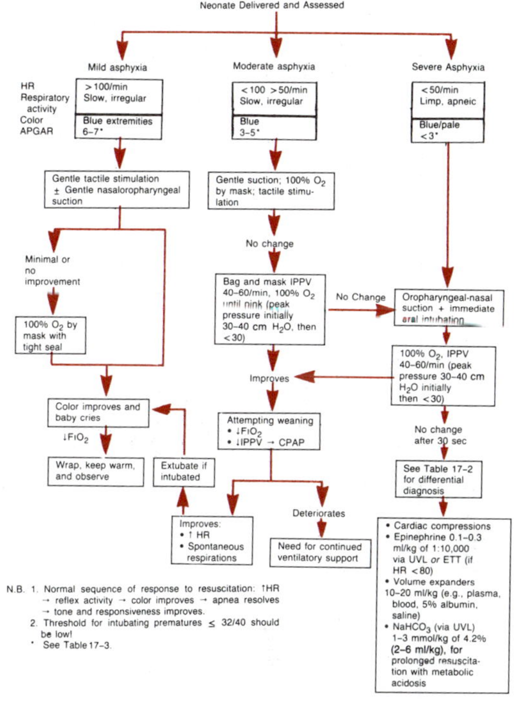

Figure 17–4 Guide to assessment and management of neonate at delivery.

TABLE 17–2 Management of Nonresponse to IPPV

Cause of Nonresponse	Diagnostic Features	Action
ETT not in correct location	Auscultate for asymmetric air entry and chest movement Chest x-ray to confirm position	When in doubt, reintubate and reassess
Tension pneumothorax	Displaced apex beat ± hemodynamic compromise Decreased or unequal air entry Chest x-ray to confirm or trans-illuminate	Drain with butterfly needle until stable; then insert chest tube
Massive meconium aspiration	History of fetal distress and "pea soup" liquor staining Chest x-ray characteristic	Suction airways Intubate, ventilate ± sedation and paralysis Watch for pneumo-thorax

Diaphragmatic hernia	Scaphoid abdomen noted at birth ± resp. distress Bowel sounds heard over chest Chest x-ray diagnostic	Pass N/G tube and connect to low-gomco Intubate → IPPV and transfer to tertiary center ASAP ↑ risk of PFC
Hypoplastic lungs	H/O oligohydramnios ± PROM ± Potter's facies Chest x-ray characteristic	Urgent intubation Require high peak pressures ± IMV
Sepsis neonatorum ± congenital pneumonia	Maternal H/O PROM or fever Chest x-ray suspicious, but may look like RDS Cultures may be positive	Antibiotics Ventilatory support ± Volume expanders ± Inotropes

TABLE 17–3   Apgar Score*

Apgar	Sign	0	1	2
Appearance	Color	Blue, pale	Body pink, extremities blue	Completely pink
Pulse	Heart rate	Absent	<100/min	>100/min
Grimace	Reflex irritability	No response	Grimace	Cry
Activity	Muscle tone	Limp, flaccid	Some flexion of extremities	Active, well flexed
Respiration	Respiratory effort	Absent	Gasping, slow irregular	Regular, good lusty cry

* N.B. An APGAR score should be done at 1 and 5 min and thereafter at 5 min intervals until a score of ≥ 7 is achieved. Modified from Ostheimer GW. Resuscitation of the newborn infants. Clin Perinatol 1982; February: 183.

Table 17–4   Thick (''Pea Soup'') Meconium Stained Liquor Noted During Delivery

Nasal suction by obstetrician when ''crowning'' occurs is recommended

Radiant heater; supine. DO NOT STIMULATE!

Intubate

Suction trachea by using ETT as suction catheter

Reintubate and suction until clear

Dry thoroughly; place dry blanket under infant. Don't wrap.

Stimulate to breathe, if necessary

O_2 by mask, keeping tight seal, to improve color if necessary (may need some IPPV)

Aspiration of stomach *early* to avoid further aspiration of swallowed meconium

(Modified from Merritt TA. Respiratory distress. In: Ziai M, Clarke TA, Merritt TA, eds. Assessment of the newborn. Boston: Little, Brown, 1984:167–168.)

Neonatal Seizures

General Considerations

- Multifactorial etiologies are most frequently associated with neonatal seizures (Table 17–5)

Clinical Features

- Signs and symptoms of seizures in newborns are often subtle—e.g., apnea, eye deviation, tonic posturing, bicycling leg movements, ''sucking''
- Do not confuse with jitteriness (these movements cease when limb is held or flexed); i.e., jitteriness is stimulus sensitive

Management

- Investigations
  1. Biochemical: electrolytes, Ca^{2+}, Mg^{2+}, arterial blood gas (ABG), glucose (Chemstrip bG + serum glucose), ± serum NH_4
  2. Septic screen—CBC, diff. and appropriate cultures, ± TORCH screen

TABLE 17–5   Etiology of Neonatal Seizures and their Approximate Time of Onset*

	0–3 Days	4–7 Days	After 10 Days
Brain injury[†]	+		
Complicated hypocalcemia	+		
Benign hypocalcemia		+	
Hypoglycemia	+		
Pyridoxine dependency	+	+	+
Infection (TORCH, meningitis, sepsis)	+	+	+
Malformation	±	+	+
Metabolic defects [‡]		+	+
Subdural			+
Drug withdrawal	+	+	+
IVH/SEH	+		

* Modified from Weiner HL, et al, eds. Pediatric neurology. 2nd ed. Baltimore: Williams & Wilkins, 1982:50.
[†] Most common cause (includes asphyxia, trauma).
[‡] Urea cycle disorders, MSUD, PKU, galactosemia.

386

3. Metabolic screen on plasma and urine
4. EEG, head ultrasound, $\pm$ CT SCAN
5. N.B. When etiology is obvious, many of above investigations may be bypassed

- Treatment
  1. Specific therapy
     - Treat as appropriate, e.g., D10W for hypoglycemia (see p 395) and 10% calcium gluconate for hypocalcemia (see p 398)
  2. Symptomatic therapy—drugs
     - Phenobarbitone, 10 mg/kg, slow IV push. May repeat in 20–30 min. Maximum 20–30 mg/kg in 24 hr.
       Drug level in 48 hr; then commence maintenance 4–6 mg/kg/day IV/PO. Therapeutic levels: 65–130 μmol/L (15–30 mg/L).
       N.B. May produce *apnea!*
     - Phenytoin (Dilantin)—used if phenobarbital not successful in maximal doses (20–30 mg/kg)
       Loading dose 10–20 mg/kg by *slow* IV push (not >1 mg/kg/min) divided into two doses. (N.B. Congeals when mixed with dextrose-containing solutions.) Maintenance 3–5 mg/kg/day IV (not well absorbed orally). Therapeutic level 40–80 μmol/L (10–20 mg/L)
     - Paraldehyde—for seizures resistant to above therapy. Dilute 5 ml of solution (1 gm/ml) in 95 ml of "⅔–⅓" IV solution (i.e., 3.33% dextrose in 0.3% saline). Infuse at rate of 0.5–2 ml/kg/hr. Titrate to patient response.
     - Diazepam (Valium) as continuous infusion in dosage of 0.3 mg/kg/hr (mixed with normal saline) has been found safe and effective treatment in some resistant cases (may →↑ unconjugated bilirubin)
     - Pyridoxine: 50–150 mg IM/IV under EEG monitoring is in order as a trial, if all else

fails. EEG should normalize in pyridoxine dependency.
- In persistent cases further management must be undertaken only after discussion with staff neonatologist
- N.B. *Do not overtreat*! The prognosis is related to the etiology, not to seizures per se.

- Prognosis and follow-up
  1. Duration of therapy is controversial, but dependent on etiology to some extent
  2. In most uncomplicated cases anticonvulsants could be discontinued (at least as a trial) prior to discharge from the nursery
  3. Alternatively the infant could be maintained on the same dose and allowed to be weaned by growth only, then discontinued at $\sim$ 3 mo, as long as EEG and development are normal and infant is seizure-free
  4. In general the following suggest poor prognosis:
     - Low APGAR score at 5 min or more
     - Early onset of seizures
     - Seizures that are prolonged or difficult to control
     - Abnormal EEG

NEONATAL METABOLIC PROBLEMS

Fluid and Electrolyte Problems

General Considerations

- Fluid and electrolyte requirements in neonates vary to a great extent, depending on gestational age and size. Hence careful monitoring of various parameters is frequently required. Weight is a most useful, and often underutilized parameter.

TABLE 17–6 Average Daily Electrolyte Requirements

Electrolyte	Usual Intake (mmol/kg/day)	Starting Age (hr)	Comments	Standard Solutions for Adding to IV Fluids
Na^+	1–2 (term) 3–5 (prem.)	24	Urinary losses are high and may reach 10–12 mmol/kg/day in prems Hypernatremia in early neonatal period usually indicates dehydration, especially in infants <1,000 g BW on days 1–2	3% NaCl (0.5 mmol/ml or 0.5 mEq/ml)
K^+	1–2	24—according to voiding and serum levels	Hyperkalemia may be associated with hemolysis, metabolic acidosis, hemorrhage, renal failure	2 mmol/ml KCl
Ca^{2+} LBW	1–2	6 hr	Maintenance Ca^{2+}, especially in first three days of life Watch IV site: Ca^{2+} toxic to tissues Do not mix with $NaHCO_3 \rightarrow$ chalk	10% Ca gluconate (2.24 mmol/10 ml; 9 mg elemental Ca/ml)

TABLE 17–7   Average Daily Fluid Requirements (ml/kg/day)[‡]

(Birth) Weight	Day 1	Day 2	Day 3	Day 4	Day 5	> Day 5
600–800 g[+]	80–100	100–125	130	130	150	150–200
800–1,000 g	60–100	90–115	120	130	150	150–200
1–1.5 kg	60	70	100	120	150	150–200
1.5–2.0 kg	60	70	100	120	140	150–180
>2.0 kg	60	75	90	120	140	160–180

[‡] These are only guidelines; adjust as per urine output, weight changes, electrolytes and such.

[+] This is still being defined for this weight group. Because of extremely high insensible water loss, fluids must be individually tailored, by watching above parameters (e.g., u/o, Na^+).

N.B. 1. Add 30–50% for radiant heaters.
2. Add 10–50% for phototherapy.
3. Subtract ~ 10% for Saran Wrap and heat shields.
4. Subtract ~ 20–30% for endotracheal intubation and assisted ventilation.
5. <600 g—start at rates as per 600–800 g infant and adjust as appropriate.

Monitoring for Fluid and Electrolyte Regimens

- Intake and output charting—accurate; hourly in small neonates, at least
- Body weight daily (expect ~ 10 g/kg/day loss for first 5–10 days)
- Urine specific gravity ~ q8h (normal range, 1.003–1.015)
- Urine glucose tid–qid in smaller neonates
- Serum electrolytes, urea (or BUN) daily (less frequently in stable infants)
- Urine electrolytes when indicated
- Diuresis may signal improvement in respiratory status in RDS
- Infants on high fluid volumes (especially smaller infants <1,000 g) are at increased risk of developing clinically significant PDA!
- Usual water losses: ~ 85–170 ml/kg/day in infant <1,500 g, ~ 70–145 ml/kg/day in infant 1,500 to 2,500 g

Specific Electrolyte Derangements

Hyponatremia
General Considerations

- Definition: Na <130 (all gestations)
- Two main causes
  1. Excess Na vs H_2O loss
     - Renal tubular immaturity (especially <32/40 gestation)
     - Hypoxic insult to renal tubules causing decreased conservation of Na
     - Diuretics, especially loop diuretics
     - GI losses, plus congenital adrenal hyperplasia (↓Na, ↑K)
  2. Water retention
     - Iatrogenic pre- (to mother) or postnatal (to baby)
     - SIADH
     - CHF
     - Post indomethacin therapy

Management

- In (1)—replace Na losses: (Na desired − actual Na) × wt (kg) × 0.6, over 24–48 hr. More rapid replacement with 3% NaCl if symptomatic (seizures, apnea, hypotonia), e.g., 4–6 ml/kg over 1½–2 hr.
- In (2)—fluid restriction mainly (½–⅔ maintenance), unless symptomatic →give 3% NaCl ± diuretics

Hypernatremia

General Considerations

- Definition: Na >150
- Two main causes
  1. Excess H_2O vs Na loss
     - Dehydration from ↑ insensible water loss, e.g., under radiant warmer (most common)
     - Diarrhea and vomiting
     - Necrotizing enterocolitis
     - Osmotic diuresis, e.g., hyperglycemia (rare)
  2. Excess Na administration: $NaHCO_3$ for acidosis

Management: Dependent on (Body) Weight

- Infants <2.5 kg
  1. Calculate excess Na thus: (observed Na − 145) × body wt (kg) × 0.6
  2. Aim to correct serum Na slowly, e.g., not to fall at a rate >10 mmol (mEq)/L/24 hr
  3. If ↑Na^+ is secondary to dehydration, assume fluid deficit 10–15% (100–150 ml/kg) and correct so as not to → precipitous ↓ in Na. N.B. If patient "shocky," treat with 5% albumin *or* FFP *or* normal saline (10–15 ml/kg). Then, if stable, continue as above. Too rapid hydration + Na correction → cerebral edema + seizures!
  4. If initial Na >160, use normal saline to

replace *deficit* (but use the usual Na intake of $\sim$ 3 mmol (mEq)/kg/day in appropriate fluid volume for maintenance)
   5. If initial Na <160, use D5W + 0.45% saline to replace fluid *deficit*
- Infants <1.5 kg
   1. Above formulas invalid for VLBW infants. Fluid deficits may be 20–25% of body weight
   2. Initially use D5W or D5:0.2% saline for replacement of deficit, and monitor serum Na, weight, u/o, and urine Na^+ losses at frequent intervals, adjusting IV fluid volume and content appropriately

Hypokalemia

- Most commonly iatrogenic, e.g., inadequate intake, excessive urinary losses from diuretic therapy, or respiratory alkalosis

Hyperkalemia

General Considerations

- Definition: K^+ > 7.0 mmol/L (mEq/L)
- Causes
   1. ↑ Input (usually IV)
   2. Cellular leak (sick cell syndrome, cell necrosis, blood resorption)
   3. Renal failure
   4. Adrenal insufficiency (CAH; bilateral adrenal hemorrhages, infarcts)
- Always obtain EKG. Monitor continuously. The first three causes are common in VLBW infants.

Management: Ensure That Blood Sample is Not Hemolyzed!

- If K^+ >8 mmol/L + EKG changes or arrhythmia present
   1. 10% Ca gluconate 0.5–1.0 ml/kg over 2–3 min with EKG monitoring

2. Ion exchange resin, e.g., Kayexalate, 1 g/kg pr
   (may be started at lower K^+, e.g., ≥ 7.0).
   Avoid oral route in small infants!
3. Alkalinize with $NaHCO_3$, 1.5–2.0 mmol/kg
   over 10–15 min IV
4. Consider glucose/insulin: 0.5–1.0 g/kg glucose, 0.1–0.25 U/kg insulin, IV over 30 min
- If renal failure exists, consider peritoneal
  dialysis

Acid-Base Status

Respiratory Acidosis

- Corrected by ventilation, *not* bicarbonate

Metabolic Acidosis

General Considerations

- Definition: bicarbonate < 20.0 mmol/L
- May have element of respiratory compensation
  affecting pH. Look for a cause! These include
  1. Sepsis
  2. Hypoxia and shock
  3. PDA and cardiac failure
  4. Renal losses of bicarbonate (RTA)
  5. Metabolic disorders: organic acidemias and
     amino acidurias, congenital lactic acidosis
  6. Excessive protein load
  7. Subependymal hemorrhage (SEH) or
     intraventricular hemorrhage (IVH)
- N.B. In severe RDS usually $\rightarrow$ mixed metabolic
  respiratory acidosis

Management

- The underlying cause should be identified and
  treated first, unless acidosis is severe; e.g., in
  hypovolemia, give volume
- $NaHCO_3$ is administered to correct acidosis
  when pH < 7.25 and base excess ≥ -10

- ½ correction = base deficit × wt (kg) × 0.3
  (½ of this given stat if considered urgent). Two
  mmol/kg expected to increase pH by ~ 0.1
  unit. Give as slow infusion over 1–4 hr unless
  severe. (*Do not* infuse with Ca^{2+}-containing solution.)

Respiratory Alkalosis

- If occurs while on mechanical ventilation, this
  may be an indication to reduce ventilation.
- N.B. Marked respiratory alkalosis with
  pH >7.50 may decrease cerebral blood flow
  (? ↑ risk of periventricular leucomalacia)

Metabolic Alkalosis

- Causes include
    1. Hypochloremia
    2. Excessive bicarbonate therapy
    3. Hypokalemia
    4. Phosphate excess
    5. Postexchange transfusion

Other Metabolic Disorders

Neonatal Hypoglycemia

General Considerations and Clinical Features

- Normal glucose requirements in neonates 5–7
  mg/kg/min (see Figure 17–5)
- Symptoms of hypoglycemia include jitteriness,
  apnea, unconsciousness, seizures, lethargy,
  poor feeding, cyanosis, CHF, hypothermia
- Definition: blood glucose <2.2 mmol/L (40
  mg/dl) in all newborn infants regardless of
  gestation
- Classification
    1. Simple (isolated)
        - Transient
            a. Bolus glucose → rebound phenomenon
            b. IDM (infant of diabetic mother)
            c. SGA/propranolol infant (maternal ↑ BP)

d. Preterm infant
e. Post-term infant
f. ± Asphyxiated infant
- Permanent
a. Panhypopituitarism (midline defects, micropenis, hypoglycemia)
b. Nesidioblastosis ⎫ Pancreatic
⎬ dysmaturity
c. Beckwith-Wiedemann ⎭ syndrome
syndrome
2. Complex—associated with metabolic acido-sis, hepatomegaly

Management

- Investigations
1. Blood sugar (to confirm Dextrostix)
2. If hypoglycemia persistent or recurrent
   - 3-OH butyrate (plasma)
   - Insulin level (plasma)
   - GH (plasma)
   - Cortisol (plasma)
   - Ketone bodies and urine for organic acids—all done while patient is hypoglycemic if possible

- Therapy
1. Transient hypoglycemia
   - Goal of therapy should be anticipation and prevention
   - Early introduction of oral feeds (if feasible). Feed frequently (q2–3h) in predisposed infants.
   - Frequent monitoring of Chemstrips bG (Dextrostix) in susceptible infants (prior to feeds in patients being fed or when symptomatic)
   - In patients NPO, glucose 5–7 mg/kg/min as D10W should be started (see Fig. 17–5), as continuous infusion
2. If patient presents with hypoglycemia (symptomatic)

- 0.1–0.2 g/kg (1–2 cc/kg of D10W) glucose is given IV STAT, followed by 5–7 mg/kg/min
- Check Chemstrip bG at ½ hr and 1 hr, then every 2 hr until stable
- Aim to maintain blood glucose at 3.5–5.0 mmol/L (65–90 mg/dl)
- If patient remains hypoglycemic or needs >10 mg/kg/min of glucose, commence glucagon 1 mg/24 hr (or 0.3 mg/kg/24hr) as continuous infusion
- Infants with transient hypoglycemia rarely require glucagon

3. Persistent hypoglycemia
   - Inability to reduce glucagon infusion after 10–14 days suggests "pancreatic dysmaturity syndrome," and treatment with diazoxide may be tried (5–20 mg/kg/day). If this fails, total pancreatectomy is the treatment of choice
   - Steroids or growth hormone treatment is used only for specific indications, e.g., panhypopituitarism

4. N.B. *All patients with persistent hypoglycemia should be cared for in a tertiary pediatric center*

Hyperglycemia

General Considerations

- Definition: blood glucose (BG) >10 mmol/L (180 mg/dl), often associated with glycosuria
  1. Commonly secondary to ↑ glucose load in TPN or parenteral glucose infusions, especially in VLBW infants
  2. Consider sepsis in diagnosis, especially if occurs suddenly

Management

- Confirm Chemstrip with blood glucose
- Decrease IV glucose infusion or concentration

of glucose in TPN, e.g., D7.5 or D5 from D10W
- Monitor weight, input + output, and urine glucose
- ± Septic screen
- *Rarely* requires insulin treatment

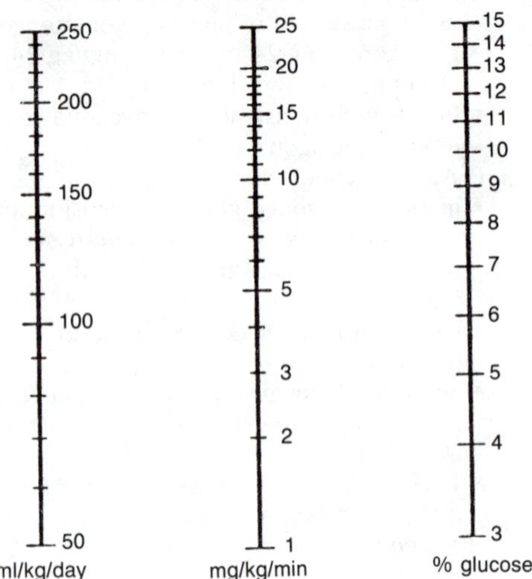

Figure 17–5   Glucose rate calculator. (From Klaus MH, Fanaroff AA, eds. Care of the high risk neonate. Philadelphia: W.B. Saunders, 1979:430.)

Hypocalcemia

General Considerations

- Definition
  1. Full term: Ca <1.9 mmol/L (7.5 mg/dl) } Ionized Ca^{2+} <0.75 mmol/L (3 mg/dl)
  2. Preterm: Ca <1.75 mmol/L (7.0 mg/dl)

- Etiology (Table 17–8)

TABLE 17–8   Etiology of Neonatal Hypocalcemia

Early (24–72 hr)	*Late (7–10 days)*
Prematurity/LBW	Vitamin D deficiency
Birth asphyxia	High phosphate formulas
IDM	Rare now
DiGeorge syndrome	Others:
Infection (sepsis)—severe	Drug induced e.g.,
Intracranial hemorrhage	Furosemide, steroids
Hyperparathyroid mother	Alkalosis, exchange
Inadequate calcium	transfusions (citrate)
intake	Renal disease

Management

- Anticipation and prevention are the best (ideal) management
- Serum calcium measurements should be determined regularly in high risk infants
- 25–45 mg elemental Ca/kg/day IV (3–5 ml/kg/day of 10% Ca gluconate) prophylactically offsets early onset hypocalcemia in most susceptible infants, when given as continuous infusion for the first 48–72 hr of life
- Orally 75 mg/kg/day with feeds is recommended. (Recall: 10% Ca gluconate = 9% elemental Ca = 9 mg/ml)
  1. Symptomatic hypocalcemia (irritability, jitteriness, cyanosis, seizures, stridor, brisk reflexes, dysrhythmias, increased QT interval)
     - Seizures often multifocal and migratory and patient may be alert between spells
     - Immediate treatment: 1–2 ml (100–200 mg)/kg of 10% Ca gluconate (9–18 mg/kg elemental Ca^{2+}) by slow IV infusion (peripheral vein or UVL) over 10 min, under EKG monitoring (bradycardia/asystole)
     - Follow with parenteral therapy as for

"prophylactic group" above until normocalcemia maintained. In some infants,
this dose can be halved and then maintained for 72 hr post birth.
2. Asymptomatic group: Treat when Ca <1.8
mmol/L (7.2 mg/dl). If patient able to feed,
supplement oral feeds with calcium; 75
mg/kg/day elemental calcium is the recommended daily dosage. (Calcium lactate or
gluconate can be used.) In infant NPO,
35–45 mg/kg/day elemental Ca^{2+} IV by continuous infusion is recommended.
- Points to note
1. All patients receiving Ca^{2+} infusions should
be on a cardiac monitor!
2. The IV site should be closely observed for
extravasation. Ca^{2+} produces severe interstitial
necrosis!!
3. All hypocalcemic infants should have a Mg^{2+}
level measured simultaneously. Hypo-Mg^{2+}
may coexist with hypo-Ca^{2+}.
4. Vitamin D supplementation is often also added to the therapy of high risk infants (e.g.,
premature infants on "special care" formulas). Usual dosage: vitamin D_3 ~ 700 IU/day.

Unusual Metabolic Disorders with Acute Presentation

General Considerations and Clinical Features

- Three major categories
1. Neurologic symptoms predominate: maple
syrup urine disease (MSUD), hyperammonemia, nonketotic hyperglycinemia
2. Acidosis predominates: lactic acidosis;
organic acidemias; glycogen storage disease
(GSD), type I*
3. Liver involvement: galactosemia, fructosemia,*
tyrosinemia*

* These tend to present late in neonatal period

- Basically, most metabolic conditions in the newborn present like other catastrophic events, e.g., sepsis, IVH, with lethargy, poor feeding, hypotonia or hypertonia, seizures. May or may not be associated with acidosis or hypoglycemia. There is often unexplained deterioration in clinical status. NOTE: The following is a brief list of some metabolic disorders:
  1. Hyperammonemia
     - Urea cycle defects (UCD)
     - Transient hyperammonemia of newborn (THAN)
     - Organic acidopathies (OA)
     Features
     - Lethargy, vomiting, seizures, and respiratory acidosis
     - Metabolic acidosis with OAs but later in UCD and THAN (usually prems with asphyxia)
     - Moderate hepatomegaly with mild cerebral edema
     - Coma develops rapidly and early in most cases
  2. Maple syrup urine disease (MSUD)
     - Symptoms due to increasing cerebral edema over first week of life
     - Acidosis and ketosis frequently not evident
     - Smell the urine—may be quite characteristic
  3. Nonketotic hyperglycinemia (NKH)
     - "Rag doll" extreme floppiness, then intractable seizures
     - Hiccoughs
     - ↑ CSF glycine required for diagnosis
  4. Organic acidopathies
     - Congenital lactic acidosis
     - Methylmalonic aciduria, propionic acidemia
     - Others

- Account for anion gap >20 with blood lactate (and urine organic acids)
      - Variable pancytopenia
      - *Neonatal ketonuria is a medical emergency*
5. Galactosemia
      - Inexplicable hepatomegaly and jaundice
      - Reducing substances in urine (Clinitest)
      - ± Gram negative sepsis (generalized)
      - Get galactosemia screen off *before* giving blood transfusion

Management

- All such infants should therefore have the following screening tests done immediately:
   1. ABG, electrolytes, NH_3, Ca^{2+}, glucose, Mg^{2+}, urea, lactate
   2. Urine for ketones, metabolic screen, amino and organic acids
   3. Sepsis work-up if not already done (keep sample of CSF)
   4. Calculate anion gap (normal = 15–20 in neonate)
   5. Galactosemia screen (before transfusion)
- It is sometimes useful to smell the urine (boiled or frozen), as it may be helpful in the diagnosis (e.g., burnt sugar–almond smell in MSUD).
   1. Basic therapy: mainly supportive initially
      - NPO (at least initially)
      - Start on parenteral glucose containing solution, e.g., D10W (except for lactic acidosis)
      - Treat acidosis with bicarbonate and hyperammonemia with peritoneal dialysis ± exchange transfusions
      - ± Ventilatory support
   2. Specific therapy: when diagnosis available
      N.B. *Early consultation with metabolic service is recommended*

NEONATAL RESPIRATORY DISORDERS

Respiratory Distress

General Considerations

- Respiratory distress may present in many different ways in the newborn and management is therefore varied, depending on the cause (see Table 17–9 and Fig. 17–6).

Differential Diagnosis

- See Table 17–9

Management

- Goals of therapy
  1. To maintain Pco_2 < 50 torr
  2. To maintain Po_2 between 50–70 torr
  3. To maintain pH > 7.25
  4. *All term newborn infants with respiratory distress should be treated as sepsis with antibiotics (see* Sepsis Neonatorum*) until ruled out.* (Details of ventilation can be sought in neonatology texts, journals, or handbooks, such as those recommended at the end of this chapter.)
- Specific criteria for mechanical ventilation
  1. Marked hypoxia (Po_2 < 50 mm Hg with > 25% FiO_2) in infant < 1,250 g
  2. Rising Pco_2
  3. Shock with poor perfusion and hypotension, irrespective of ABG values
  4. Frequent apnea not responding to other forms of treatment (e.g., caffeine, CPAP)
  5. Infant > 35 wk with PaO_2 < 60 torr in $FiO \geq$ 60%

Apnea of Prematurity

General Considerations

- Definition: cessation of respiration of > 15–20

TABLE 17–9 Differential Diagnosis of Respiratory Distress in Newborn Period*

Pulmonary Disorders	
Common	Less Common
Respiratory distress syndrome	Pulmonary hypoplasia
Transient tachypnea (TTN)	Upper airway obstruction
Meconium Aspiration	Rib cage abnormalities
Pneumonia	Space occupying lesions
Pneumothorax	(e.g., diaphragmatic hernia)
	Pulmonary hemorrhage
	Immature lung syndrome

Extrapulmonary Disorders		
Vascular	Metabolic	Neuromuscular
Persistent fetal circulation (PFC)	Acidosis	Cerebral edema
Congenital heart disease	Hypoglycemia	Cerebral hemorrhage
Hypovolemia-anemia	Hypothermia	Muscle disorders
Polycythemia		Spinal cord problems
		Phrenic nerve palsies
		Drugs

* Presentation ± cyanosis ± grunting ± retractions ± tachypnea ± apnea ± shock ± lethargy.
Modified from Klaus MH, Fanaroff AA, eds. Care of the high risk neonate. Philadelphia: W.B. Saunders, 1986:179.

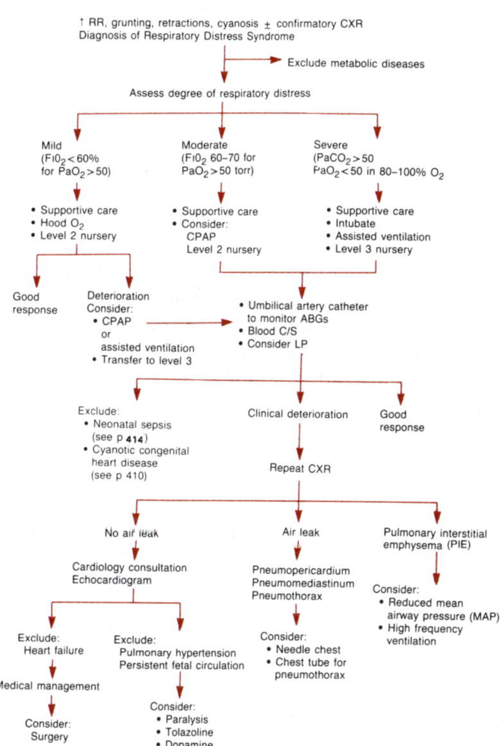

Figure 17–6 Initial management of respiratory distress syndrome. (Modified from Berman S, ed. Pediatric decision making. Toronto: B.C. Decker, 1985:219.)

sec duration, with fall in heart rate to <100/min (bradycardia) or cyanosis. After 30–45 sec of apnea, pallor and hypotonia will occur. Apnea may be central, obstructive, or mixed

- *Do not* attribute apnea automatically to prematurity, especially in infants of gestational age >30/40
- Always exclude secondary causes

Management

- See Table 17–10

NEONATAL CARDIOLOGY

General Considerations

- Cardiovascular disorders in the neonate may present in one or all of the following ways:
1. Heart murmur found on routine examination
2. Central cyanosis (Fig. 17–7)
3. Congestive heart failure (CHF)
4. Dysrhythmias

Cyanotic Newborn

- To exclude cyanotic cardiac disease, place in 100% FiO_2 (hyperoxic test) with $TcPO_2$ monitor in situ for 10–15 min or until $TcPO_2$ >250
- Failure to produce a definite increase in $TcPO_2$ (usually >100 torr) is highly suggestive of cardiac R to L shunting
- In pulmonary disease, a reading of 250–300 torr (sometimes after some IPPV is added) is usual, in 100% O_2
- N.B. "Normal" hyperoxic test →PaO_2 >500 torr. However, normal "physiologic shunt" may → PaO_2, 450–500 torr.

Congestive Heart Failure

- See Table 17–11
- For management see cardiology section, p 41

Dysrhythmias

- The most common in the neonatal period are
1. Supraventricular tachycardias—may be cause of intrauterine CHF or hydrops

TABLE 17–10 Management of Apnea

Immediate Resuscitation

Proceed as necessary
1. Surface stimulation
2. Gentle nasopharyngeal
   suction
3. Ventilation with inflating
   bag and mask
4. Intubation and IPPV

Review Possible Causes Needing Specific Therapy

	Cause	Action
1. Infection	Neonatal sepsis	Infectious screen including LP
	Meningitis	Consider antibiotics
	Necrotizing enterocolitis (NEC)	
2. Thermal instability	Hypo/hyperthermia	Assess body and isolette temperature
3. Metabolic disorders	Hypoglycemia	Dextrostix $\pm$ blood glucose
	Hypocalcemia	Serum Ca^{2+}, EKG ($\uparrow$ QoTc interval)
	Hypo/hypernatremia	Electrolytes, urea, review intake/output, wt.
	Hyperammonemia	Serum $NH_4{}^+$

TABLE 17–10 Continued

4. CNS problems	Asphyxia	Observation of "spells,"
	Intracranial hemorrhage	EEG, fontanelle tension, $\pm$ LP,
	Cerebral malformation	head U/S $\pm$ CT scan
	Seizures	Consider anticonvulsants
5. Decreased O_2 delivery	Hypoxemia	CXR, ABG; check location of
	Worsening RDS $\pm$ complication	ETT and patency
	Anemia/shock	CBC, electrolytes, urea
	L to R shunt (PDA)	2D-ECHO, ECG
6. Upper airway	Choanal atresia	Attempt passage of N/G tube
obstruction	Large tongue	Oropharyngeal airway
	Reflux	CXR for aspiration
7. Drugs	Maternal	Drug-toxic screen
	Fetal	

Continuing Management to Prevent Recurrences, and Monitoring

Consider:
  Continuous $TcPO_2$ monitoring. Adjust FIO_2 appropriately.
  Minimize handling of small infants
  $\pm$ "Rocking mattress" stimulation
  ? Alter feeding pattern, e.g., slow continuous orogastric, or IV

Continued next page

Drug therapy: (i) Caffeine citrate, 10 mg/kg loading → 2.5 mg/kg/day. Therapeutic range = 30–70 μmol/L (5–20 μg/ml). Lower incidence of side effects with caffeine vs. aminophylline. (ii) Aminophylline, 6 mg/kg loading → 1.5–2 mg/kg/dose q8–12h. Therapeutic range, 11–55 mmol/L (3–10 mg/L).

Repeated attacks: Use assisted ventilation for several days:

- NPT or nasal prong CPAP
- ETT CPAP
- IPPV (often need only *slow* rate)

Modified from Forfar JL, Arneil GC. Textbook of paediatrics. 2nd ed. New York: Churchill Livingstone, 1978:156.

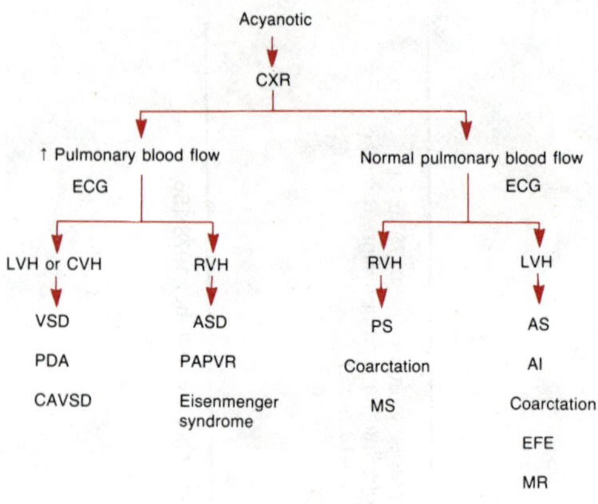

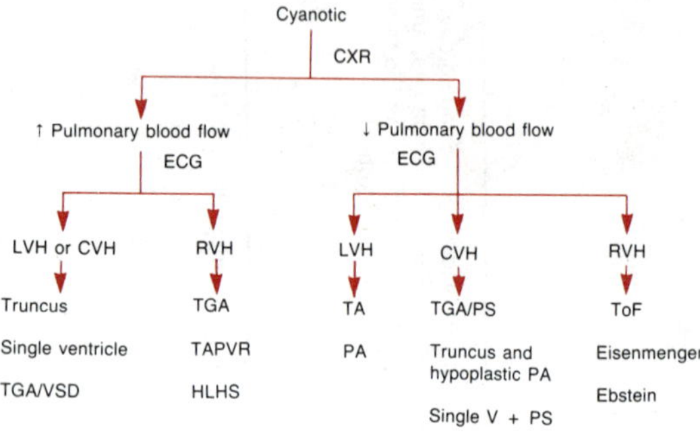

Figure 17–7 Differential diagnosis of congenital heart disease. LVH = L ventricular hypertrophy. CVH = combined vent. hypertrophy. RVH = R ventricular hypertrophy. CAVSD = combined atrioventricular septal defect. PAPAVR = partial anomalous pulmonary venous return. AS = aortic stenosis. AI = aortic incomp. PS = pulmonary stenosis. MS = mitral stenosis. MR = mitral regurgitation. EFE = endomyocardial fibroelastosis. TGA = transposition of great vessels. HLHS = hypoplastic left heart. ToF = Tetralogy of Fallot. TA = tricuspid atresia. PA = pulmonary atresia.

Onset of CHF Related to Mechanism

a. Birth	b. Day 1
Arrhythmias	As at birth, plus...
Anemias	Hypoplastic ''L'' heart
A-V fistula	Metabolic abnormalities
Perinatal asphyxia	Tricuspid atresia/Ebstein's
	Critical pulmonary stenosis
c. Weeks 1 and 2	d. Weeks 2 to 4
Arrhythmias	As in (c) plus...
Coarctation	TAPVD (unobstructed)
TGA with VSD	Truncus arteriosus
TAPVD (obstructed)	A-V canal
Myocarditis	
Fibroelastosis	
Pompe's disease	
PDA in premature	

2. Bradycardia—may be secondary to congenital complete heart block (? maternal lupus)

- For management of dysrhythmias see cardiology section, p 50

Common Neonatal Cardiovascular Lesions

Patent Ductus Arteriosus

General Considerations

- A common association with RDS (HMD) in the premature infant. Occurs in ~ 80% of infants <1,000 g and ~ 20% of all premature infants
- Characteristic murmur and hyperdynamic circulation ± signs of CHF may be present. (May have "silent ductus.")

Management

- Fluid restriction ~ ⅔–¾ maintenance, while avoiding dehydration and catabolic state
- If above not sufficient, add furosemide (Lasix),

1–2 mg/kg/dose
- Transfuse to maintain hematocrit $\geq$ 45%
- Indomethacin: dosage 0.2 mg/kg/dose q8–12h × three doses or less. Maintain ⅔ fluid maintenance fluids during treatment. Success after first dose ~ 80%; ~ 25% reopen but ~ 18% reclose without further treatment. Contraindications to indomethacin therapy: creatinine >160 mmol/L (1.8 mg/dl), urea >9.0 mmol/L (BUN >25 mg/dl), oliguria <0.5–1 ml/kg/hr, NEC, thrombocytopenia <80,000 ± hyperbilirubinemia, ± IVH.
- Treatment with indomethacin should indicate that sufficient significance is given to the PDA, such that surgical ligation will be undertaken if treatment fails.
- N.B. *The presence of a duct dependent lesion should always be seriously considered if there is deterioration following indomethacin therapy! (Can be avoided by doing ECG, CXR ± 2D–ECHO prior to treatment.)*

Duct Dependent Lesions

Management

- Lesions include interruption of aortic arch, coarctation or severe narrowing of aortic isthmus, severe ToF, pulmonary atresia, tricuspid atresia, TGA, severe Epstein's anomaly. Therapy geared toward maintaining ductal patency.
  1. Prostaglandin E_1, 0.05–0.1 μg/kg/min, while monitoring $TcPO_2$ or O_2 saturation to ensure PO_2 >30 torr
  2. Side effects include apnea, hyperthermia, jitteriness, flushing, lethargy, diarrhea. Most of these are tolerable and require minimal intervention. *Always be prepared to intubate in case of apnea! These patients must be transferred to a tertiary pediatric center.*

Persistent Pulmonary Hypertension (PPH)

General Considerations and Clinical Features

- Condition with right to left shunting through the foramen ovale, or PDA associated with pulmonary arteriolar spasm or thickening (primary). May be primary or secondary. Most infants with primary PPH are term or post-term. Secondary causes or associated conditions include
  1. Meconium aspiration syndrome
  2. Severe transient tachypnea of the newborn (TTN)
  3. Hyaline membrane disease
  4. Group B streptococcal pneumonia or sepsis
  5. Pulmonary hypoplasia $\pm$ diaphragmatic hernia
  6. Severe asphyxia (any cause)
  7. Polycythemia
- Marked cyanosis, acidosis, and R ventricular heave are frequent findings.

Management

- Investigations
  1. In 100% O_2, PO_2 rarely >20–30 torr
  2. Chest x-ray: oligemic lung fields, or consistent with underlying disease (e.g., group B strep., meconium aspiration). Cardiomegaly also seen on CXR.
  3. ECG: right ventricular strain
- Therapy
  1. Each patient may have a "critical PCO_2 level" below which PO_2 begins to rise. This may therefore be tested by "rapid rate" ventilation, 100–150/min, to achieve PCO_2 20–30 torr (pH 7.45–7.55). High frequency oscillation if high PIP required to achieve PCO_2.
  2. Treat primary disorder, e.g., sepsis
  3. Drug therapy—none are proven effective, but the following occasionally seem to help some patients:

- Tolazoline 2 mg/kg IV bolus; then 1–2 mg/kg/hr after correction of acidosis. (May → hypotension; therefore need arterial BP transducer line.)
- Dopamine, 2–5 μg/kg/min *increasing to 10–15 μg/kg/min to counter systemic hypotension resulting from tolazoline. Volume expanders may also be used.*
- Labile patients may be sedated $\pm$ paralyzed (morphine $\pm$ pancuronium)

Prognosis

- Poor prognosis associated with
  1. Severe pulmonary hypoplasia and inability to decrease PCO_2 with ventilation
  2. Requirement of PIP >35–40 cm H_2O
  3. Requirement of PCO_2 <20 torr to keep PO_2 >50 torr
  4. Marked PO_2 lability
  5. Group B strep. sepsis

SEPSIS NEONATORUM

General Considerations

- Risk factors: sepsis should be considered in any sick newborn infant! High risk factors include
  1. Prematurity
  2. Prolonged rupture of membranes (≥ 24 hr) $\pm$ maternal chorioamnionitis
  3. *Early onset respiratory distress esp. in full term*
  4. Maternal fever, sepsis, urinary tract infection
  5. Neonatal manipulation or instrumentation

Clinical Features

- Often nonspecific and include poor feeding, weak suck, lethargy, cyanosis, temperature instability, respiratory distress, jaundice, sclerema, tachycardia, poor perfusion, hypotension

Management

- Investigations include
  1. Blood cultures; spinal fluid for c+s; urine for c+s in all infants
  2. Also CBC, differential white cell count, platelets; CXR; latex agglutination (or CIE) on urine/CSF/blood; C reactive protein (CRP)
  3. In immediate neonatal period the following are especially useful:
     - Tracheal aspirate (done under direct vision) for Gram stain and c+s
     - Gastric aspirate (Gram stain and c+s)
     - ± Surface cultures (e.g., ear, umbilicus)
     - High vaginal swabs on mother may yield useful information
     - Histologic examination of umbilical cord and placenta
- Treatment
  1. General—remove all indwelling catheters (arterial, venous, or bladder)
  2. Antibiotics
     - A combination of ampicillin and an aminoglycoside (e.g., gentamicin, amikacin) is the most common first line choice
     - Ampicillin and a third generation cephalosporin (e.g., cefotaxime) are a good second line choice
     - Third generation cephalosporins *alone* are sometimes used preferentially for proven gram negative sepsis or meningitis
     - Clindamycin may be added if necrotizing enterocolitis (NEC) is suspected
     - Vancomycin may be added for suspected *Staphylococcus epidermidis* sepsis
  3. Supportive therapy: If signs of shock or poor perfusion present, may need colloids ± inotropes
  4. Duration of therapy
     - Proven septicemia: 10 days minimum
     - Meningitis: 2–3 wk minimum. LP after dis-

continuation of therapy.
- Negative cultures but strong suspicion of sepsis: 5–10 days therapy

NEONATAL JAUNDICE

General Consideration

- Causes can be categorized by age of first appearance
  1. <24 hr
     - Hemolytic disease until proven otherwise
     - Sepsis or TORCH also possible causes
  2. 24–72 hr
     - Mostly "physiologic" (Table 17–12)
     - Nonmajor blood group hemolytic (e.g., G6PD deficiency, PK deficiency, sphero-cytosis, Duffy, Kell)
     - Polycythemia (SGA; late clamping of the cord; maternal-fetal and fetofetal trans-fusions)
     - Sepsis or TORCH
     - Bruising or hemorrhage, or swallowed blood
  3. 72–96 hr
     - "Physiologic" ± breast milk jaundice most common
     - Infection—sepsis (including UTI) or hepati-tis (TORCH)
     - GI obstruction (↑ enterohepatic circulation)
  4. > 1 wk (prolonged neonatal jaundice) Consider
     - Hypothyroidism (may not have typical features)
     - Galactosemia
     - Breast milk (benign)
     - Prolonged physiologic (e.g., preterm)
     - Crigler-Najjar syndrome, Gilbert's disease
     - Obstructive jaundice (e.g., "hepatitis," biliary atresia, inspissated bile syndrome, choledochal cyst, α_1-antitrypsin deficiency)

TABLE 17–12   Nonphysiologic Jaundice (Jaundice Requiring Investigation or Treatment)

Clinically apparent jaundice in first 24 hr of life
Increase in total serum bilirubin concentration of >85 μmol/L (5 mg/dl) per day
Total serum bilirubin concentration >220 μmol/L (13 mg/dl) within the first 4 days of life in term infants
Direct serum bilirubin concentration higher than 34 μmol/L (2 mg/dl)
Visible jaundice lasting >1 wk in term infants or 2 wk in premature infants

Modified from Foetus and Newborn Committee, Canadian Paediatric Society. Use of phototherapy for neonatal hyperbilirubinemia. Can Med Assoc J 1986; 134:1237–1245.

Clinical Features and Investigations

- Jaundice occurring <1 wk of age
  1. Family history of jaundice; maternal history—blood group and Rh status, previous pregnancies, transfusions, Rhogam
  2. Physical findings—hepatosplenomegaly, enclosed hemorrhage
  3. Infant's blood group and Rh status; Coomb's test (DCT) on infant. Negative Coomb's test does not rule out hemolytic anemia, e.g., ABO incompatibility.
  4. Total bilirubin (BR) or microbilirubin (MBR)
  5. CBC, hematocrit, $\pm$ reticulocyte count, blood smear
  6. Blood, urine, and CSF cultures
  7. N.B. In most cases the latter two lines of investigation (CBC, cultures) are not required. The presence of clinical signs and symptoms may dictate appropriate (further) investigations.
- Prolonged jaundice (> first week)
  1. Above features and investigations plus
     - Thyroid function (T_4, TSH)
     - Galactosemia screen—for galactose-1-phosphate uridyl transferase; screen urine

for galactose, if being fed lactose
- Total and direct bilirubin
- Liver function tests
- Further investigations as appropriate, e.g., phenobarbital stimulation test for Crigler-Najjar syndrome type II, withdrawal of breast milk (BM) × 24–48 hr for BM jaundice.
- N.B. Premature infants—later onset (6th–7th day) of "physiologic" jaundice, and of longer duration (up to 14th day)

Management

Phototherapy (for *specific* guidelines see Tables 17–13 and 17–14 and Fig. 17–8)

1. Usually initiated when unconjugated bilirubin level is ½–⅔ the exchange level, depending on rate of rise, independent of etiology
2. More effective when combined with oral feeds and functioning GIT
3. More effective in stabilizing bilirubin levels, in high risk situations, at low levels, than in abruptly reducing established high levels
4. Blue light most effective, *but* affects ongoing assessment of infant by altering observer perception
5. May use either continuous or intermittent (6 hr on, 6 hr off) with similar efficacy
6. "Double" phototherapy indicated when bilirubin levels approach within 35 μmol/L (2 mg%) of exchange level (but may be initiated earlier)
7. Insensible fluid loss may increase ~ 35% necessitating increased fluid intake, especially in VLBW infants
8. Serum bilirubin levels should be followed every 6 hr or less, depending on level and etiology
9. Delaying initiation of phototherapy until

bilirubin levels are >200 μmol/L (12 mg/dl) by 24 hr after birth may significantly reduce the number of infants receiving phototherapy for ABO incompatibility without increasing the need for exchange transfusions (assuming no other high risk factor present, e.g., preterm)

10. *Exclude* treatable causes of jaundice (e.g., sepsis, metabolic). Many of these causes of jaundice may initially respond to phototherapy, and delay primary treatment.

11. Phototherapy treatment can be used prophylactically in high risk infants, e.g., markedly bruised prems (controversial), and as an adjunct but not replacement for exchange transfusion

12. Contraindicated in the presence of conjugated hyperbilirubinemia ($\rightarrow$ "bronzed" baby)

13. Complications and side effects
    - Hypernatremic dehydration
    - Hyperthermia
    - Masking potentially serious causes, e.g., sepsis
    - "Bronzing"—if $\uparrow$ direct bilirubin
    - ? Retinal damage—if eyes uncovered
    - Transient rashes
    - Loose stools (desirable)

- Exchange transfusion
  1. Indications in hemolytic disease of newborn
     - Cord hemoglobin <120 g/L (12 g/dl) or cord BR > 80 μmol/L (5 mg/dl)
     - Postnatal rate of rise of unconjugated BR >17 μmol/L (1 mg/dl)/hr in ABO incompatibility (but >0.5 mg/dl/hr in Rh)
     - Serum unconjugated BR >340 μmol/L (20 mg/dl) in first 48–72 hr of life (controversial)
     - Rapid progression of anemia despite satisfactory control of jaundice

TABLE 17–13   Suggested Values of Serum Unconjugated Bilirubin at Which Phototherapy Should Be Considered for Neonatal Hyperbilirubinemia

Birth Weight (g)	Bilirubin level, μmol/L (mg/100 ml)	
	Uncomplicated Course	Complicated Course[*]
<1,250	136 (8)	85 (5)
1,250–1,499	170 (10)	136 (8)
1,500–1,999	205 (12)	170 (10)
2,000–2,499	220 (13)	205 (12)
≥2,500	255 (15)	220 (13)

[*] Includes asphyxia neonatorum, prolonged hypoxemia, severe acidosis, hypothermia (rectal temperature less than 35° C), septicemia, meningitis, deterioration of or insult to central nervous system, and birth weight less than 1,000 g.
Foetus and Newborn Committee, Canadian Paediatric Society: Use of phototherapy for neonatal hyperbilirubinemia. Can Med Assoc 1986; 134:1239.

- Hydrops fetalis (may be incorporated into above) requires immediate exchange transfusion with packed cells to correct anemia (see below)
- N.B. Postexchange (30–60 min) anticipate "rebound" rise in BR due to redistribution (of bilirubin)
- Much controversy exists about safe or critical levels of unconjugated BR, and they are currently ill defined. However, the threshold for intervention in the "sick," LBW, or VLBW infant should be low

2. Procedure
- Volume of exchange—preferably double volume (e.g., 160–170 ml/kg) → removal of 85% of fetal RBCs
- Type of blood—fresh and compatible with RBCs and plasma of infant. Choice of anti-

TABLE 17–14   Guidelines for Therapy for Jaundice

Indirect Serum Bilirubin	Birth Weight	<24 Hr	24–48 Hr	49–72 Hr	>72 Hr
(<5 mg/dl) <85 μmol/L	All				
(5–9 mg/dl) 85–155 μmol/L	All	Phototherapy if hemolysis			
(10–14 mg/dl)	<2,500 g	Exchange if hemolysis	←————— Phototherapy —————→		
170–240 μmol/L	>2,500 g			Investigate if bilirubin >204 μmol/L (12 mg/dl)	
(15–19 mg/dl)	<2,500 g	←————— EXCHANGE —————→		Consider exchange	
255–325 μmol/L	>2,500 g			Phototherapy	
(≥ 20 mg/dl) ≥ 340 μmol/L	All	←————————— EXCHANGE —————————→			

Key: ☐ Observe   ▨ Investigate jaundice

In presence of (1) perinatal asphyxia, (2) respiratory distresss, (3) metabolic acidosis (pH ≤ 7.25), (4) hypothermia (<35° C), (5) ↓ serum protein, (6) BW <1,500 g, (7) CNS deterioration, (8) sepsis, treat as in next higher bilirubin category.

Modified from Maisels MJ. Neonatal jaundice. In: Avery GB, ed. Neonatology. 2nd ed. Philadelphia: J.B. Lippincott, 1981.

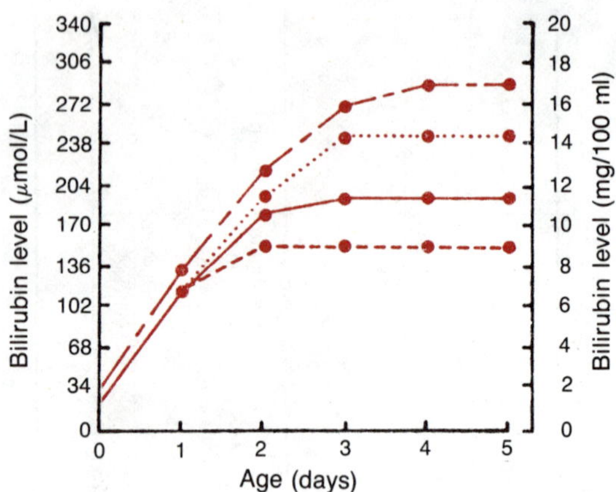

Figure 17–8 Suggested guide for initiation of phototherapy in neonatal hyperbilirubinemia. Curves represent serum unconjugated bilirubin level at which phototherapy should be considered. •— · —• = birth weight >2,500 g; •·····• = 2,001–2,500 g; •—• = 1,500–2,000 g; •---• = <1,500 g. (From Foetus and Newborn Committee, Canadian Paediatric Society. Use of phototherapy for neonatal hyperbilirubinemia. Can Med Assoc J 1986; 134:1238.)

coagulant (heparin, citrate phosphate dextrose) is variable, dependent on reason for exchange and preference of Center. Semi-packed (Hct 40–42%) cells preferable except in hydrops (see below). Blood should be prewarmed to ~ 35° C
- Rate of exchange: 5 ml aliquots—infants <1,000 g; 10 ml aliquots—infants 1,000–2,500 g; 15 ml aliquots—infants 2,500–3,000 g; up to 20 ml aliquots—infants ≥4,000 g
- "Slow" exchanges are preferable as they are safer and the "rebound" is less (e.g., each cycle should be at least 2 min)

- Prior to exchange, blood should be drawn for CBC, electrolytes, Ca^{2+}, and bilirubin. If indicated, blood for galactosemia screen, enzyme assays (e.g., pyruvate kinase), and TORCH(S) should also be drawn
- In hydropic infants (edema $\pm$ high output CHF with Hb $<$ 80 g/L [8 g/dl]), prompt restoration of Hb is essential: 50 ml/kg packed cells exchanged for same volume of infant's blood prior to complete double exchange (when patient stable). Most infants require one or more further exchanges
- Prior to exchange, insert an NG tube, empty stomach, and leave NG tube open to air
- During exchange, monitor temperature, EKG, RR, and acid-base status. CVP (N $<$ 10 cm H_2O) may also be monitored
- Volumes of blood, cycles of exchange, and vital signs are to be recorded on a special form by an observer (e.g., nurse)
- When exchange transfusion is indicated for severe chronic anemia, e.g., fetomaternal transfusion, the required exchange volume can be estimated as follows:

$$\text{Exchange volume (ml)} = \text{Total blood volume (85 ml} \times \text{BW [kg])} \times \left(\frac{\text{Desired Hct - Initial Hct}}{\text{Hct of donor blood}} \right)$$

  - Partial exchanges can be performed for marked polycythemia:

$$\text{Exchange volume (ml)} = \text{Total BV} \times \frac{\text{Initial Hct - Desired Hct}}{\text{Initial Hct}}$$

  (N.B. FF plasma is used here)
3. Complications of exchange transfusions
   - Embolization of air bubbles, or small clots
   - Hypocalcemia, hypoglycemia, acidosis, and hyperkalemia
   - Hypo- or hyperthermia
   - Sepsis (viral or bacterial)

• Cardiac arrhythmias, volume overload
• Others (see Suggested Reading)
• Phenobarbitone prophylaxis
  1. Some authors recommend use of phenobarbitone—given to mother in late pregnancy—in certain high risk circumstances, e.g., Rh isoimmunization. (See Suggested Reading for details.)

TEMPERATURE CONTROL IN PREMATURE INFANTS

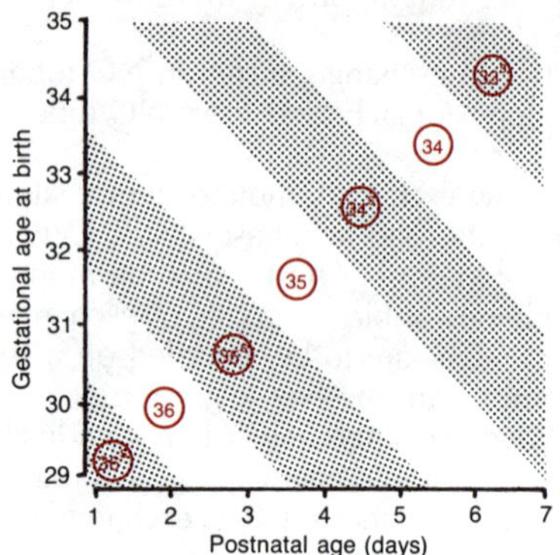

Neutral thermal environment during the first postnatal week for infants of 26–35 wk gestation.

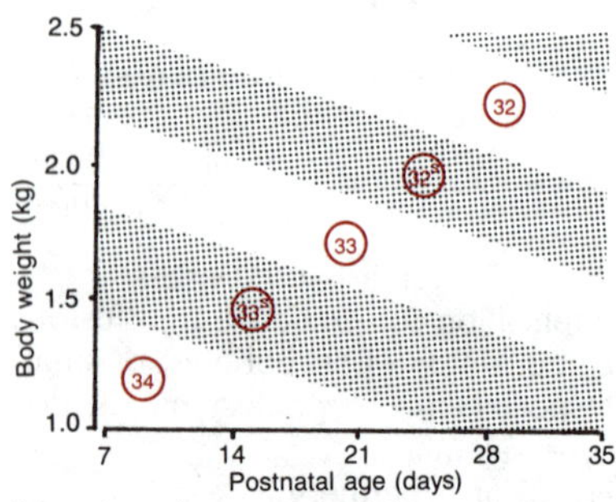

Neutral thermal environment for infants 26–35 wk gestation between 1–5 postnatal wk.

Figure 17–9   Neutral thermal environment for premature infants. The charts indicate the neutral thermal environment and are used as guidelines to set incubator temperature. The charts relate to infants of 26–35 wk gestation. No data are available for infants <26 wk. For naked infants >35 wk and >1 wk postnatal age in the incubator, the neutral thermal environment is 32.0° C. Axillary temperature of 36.7° C to 37.2° C is accepted as normal. If incubator temperature required to maintain this axillary temperature differs from that indicated in the guidelines, consider the possibility of: *A*, artefact, e.g., error in measurements of either incubator or axillary temperature, or lack of humidity, or *B*, disturbed homeostasis for age, e.g., illness. (Modified from Sauer PJJ, Dane HJ, Visser HKA. New standards for neutral thermal environment of healthy very low birthweight infants in week one of life. Arch Dis Child 1984; 59:19.)

Suggested Reading

1. Cloherty IP, Stark AR, eds. Manual of neonatal care. Boston: Little, Brown, 1985.
2. Finer NN, Kelly MA. Optimal ventilation for the neonate. Part II. Mechanical ventilation. Perinatol Neonatol 1983; 63–70.
3. Fox WW, Duara S. Persistent pulmonary hypertension in the neonate: diagnosis and management. J Pediatr 1983; 103:505–514.
4. Klaus MH, Faranoff AA, eds. Care of the high risk neonate. Philadelphia: W.B. Saunders, 1986.
5. Nelson NM. Current therapy in neonatal-perinatal medicine. Toronto: B.C. Decker, 1985–1986.

18   NEPHROLOGY

ACUTE RENAL FAILURE

General Considerations

- Definition: sudden decrease in renal function with a disturbed water and electrolyte balance and retention of nitrogenous wastes
- Oliguria: <300 ml/m²/day urine output. This is the minimum volume necessary to excrete the daily solute load of ~ 500 mOsm/24 hr. In neonates oliguria is <0.5 ml/kg/hr.
- Anuria: <1 ml/kg/24 hr (this fluid is from bladder secretions). Causes include
  1. Bilateral urinary tract obstruction
  2. Bilateral renal vein thrombosis
  3. Cortical necrosis
  4. Severe glomerulonephritis
  5. Hemolytic uremic syndrome

Management

- Rule out postrenal (obstructive) causes (ultrasound most useful)
- Differentiate prerenal from (intrinsic) renal causes
  1. "Laboratory" differentiation (Table 18–1)
  2. "Therapeutic challenge" to differentiate (Fig. 18–1)
     - Preferably carried out in ICU setting where CVP monitoring can be instituted
     - Fluid challenge: Give a test dose of normal saline, Ringer's lactate, or a colloid solution (10 or 20 ml/kg over 1–2 hr)
     - Diuretic challenge (use cautiously)
       a. To be used once prerenal factors have been corrected

b. Lasix 1–2 mg/kg/dose IV × 2 maximum (4 hr apart), ± mannitol 0.5–1 g/kg IV × 1

(N.B. Mannitol may →↑ blood volume + pulmonary edema; therefore it is not recommended in CHF. Furosemide may exacerbate renal failure and may cause ototoxicity, especially when given in large amounts in the presence of metabolic acidosis.)

- This *may* convert oliguric to nonoliguric ATN, which has a lower morbidity and mortality
- Clear response defined as urine output >2 ml/kg/hr post challenge in prerenal azotemia. However, even with a diuretic response, improvement in renal function does not always follow.

3. N.B. *All these methods must be used with caution to avoid overloading or dehydration*

TABLE 18–1 Differentiation of Prerenal from Intrinsic Renal Disorders as Causes of Acute Renal Failure

	Prerenal	Renal (Intrinsic)
Urine specific gravity[*]	>1.020	$<1.010–1.015$
Urine Na$^+$ (mmol/L)	<10	>25
Urine/plasma osmolality	>1.3	<1.1
Sediment	Hyaline and fine granular casts	Renal tubular cells and casts

[*] These values are not useful if diuretics have been used.
NB: False ↑ specific gravity with proteinuria, glycosuria, mannitol, and radio-opaque dyes.

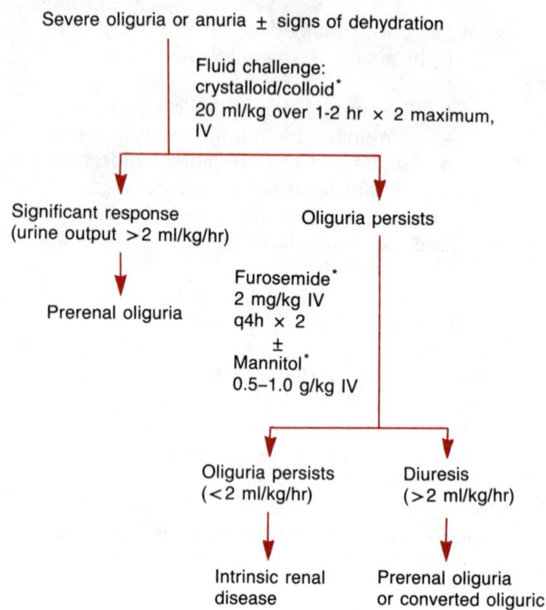

*See text for cautions!

Figure 18–1   Differentiation of prerenal from intrinsic renal causes of acute renal failure.

- Fluid management
  1. Prerenal
     Adequate rapid rehydration with an appropriate solution (saline, Ringer's lactate, blood, albumin, plasma). (See preceding section.) Once renal failure is established, treat as for renal parenchymal disease (following).
  2. Renal
     - Insensible losses (300–400 ml/m²/day, or 20 ml/kg/day), plus...
     - Urine losses, plus...

- Replace other losses (blood, GI)
- Increase 12% for each 1° C rise in temperature
3. NOTES:
  - *Monitor* with frequent weights and electrolyte and acid-base assessment (a fluid flow chart can be useful here)
  - CVP monitoring may be necessary (see following)
  - Infection is the major cause of death in ARF. Therefore avoid unnecessary instrumentation at all costs!
- Management of specific complications
  1. Acidosis (metabolic): see p 141
  2. Hypertension: see p 443
  3. Hyperkalemia
     - Investigations
        STAT ECG: tall peaked T waves, widening of QRS, ↑ PR interval, ↓ size of P and R waves, ST segment depression, and gradual prolongation of QT interval
     - Treatment
        a. $Na^+ - K^+$ exchange resin, e.g., kayexalate 1 g/kg orally (except in prematures) or rectally q1–2h prn. (Rectal administration more rapidly effective [~ 30 minutes], whereas oral administration may take ~ 12 hr to have effect.)
        b. If K^+ >7.0 mmol(mEq)/L, in addition to preceding give:
           - $NaHCO_3$ 1–3 mmol(mEq)/kg IV (shifts K^+ into cells), but beware if ↓ Ca^{2+} present, as may precipitate tetany. For each 0.1 pH ↓, plasma K^+ ↑ ~ 0.6 mmol(mEq)/L.
           - Dextrose 0.5 g/kg/hr until blood sugar 14 mmol/L (250 mg/dl). This shifts K^+ into cells (see following).

c. If ECG changes present
  - 10% calcium gluconate 0.5 ml/kg IV over 3–5 min causes rapid reversal of ECG changes by antagonizing effect of ↑ K^+
  - Note that calcium gluconate does not affect K^+ levels; hence must be combined with preceding therapy. (*Do not use simultaneously with $NaHCO_3$!*)
  - Insulin (exogenous) may be used with glucose infusion, but should be avoided if possible (usual dose=1 unit regular insulin/5 g of glucose)

d. Dialysis—specific indications
  - Fluid overload uncontrollable with preceding treatment and causing hypertension or pulmonary edema
  - Uncontrolled hyperkalemia
  - Severe uncontrolled metabolic acidosis
  - Clinical signs of progressive uremia (CNS)
  - Dialysable nephrotoxin
  - Hyperammonemia
  - N.B. *The duration of action of bicarbonate, Ca^{2+}, glucose, and insulin is short, and dialysis should be started early to remove K^+ from the body rather than redistributing it intracellularly!*
  - Dialysis may also facilitate early introduction of aggressive nutritional therapy

URINARY TRACT INFECTIONS (UTI)

General Considerations

- Definition: significant bacteriuria with pyuria
  1. Two clean voided urine specimens showing $\geq 10^5$ pure colonies/ml of same organism (90–95% probability of a UTI) or
  2. $>10^3$ pure colonies/ml in a catheter specimen or
  3. Any concentration in a suprapubic specimen
- Predisposing factors include
  1. Sex–males predominate in neonatal period; females predominate thereafter
  2. Congenital structural anomalies (e.g., posterior urethral valves, duplications, fistulas, hypospadias, ureteroceles)
  3. Foreign bodies, e.g., indwelling catheter
  4. Neurologic conditions, e.g., meningomyelocele, tumor, tethered cord
  5. Genital abuse should be considered
  6. In females also consider severe constipation, pinworms, incorrect voiding pattern with holding back, bubble bath, improper wiping
- Etiologic agents
  1. *E. coli* accounts for $>85\%$ of UTIs in girls. Proteus accounts for the majority in males.
  2. Also consider *S. fecalis,* Klebsiella, Pseudomonas, *S. epidermidis*
- Differential diagnosis of pyuria
  1. Bacterial UTI
  2. Viral cystitis (adenovirus causes hemorrhagic cystitis)
  3. Fever or dehydration
  4. Mycoplasma/tuberculosis
  5. Appendicitis

Management

- Investigations
  1. Urine for culture and sensitivity (clean catch, catheter, or suprapubic)
  2. Urine for microscopy (see p 460)
  3. Blood culture and CBC in neonate (as usually systemic infection)
  4. Screening tests, e.g., nitrite or dipslides (Uricult), may be used in the office (see p 463) or at home
- Treatment
  1. Maintain adequate fluid intake
  2. Antibiotic therapy
     - Oral therapy, e.g., amoxicillin, trimethoprim-sulfamethoxazole (TMP-SMX), nitrofurantoin, sulfisoxazole, and cephalosporins, is usually adequate for acute uncomplicated UTI, with or without symptoms
     - Parenteral therapy, e.g., ampicillin plus gentamicin (or other aminoglycoside), is usually recommended in ill child
     - A simple (uncomplicated) infection is usually treated for 7–10 days. (Single dose therapy controversial in children.)
     - Complicated (upper tract) infections usually treated for 10–14 days
     - Antibiotic sensitivities should be checked and treatment adjusted accordingly

Follow-Up

- Cultures
  1. In 48 hours should be sterile
  2. 2–3 days following cessation of therapy to exclude early reinfection
  3. Rates of recurrence (same organism) of UTI directly related to number of previous episodes
  4. May need follow-up cultures or nitrite sticks

- Radiologic evaluation
    1. Indicated after a first UTI in all males, and in females <13 yr (not sexually active)
    2. Intravenous pyelogram (IVP) (or ultrasound) and voiding cystourethrogram (VCUG) to determine vesicoureteral reflux and obstructive or potentially obstructive lesions
    3. Follow-up studies if reflux present
- Indications for chemoprophylaxis (e.g., small dose TMP-SMX, or nitrofurantoin)
    1. Visicoureteral reflux, until free of reflux for at least 1 yr
    2. Obstructive uropathy (anatomic or neurogenic)
    3. Normal anatomy, but $\geq$ three UTIs/yr
- Surgery (may be) indicated for
    1. Anatomic anomaly
    2. Antireflux procedure
- Development and growth
    1. Follow child's growth, development, blood pressure, and renal function if indicated

CHRONIC RENAL FAILURE

General Considerations and Clinical Features

- There is chronic reduction of renal function with a decrease in GFR resulting in clinical and biochemical disturbances
- Onset is gradual with initial biochemical abnormalities asymptomatic
- Progresses to nonspecific symptoms of fatigue, malaise, anorexia, and headaches
- With progressive disease, more systemic involvement emerges (Table 18–2)

TABLE 18–2 Important Clinical Features of Chronic Renal Failure

Growth Failure and Delayed Puberty
  Inadequate caloric intake (anorexia)
  Acidosis
  Renal osteodystrophy
  Steroid therapy
  Hormonal disturbances
Fluid Balance-Biochemical Derangement
  Na^+ and H_2O retention→edema and circulatory congestion
  ↑ BP and CHF
  ↑ K^+ ± dysrhythmias
  Metabolic acidosis—impaired NH_3 production and acid metabolite excretion
  ↑ urea and creatinine; ↓ creatinine clearance
  ↑ urate and triglycerides
Neurologic Dysfunction
  Encephalopathy
  Seizures
  Peripheral neuropathy
Renal Osteodystrophy
  ↓ Phosphate (P) excretion →↑ P, binds Ca^{2+} →↑ PTH
  Impaired hydroxylation $25(OH)D_3$→↓ Ca^{2+} GI absorption →↑ PTH
  Radiologic changes
    ↓ Bone age
    Subperiosteal bone resorption on radial aspect of phalanges
    Rachitic changes
Hematologic
  Anemia (usually normochromic normocytic)
  Bone marrow suppression
  ↓ Erythropoietin
  ↓ Folate/Fe, etc.
Bleeding
  Platelet dysfunction

Management

- General
  1. Monitor biochemical and hematologic parameters regularly
  2. Psychological and educational support
- Dietary
  1. A dietician should be consulted for all patients
  2. If possible, avoid stringent unpalatable diets
  3. Ensure adequate caloric intake
  4. Ensure high quality protein and essential amino acid intake, although total protein intake should be decreased
  5. Diet low in K^+, phosphate (P), Na^+
  6. Infants may need to be gavage fed (or have gastrostomy inserted) if oral intake is poor
  7. Multivitamin supplements
  8. Oral phosphate binders, e.g., calcium carbonate (OSCAL). Avoid aluminium preparations in children.
  9. Adequate dietary calcium with supplementary vitamin D (dihydrotachysterol or $1,25(OH)_2D_3$)
- Fluid and electrolytes
  1. Restrict fluid if edema, ↑ BP, CHF present
  2. Diuretics may be indicated
  3. Antihypertensives as required (see p 453)
  4. Kayexalate orally or per rectum for hyperkalemia (see p 429 for acute management)
  5. Bicarbonate for metabolic acidosis
- Anemia
  1. This is well tolerated. Transfuse slowly and with small volumes if patient is symptomatic.
- Other
  1. For end stage renal failure, one needs to consider dialysis or renal transplantation

GLOMERULONEPHRITIS

General Considerations and Clinical Features

- May be characterized by
  1. Nephritic syndrome
     - Oliguria (< 300 ml/m²/day)
     - Hematuria (gross or microscopic)
     - Edema
     - ↑ BP
  2. Or nephrotic syndrome (to follow), or a mixture of both
- Etiology: see Table 18–3

TABLE 18–3 Etiology of Glomerulonephritis (GN)

↓ C_3	Normal C_3
Poststreptococcal (PSAGN)	IgA nephropathy (Berger's)
Membranoproliferative GN, types I and II	Hereditary nephritis (Alport's)
	Rapidly progressive GN
Systemic lupus (SLE)	Henoch-Schönlein purpura (HSP)
Bacterial endocarditis (SBE)	
Shunt nephritis	Goodpasture's syndrome and anti-GBM disease
	Membranoproliferative GN, type I

Management

- Investigations and work-up
  1. Family history—deafness (high frequency) and hematuria
  2. General investigations
     - Urinalysis for protein, blood, microscopy (casts—hyaline, granular, and cellular)
     - Total hemolytic complement and C_3 (remains low for about 2–6 wk in PSAGN)
     - Electrolytes, urea (BUN), creatinine, acid-base status

- CBC and smear, ESR
  - Protein electrophoresis and cholesterol if
    significant edema
  - Chest x-ray ($\pm$ cardiomegaly $\pm$ pulmonary
    edema $\pm$ effusion)
3. Specific investigations
  - Throat swab (or swab of impetigo if
    present), antistreptolysin-O titer (ASOT),
    antihyaluronidase titer
  - Renal biopsy may be indicated
- Treatment—General
  1. Hospitalization usually necessary, in view of
     unpredictable severity of acute phase, to ob-
     serve for
     - Renal failure
     - Circulatory overload (with ↑ BP, pulmonary
       edema, encephalopathy)
     - Electrolyte and acid-base disturbances
  2. Fluid management: restrict for oliguria,
     hyponatremia, circulatory overload (insensi-
     ble water loss [400 ml/m²/24 hr] + urine
     output)
  3. Dietary therapy: low salt (if hypertensive),
     low K⁺ (if ↑ K⁺), normal protein
  4. Hyponatremia: fluid restriction (hypertonic
     saline *only* if symptomatic; see p 136 and 139)
  5. Positive bacterial cultures: penicillin or as ap-
     propriate
  6. See relevant sections for management of
     hyperkalemia (p 429), acidosis (p 141),
     hypertension (p 443), and cardiac failure (p
     41 and 42)

HEMOLYTIC UREMIC SYNDROME

General Considerations

- Acute onset of microangiopathic hemolytic anemia, thrombocytopenia, and acute renal failure
- Usually infants; often a diarrheal prodrome
- Acute onset; usually good prognosis
- Predominantly glomerular involvement may follow a viral (coxsackie, arbovirus) or bacterial (group A β-hemolytic strep, Salmonella, Shigella) infection
- Typical case is secondary to a particular *E. coli* that produces a verotoxin
- Nonepidemic forms (sporadic form, familial form) exist—with a worse prognosis and more vascular involvement

Clinical Features

- Prodromal illness: days to 2 wk before presentation
- Acute onset of irritability, lethargy, coma, severe pallor, purpura, bruising, oliguria, and often anuria
- Jaundice and pancreatic dysfunction may be noted, and renal failure may lead to hypertension, seizures, and circulatory overload
- Acute phase may last weeks to months and in some the course is progressive with chronic renal failure

Management

- Investigations
  1. CBC and smear: ↓Hb, anisocytosis, fragmented, helmet shaped and burr cells; ↑reticulocytes; platelets normal early, then ↓
  2. Urinalysis (if not anuric): hematuria, proteinuria, RBC and granular casts on microscopy
  3. Stool cultures (e.g., Shigella, *E. coli*)

PROTEINURIA

General Considerations

- Definition: >150 mg/24 hr, or >140 mg/m² in small children
- Classification of proteinuria
  1. Glomerular
     - ↑ Capillary permeability to protein
     - Examples include primary nephrotic syndrome, membranous GN, poststreptococcal GN, drugs, diabetes
  2. Tubular: ↓ reabsorption from filtrate, e.g., Fanconi's syndrome, interstitial nephritis
- Causes of proteinuria
  1. Intermittent proteinuria
     - Functional, e.g., related to strenuous exercise, fever, extreme cold
     - Orthostatic
       a. Occurs only when person is upright
       b. Good prognosis
       c. May be seen in resolving pyelonephritis or glomerulonephritis
       d. Tends to disappear slowly
     - Transient but not orthostatic
       a. Excellent prognosis
       b. Often idiopathic
  2. Persistent proteinuria
     - Non-nephrotic:
       or
     - Nephrotic:

     ↑ risk of development of ↑BP, CRF. Renal biopsy may → minimal lesion nephrotic syndrome, focal segmental glomerulosclerosis, membranoproliferative GN, membranous nephropathy, Berger's disease

Management

- Exclude transient proteinuria
- Exclude orthostatic
    1. Test urine sample *immediately* upon rising, and another after walking or standing for 2 hr or more. (Repeat × 2.)
    2. 2 × 12 hr urine collections (12 hr while ambulant, 12 hr while recumbent)
- History
    1. Family history of renal disease, deafness
    2. Medications, e.g., gold, penicillamine, probenecid, amphotericin
    3. Other symptoms related to urinary tract or other systemic diseases
- Physical signs: height, weight, and BP
- Complete urinalysis (including specific gravity [SG])
- Renal function
    1. 24 hr urine collection for protein, and creatinine clearance
    2. Urea, creatinine, electrolytes
- Further work-up if associated features dictate (e.g., protein electrophoresis, C_3, serum lipids)
- Renal biopsy may be indicated (see below)

NEPHROTIC SYNDROME

General Considerations

- Characterized by
    1. Proteinuria (>50 mg/kg/day or >40 mg/m²/hr)
    2. Hypoproteinemia (often <25 g/L [or 2.5 g/dl] albumin)
    3. Edema
    4. Hyperlipidemia
- Etiology: may be primary or secondary; see Table 18–4

- Indications for renal biopsy
    1. Age <1 yr
    2. Marked nephritic syndrome components ($\uparrow$
       BP, renal failure, gross hematuria) and etiol-
       ogy not known
    3. Low C_3
    4. No response *once on steroid therapy* for 4–8
       wk
- Complications
    1. Diminished resistance to infection (pneu-
       mococcus, *H. influenzae*, coliforms), espe-
       cially peritonitis
    2. Hypovolemia, with postural hypotension, cir-
       culatory collapse, renal failure (in minority of
       patients with minimal change lesion)
    3. Protein depletion
    4. $\uparrow$ Coagulability of blood, leading to thrombo-
       sis (especially of renal vein)
    5. Complications of therapy (diuretics, steroids,
       cytotoxics)

Management

- General
    1. Diet
        - Protein normal, unless in renal failure
        - Low Na^+
        - Decrease fluid intake if edema severe and
          progressive
    2. Exclude bacterial infection, e.g., peritonitis,
       and treat appropriately if present
    3. Guard against skin breakdown
    4. Psychological support
- Edema
    1. For respiratory distress, impending skin
       breakdown, or marked ascites
        - Infuse 1 g/kg of salt-poor 25% albumin IV
          over $\sim$ 1–2 hr, followed by IV furose-
          mide, 1–2 mg/kg

2. Avoid too aggressive efforts at diuresis, as this may produce intravascular depletion and further aggravate oliguria and hypercoagulable state
- Specific therapy
  1. Remission induction
     - Prednisone 2 mg/kg/day (60 mg/m²/day) in 3–4 doses (maximum 80 mg/day)
     - Treat until urine negative for 5 days, or for a total of 28 days
     - If no remission in 28 days, consider biopsy. If biopsy consistent with steroid responsive type, resume therapy for another 28 days, or alternatively consider addition of cyclophosphamide. If compatible with steroid resistant type, treat with appropriate therapy, if available or applicable.
  2. Maintenance therapy
     - Prednisone 1.5–2.0 mg/kg (45–60 mg/m²/day)—single dose (maximum 80 mg/day), alternate days for 28 days; then reduce quickly
     - Alternatively reduce by 10 mg q2–4wk to 30 mg; then ↓ by 5 mg q2–4wk until discontinued
     - Monitor first morning void for albumin at home
  3. Relapse (~ two-thirds of patients)
     - 2+ or heavier proteinuria for 7 consecutive days
     - Treat as above to induce remission; then give alternate day treatment
     - Cytotoxic drugs (e.g., chlorambucil, cyclophosphamide) are used for steroid dependent, steroid resistant cases or frequent relapsers, but because of serious potential side effects this should be done in consultation with a nephrologist
     - Steroid resistant cases should be considered for renal biopsy

TABLE 18–4   Causes of Nephrotic Syndrome in Children

Primary (90%)	Secondary (10%)
Minimal lesion (~70%)	Lupus erythematosus (SLE)
Focal glomerulosclerosis	Anaphylactoid purpura
Diffuse mesangial proliferation	Infections—malaria, hepatitis B, congenital syphilis
Membranous glomerulopathy	
Membranoproliferative GN	Lymphoproliferative disorders
Congenital nephrosis	Drugs, e.g., mercury, gold, bismuth

HYPERTENSION

General Considerations

- Etiology (Table 18–5)
  1. Secondary hypertension more likely if
     - Onset <13 yr
     - Diastolic pressure ≥120 mm Hg
     - Abnormal urinalysis or renal function
  2. Essential or primary probably less common
- Normal BP values dependent on age (see Figs. 18–2, 18–3)

Management

- Acute hypertensive crisis
  1. Ensure that proper BP cuff size is used, and repeat BP 2–3 × prior to treatment, unless symptomatic (e.g., seizures ± papilledema). Check BP in lower limbs as well.
  2. For malignant or accelerated (± hypertensive encephalopathy ± L ventricular failure ± marked acute elevation in BP, e.g., 160/110) hypertension, urgent drug therapy is warranted (Table 18–6)

TABLE 18–5   Etiology of Hypertension

- Primary or essential
- Secondary
  1. Cardiovascular—coarctation
  2. Renal and vascular
     Congenital (polycystic, hydronephrosis)
     Glomerulonephritis—acute or chronic
     Reflux nephropathy
     Pyelonephritis
     Renal artery stenosis (2° causes include
       neurofibromatosis)
     Renal vein thrombosis
     Renal tumors (e.g., Wilm's, sarcoma)
  3. Endocrine
     Pheochromocytoma
     Cushing's
     Hyperaldosteronism
     Adrenal carcinoma
     Hyperthyroidism
     Congenital adrenal hyperplasia
  4. Miscellaneous
     Drugs (steroids, oral contraceptives)
     ↑ Intracranial pressure
     Burns
     Autonomic (Guillain-Barré, Riley-Day, polio)
     Lead nephropathy
     Hypercalcemia
     Immobilization
     Post surgery with inflammatory bowel disease

3. Once the acute "crisis" is over, attempts must be made to find an etiology, if not already known. Therapy can then be directed at the primary cause (if possible) or at preventing a recurrence of the "crisis" with maintenance (drug) therapy (Table 18–7).

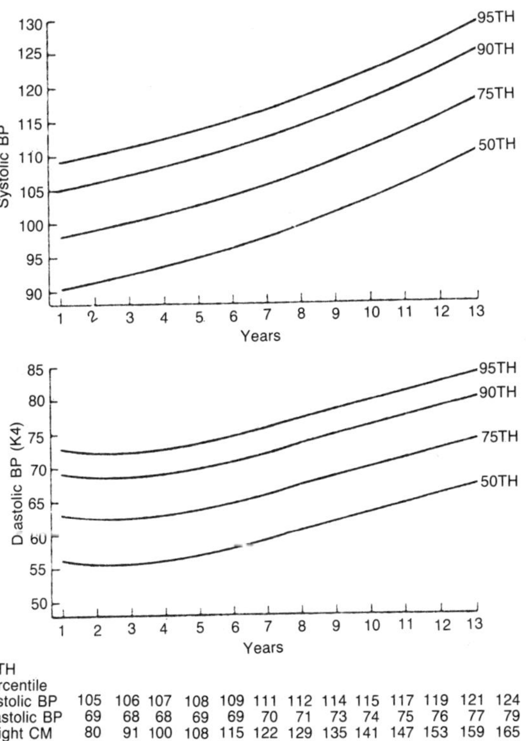

90TH Percentile												
Systolic BP	105	106	107	108	109	111	112	114	115	117	119	121	124
Diastolic BP	69	68	68	69	69	70	71	73	74	75	76	77	79
Height CM	80	91	100	108	115	122	129	135	141	147	153	159	165
Weight KG	11	14	16	18	22	25	29	34	39	44	50	55	62

A. Boys: 1–13 yr of age

Figure 18–2   Percentiles of blood pressure measurement in boys and girls. (From Report of the Second Task Force on Blood Pressure Control in Children—1987. Pediatrics 1987; 79:5–6.)

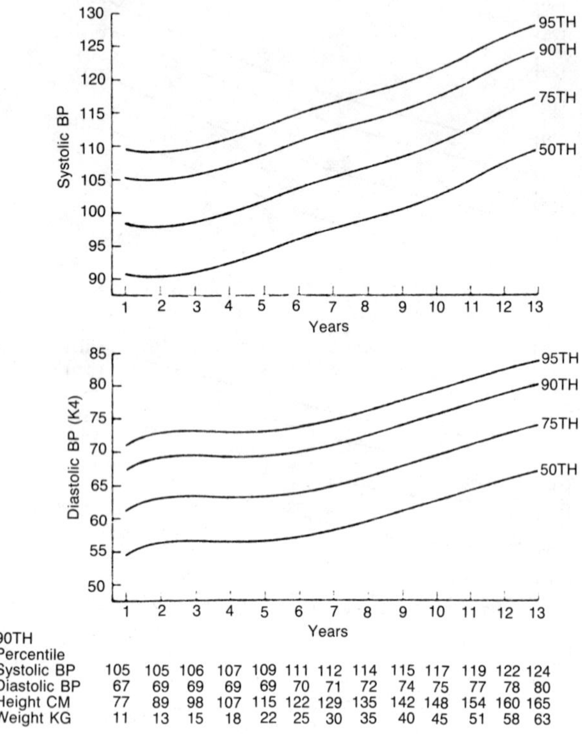

90TH Percentile													
Systolic BP	105	105	106	107	109	111	112	114	115	117	119	122	124
Diastolic BP	67	69	69	69	69	70	71	72	74	75	77	78	80
Height CM	77	89	98	107	115	122	129	135	142	148	154	160	165
Weight KG	11	13	15	18	22	25	30	35	40	45	51	58	63

B. Girls: 1–13 yr of age

Figure 18–2 Continued.

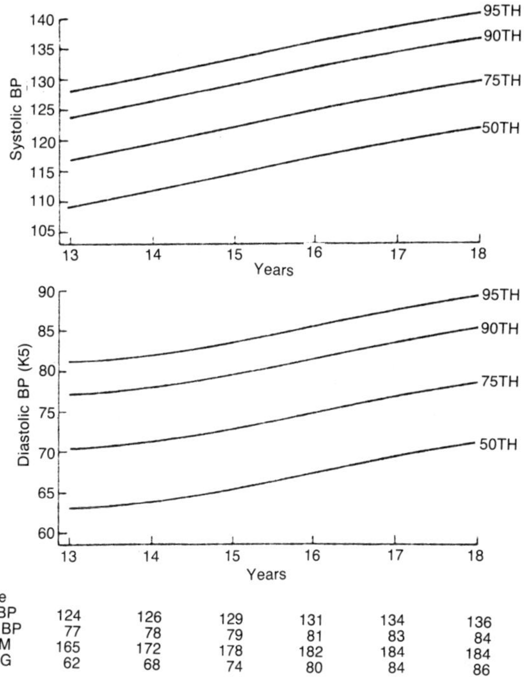

90TH Percentile						
Systolic BP	124	126	129	131	134	136
Diastolic BP	77	78	79	81	83	84
Height CM	165	172	178	182	184	184
Weight KG	62	68	74	80	84	86

C. Boys: 13–18 yr of age

Figure 18–2 Continued.

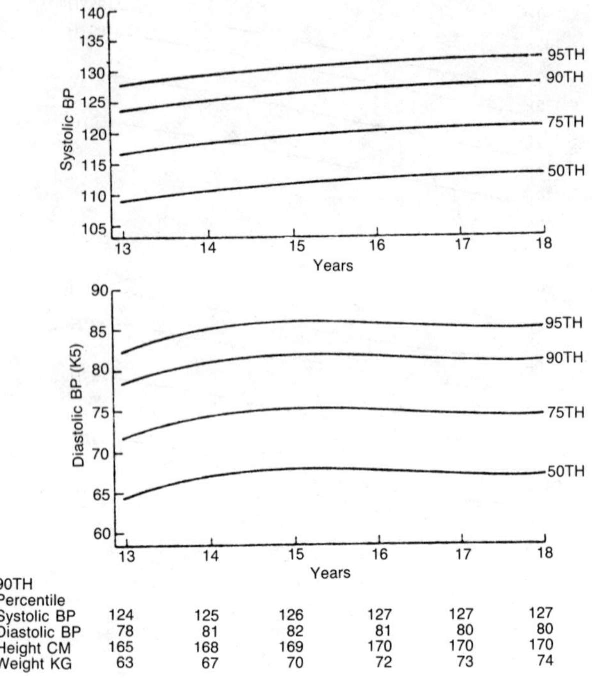

90TH Percentile						
Systolic BP	124	125	126	127	127	127
Diastolic BP	78	81	82	81	80	80
Height CM	165	168	169	170	170	170
Weight KG	63	67	70	72	73	74

D. Girls: 13–18 yr of age

Figure 18–2 Continued.

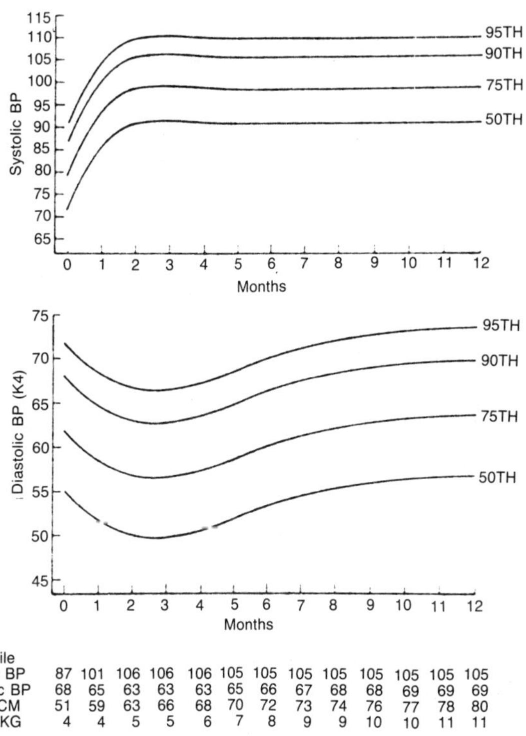

OTH Percentile													
ystolic BP	87	101	106	106	106	105	105	105	105	105	105	105	105
iastolic BP	68	65	63	63	63	65	66	67	68	68	69	69	69
eight CM	51	59	63	66	68	70	72	73	74	76	77	78	80
/eight KG	4	4	5	5	6	7	8	9	9	10	10	11	11

A. Boys

Figure 18–3 Percentiles of blood pressure in infants awake, (birth to 12 months of age). (From Report of the Second Task Force on Blood Pressure Control in Children—1987. Pediatrics 1987; 79:5–6.)

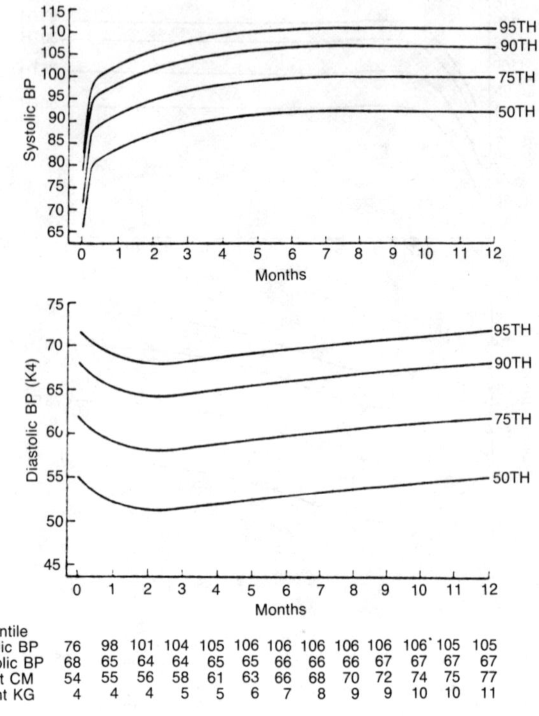

90TH Percentile												
Systolic BP	76	98	101	104	105	106	106	106	106	106	106	105	105
Diastolic BP	68	65	64	64	65	65	66	66	66	67	67	67	67
Height CM	54	55	56	58	61	63	66	68	70	72	74	75	77
Weight KG	4	4	4	5	5	6	7	8	9	9	10	10	11

B. Girls

Figure 18–3 Continued.

TABLE 18–6 Emergency Drug Therapy in Hypertensive Emergencies

Drug: Dosage	Duration	Side Effects
Vasodilators		
Diazoxide: 1–2 mg/kg/dose IV bolus (over 30 sec) q5–15 min until BP controlled (onset within minutes → arteriolar dilation)	Up to 24 hr (mean ~ 5 hr)	Acute hypotension, ↑ glucose, tachycardia, Na^+ and fluid retention, headache
Nitroprusside: 0.5–8.0 μg/kg/min IV, titrated to response (immediate onset → arteriolar and venous dilation)	During infusion only	Hypotension, tachycardia, headache, nausea, chest pain; *↑ risk of cyanide poisoning if used >48 hr!*
Hydralazine 0.2–0.5 mg/kg IV (max. 25 mg IV) (arteriolar dilation—onset within 30 min)	4–12 hr	Hypotension, tachycardia, fluid retention, vomiting, lupus-like syndrome
Sympathetic Blocking Agents		
Labetalol 1–3 mg/kg IV (α and β blocker—onset within minutes)	Up to 24 hr	GI upset, headache, dizziness
Phentolamine 0.1–0.2 mg/kg IV (α-blocker used in pheochromocytoma → immediate onset)	30–60 min	Tachycardia, ↓ BP, nausea, vomiting, abdominal pain

Continued next page

TABLE 18–6 Emergency Drug Therapy in Hypertensive Emergencies (Continued)

Drug: Dosage	Duration	Side Effects
Others		
*Captopril: 0.3–2 mg/kg per dose PO (angiotensin converting enzyme inhibitor—onset within 15 min)	8–12 hr	Neutropenia, proteinuria, reversible renal failure in renovascular disease, rash
*Nifedipine: 0.25–0.5 mg/kg sublingually: maximum 20 mg (calcium channel blocker—onset within 20–30 min)	6 hr	Dizziness and facial flushing
*Clonidine: 2–6 μg/kg IV (central α adrenergic stimulation—onset within 30 min)	8 hr	Sedation, dry mouth, rebound ↑ BP

* 2nd line drugs.

TABLE 18–7 Drug Therapy for Nonemergent Hypertension

Diuretics
  Hydrochlorothiazide
  Spironolactone: Caution in CRF→ ↑ K^+
  Furosemide
β-Blockers
  Propranolol: Avoid in asthmatics, diabetics, Raynaud's, CHF
  Metoprolol: → headache, bronchospasm, fatigue, dizziness
  Nadolol (Corgard): Advantage—once daily use (side effects as per propranolol)
Vasodilators
  Hydralazine
  Minoxidil: → hirsutism, Na^+ and fluid retention
  Prazosin: α-blockade as well (may → +ve ANA)
Sympathetic inhibitor and peripheral norepinephrine depletion
  α-Methyl-dopa: may → Coomb's positive hemolytic anemia, ↑ liver enzymes
Calcium channel blockers
  Nifedipine: Dosage not yet established in pediatric age group (may → peripheral edema, dizziness, headache, nausea and vomiting)
Angiotensin converting enzyme inhibitor
  Captopril: See formulary for dosages and side effects
  Enalapril (Vasotec): Dosage not yet established in pediatric age group; advantage—once daily use (side effects as per captopril)

Notes: 1. Dosages are in formulary.
2. All vasodilators are associated with fluid retention; therefore, it is often necessary to combine with a diuretic.
3. Drug therapy often starts with diuretics, then sympatholytics (e.g., β-blockers, α-methyl-dopa) and vasodilators are added systematically. This approach, however, may be modified according to etiology (e.g., captopril in patients with "renal" hypertension may be introduced earlier in certain situations).

- ''Work-up'' of hypertension should include
  1. Confirmation of BP by frequent measurement
     with an appropriate sized cuff (two-thirds of
     arm, and bladder to completely encircle arm)
  2. Investigation for etiology, the sequence of
     which is determined by the clinical findings
     - Renal
       a. Urinalysis and urine specific gravity
       b. Urine culture
       c. Plasma electrolytes, urea, creatinine,
          blood acid-base status, uric acid
       d. Creatinine clearance
       e. Ultrasound of abdomen (anatomy of GU
          system)
       f. IVP, renal scan
       g. Renins (peripheral $\pm$ renal vein)
       h. $\pm$ Arteriogram
     - Cardiac
       a. CXR, ECG
       b. Echocardiogram
     - Endocrine
       a. 24 hr urine for VMA and catecholamines
       b. Cortisol, aldosterone, renin (plasma)
       c. Thyroid function tests
- Treatment of hypertension
  1. General
     - Low Na^+ diet, no added salt
     - Weight reduction and control
     - Physical activity (dynamic or aerobic ex-
       ercise)
     - Avoid smoking
  2. Drug therapy
     - If symptomatic
     - If target organ damage
     - If BP persistently >95th percentile
     - For specific medications, see Table 18–7.
       For dosages, see formulary.

NOCTURNAL ENURESIS

General Considerations

- Definition: the involuntary emptying of the bladder at night after the age when bladder control is expected
- Can be considered a normal variation of bladder control rather than a disease state
- 10% of enuretics have daytime wetting
- Occurrence: ~ 30% at age 4 yr, ~ 10% at age 6 yr, 3% at age 12 yr, and 1% at age 18 yr. Spontaneous ''cure'' rate ~ 15%/yr.
- Proposed predisposing factors
  1. Genetic predisposition (delayed maturation)
  2. Slight male preponderance
  3. Small functional bladder capacity
  4. Inappropriate toilet training may be contributory
  5. Precipitation by stressful environmental events may cause regressive enuresis (e.g., divorce, new sibling)
  6. Organic etiology (UTI, diabetes mellitus-insipidus, chronic renal failure) in small minority

Management

- Remember that the problem is usually benign and self-limiting
- All enuretics should have the following basic screening evaluations done:
  1. Simple urinalysis (protein, glucose, specific gravity) ± urine culture
  2. Growth chart (height, weight) should be plotted
- Therapeutic approaches
  1. Bedtime routine
     - Restrict fluids 2–3 hr before bedtime
     - No diapers or plastic pants after age 4 yr
     - Double voiding at bedtime

2. Reassure child about etiology and prognosis
3. Positive reinforcement techniques (e.g., Star chart) and no punitive action by caregivers
4. Bladder exercises
5. Drugs: imipramine is a potentially lethal drug and should be used with caution for a limited period after other modalities have failed (high relapse rate)
6. Enuresis alarms
   - These should be used on a motivated child, not before 8 yr of age
   - Cures are attained slowly, but the success rate is higher than with other modes of therapy alone

PERITONITIS IN CHRONIC AMBULATORY PERITONEAL DIALYSIS (CAPD)

General Considerations

- Etiologic agents: *Staphylococcus epidermidis, Staphylococcus aureus, Streptococcus viridans,* gram negative organisms, e.g., *E. coli*, Pseudomonas

Management

- Investigations
  1. Clinical diagnosis
     - Cloudy effluent
     - Abdominal pain
     - Fever
  2. Laboratory diagnosis
     - Dialysate WBC >100/mm^3 with >50% polymorphonucleocytes (PMN) ± positive Gram stain
     - Positive culture

- Treatment
  1. Using 1.5% dianeal, do three exchanges (in and out) with heparin (500 units/L) added
  2. Save the initial cloudy bag. Refrigerate until it can be taken to a laboratory for culture.
  3. To the fourth bag add
     - Cefazolin (Ancef, Kefzol), 500 mg/L
     - Tobramycin, 1.7 mg/kg/bag
     - Heparin, 500 U/L
  4. To subsequent bags add
     - Cefazolin, 250 mg/L
     - Tobramycin, 8 mg/L
     - Heparin, 500 U/L. If bag still cloudy, continue heparin until bag clears.
  5. Antibiotics to be adjusted pending sensitivities
  6. *Staphylococcus aureus* peritonitis
     - Cloxacillin: loading dose 1 g/L, then maintenance 100 mg/L, added to each bag.
     - Rifampin 10–20 mg/kg/day divided bid PO
  7. Continue therapy for minimum of 2 wk for proven cases; resistant cases may need longer therapy

RENAL FUNCTION TESTS
Creatinine Clearance (C_{cr})

- A fairly good measure of GFR; approximates inulin clearance in the normal ranges of GFR
- Limitations
  1. Creatinine production can vary, especially with severe illness
  2. Some secretion occurs, particularly when renal function is markedly reduced
  3. The consumption of red meat can ↑ serum creatinine

4. A 24 hr urine volume <1 L usually gives a
   falsely low reading in older children or
   adults
- Calculation of C_{cr}:

$$C_{cr} = \frac{U \times V}{P \times t} \times \frac{1.73}{SA}$$

where: U =urine concentration in mg/dl
         or μmol/L
       V =total volume of urine in 24 hr
         (in ml)
       t   =time of collection of urine
         (24 hr=1,440 min=86,400 sec)
       P =serum creatinine (mg/dl or μmol/L)
       SA =surface area (m²)

- Normal production of creatinine by body
  1. Adult females and children: 135–175
     μmol/kg/day (15–20 mg/kg/day)
  2. Adult males: 175–220 μmol/kg/day (20–25
     mg/kg/day)
- GFR also can be very accurately determined
  (especially in decreased renal function) by renal
  scan, using [99M]Technetium-labeled DTPA

ROUTINE URINALYSES

Glucose and Reducing Substances

- Clinistix—specific for glucose (glucose oxidase
  test)
- Clinitest tablets
  1. Interpretation of results: see Table 18–8
  2. Positive in the presence of the following:
     - Glucose
     - Nonglucose reducing substances, e.g., fruc-
       tose, galactose, lactose, ascorbic acid,
       homogentisic acid, pentose, tyrosine, chlo-
       ramphenicol, chloral hydrate, sulfonamides,
       salicylate metabolites

TABLE 18–8   Interpretation of Results Using Clinitest Tablets

Color	Glucose	Color	Glucose
Blue	Negative	Green-brown	1.0%
Blue-green	Trace	Yellow	1.5%
Green	0.5%	Yellow-orange	2.0%

3. Method: add 2 drops urine to 10 drops water; then add tablet (Clinitest)

Proteinuria (i.e., Albuminuria)

- Commercial reagent strips available, e.g., Albustix, Hemacombistix. Useful for screening and follow-up.
- 24 hr urine protein usually <0.10 g/m²/day over 1 yr of age
- See p 439 for interpretation and evaluation of proteinuria

Hematuria

- Microscopy for RBCs
- Dipstix (Hemastix or Hemacombistix) or Hematest tablet

Interpretation

- Hemastix positive: hematuria, hemoglobinuria, myoglobinuria
- Hemastix negative:
    1. "Red diaper syndrome," e.g., urates, Serratia
    2. Dyes, drugs
    3. Alkaptonuria (black)

Differential Diagnosis of Hematuria

- R/O menses
- Infections: viral or bacterial of urinary tract
- Familial: benign recurrent, Alport's
- Anatomic: stones, tumors, obstruction
- Trauma: remember child abuse
- "Metabolic": hypercalciuria (very common)
- Glomerular: glomerulonephritis (see p 436)
- Vascular: renal vein thrombosis; cortical and medullary necrosis
- Hematologic: sickle cell disease, bleeding diathesis
- General: exercise induced, drugs (e.g., aspirin, dipyridamole)

Ketonuria

- Ketostix or Acetest tablet: tests only for acetone, not 3-hydroxybutyrate. Positive in starvation, diabetic ketoacidosis, and organic acidopathies, among others.

Myoglobinuria

- Dissolve 2.8 g ammonium sulfate in 2 ml urine. Hb is precipitated, while myoglobin stays in solution. Many false positive results.
- Spectrophotometric methods more accurate
- Positive in postseizure state, after exercise (strenuous), McArdle's disease, crush injuries, hyperthermia. Risk of acute tubular necrosis.

Microscopy

- See Figure 18–4
- Unspun urine—to look for WBCs and bacteria
- Spun urine—to look for formed elements, e.g., casts (centrifuge at 2,000–3,000 rpm for 1–2 min)

Screening Tests for UTIs

- Nitrite: urinary pathogens reduce nitrate to nitrite. Urine should be in the bladder for at least 4–6 hr. When the colony count is $\geq 10^5$ col/ml, it will pick up $\sim$ 85–90%. The test does not detect gram positive organisms.
- Bacterial culture
    1. Dipslide (Uricult): very few false negatives or positives ($<$1%); simple and cheap
    2. Dehydrated media (Microstix): 10% false negative, 1% false positive

Bilirubinuria

- Ictotest tablet

Urobilin

- Removal of bilirubin if present: 10 ml urine plus 5 ml 10% aqueous BaCl solution; filter solution
- 5 ml urine filtrate added to 5 ml alkaline zinc acetate solution + 3 drops Lugol's iodine solution. This is then mixed, filtered, and transilluminated with flashlight
- Interpretation
    1. Slight green fluorescence = normal
    2. No fluorescence = no urobilin $\Big\}$ Abnormal
    3. Increased fluorescence— proportionate to urobilinuria

Ferric Chloride Reaction

- Add 6 drops of 5% ferric chloride ($FeCl_3$) solution to 0.5 ml (10 drops) of fresh urine, and mix well
- Observe color and compare with chart (Table 18–9); disregard color appearing after 10–20 sec
- Positive tests must be followed by quantitative tests to characterize nature of compound

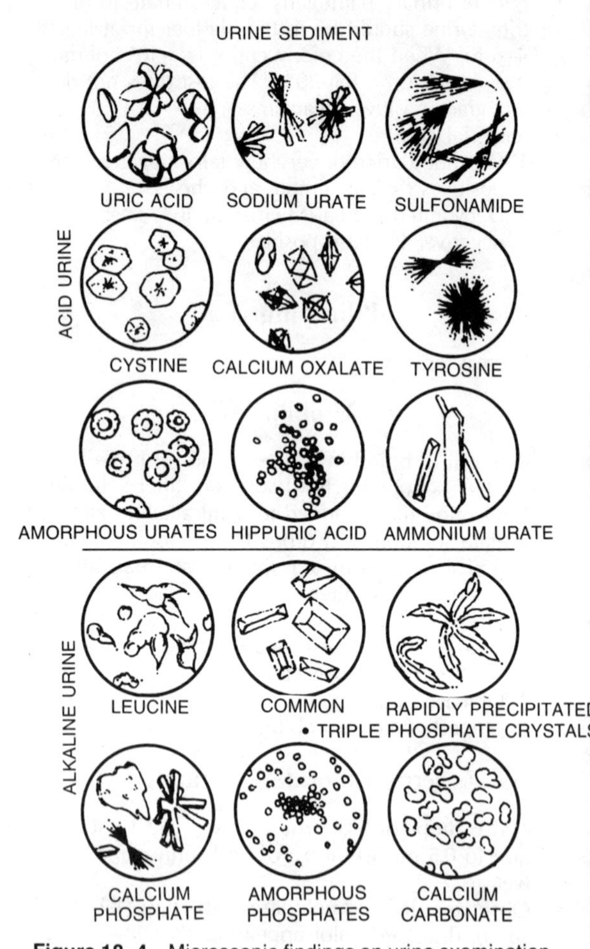

Figure 18–4   Microscopic findings on urine examination.

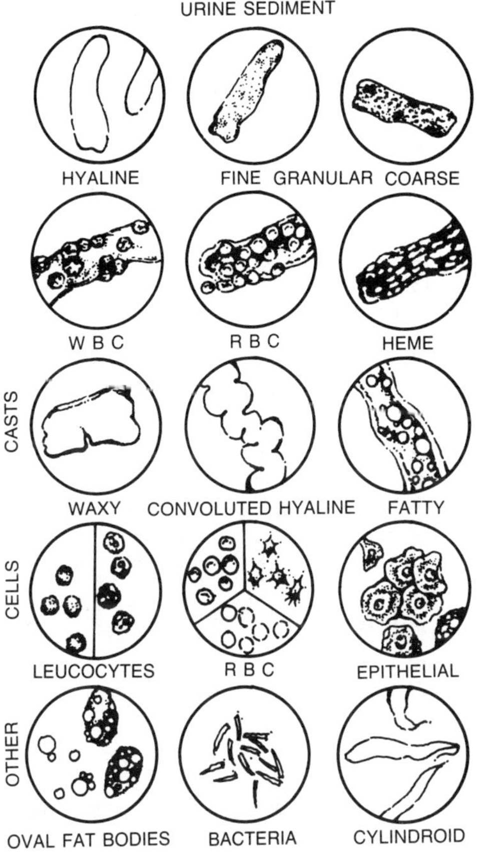

URINE SEDIMENT
HYALINE
FINE GRANULAR
COARSE
W B C
R B C
HEME
CASTS
WAXY
CONVOLUTED HYALINE
FATTY
CELLS
LEUCOCYTES
R B C
EPITHELIAL
OTHER
OVAL FAT BODIES
BACTERIA
CYLINDROID

TABLE 18–9 Interpretation of Ferric Chloride Reaction

Inborn Errors of Metabolism That Produce a Positive Ferric Chloride Reaction

Condition	Compound in Urine	Color
Phenylketonuria	Phenylpyruvic acid	Blue-green (fades)
Histidinemia	Imidazole acetic acid	Blue-green (fades)
Maple syrup urine disease	Keto analogues of branched chain amino acids	Gray-green
Hereditary tyrosinemia and tyrosinosis	p-Hydroxyphenyl compounds	Green (fades quickly)
Alkaptonuria	Homogentisic acid	Green (fades quickly)
Oasthouse disease	Alpha-hydroxybutyric acid and phenylpyruvic acid	Green

Nonhereditary Conditions in Which Urinary Metabolites Produce a Positive Ferric Chloride Reaction

Condition	Compound in Urine	Color
Transient tyrosinemia of newborn	p-Hydroxyphenyl compounds	Green (fades quickly)
Melanoma	Melanin	Gray-black
Pheochromocytoma	Catecholamines	Blue-green
Carcinoid syndrome	5-Hydroxyindolacetic acid	Blue-green or dark green
Liver disease	Bilirubin	Blue-green (may fade)
Diabetic acidosis	Acetoacetic acid	Purple or cherry red

Positive Urinary Ferric Chloride Reactions in Persons Ingesting Drugs

Drug	Color of Urine Test
Salicylates	Purple
Phenothiazines	Purple
Antipyrine	Red
Isoniazid	Yellow-green to brown
L-Dopa	Green
Iodochlorohydroxyquin	Blue-green

From Rudolph AM, ed. Pediatrics. 17th ed. Norwalk: Appleton-Century-Crofts, 1982:254.

Phenylketones

- Phenistix
  1. Gives results similar to those with ferric chloride solutions
  2. Also positive with salicylates and phenothiazines

Dinitrophenylhydrazine (DNPH) Test for Ketoacids

- Dissolve 100 mg 2,4-DNPH in 100 ml 2N HCl. Refrigerate reagent.
- Add 10 drops of DNPH reagent to 1 ml urine (at room temp)
- A positive result occurs if a yellow or chalky precipitate forms within 10 min
- A positive test may occur in MSUD, PKU, ketotic hyperglycinemia, methylmalonicaciduria, and many other conditions with α-ketoaciduria

Cyanide Nitroprusside Test

- Used as screen for cystinuria and homocystinuria
- See metabolic or pediatric texts for details

Suggested Reading

1. Edelmann CM, ed. Pediatric kidney disease. Vols. I, II. Boston: Little, Brown, 1978.
2. Fine RN, ed. Pediatric nephrology. Pediatr Clin North Am 1982; 29 (August): whole volume.
3. Fine RN, Gruskin AB, eds. End stage renal disease in children. Philadelphia: W.B. Saunders, 1984.
4. Postlethwaite RJ, ed. Clinical paediatric nephrology. Bristol: John Wright, 1986.
5. Task Force on Blood Pressure Control in Children. Report of the Second Task Force on Blood Pressure Control in Children—1987. Pediatrics 1987; 79:1–25.

NEUROLOGY AND NEUROSURGERY

SEIZURES AND STATUS EPILEPTICUS

Classification

TABLE 19–1 Classification of Seizures

Partial Seizures	Generalized Seizures
Simple partial (consciousness not impaired)	Absence (petit mal)
Motor: focal, adversive, jacksonian	Tonic-clonic (grand mal)
Sensory: tingling, light flashes, buzzing, foul smell, vertigo	Tonic or clonic
Autonomic: pallor, flushing, pupillary dilation	Myoclonic
Psychic: déja vu, fear, forced thinking, macropsia, micropsia, music, scenes	Atonic
	Infantile spasms
Complex partial (consciousness impaired; psychomotor or temporal lobe)	
Impairment of consciousness at onset	
Without impairment of consciousness at onset (simple partial onset)	
Partial seizures evolving to generalized tonic-clonic seizures	

TABLE 19–2   Differentiation: Seizure, Syncope, Breath Holding

Symptom	Seizure (Generalized Type)	Syncope	Breath Holding	
			"Blue"	"White"
Precipitating event	–	Usually present	Frustration	Pain
Loss of consciousness	Yes—can be prolonged	Yes—brief	May occur	May occur
Onset	Aura	Light-headed, queasy, blurred vision	Frustration, crying	Pain, injury
Appearance	Rubor, cyanosis, sweating	Pale, clammy, cold	Cyanosis, holds breath in inspiration	Pale, "death white"
Motor activity	Prominent	Minimal	Can terminate (rarely) in generalized tonic-clonic seizure	
Persisting neurologic signs	±	–	–	–
EEG (between episodes)	Usually abnormal	Normal	Normal	Normal
Age	Not specific	Older child, adolescent	6 mo–4 yr	1–4 yr
Treatment	Conventional anti-convulsants if recurrent	Semiprone position	Nil	Nil

Status Epilepticus

General Considerations

- Definition of generalized convulsive status: a single generalized tonic-clonic convulsion or a series of generalized tonic-clonic convulsions lasting 30 min or longer without intervening return of consciousness
  1. Types
  - Convulsive status
    - a. Generalized: tonic-clonic status, myoclonic status, tonic status
    - b. Focal: focal motor status (jacksonian status), epilepsia partialis continua
  - Nonconvulsive status: petit mal status, complex partial status (psychomotor status)

Management

- Stabilization: 0–10 min
  1. Secure airway, blood pressure, nasal O_2; intubate as occasion arises
  2. Blood for CBC, electrolytes, BUN, drug levels, calcium, magnesium, toxic screen, glucose (Dextrostix)
  3. Start intravenous infusion with 5% dextrose in normal saline (if indicated, use 25% dextrose, 2 ml/kg)
  4. Blood gases; if pH <7.1 give bicarbonate
  5. Monitor respirations, blood pressure, and ECG
- Control of seizures
  1. 10–25 min
    - Diazepam, 0.1–0.3 mg/kg IV (maximal dose ≤5 yr—5 mg, >5 yr—10 mg) to be given no faster than 2 mg/min; may repeat if necessary every 10 min for maximum of three doses. If unable to start intravenous

line, may give one dose of rectal diazepam (same preparation as is given parenterally) 0.3–0.5 mg/kg/dose (maximal dose ≤ 5 yr—5 mg, >5 yr—10 mg). Draw up in tuberculin syringe. Remove the needle, insert syringe into rectum, and give solution as bolus.

- Alternative: lorazepam 0.05 mg/kg/dose IV to be given no faster than 2 mg/min. Should not be repeated more than once (maximum 4 mg/dose, 8 mg/12 hr).
- *Be prepared to intubate patient* (diazepam and lorazepam can cause apnea)
- Start phenytoin after first dose of diazepam; give 20 mg/kg IV (maximum 1 g), no faster than 50 mg/min. If bradycardia or hypotension occur, slow infusion rate.

2. 25–40 min: If seizures persist, intubate and ventilate child; complete phenytoin infusion if not already finished
3. 40–60 min: If seizures continue, start infusion of phenobarbital, loading dose of 20 mg/kg IV, no faster than 60 mg/min; monitor respirations and blood pressure
4. 60–90 min: If phenobarbital has not terminated seizures, start thiopentone; EEG monitoring; keep EEG near flat for 12–24 hr using thiopentone infusion (child must be intubated and ventilated in an ICU setting while receiving thiopentone)

- Diagnostic evaluation: Should coincide with control of seizures; detailed history, physical examination, and consideration of further diagnostic work-up with special consideration of treatable diseases (e.g., hypoxia, meningitis, encephalitis, metabolic disorders, drug overdose, mass lesions with cerebral edema, and intracerebral bleeding)

Febrile Convulsions

Clinical Features

- The following features suggest benign type:
  1. Age 6 mo–4 yr
  2. Duration—less than 5 min
  3. Seizure is symmetric
  4. Child is neurologically normal before and after convulsion
  5. Onset of seizure during first 24 hr of fever; occurrence of only a single seizure during the first 24 hr
  6. Positive family history of febrile seizures only and negative family history of epilepsy
- Increased predisposition to subsequent epilepsy if
  1. Antecedent neurologic or developmental abnormality
  2. Generalized or focal convulsions of longer than 15 min or more than one seizure in 24 hr
  3. Onset prior to 1 yr of age
  4. Multiple recurrences
  5. Positive family history of epilepsy

Management

- Acute management
  1. Place child in semiprone position to prevent aspiration of vomitus and maintain adequate oxygenation
  2. Most febrile seizures end spontaneously before an intravenous line is established
  3. If seizure continues, treat as for convulsive status (see p 469) but omit phenytoin and give phenobarbital loading dose instead (be prepared to intubate if there is respiratory depression)
  4. When convulsions have ceased, completely undress child and cover with a light sheet. If

temperature $>38.5^\circ$ C, give acetaminophen
(rectal or oral).
- Investigations
  1. Lumbar puncture if meningitis is suspected;
     higher index of suspicion in
     - The young child (<1 yr)
     - The child in whom no reasonable explanation can be found for the fever
     - An atypical febrile convulsion
  2. CBC, urinalysis, $\pm$ blood culture
  3. Of limited value—EEG, electrolytes, glucose,
     urea, calcium, and phosphorus (only if
     specific clinical suspicion)
  4. Of no value—skull x-ray
- Treatment
  1. Hospitalization rarely necessary!
  2. Conditions to be met before discharge from
     emergency room
     - The child is alert and completely recovered
       from the seizure
     - All indicated investigations have been
       carried out
     - The parents are capable of following
       instructions for control of the fever, giving
       medication, and emergency care of
       recurrent seizures
     - Follow-up is assured as an outpatient
  3. Benefits of hospitalization
     - Reassurance to overwrought parents
     - Close observation and initial treatment
       pending cultures if meningitis is questioned
  4. Risks of hospitalization: unnecessarily
     reinforce idea that child is abnormal
  5. Indications for admission
     - Prolonged, unilateral, or repeated seizures
     - If meningitis or other life threatening
       disease cannot be excluded
     - Social factors

- Discuss with parents
  1. Risks of seizures
  2. Management of a recurrent seizure: If a seizure lasts >10 min, take child to a facility where intravenous medication can be utilized, or give rectal medication at home. (Give instructions to parents about use of rectal diazepam [see p 470]. Rectal paraldehyde can also be used [see below].)
  3. Consideration of chronic prophylaxis for children with one or two of these risk factors:
     - Family history of afebrile seizures
     - Suspect or abnormal neurologic development prior to first febrile seizure
     - Atypical febrile seizures—longer than 15 min, focal, multiple in 1 day, transient or persistent neurologic abnormality
     - First febrile seizure occurs before 1 yr of age
     - Recurrent febrile seizures
     - High level of parental anxiety
- Specific anticonvulsant therapy if indicated
  1. Continuous daily administration—phenobarbital: 3–5 mg/kg/day PO once daily or valproic acid (see p 850)
  2. Intermittent therapy. For acute convulsion: home use of rectal diazepam (see p 470) or rectal paraldehyde, 300 mg/kg (0.3 ml of undiluted paraldehyde/kg) diluted in equal amount of mineral oil and administered by syringe and nasogastric tubing

ACUTE ATAXIA

Differential Diagnosis

- Acute cerebellar ataxia (infectious or post-infectious)
  1. Varicella

2. Mumps
3. Influenza A and B
4. ECHO and Coxsackie
5. Mycoplasma
- Intoxication—drugs, alcohol
- Posterior fossa mass
  1. Tumor
  2. Subdural, epidural
- Myoclonic encephalopathy (opsoclonus-myoclonus syndrome)—frequently associated with neuroblastoma
- Metabolic disorders
  1. MSUD (intermittent form)
  2. Hartnup disease
  3. Pyruvate decarboxylase deficiency
  4. Argininosuccinic aciduria
- Benign paroxysmal vertigo of childhood (migraine variant)
- Polyradiculoneuritis (Guillain-Barré syndrome)
- Acute labyrinthitis
- Frequent minor motor seizures

Management (Initial)

- History, physical and neurologic examinations
- Consider (in emergency room)
  1. Urgent CT scan if indicated, e.g., signs of ↑ ICP
  2. CSF examination
  3. Toxic screen
  4. Serum ammonium and amino acid levels
  5. EEG

ACUTE HEMIPLEGIA

Definition

- Postnatally acquired hemiplegia (usually of sudden onset) in a child apparently neurologically unimpaired at birth

Differential Diagnosis

- Trauma
  1. Head injury
  2. Intraoral—damage to carotid artery (history of fall with object in mouth 3–24 hr prior to hemiplegia, ecchymoses of posterior pharynx)
  3. Fractures—air, fat embolism
- Infection
  1. Meningitis
     a. Early—cortical venous thrombosis, subdural hygroma
     b. Late—abscess, epidural empyema
  2. Focal encephalitis—herpes simplex, less commonly Coxsackie A9
  3. Postinfectious
  4. Fungal, parasitic abscesses
- Cardiac disease
  1. Cyanotic CHD
     a. Less than 2 yr—cerebral thrombosis (risk factors—polycythemia and hypoxemia)
     b. Greater than 2 yr—brain abscess
  2. Arrhythmias—mural thrombosis
  3. Bacterial endocarditis
- AVM
- Occlusive cerebrovascular disease
  1. Moya-moya syndrome
  2. Carotid arteritis, PAN, SLE
  3. Hyperlipidemia
- Systemic illness
  1. Hematologic
     - Hemorrhage in association with leukemia, hemophilia, ITP
     - Sickle cell anemia and other hemoglobinopathies—hemorrhage and occlusive disease
     - Hypercoagulable states—polycythemia
  2. Metabolic
     - Dehydration—dural sinus and cerebral venous thrombosis

- • Diabetes mellitus
  - • Homocystinuria
  - • MELAS (mitochondrial encephalo-myopathy, lactic acidosis, and strokelike episodes)
- Status epilepticus
- Space occupying intracerebral mass with acute hemorrhage
- Hypertension
  1. Infarct
  2. Hemorrhage
- Hemiplegic migraine

Management

- History, physical and neurologic examinations
- CBC, WBC, differential, ESR, platelets, PT, PTT, sickle cell prep. (when appropriate), glucose, electrolytes, lipid profile
- Emergency CT scan when indicated
- If CT negative, consider CSF examination
- Additional laboratory investigations
  1. EEG
  2. ECG and 2-D echocardiogram
  3. Arterial blood gases, and serum and CSF lactate and amino acids if MELAS is considered
  4. Urine nitroprusside test for homocystinuria
  5. Cerebral arteriography when indicated

INTRACRANIAL MASS LESIONS AND INCREASED INTRACRANIAL PRESSURE

Clinical Features and Differential Diagnosis

- ''Axial'' syndrome
  1. Features
     - • Morning headache
     - • Vomiting

- Drowsiness
    - Altered visual fixation (diplopia)
    - Papilledema
    - Enlargement of head
  2. Diagnostic considerations
    - Head injury, trauma
    - Infection—cerebral abscess
    - Cerebral neoplasm
    - Subdural effusion
    - Hydrocephalus or blocked shunt
- Herniation syndromes
  1. Uncal (lateral) syndrome—unilateral dilated pupil with contralateral hemiplegia → increasing stupor, bilateral hemiplegia with bilateral Babinski responses → brain stem dysfunction (absent oculocephalic responses, abnormal ice water calorics)
  2. Central syndrome—change in alertness or behavior; progression to decorticate posturing → dilation of pupils and impaired oculo-vestibular responses → loss of brain stem function

Management

- Investigation
  1. History, physical and neurologic examinations
  2. Urgent CT scan with AP and lateral skull films. If mass lesion; depending on location, may require further diagnostic studies, e.g., arteriography.
  3. Sellar-parasellar lesions—neuroendocrine assessment essential
  4. Visual and oculomotor disorders—neuro-ophthalmologic assessment
  5. No LP unless CNS infection is suspected and CT scan is *normal* (LP contraindicated in presence of significantly elevated ICP and absolutely contraindicated if evidence of a mass lesion). If infection is seriously consi-

dered, begin treatment with IV antibiotics
while awaiting CT scan.
- Acute treatment of ↑ ICP
  1. Admission to ICU—intubation → hyperventi-
     lation (keep $PaCO_2$ 30–35 mm Hg)
  2. Fluid restriction (30% of maintenance fluids)
  3. Keep mean arterial blood pressure ≥65 mm
     Hg to maintain adequate cerebral perfusion
     (if unable to keep intracranial pressure <20,
     may need higher arterial blood pressure to
     maintain perfusion)
  4. Do not allow temperature to go above 37º C
  5. Avoid unnecessary stimulation of patient (e.g.,
     aggressive physiotherapy)
  6. With intracranial pressure monitoring equip-
     ment in place
     - Keep ICP <20 mm Hg
     - Mannitol 20%—0.2–0.5 g/kg IV over 10–30
       min (insert indwelling urinary catheter).
       May repeat q2h prn. If no sustained
       response after 3–4 doses, consider alterna-
       tive methods for decreasing ICP.
     - If no response to mannitol, consider use of
       thiopentone (loading dose of 2–3 mg/kg IV
       bolus followed by continuous infusion of
       1–2 mg/kg/hr; may use up to 5 mg/kg/hr if
       necessary). Monitoring of serum drug con-
       centrations is recommended.

ACUTE HEAD INJURY

Emergency Management

- The initial attention of medical staff should be
  directed toward basic resuscitation with maintenance of the airway, breathing, and circulation (see p 652)
- High index of suspicion for cervical spinal
  fracture!
- Initial patient evaluation:
  Glasgow coma scale (see p 481); severe =
  3–8, moderate = 9–12, minor = 13–15

- Intubation and hyperventilation if Glasgow coma score ≤ 7
- See p 662 for management of trauma
- Transport to center with neurosurgical resources

Further Investigations

- CT scan with bone windows (can use "one slice")
- A normal skull x-ray does not imply that the patient has not suffered a severe head injury. May be a useful screening procedure for
  1. Clinical evidence of basilar skull fracture
  2. Age <2 yr
  3. Cephalohematoma
- MRI (magnetic resonance imaging) assessment of isodense bilateral subdural hematoma, extracerebral traumatic lesions
- Multimodal evoked potentials

Treatment

- Treat ↑ ICP
  1. As noted above. Mannitol is used only to gain time while patient and operating room are readied for surgery or diagnostic studies are being performed *or* under ICU conditions with ICP monitoring.
  2. Recent studies *do not* support the use of steroids to treat ↑ ICP in patients with head injuries
  3. Keep $PaCO_2$ 30–35 mm Hg
  4. Do not allow temperature to go above 37° C
- Do not give ASA to treat fever in any neurosurgical patient (because of its interference with normal clotting)
- Narcotics are contraindicated in all head injury patients (they obscure estimation of the Glasgow coma score)
- Post-traumatic seizure soon after head injury is common. Unless the seizure is prolonged, anti-

convulsant therapy is not required. There is controversy with regard to the value of prophylactic anticonvulsants.
- Compound brain wound: Apply sterile dressing, start prophylactic antibiotics, obtain plain films of skull, and take patient to operating room as soon as possible.

COMA (NONTRAUMATIC) AND ASSESSMENT OF CHILD WITH ALTERED LEVEL OF CONSCIOUSNESS

Pediatric Coma Scale

- See Table 19–3

Emergency Management and Assessment

- Stabilize vital signs
- Obtain history
- Brief emergency room examination
- Investigations: CBC, electrolytes, creatinine, blood gases, glucose (Dextrostix), LFTs, PT, PTT, ammonium, toxic screen, save 5 ml of heparinized blood (for metabolic studies if required later)
- Any child with a Glasgow coma score ≤ 7 (see p 481) should be intubated and hyperventilated
- Consider giving glucose (2 ml/kg of 25% dextrose) if Dextrostix or results of blood glucose are not immediately available

After Stabilization

- Full examination
- Diagnostic considerations
  1. Structural—supratentorial destructive or mass lesion, infratentorial lesion
  2. Toxic, metabolic, or infectious

TABLE 19–3 Pediatric Coma Scale (Modification of Glasgow Coma Scale)

		>1 yr	<1 yr	
Eyes opening	4	Spontaneously	Spontaneously	
	3	To verbal command	To shout	
	2	To pain	To pain	
	1	No response	No response	
		>1 yr	<1 yr	
Best motor response	6	Obeys		
	5	Localizes pain	Localizes pain	
	4	Flexion-withdrawal	Flexion-withdrawal	
	3	Flexion-abnormal (decorticate rigidity)	Flexion-abnormal (decorticate rigidity)	
	2	Extension (decerebrate rigidity)	Extension (decerebrate rigidity)	
	1	No response	No response	
		>5 yr	2–5 yr	0–23 mo
Best verbal response	5	Orientated and converses	Appropriate words and phrases	Smiles, coos, cries appropriately
	4	Disorientated and converses	Inappropriate words	Cries
	3	Inappropriate words	Cries or screams	Inappropriate crying or screaming
	2	Incomprehensible sounds	Grunts	Grunts
	1	No response	No response	No response
Total	3–15			

481

Principles of Management

- Intubation and hyperventilation if Glasgow coma score ≤ 7
- Maintenance of optimal heart rate, systemic BP, respiratory status
- Correct systemic glucose, acid-base, fluid-electrolyte imbalance
- Management of hypo- or hyperthermia
- Treatment of ↑ ICP (see p 478)
- Treatment of seizures
- Identify cause and treat

ASSESSMENT FOR BLOCKED SHUNT SYSTEM

Clinical Features

- Progressive history of increasing lethargy, vomiting, and headache
- May be associated with abdominal pain or fever
- Most useful indication of shunt malfunction is the history from the parent that child's symptoms are identical to those at the time of the last malfunction

Management

- Determine shunt patency by depressing subcutaneous pump: should depress easily and refill within 5–15 sec
- X-rays of skull, chest, abdomen rarely useful; only to determine whether tubing is intact throughout its length
- If symptoms are intermittent or associated with abdominal pain and fever—sample CSF through subcutaneous reservoir for culture. Can combine procedure with radionuclide shunt scan.

ACUTE SPINAL CORD COMPRESSION

Clinical Features

- This is a neurosurgical emergency!
- Early signs and symptoms
  1. Back pain
  2. Alteration in bladder (more or less frequent urination) or bowel (constipation) function
  3. Weakness in lower extremities
  4. Loss or alteration of pinprick sensation in lower extremities
  5. Loss of position or vibration sense in feet
  6. Hyperreflexia in lower extremities
  7. Tenderness over spine

Management

- Careful neurologic examination (determine level of cord lesion)
- Check for primary tumor sites—CXR, CBC, abdominal examination
- Neurosurgical consultation and proceed to myelogram (and CSF examination) or MRI (if feasible)

"OPEN" MYELOMENINGOCELE

Initial Evaluation and Treatment

- Examination (brief) to determine size of lesion, distal motor paralysis of legs and sphincters, associated neurogenic foot deformities, and presence of hydrocephalus
- Transport for neurosurgical management. Keep patient prone with moistened sterile saline dressings applied to open defect (must be kept wet at all times and changed as necessary).

Treatment

- Operative repair ± ventriculoperitoneal shunt
- Urologic and orthopaedic assessment

REYE SYNDROME

Clinical Features

- Antecedent viral illness
- Pernicious vomiting followed by combative behavior, irritability, and lethargy
- Encephalopathy lasts 24–96 hr
- Hyperammonemia, hypoprothrombinemia, ↑ serum transaminases
- Hypoglycemia (in children <3 yr)

Management

- Investigation
  1. Assess stage (Lovejoy)
     - Stage I: Vomiting, lethargy, and sleepiness
     - Stage II: Disorientation, delirium and combativeness, hyperventilation, hyperactive reflexes, appropriate response to noxious stimuli
     - Stage III: Obtunded, coma, hyperventilation, decorticate rigidity
     - Stage IV: Deepening coma, decerebrate rigidity, loss of oculocephalic reflexes (often asymmetric), large fixed pupils, disconjugate eye movements in response to cold caloric stimulation
     - Stage V: Seizures, loss of deep tendon reflexes, respiratory arrest, flaccidity
  2. Initial investigations: AST (SGOT), ALT (SGPT), PT, PTT, electrolytes, glucose, ammonium, plasma salicylate level, quantitative plasma amino acids (↑ lysine in Reye syndrome), urinary organic acids (to rule out

organic acidopathy mimicking Reye
syndrome)
3. BECAUSE OF THE INCREASED ICP A
LUMBAR PUNCTURE SHOULD BE
AVOIDED IF POSSIBLE
4. Liver biopsy is mandatory to confirm
diagnosis
- Treatment
  1. Stage I
     - Fluid restriction, monitor blood glucose,
       PT, and PTT
     - Closely monitor level of consciousness
  2. If progression to stage II or greater
     - Monitor blood glucose, PT, and PTT
     - ICU admission with monitoring and treat-
       ment of ↑ ICP (see p 478)
     - In Reye syndrome, phenobarbital is used in
       addition to standard treatment of ↑ ICP:
       phenobarbital 20 mg/kg IV loading dose
       and then 10–20 mg/kg/day IV ÷ TID (aim
       for phenobarbital levels 215–430 μmol/L
       [50–100 mg/L])

HEADACHE

Muscle Contraction and Tension

Clinical Features

- No prodrome
- Bilateral, usually continuous, bandlike
- Often chronic, difficult to treat
- Usually accompanying anxiety or depression

Management

- Analgesics—ASA, acetaminophen
- Identification and alleviation of underlying
  stress

Migraine

Clinical Features

- At least three of the following
  1. Aura (most often visual)—rare in children
  2. Unilaterality of headache
  3. Throbbing pulsatile quality
  4. Nausea, vomiting, abdominal pain
  5. Relief after vomiting or falling asleep
  6. Family history of migraine in parents or siblings
  7. Transient neurologic deficit(s)
- Classification
  1. Classic
  2. Common
  3. Complicated—hemiplegic, ophthalmoplegic, basilar, acute confusional
  4. Migraine equivalents—cyclic vomiting, periodic syndrome (abdominal pain), paroxysmal vertigo, paroxysmal torticollis
  5. Cluster

Management

- Acute attack
  1. Dark quiet room
  2. Analgesics—ASA, acetaminophen
  3. Antiemetics—chlorpromazine, dimenhydrinate
- To abort acute attack
  1. ASA in aura
  2. Ergotamine—usually not effective in children (contraindicated in complicated migraine)
- Prophylaxis
  1. Remove triggering factors and events
  2. Propranolol
  3. Anticonvulsants (e.g., phenobarbital or phenytoin)
  4. Biofeedback

Monitoring of Child with Confirmed Guillain-Barré Syndrome

- Airway protection and ventilation
  1. Intubation (in order to protect the airway) is necessary if
     - Signs of bulbar involvement (e.g., dysphagia, dysarthria, hoarseness, weak cough)
     - Deteriorating vital capacity
     - Cardiovascular instability
  2. Do not wait for abnormal blood gases to intubate; child may require intubation and ventilation despite relatively normal blood gases
- Plasmapheresis may be helpful if
  1. Rapidly progressive disease
  2. Worsening respiratory status
- Monitor for autonomic instability
  1. Cardiac arrhythmias
  2. Blood pressure instability (hypo- or hypertension)

PRIMITIVE AND PROTECTIVE REFLEXES

TABLE 19–4　Primitive and Protective Reflexes

Primitive reflexes—present at birth, disappear at $\sim$ 3–4 mo
Local
Head: righting response
Upper limbs: primitive finger grasp, arms brought forward when placed prone
Lower limbs: primitive toe grasp, placing, supporting, primary stepping
General
Asymmetric tonic neck (never obligatory)
Moro response
Secondary reflexes—appear at 4–9 mo
Rolling
Balancing
Protective: downward parachute (appears at $\sim$ 4 mo), lateral propping (appears at $\sim$ 6–7 mo), forward parachute (appears at $\sim$ 9 mo)

Suggested Reading

1. Barbosa E, Freeman JM. Status epilepticus. Pediatr Rev 1982; 4:185–189.
2. Fenichel GM. Migraine in children. Neurol Clin 1985; 3:77–94.
3. Golden GS. Stroke syndromes in childhood. Neurol Clin 1985; 3:59–75.
4. Rockoff MA, Pascucci RC. Reye's syndrome. Symposium on pediatric emergencies. Emerg Med Clin North Am 1983; 1:87–100.
5. Schaffer L, et al. Aspects of evaluation and treatment of head injury. Neurol Clin 1985; 3:259–273.
6. Vining PG, Freeman JM. Epilepsy in children. Pediatr Ann 1985; 14:705–770.

INFANT FEEDING

Breast Feeding

Advantages

- Protection against respiratory and GI infection (contains IgA, macrophages, lysozyme, lactoferrin) } Major advantage in developing countries
- Sterile
- Inexpensive
- Easily digested protein content (casein/whey ratio equals 30/70)
- ↑ Bioavailability of iron
- ↓ Risk of overfeeding
- Low renal solute load
- ↑ Maternal infant bonding
- ? Protection against atopic disease

Comments

- Breast milk jaundice can occur
- Environmental contamination can occur (↑ secretion in breast milk of insecticides, PCBs)
- Vitamin D supplement may be required
- If mother is a strict vegetarian, breast milk may be deficient in vitamin B_{12}. Other vitamin deficiencies may occur, depending on specific diet of mother.
- Initially a breast-fed infant may have a watery stool after every feeding. However, after a few weeks a breast-fed infant may only have a soft stool every few days.

Contraindications

- Inborn errors of metabolism (e.g., galactosemia)

- Mother with sputum positive TB
- Specific maternal drugs (see p 876–877)
- HBsAg positive mother (relative contraindication to breast feeding in developed countries; not a contraindication to breast feeding in underdeveloped areas)

Treatment of Common Problems

- Engorgement
  1. Occurs most often in first week post partum
  2. Best treated by frequent nursing and application of heat to breast prior to nursing
- Sore nipples
  1. Ensure correct position of infant on breast
  2. Allow nipples to air dry after each feed
  3. Avoid breast shields with plastic or rubber liners
  4. Check for thrush
- "Not enough milk"
  1. Assess hydration of infant (e.g., 6–8 wet diapers/day and several stools indicate the infant is well hydrated)
  2. Adequate weight gain is best way to assess adequacy of milk supply
  3. Increase frequency of feeds
  4. Avoid supplementary bottles
  5. Encourage mother to drink plenty of fluids for proper fluid balance
- Nipple confusion
  1. Avoid exposure to bottle nipples and pacifiers at least until infant is 4–6 wk of age, as breast feeding requires different sucking mechanism
- Mastitis, breast abscess
  1. Most common pathogen is *S. aureus*
  2. Continue to nurse on both breasts if mastitis is present
  3. Avoid nursing from involved breast if breast abscess is present

4. The mother may require antibiotics (e.g., cloxacillin). If she develops an abscess, incision and drainage may be necessary.

Bottle Feeding

General Considerations

- If breast milk is not available, use humanized formulas (e.g., Similac, SMA, Enfalac)
- Whole cow's milk and goat's milk are not suitable for infants less than 6 mo old; 2% milk should not be given before 12 months
- Formulas using evaporated whole cow's milk are not as suitable as humanized formulas
- Incorrectly prepared formulas can lead to FTT (too dilute) or hypernatremia (too concentrated)

Forms Available

- Liquid concentrate
- Ready to feed
- Powdered concentrate

Preparation (Aseptic Method)

- Prepare formula for a 24 hr period
- Wash bottles, nipples, caps, and any equipment to be used in hot soapy water. Rinse well and then sterilize by boiling for 5 min in a covered pot.
- Sterilize water needed for formula dilution by boiling in a covered pot for 5 min
- Using sterilized tongs, remove sterilized bottles and equipment from pot
- Rinse top of formula can with boiling water. Open with sterilized can opener.
- Pour cooled (adding hot water to formula may cause destruction of heat-sensitive vitamins), sterilized water into bottles or sterilized pitcher, and add required amount of liquid or powdered concentrate (see directions on package). Mix

well. Pour into bottles if using pitcher. (Ready-to-feed formula can be poured directly into sterilized bottles.)
- Using tongs, put nipples and caps on bottles
- Refrigerate and use within 24 hr

Supplements

- Vitamin D, 400 IU/day, for breast fed infants who do not have exposure to sunlight
- Iron supplement for breast fed infants required at 6 mo (e.g., infant cereals); formula fed infants should receive iron-fortified formula from birth
- Fluoride supplement (Table 20–1) required in areas where community water supply contains <0.3 ppm fluoride (not necessary in Canada if using ready-to-feed formula)
- Goat's milk is not recommended for infants under 6 mo of age, but if used requires supplementation of fólate and vitamins C and D. Canned evaporated goat's milk may or may not already be enriched with vitamins C and D and folate.

Introducing Solids

- Six to 9 mo is a critical period for learning how to chew and for development of taste and texture preferences; therefore the introduction of solids should not be delayed beyond 6 mo of age (Table 20–2)
- Introduce new foods one at a time with a separation of 1 wk
- Do not use honey or corn syrup in infants under 1 yr of age (risk of infant botulism)
- Offer foods from a spoon. Do not add them to bottle.

TABLE 20–1 Daily Fluoride Supplement for Breast and Formula Fed Infants[*]

Fluoride Content of Drinking Water (ppm)	2 wk to 2 yr	2 to 3 yr	3 to 16 yr
<0.3	0.25 mg	0.5 mg	1.0 mg
0.3–0.7	0	0.25 mg	0.5 mg
>0.7	0	0	0

[*] 2.2 mg sodium fluoride contains 1 mg fluoride.
Modified from Forbes GB. Pediatric nutrition handbook. 2nd ed. Elk Grove Village, IL: American Academy of Pediatrics, 1985:171.

TABLE 20–2 Timing of Introduction of Various Food Groups

Age	Food	Comments
0–4 mo	Breast milk, formula	Will meet nutritive needs exclusively until 6 mo of age
3–6 mo	Iron-enriched cereal	Introduce rice cereal first (least allergenic) Delay gluten (i.e., wheat cereals) until 6 mo of age
4–7 mo	Pureed vegetables	Yellow-orange vegetables first, green last (more bulk) Do not give high nitrate-nitrite containing vegetables (beets, spinach, turnips) until 12 mo of age Introduce vegetables before fruit (less chance of "sweet tooth")
6–9 mo	Pureed fruits and juices	Avoid "desserts" and fruit mixtures
6–9 mo	Pureed meats, fish, and poultry, egg yolk	Do not give egg white until 12 mo of age (risk of allergy)
9–12 mo	Finger foods, peeled fruit, cooked vegetables, cheese	Should be without added sugar, fat, salt, or seasonings Introduce varied food texture and encourage chewing

Foods to Avoid

- A variety of small food items or chewed vegetable matter can lead to choking, aspiration, or even asphyxia. Toddlers should be fed sitting down, in a quiet location and with an adult present.
- Raw vegetables such as carrot sticks are not appropriate for teething, because the partially chewed bolus can be aspirated if the child is moving about
- Weiners should not be given to children under 3 yr unless cut up lengthwise so that they do not create a plug
- Peanut butter must never be given by itself, because it produces a sticky bolus that can compromise the airway
- Caution parents about the danger of nuts, popcorn, small candies, raw peas and beans, grapes, and seeds of any type, especially before the age of 3 yr. Nuts (including peanuts) are especially dangerous.
- Children should not be put to sleep with a bottle containing any sugar-containing fluid. This includes milk and apple juice. If a child requires a bottle in bed to calm, any liquid but water can lead to serious dental decay.

Vegetarian Diets

- High in bulk, low in calories, vitamin B_{12}, vitamin D, and possibly protein
- Can develop protein-calorie malnutrition, rickets, vitamin B_{12} deficiency, and multiple other deficiencies
- Need dietitian's supervision
- Not recommended for preschool children

FAILURE TO THRIVE

General Considerations

Infants who fail to gain weight adequately (e.g., below the 3rd percentile, or a fall over two major percentile lines) are considered as failing to thrive

Psychosocial Deprivation

- Majority of children with FTT have this diagnosis
- Diagnosis should be a positive one (e.g., abnormalities found in psychosocial history)
- These children are watchful, have decreased vocalization and minimal smiling, and often have developmental delay in language and social-adaptive areas

Differential Diagnosis

- The differential Dx of FTT is extensive
- Various categories include
    1. Inadequate caloric intake
    2. Inadequate absorption and assimilation
    3. Failure of utilization or increased metabolism
    4. Understimulation, deprivation

Management

- With an organic cause of failure to thrive, the history and physical give a clue to the diagnosis in >90% of the cases
- If there is no indication of organic disease on history or physical, defer investigations for 1 wk and initiate trial of therapy
- Trial of therapy
    1. Determine ideal weight for actual height, and use this to calculate caloric needs
    2. Provide adequate calories (~150% of normal requirements)

3. Keep record of daily weight, daily calorie counts
4. Establish a program of environmental stimulation

- If there is no response to trial of therapy, reevaluate for organic disease; the following minimum laboratory investigations should be considered:
  1. CBC, ESR, electrolytes, BUN, creatinine, venous gases, Ca, P, glucose, thyroid function tests
  2. Urine—microscopy, specific gravity, culture, metabolic screen
  3. Stool—microscopy (fat, white cells), occult blood
  4. 3–5 day fecal fat collection
  5. Sweat chloride
  6. CXR
- Depending on clinical suspicion, the following tests may be indicated:
  1. Liver function tests
  2. Immunoglobulins
  3. Chromosomes
  4. Radiologic investigation
     - Skeletal survey
     - Bone age
     - Skull x-ray
     - Abdominal and head ultrasound

Follow-Up

- After therapy has been instituted, it is essential to assess growth parameters and development over an extended period of time

PROTEIN ENERGY MALNUTRITION

General Considerations

- World Health Organization defines protein

energy malnutrition as a range of pathologic
conditions arising from lack, in varying
proportions, of protein and calories, occurring in infants and children and most commonly associated with infection
- Major deficiencies are in protein and calories,
  but one should also consider deficiencies of
  Ca, Zn, Mg, P, and vitamins, e.g., riboflavin,
  nicotinic acid, and vitamin A
- Table 20–3 is a classification of nutritional
  status in childhood

Clinical Features

- Marasmus and kwashiorkor are two classic disease syndromes, but represent a spectrum of
  protein energy malnutrition
  1. Marasmus
     - Growth failure
     - Loss of subcutaneous tissue
     - Muscle wasting
     - Wizened facies
  2. Kwashiorkor
     - Growth failure
     - Preservation of subcutaneous tissue
     - Edema
     - Skin and hair changes
     - Apathy, altered mentation

Management

- Investigations
  1. Dietary history, social economic status
  2. Biochemical parameters (e.g., CBC, electro-
     lytes, Ca, Mg, P, BUN, creatinine, venous
     gases)
  3. Anthropometry
     - Weight, height, head circumference, skin-
       fold thickness, midarm circumference
     - Weight for height (one of the better meas-
       urements to use in developing countries as

TABLE 20–3 Classification of Nutritional Status in Childhood

Classification	Observed Weight as % of Ideal Weight/Length
Overweight	>110
Normal range	90–110
Mild PEM*	85–90
Moderate PEM	75–85
Severe PEM	<75

* PEM = protein energy malnutrition.
Modified from McLaren DS, Read WWC. Classification of nutritional status in early childhood. Lancet 1972; 2:146.

     it is simple, reproducible, and age-sex independent)
4. Assess hydration status
5. Search for sepsis, infection
- Treatment
  1. Admit to hospital
  2. Rehydrate with an oral balanced electrolyte solution, e.g., WHO oral rehydration solution
  3. Diet
     - Protein: 3–4 g/kg/day (use lactose-free formula if available)
     - Calories: 90–200 kcal/kg/day (start low, e.g., 90 kcal/kg/day, and build up gradually)
     - Multivitamin (especially vitamin A) and iron supplement
     - Cu, Zn, Mg, P supplement

     It may be necessary to supplement beyond the amounts present in the formula

  4. Treat intestinal parasites
  5. Watch for complications (diarrhea, CHF, infections, bleeding, seizures, hypothermia, hypoglycemia)

TOTAL PARENTERAL NUTRITION

General Considerations

- Indicated when enteric route insufficient to provide total nutritional needs
- Use a central line (CVL) when peripheral line inadequate for:
  1. Nutrient intake: e.g., difficult venous access
  2. Expected length of TPN: dependent on circumstances
  3. Osmolality of solution required: >125 g/L (12.5%) glucose

Catheter Care

- Must be inserted by experienced personnel under sterile technique
- Peripheral line should be changed frequently (every 3 days) to prevent significant bacteremia
- Infusion sets to be changed every 2 days

Ordering TPN

- General
  1. Usually TPN is given as two solutions: one solution with amino acids, glucose, electrolytes, and minerals, and a second solution of lipids
  2. Table 20–4 contains examples of HSC solutions
  3. In most instances, ordering a solution with the appropriate concentrations of the components noted in Table 20–4 at maintenance fluid rates (see pp 129 and 390) provides adequate nutrient intake
  4. Ensure that you provide the appropriate caloric requirements for age (see Tables 20–4, 20–5)
  5. To give more calories, ↑ lipid or ↑ glucose (see cautionary notes under Lipid and Carbohydrate, to follow)

6. When weaning off TPN, decrease rate in a stepwise fashion over 1–2 hr to avoid hypoglycemia
7. For infants and children who have excessive fluid requirements, use an ordinary IV solution to make up the difference, rather than TPN
8. Using TPN without a lipid solution leads to essential fatty acid deficiency
9. Monitor child while on TPN (see p 505)

- Protein
  1. Start protein at 2 g/kg/day. This may be increased to a maximum of 4 g/kg/day.
  2. Optimal range: <1 yr=2.0–2.5 g/kg/day
  >1 yr=1.0–2.5 g/kg/day
  3. May need to give increased amount of protein in protein-losing illnesses
- Lipid
  1. Start lipid at 1 g/kg/day. Increase to a maximum of 4 g/kg/day.
  2. Optimal range: 2–4 g/kg/day.
  3. Caution when using with drugs—may not be compatible in solution
  4. Relative contraindication to use in the following situations:
     - Neonatal indirect hyperbilirubinemia (free fatty acid component may compete with albumin binding sites for bilirubin)
     - Thrombocytopenia (lipid overload may interfere with platelet function)
     - Respiratory distress (lipid overload may interfere with gas exchange; normal lipid levels do not interfere)
     - Sepsis (lipid intolerance—increased lipid levels—may occur with untreated sepsis; withhold lipids for 24 hr upon recognition of sepsis)
- Carbohydrate
  1. Start carbohydrate as a 100 g/L (10%) solution. Carbohydrate solutions containing more

than 125 g/L (12.5%) should be used via central venous access only. Danger of sclerosing vein if >125 g/L (12.5%) solution used peripherally. Usually a 200 g/L (20%) solution is used when central venous access is available. In special circumstances, one may increase to 250–300 g/L (25–30%), e.g., significant fluid restriction.

2. Glucose tolerance is monitored via urinary glucose and occasional serum glucose. If glucose intolerance occurs
   - ↓ TPN infusion rate
   - Consider sepsis as a cause of glucose intolerance
   - May need to ↓ glucose concentration
   - May rarely require insulin

- Electrolytes, trace metals, vitamins
  1. Electrolyte requirements vary with age and condition
  2. See Table 20–4 for examples of appropriate electrolyte concentrations in solution
  3. Ca, P, Mg, Zn, Cu, Mn, Cr, I, and Se must be present in TPN solution
  4. Fe must be present in TPN solution except for the premature infant less than 1 mo of age
  5. All vitamins need to be supplemented. An example of total vitamin supplementation is *MVI Pediatric*.

Complications

- Problems with catheters
  1. Venous thrombosis, infection—sepsis, catheter malfunction, leakage, uncoupling, dislodgment, extravasation
- Metabolic
  1. Hyperglycemia

TABLE 20–4 Composition of VAMIN-N Based Standard Solutions (per L)[*][†]

	Premature Infants				Infants, Children, and Adolescents	
	P–5	P–7.5	P–10	PI–10	I–10	I–20[‡]
Protein (g)	15	15	20	20	30	30
Glucose (g)	50	75	100	100	100	200
Energy (kcal)[§]	248	340	455	455	495	870
Na (mmol)	20	20	14.3	30	30	30
K (mmol)	20	20	18.9	30	30	30
Cl (mmol)	21.1	21.1	15.7	31.3	32.1	32.1
Ca (mmol)	9	9	9	9	9	9
P (mmol)	9	9	9	9	9	9
Mg (mmol)	3	3	4	4	4	4
Zn (μmol)	46	46	46	46	46	46
Cu (μmol)	6.3	6.3	6.3	6.3	6.3	6.3
Mn (μmol)	1.8	1.8	1.8	1.8	5.0	5.0
I (μmol)	0.47	0.47	0.47	0.47	0.47	0.47
Cr (μmol)	0.076	0.076	0.076	0.076	0.076	0.076

| Se (μmol) | 0.25 | 0.25 | 0.25 | 0.25 | 0.25 | 0.25 |
| Fe (μmol)[#] | -- | -- | -- | -- | 18 | 18 |

* Modified from Guidelines for total parenteral nutrition. Toronto: The Hospital for Sick Children, 1986.
Fat emulsion 10%—1100 kcal/L, 100 g fat/L, 47 g linoleic acid/L
Fat emulsion 20%—2000 kcal/L.

† P solutions are for premature infants who are not fluid restricted.
I solutions are for premature infants who are fluid restricted and for children and infants.

‡ I–20 is intended for central venous line therapy only.

§ Energy unit: 1 kcal = 4.2 kJ. The energy content includes the potential energy from the protein as well as that from the glucose.

Iron can be included in the "P" solutions in neonates who have been receiving TPN for 1 mo or more and should therefore be ordered.

TABLE 20-5 Summary Examples of Recommended Nutrient Intakes for Canadians[*†‡]

Age	Sex	Energy (kcal/kg/day)	Protein (g/kg/day)	Fat-Soluble Vitamins			Water-Soluble Vitamins			Minerals				
				Vitamin A (RE/day)	Vitamin D (μg/day)	Vitamin E (mg/day)	Vitamin C (mg/day)	Folacin μg/day	Vitamin B_{12} (μg/day)	Calcium (mg/day)	Magnesium (mg/day)	Iron (mg/day)	Iodine (μg/day)	Zinc (mg/day)
Months														
0-2	Both	100-120	2.4	400	10	3	20	50	0.3	350	30	0.4	25	2
3-5	Both	95-100	2.0	400	10	3	20	50	0.3	350	40	5	35	3
6-8	Both	95-97	2.0	400	10	3	20	50	0.3	400	50	7	40	3
9-11	Both	97-99	1.9	400	10	3	20	55	0.3	400	50	7	45	3
Years														
1	Both	101	1.7	400	10	3	20	65	0.3	500	55	6	55	4
2-3	Both	94	1.5	400	5	4	20	80	0.4	500	70	6	65	4
4-6	Both	100	1.4	500	5	5	25	90	0.5	600	90	6	85	5
7-9	M	88	1.2	700	2.5	7	35	125	0.8	700	110	7	110	6
	F	76	1.2	700	2.5	6	30	125	0.8	700	110	7	95	6
10-12	M	73	1.1	800	2.5	8	40	170	1.0	900	150	10	125	7
	F	61	1.1	800	2.5	7	40	180	1.0	1000	160	10	110	7
13-15	M	57	1.0	900	2.5	9	50	150	1.5	1100	210	12	160	9
	F	46	0.89	800	2.5	7	45	145	1.5	800	200	13	160	8
16-18	M	51	0.88	1000	2.5	10	55	185	1.9	900	250	10	160	9
	F	40	0.81	800	2.5	7	45	160	1.9	700	215	14	160	8
19-24	M	42	0.82	1000	2.5	10	60	210	2.0	800	240	8	160	9
	F	36	0.74	800	2.5	7	45	175	2.0	700	200	14	160	8
Pregnancy (additional)		(kcal/day)	(g/day)											
1st Trimester		100	15	100	2.5	2	0	305	1.0	500	15	6	25	0
2nd Trimester		300	20	100	2.5	2	20	305	1.0	500	20	6	25	1
3rd Trimester		300	25	100	2.5	2	20	305	1.0	500	25	6	25	2
Lactation (additional)		450	20	400	2.5	3	30	120	0.5	500	80	0	50	6

* Modified from Bureau of Nutritional Sciences. Recommended nutrient intakes for Canadians: 1983:179-180.

† The figures for energy are estimates of average requirements for expected patterns of activity. For nutrients not shown, the following amounts are recommended: thiamin, 0.4 mg/1000 kcal (0.48 mg/5000 kJ); riboflavin, 0.5 mg/1000 kcal (0.6 mg/5000 kJ); niacin, 7.2 NE/1000 kcal (8.6 NE/5000 kJ); vitamin B_6, 15 μg, as pyridoxine, per gram of protein; phosphorus, same as calcium.

‡ Recommended intakes during periods of growth are taken as appropriate for individuals representative of the mid-point in each age group. All recommended intakes are designed to cover individual variations in essentially all of a healthy population subsisting upon a variety of common foods available in Canada.

    2. Hypoglycemia upon withdrawal or decreased rate
    3. Mild aminoaciduria or aminoacidemia
    4. Electrolyte abnormalities
    5. Mild liver function abnormalities
    6. TPN associated cholestasis
    7. Eosinophilia—benign
- Infections
  1. Thrombophlebitis
  2. Bacteremia
  3. Fungemia
  4. Sepsis and seeding of infection peripherally

Monitoring

- Growth parameters
- Fluid balance
- Urine for glucose daily and with solution changes or sepsis
- CBC, BUN, P, Ca, bilirubin, albumin, Mg once a week
- Electrolytes, glucose twice a week
- Liver function tests, creatinine as necessary
- All the preceding prior to start of therapy
- Lipid levels twice weekly and with solution changes or sepsis

---

See also Table 20–5 Summary Examples of Recommended Nutrient Intakes for Canadians; Table 20–6 Vitamin Deficiencies; and Table 20–7 Composition of Formulas

Suggested Reading

1. Goldbloom RB. Failure to thrive. Pediatr Clin North Am 1982:29.
2. Kramer MS. Breast feeding: current concepts and recent developments. In: Moss AJ, ed. Pediatrics update: review for physicians 1985. New York: Elsevier, 1985:167–186.
3. Pencharz PB, ed. Symposium on nutrition. Pediatr Clin North Am 1985:32(2).
4. Walker WA, Watkins JB. Nutrition in pediatrics: basic science and clinical application. Boston: Little, Brown, 1985.

TABLE 20–6   Vitamin Deficiencies

Vitamin	Signs and Syndromes	
A: rare, defective diet for many months	Night blindness Corneal xerosis Keratomalacia	Follicular hyperkeratosis ↑ ICP Poor growth
Thiamin (B_1): beriberi, common in alcoholics	Restlessness Ascending bilateral polyneuritis Wernicke's syndrome Korsakoff's psychosis	Tender muscles Anorexia CHF Edema
Riboflavin (B_2): rare	Cheilosis Glossitis	Corneal vascularization Seborrhea
Niacin: pellagra, rare	Dermatitis (in sun exposed areas) Dementia Diarrhea	Weakness Angular stomatitis
Pyridoxine (B_6)	Infantile seizures Peripheral neuritis Seborrhea	Glossitis Hypochromic microcytic anemia

Folic acid	Megaloblastic anemia Stomatitis	Weight loss Glossitis
B_{12}	Pernicious anemia Optic atrophy Retinitis	Neuropathy $\rightarrow$ sensory loss, $\downarrow$ reflexes, $\uparrow$ incoordination
C: scurvy	Petechial hemorrhage of skin and mucous membranes Delayed wound healing Gums (only if teeth are present): bluish, swollen, spongy, and bleeding	Sicca syndrome of Sjögren: xerostomia, enlarged salivary glands Orbital hemorrhage Generalized tenderness Subperiosteal hemorrhage (very painful) Scorbutic rosary (sharper than rachitic)
D: rickets in growing child, osteomalacia in adult	Craniotabes Enlarged epiphyses Rachitic rosary	Harrison's groove Delayed tooth eruption Enamel defects
E	Hemolytic anemia in newborn Neuropathy: atrophy of long tracts	? Retinitis pigmentosa Seborrheic dermatitis
K	Signs of generalized bleeding disorder (ecchymoses, hematuria, melena, subdural hematoma)	Hemorrhagic disease of newborn

TABLE 20–7   Composition of Formulas

Owing to changes in formulation, all data subject to change.
Non-Canadian formulations may vary.
Liquid feedings, unless otherwise specified, per 1 L normal dilution.

	Energy (kcal)*	Protein g	Protein Type or Casein/ Whey	CHO g	CHO Type	Fat g Type	Ca (mg)	P (mg)	Fe (mg)	Na (mmol)	Cl (mmol)	K (mmol)	GI Solute Load[†] (mmol/kg H_2O)	Vit.D (IU)
Infant Feedings														
Milks														
1. Human milk, mature	620	13	30/70	65	Lactose	31	260	130	tr	11	13	15	300	60
2. Milk, cows whole**	628	32	82/18	48	Lactose	36	1220	930	tr	22	27	40	315	360[§]
3. Milk, cows 2%	516	36	82/18	48	Lactose	20	1260	950	tr	22	28	41	-	360[§]
4. Milk, cows skimmed	360	36	82/18	52	Lactose	tr	1270	950	tr	23	29	44	-	360[§]
5. Whole goat's milk (folate and vitamin D deficient)	708	36	-	44	Lactose	44	1370	1110	tr	22	37	53	-	24
Milk based formulas														
1. Enfalac/Enfalac with iron (Enfamil in the U.S. is identical to Enfalac in Canada)	670	15	40/60	69	Lactose	38	460	320	1/13	8	12	18	300	400
2. SMA/SMA with iron	680	15	40/60	72	Lactose	36	440	300	2/13	7	11	14	300	420

3. Similac/Similac with iron	676	15	82/18	72	Lactose	36	520	390	2/12	10	14	17	290	400
4. Similac with whey/ Similac with whey and iron	676	15	40/60	72	Lactose	36	400	300	2/12	9	13	17	300	400
5. Similac PM 60/40 (low phosphorus)	676	16	40/60	69	Lactose	38	380	190	2	7	11	15	260	400
Soy based formulas														
1. Isomil	676	18	Soy	68	Glucose polymers and sucrose	37	700	500	12	13	15	18	250	400
2. ProSobee	670	20	Soy	68	Glucose polymers	36	630	500	13	13	14	20	200	400
3. Nursoy	670	21	Soy	69	Glucose polymers and sucrose	36	630	450	13	9	11	19	296	420
Low birth weight formulas														
1. Enfamil premature														
20 kcal/oz	680	20	40/60	74	Glucose polymers and lactose	34	800	400	1	12	16	19	244	430
24 kcal/oz	805	24		89		41	950	480	1	14	19	23	300	510

TABLE 20–7
Continued

	Energy (kcal)*	g	Protein Type or Casein/ Whey	g	CHO Type	Fat g Type	Ca (mg)	P (mg)	Fe (mg)	Na (mmol)	Cl (mmol)	K (mmol)	GI Solute Load[†] (mmol/kg H_2O)	Vit.D (IU)
2. Similac special care														
20 kcal/oz	676	18	40/60	72	Glucose	37	1100	600	3	13	15	21	250	420
24 kcal/oz	812	22		86	polymers and lactose	44	1320	720	3	15	18	26	300	500
3. "Preemie" SMA														
20 kcal/oz	675	20	40/60	70	Glucose	35	750	380	3	14	15	19	268	510
24 kcal/oz	810	20		86	polymers and lactose	44	750	400	3	14	15	19	268	510
Special formulas														
1. Lamb base (24 kcal/oz) including added glucose, corn oil, Ca(CO_3)_2, and mineral mix Vitamin and Fe deficient Values vary with recipe For multiple intolerances	780	26	Lamb	72	Glucose	43 Lamb and corn oil	820	340	2	14	16	19	-	-
2. Lofenalac (low phenylalanine)—for PKU	677	22	Hydrolysed casein	88	Glucose polymers	26 Corn oil	630	480	13	14	14	18	360	420

3. Nutramigen—for intolerance to intact protein	670	19	Hydrolysed casein	91	Glucose polymers	26	Corn oil	630	420	12	14	16	19	320	360
4 Portagen[++]—for fat malabsorption	670	24	Casein	78	Glucose polymers and sucrose	32	MCT and corn oil	630	470	13	13	16	21	220	190
5. Pregestimil—for fat and protein malabsorption or intolerance to intact protein	670	19	Hydrolysed casein	91	Glucose polymers	27	Corn oil and MCT	630	420	13	14	16	19	350	420
6. RCF (carbohydrate free) For carbohydrate intolerance. This is not a complete formula. One must specify type and amount of carbohydrate to be added (usually up to 70 g/L)	405	20	Soy	0		36	Soy oil and coconut oil	710	510	2	14	17	20	64	410

Complete Liquid Feedings

General
1. Enrich (with fibre)	1100	40	Casein and soy	163	Glucose polymers, sucrose, and soy polysaccharides	38	Corn oil	720	720	13	37	41	40	480	290

TABLE 20–7
Continued

	Energy (kcal)*	g	Protein Type or Casein/ Whey	g	CHO Type	g Fat Type	Ca (mg)	P (mg)	Fe (mg)	Na (mmol)	Cl (mmol)	K (mmol)	GI Solute Load[†] (mmol/kg H$_2$0)	Vit.D (IU)
2. Ensure	1060	37	Casein and soy	145	Glucose polymers and sucrose	37 Corn oil	500	500	10	30	31	31	450	210
3. Ensure plus	1500	58	Casein and soy	199	Glucose polymers and sucrose	54 Corn oil	600	600	14	48	45	49	600	200
4. Isocal	1060	34	Casein and soy	133	Glucose polymers	44 Soy oil and MCT	630	530	10	23	30	34	300	210
5. Meritene	960	58	Skim milk and casein	110	Glucose polymers and sucrose	32 Corn oil	1200	1200	14	38	45	41	505 (varies with flavor)	320
6. Osmolite HN	1064	45	Casein and soy	142	Glucose polymers	37 MCT, corn oil, and soy oil	770	770	14	41	41	40	300	310
7. Sustacal, liquid	1020	61	Skim milk, casein, and soy	140	Sucrose and glucose polymers	24 Soy oil	1300	1160	17	48	51	45	625 (varies with flavor)	300

Elemental

1. Vital HN	1000	42	Hydro-lysed whey, meat, and soy; amino acids	185	Glucose polymers and sucrose	11	Saf-flower oil and MCT	670	670	12	20	25	34	460	270
2. Vivonex standard	1000	20	Amino acids	231	Glucose polymers	2	Saf-flower oil	560	560	10	20	20	30	550 (varies with flavor)	220

Incomplete Liquid Feedings

1. Amin-Aid (essential amino acids)—does not contain vitamins or minerals	1956	19	Essential amino acids plus histidine	366	Glucose polymers and sucrose	46	Soy cil	-	-	-	<15	-	<6	1095	-
2. Citrotein	660	41	Egg white	122	Sucrose and glucose polymers	2	Soy oil	1060	1060	38	31	27	18	480 (varies with flavor)	420

TABLE 20-7
Continued

	Energy (kcal)*	Protein g	Protein Type or Casein/ Whey	CHO g	CHO Type	Fat g Type	Ca (mg)	P (mg)	Fe (mg)	Na (mmol)	Cl (mmol)	K (mmol)	GI Solute Load† (mmol/kg H₂0)	Vit.D (IU)
Formula Modules														
Carbohydrate (per 100 g)														
1. Caloreen	400	-	-	96	Glucose polymers	-	-	-	-	<2	-	tr	-	-
2. Polycose														
Powder	380	-	-	94	Glucose	-	<30	<5	-	<5	<7	tr	-	-
Liquid (per 100 ml)	200	-	-	50	polymers	-	<20	<3	-	<3	<4	tr	900	-
Fat (per 100 ml)														
1. Corn oil	820	-	-	-	-	93	-	-	-	-	-	-	-	-
2. MCT	765	-	-	-	-	93 Modified coconut oil	-	-	-	-	-	-	-	-
3. Microlipid	450	-	-	-	-	50 Safflower oil	-	-	-	-	-	-	80	-
Protein (per 100 g)														
1. RDP (rapidly dispersing protein)	360	75	Whey	5	Lactose	4	370	320	2	10	7	21	35	-
2. Propac	400	77	Whey	5	Lactose	8	600	310	-	10	2	13	-	-

* 1 kcal = 4.2 kJ.

† Renal solute load can be estimated using the following formula:
  Renal solute load (mmol/L) = 4 × protein (g/L) + Na (mmol/L) + K (mmol/L) + Cl (mmol/L).

** Fat content of whole cows milk varies with location.

§ In Canada, commercial cows milk is fortified to 360 IU/L.

++The values listed are for a formulation diluted to 670 kcal/L (used for infants). Following instructions on the label will create a 1000 kcal/L

21 OPHTHALMOLOGY

EYE EXAMINATION IN INFANTS

Basic Approach

- Infant should be maintained in a quiet, content, and alert mood
- By simple observation, without touching, note
  1. Anatomic integrity of globes and surrounding tissues
  2. How child responds visually to environment
  3. Presence or absence of nystagmus
  4. Relative straightness of eyes
- Comparison of the corneal light reflexes from a hand light demonstrates the presence or absence of strabismus (see under Strabismus)
- Vision is assessed in terms of the child's being able to fixate on objects with the eyes central, steady, and maintaining fixation
- Visual fields can be tested by "wiggling" an object or a light in each quadrant of the peripheral field binocularly and observing the child's refixational movements to fixate the object
- Poor vision is evidenced by
  1. Obvious media problems, e.g., cataracts
  2. Roving nystagmus
  3. Inability to fixate on a visual object
  4. Absence of any spontaneous visual response to the environment
- As many observations as possible should be made before the child is actually touched
- A cover test demonstrates the presence or absence of strabismus (see appropriate section)
- The ocular globes can be examined more carefully

1. The corneal sheen should be intact, without any breaks, as due to abrasions
2. The pupils should be equal and reactive to light
3. A clear red reflex should be ascertained bilaterally
4. Look for evidence of Horner's syndrome (miosis, ptosis, anhidrosis, and heterochromia)

- The pupils can be dilated for funduscopy as follows:
  1. 1% Mydriacyl, 1–2 drops in each eye, followed in 5–10 min by
  2. 1% Cyclogyl, 1–2 drops in each eye or 2.5% Neo-Synephrine, 1–2 drops in each eye
- In neonates, the following is recommended:
  1. 2.5% Neo-Synephrine, 1–2 drops in each eye, followed in 5–10 min by
  2. ½% Mydriacyl, 1–2 drops in each eye
- For funduscopy, immobilization of children and infants is important to adequately visualize the posterior pole
- High refractive errors prevent accurate visualization of the fundus; in all doubtful cases, ophthalmologic consultation for indirect ophthalmoscopy should be sought

OPHTHALMOLOGIC EMERGENCIES

Neonatal Conjunctivitis

Chemical

- 1% silver nitrate is still used for gonococcal prophylaxis when applied within 1 hr after birth
- Conjunctivitis occurs within 12 hr after application
- Resolves spontaneously within 2–3 days
  N.B. Silver nitrate 1% does not prevent

chlamydial or gram negative conjunctivitis, and does not treat established gonococcal infection

Bacterial

General Considerations

- Usually *Staphylococcus aureus, Streptococcus pneumoniae*, and gram negative organisms, in addition to *N. gonorrhoeae* (GC)

Clinical Features and Investigations

- Onset usually between the 1st and 5th days in GC
- Diagnosis made by finding intracellular organisms on Gram stain and by special cultures for GC. Other organisms identified by culture.

Treatment

- GC treated by prophylaxis with 1% silver nitrate or erythromycin 0.5% ointment at birth. Established GC infection treated aggressively with systemic (IV) aqueous crystalline penicillin G plus topical tetracycline eye ointment, pending results of sensitivity studies
- Penicillinase-producing *N. gonorrhoeae* requires systemic Cefotaxime in the neonate
- Other organisms are treated with topical neomycin-polymyxin B ointment or drops. Systemic therapy only for moderate to severe infections

Chlamydial

General Considerations

- *C. trachomatis*—most prevalent identifiable infectious cause of neonatal conjunctivitis

Clinical Features and Investigations

- Onset between 5th and 14th days of life. Presentation may be variable and nonspecific.
- May have associated pneumonitis
- Diagnosis based on demonstration of inclusion bodies on Giemsa stain of scrapings (palpebral conjunctiva)

Treatment

- Topical erythromycin ointment or 10% sulfacetamide ointment or drops *plus* oral erythromycin × 14 days

Viral

General Considerations

- Herpes simplex types I and II may cause conjunctivitis in the neonate

Clinical Features and Investigations

- Onset usually between the 2nd and 14th days, but may occur any time
- Diagnosis based on high index of suspicion, plus fluorescein slit lamp examination (dendritic corneal lesion) and scrapings

Treatment

- Topical trifluridine and systemic acyclovir constitute the treatment of choice

Orbital or Periorbital Cellulitis

- See Infectious Disease Section (p 319)

Acute Hyphema

General Considerations

Definition: blood in anterior chamber of eye, usually secondary to trauma

Management

- Child must be hospitalized for mandatory bed rest as catastrophic rebleeds can occur between the 2nd and 5th days, causing glaucoma
- Ophthalmologic consultation *must* be sought to rule out other complications and to monitor therapy

Corneal Foreign Body

Clinical Features

- Produces painful, red, photophobic, tearing eye, with foreign body (FB) sensation
- Visual acuity usually normal

Treatment

- Removal may be facilitated in some cases by use of fluorescein plus topical anesthetic, with aid of slit lamp
- A cotton swab can often be used to remove FB. In some cases a hypodermic needle may be required. (*Caution*: should be done by ophthalmologist.)
- Young infants and more difficult cases may require ophthalmologic consultation and examination under anesthesia (EUA)
- Following its removal, topical antibiotic ointment *or* drops (e.g., sodium sulamyd 10%) is instilled and the eye patched
- The patient should be reviewed by ophthalmologist in 24 hr
- N.B. High velocity FB injuries require roentgenographic investigations to rule out intra-orbital FB

Corneal Abrasion

Clinical Features

- Similar to those with corneal foreign body
- Examination facilitated by use of topical anesthesia followed by fluorescein strip to lower lid
- Defect in corneal epithelium glows green with slit lamp (blue filter)
- May have accompanying iritis

Treatment

- Treat by resting the eye. Apply topical antibiotics +/− cycloplegics (e.g., homatropine 5%) with eye patch × 24 hr
- Ophthalmologic reassessment at 24 hr

Chemical Burns (e.g., Lye) of Eye

General Considerations

- A true ocular emergency!
- May result in significant visual loss, or loss of affected eye
- Alkali burns more damaging to eye than acids

Management

- Copious irrigation with water from nearest source ASAP!
- Repeat once patient arrives in emergency department, and continue × 20–30 min with normal saline (0.9%)
- Sedation ± systemic analgesia may facilitate irrigation
- Gentle debridement should be carried out to remove debris and caustic material remaining after irrigation (search under everted lid)
- A cycloplegic (e.g., atropine 1%) reduces the risk of ciliary spasm and posterior synechiae

- Finally, topical antibiotics (gram negative coverage) should be commenced
- If possible, an ophthalmologist should be involved at an early stage

NONEMERGENT OPHTHALMOLOGIC DISORDERS

Conjunctivitis (Postneonatal)

Bacterial

General Considerations

- Staphylococcal species, *Hemophilus* and *S. pneumoniae* are the most common organisms

Management

- Treatment guided by cultures
- Majority respond to topical antimicrobials, e.g., 10% sulfacetamide drops or ointment applied frequently

Viral

General Considerations and Clinical Features

- Adenovirus, measles, varicella, influenza, and mumps are implicated viruses. Herpes simplex conjunctivitis requires urgent diagnosis and therapy.
- Red, watery eye, with slight ptosis +/− preauricular adenopathy are frequent findings

Management

- May empirically start topical antibiotics pending cultures, if unsure of diagnosis
- Associated mucocutaneous vesicles implicate herpes virus (confirm with conjunctival scrapings and fluorescein slit lamp examination).

Therapy with topical trifluridine (TFT) or adeno-
sine arabinoside (ARA-A) should be instituted.
Ophthalmologic consultation is recommended.
- Topical steroids are contraindicated

Uveitis

Anterior Uveitis

General Considerations and Clinical Features

- Often associated with rheumatic or connective
  tissue disorders, e.g., JRA, ankylosing spondylitis, Behçet's; inflammatory bowel disease, e.g.,
  Crohn's; and penetrating wounds to eye, among
  other causes (herpes, sarcoid). Idiopathic in
  50%.
- Presents with red eye, photophobia, tearing and
  deep aching pain, ↓ visual acuity, and prominent perilimbal blood vessels in acute form
- Chronic form is more insidious
- Slit lamp examination reveals inflammatory cells
  ± synechiae

Management

- Team approach with ophthalmologist and pediatric specialist
- Treat underlying condition (if applicable)
- Topical steroids plus mydriatic-cycloplegics are
  effective most often
- Systemic steroids ± immunosuppressives may
  occasionally be required
- Complications include glaucoma, cataracts,
  pupillary block and band keratopathy, blindness, and ocular atrophy (phthisis)

Posterior Uveitis

- Etiology includes various infections (viral, bacterial, fungal, and protozoal, among others).
  (See pediatric or ophthalmology texts for further
  details.)

Leukocoria (White Pupil)

- This should always be considered to be pathologic and requires urgent ophthalmologic consultation
- See Table 21–1 for some important causes

Cherry-Red Spot

- A cherry-red appearance of the macula due to the contrast between the white appearance of the peripheral macula produced by the infiltrated or edematous ganglion cells and the normal red coloration of the fovea (ganglion-free)
- See Table 21–2 for a list of conditions associated with a cherry-red spot

Hordeolum (Stye)

General Considerations

- Inflammation of glands of the eyelash follicle. Infected area is usually red and swollen and points (i.e., forms a "head").

TABLE 21–1 Some Important Causes of Leukocoria

Developmental anomalies
    Persistent hyperplastic primary vitreous (PHPV)—most common *unilateral* cause of leukocoria

Retinal vascular anomalies
    Retrolental fibroplasia—complication of prematurity and oxygen toxicity

Neoplastic lesions
    Retinoblastoma—most ominous cause of leukocoria (must be ruled out!)

Infections
    Toxocariasis

Others
    Cataracts

TABLE 21–2   Metabolic Conditions Associated with Cherry-Red Spot

"Storage" disorders:
 Tay-Sach disease (GM$_2$ type I)
 Sandhoff variant (GM$_2$ type II)
 Generalized gangliosidosis (GM$_1$ type I)
 Niemann-Pick disease (sphingomyelin lipidosis)
 Gaucher's disease
 Metachromatic leukodystrophy (MLD)
 Mucopolysaccharidoses—Farber's disease, Spranger's disease

N.B. Occlusion of central retinal artery and leukemic infiltration can produce similar "cherry-red-like" spot in the retina. The former is an ophthalmologic emergency!

- *Staphylococcus aureus* is commonly implicated

Management

- Treat with warm compresses 4–6 times daily, followed by topical antibiotic drops or ointment
- Surgical incision and drainage rarely required
- Recurrences common

Chalazion

General Considerations and Clinical Features

- Granulomatous, usually nontender swelling of meibomian gland
- Localized swelling on lid appears. May become infected. Course is protracted (months).

Management

- Acute: antibiotic ointment following warm compresses
- Persistent cases: may require incision and drainage

Strabismus (Squint)

General Considerations

- Definition: any condition in which the visual axes are not parallel
- Classification
  1. Ordinary childhood strabismus (nonparalytic)
     - Angle (deviation) between visual axes remains constant in various directions of gaze
     - Majority due to extraocular muscle imbalance or problem of accommodation or refractory errors (anisometropia)
     - 99% horizontal, 1% vertical; 80% esotropia, 20% exotropia
  2. Paralytic
     - Angle between visual axes varies in different directions of gaze
     - Usually a sign of a neurologic process involving the cranial nerves (VI, IV, III) or brain stem, or extraocular muscles
     - Urgent neurologic evaluation warranted

Clinical Features

- Hirschberg test: Light (e.g., penlight) is shone into both eyes. The position of the light reflex (from *single* source) in both corneas is noted. The light reflex is not centered on the nonfixing eye.
- Cover-uncover test (in children >1 yr): The uncovered eye, if strabismus is present, changes position to focus on the light or object

Management

- Refer *all* cases of strabismus diagnosed after 12 wk of age to ophthalmologist for assessment and follow-up
- Eye patching, glasses, or surgery used as appropriate

- Need to exclude underlying conditions, e.g.,
  cataracts, refractive error, *retinoblastoma*,
  optic nerve disease, or CNS disorder

Complications and Follow-Up

- Amblyopia is the most serious (preventable)
  complication
- Head tilt or torticollis may also occur as a com-
  pensatory action
  N.B. Pseudostrabismus is often misdiagnosed as
  strabismus. Misalignment of eyes is apparent
  because of presence of epicanthic folds ±
  broad nasal bridge

Amblyopia

General Considerations

- Poor vision in eye despite correction of refractive problem (if present). A turned eye should
  be presumed amblyopic until examined.
- There are four major causes
  1. Organic, e.g., retinal problems such as
     chorioretinitis
  2. Deprivation, e.g., ptosis (total), cataracts, cor-
     neal opacity, which lead to disuse of affected
     eye
  3. Strabismic—due to suppression of affected
     eye
  4. Refractive—due to excessive myopia, farsight-
     edness, or astigmatism

Management

- Eye patching of the preferred eye for specified
  periods
- Early referral to ophthalmologist for diagnosis
  and to guide therapy
- Remove amblyogenic factors when possible

TABLE 21–3 Recommendations for Screening Children for Amblyopia and Associated Conditions

Newborn to 4 mo
  Be sure the eyes externally appear normal and exclude cataracts by eliciting a red reflex

Infants after age 4 mo
  Perform Hirschberg test (see above)
  Confirm red reflex and check fundus
  Be aware of a positive family history
  All children after 6 mo with family history of strabismus should be examined by an ophthalmologist

Age 4 yr
  Measure visual acuity in both eyes
  Ideally all children should be referred for complete eye examination and refraction (if economically feasible)

School age
  Check vision yearly

Adapted from Stager DR. Amblyopia and the pediatrician. Pediatr Ann 1983; 12:574–584.

Suggested Reading

1. Catalano JD, ed. Pediatric ophthalmology (entire issue). Pediatr Ann 1983; 12(7).
2. Catalano JD, ed. Pediatric ophthalmology (entire issue). Pediatr Ann 1983; 12(8).
3. Crawford JS, Morin JD, eds. The eye in childhood. Orlando: Grune & Stratton, 1983.
4. Nelson LB, ed. Pediatric ophthalmology (entire issue). Pediatr Clin North Am 1983; 30(6).

LOWER LIMB PROBLEMS
Intoeing

General Considerations

- Common in children learning to walk
- Mostly self-corrects, rare in adults
- Aggravated by "sitting" on feet

Clinical Features

- See Figure 22–1
  1. Establish torsional profile (Fig. 22–2)
     - Foot progression angle
     - Measure thigh-foot angle
     - Measure range of external rotation at hip
     - Measure degree of metatarsus varus
  2. Establish coordination profile
     - Jumping by age 2 yr
     - Hopping by age 4 yr

Differential Diagnosis

- Metatarsus varus
  1. Front of foot curved inward
  2. Often present at birth and possibly aggra-
     vated by sleeping prone with feet turned in
- Internal tibial torsion—thigh foot angle < -10
  degrees
- Internal femoral torsion—external rotation of hip
  <20 degrees
- Clumsy child (can be confirmed by formal
  occupational therapy assessment)

Management

- General

EXAMINATION

1

Assess
Gait
Angle

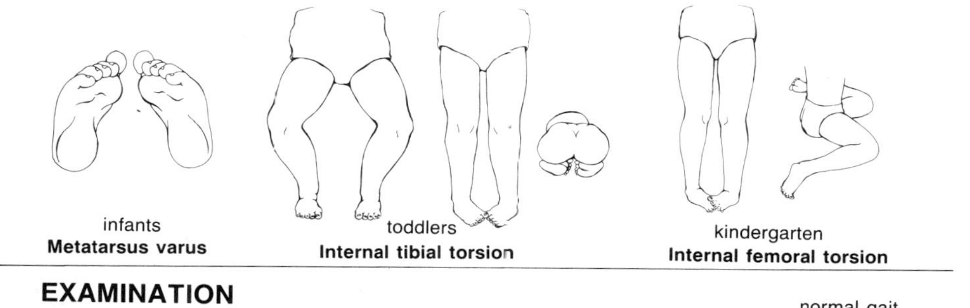

Figure 22–1 Intoeing varieties. (From The Easter Seal guide to children's orthopaedics—prevention, screening and problem solving. Ontario: The Easter Seal Society, 1982.)

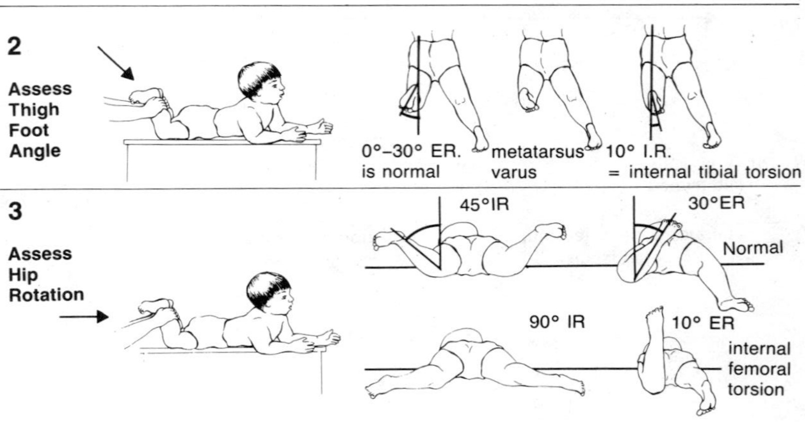

Figure 22–1 Continued

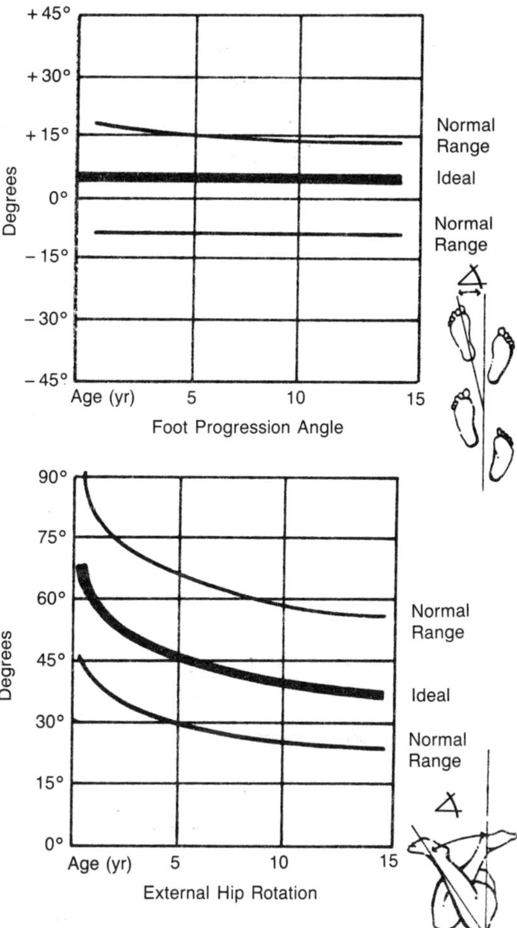

Figure 22–2 Torsional profile. The shape of the leg gradually changes as a child grows. Twists tend to disappear. This chart documents these changes. (Data based on Staheli LT, et al. Lower extremity—rotational problems in children. Normal values to guide management. J Bone Joint Surg 1985; 67A:39–47.)

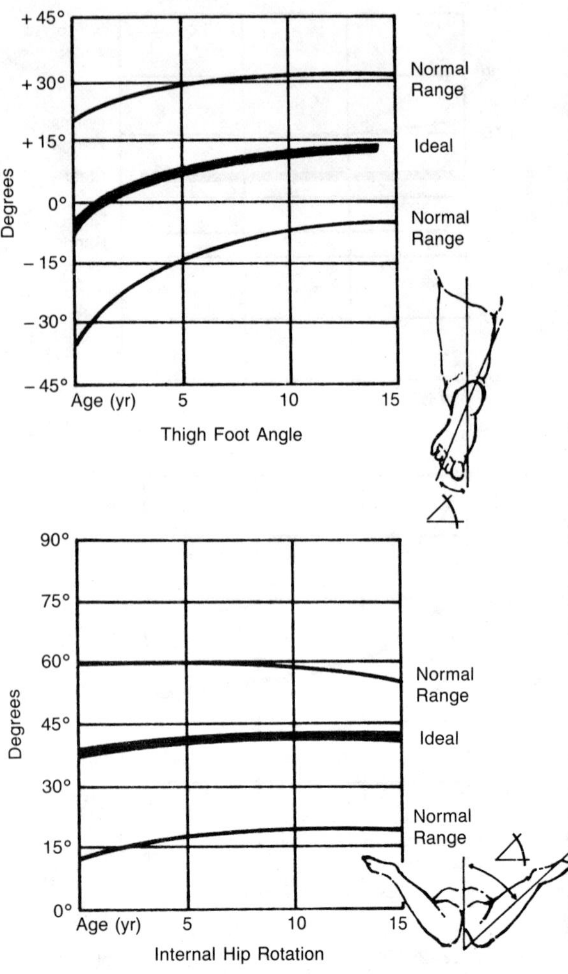
+45°
+30°
+15°
0°
- 15°
- 30°
- 45°
Degrees
Age (yr)
5
10
15
Normal
Range
Ideal
Normal
Range
Thigh Foot Angle
90°
75°
60°
45°
30°
15°
0°
Degrees
Age (yr)
5
10
15
Normal
Range
Ideal
Normal
Range
Internal Hip Rotation

1. No scientific evidence that torsion is improved by our efforts
2. Educate parents with handouts and explanations. Most, but not all, improve.
3. Suggest lotus position for sitting
- Specific therapy
    1. Metatarsus varus
        - Birth: observe
        - 3–9 mo: Wheaton splints or articulated boot
        - 9 mo–2 yr: ignore
        - 2 yr +: surgical correction
    2. Internal tibial torsion—9–18 mo: Denis-Browne night splints for 3–4 mo
    3. Internal femoral torsion
        - Splints and shoes ineffective
        - Correct sitting habits
        - If severe, consider osteotomy at 10 yr for exceptional case
    4. Clumsy child: be kind!

Out-Toeing

General Considerations

- Usually external femoral torsion
- Due to lying prone in frog position
- Self-correcting when child begins to roll over

Foot Shape Concerns

General Considerations

- Most often the degree of parental concern is out of proportion to the importance
- Occasionally a presenting complaint of cerebral palsy, muscular dystrophy

Clinical Features of Importance

- Walking: Is arch high or low? Gait abnormal?
- Test for neurologic abnormalities

TABLE 22–1   Differential Diagnosis and Management of ''Foot Shape'' Abnormalities

	Age of Presentation	Frequency	Main Feature	Treatment
Club foot	Birth	1:700	Fixed equinovarus	Serial casts at birth Operate on 80% at 3 mo
Calcaneovalgus foot	Birth	1:300	Top of foot rests on shin	Always recovers Advise stretching X-ray for congenital hip dislocation
Metatarsus varus	Birth–3 mo	1:100	Forefoot adduction	Brace at 3 mo After 2 yr requires operation
Vertical talus	Birth–3 mo	1:100,000	Rocker bottom sole	Usually requires surgical correction
Hypermobile flat foot	2 yr +	1:10	Arch appears on tiptoeing	Ignore Unaffected by attempts to treat

| Pes cavus | 10 yr + | 1:10,000 | Fixed high arch | Investigate: spinal x-ray film, nerve conduction studies, possibly myelogram
Often requires surgery |
| Toe walking | 3 yr + | 1:700 | Short calf muscle | Exclude dystrophy and cerebral palsy
If persistent, grow muscle with stretching casts |

Knee Pain

General Considerations and Management

- May be referred pain from the hip, e.g., slipped epiphysis
- Meniscal injury *rare* in children
- Main causes (and management) include
  1. Osgood-Schlatter disorder
     - Chronic stress fracture of tibial tubercle
     - Swollen and tender
     - X-ray films necessary to rule out other conditions shows enlarged and fragmented tibial tubercle
     - Treatment
       a. Explanation and reassurance
       b. Continue sports, but use basketball knee protector
       c. Expect it to last ~18 mo
  2. Peripatellar pain syndrome
     - Most frequent source of knee pain
     - Commonest in adolescent girls (athletic)
     - Pain on climbing stairs and after sitting for long time
     - Pain reproduced by compressing patella against femur
     - Probably due to overuse
     - X-ray films normal
     - Generally a protracted course, uninfluenced by our attempts to treat, but muscle stretching exercises may help
  3. Osteochondritis dissecans
     - Incomplete fracture of surface of articular cartilage of femoral condyle
     - A cause of aching knee pain and ''giving way''
     - Obvious on x-ray film
     - Tends to heal spontaneously in those still growing
     - Usually treated by observation, occasionally by immobilization, and rarely by drilling or pinning back

4. Recurrent dislocation of patella
   - With or without injury the patella starts to dislocate
   - Often pushed back by patient
   - Axial x-ray films of patella with knee flexed 40 degrees shows shallow groove
   - Treat with exercises first. Usually require surgical repair.
5. Hemarthrosis
   - When the knee swells quickly after injury, it usually is full of blood owing to a torn ligament or an osteochondral fracture
   - Arthroscopy is often the best way to plan further treatment

HIP PROBLEMS

Congenital Dislocation of Hip

General Considerations

- Sudden extension of hip at birth causes dislocation in genetically predisposed
- Most common in girls, first born, left hip, breech presentation

Clinical Features

- Stage 1. *Dislocatable*: Hip stays in joint but can be pushed out on Barlow test (Fig. 22–3). Usually recovers spontaneously after a few weeks.
- Stage 2. *Dislocated but reducible*: Positive Ortolani test (Fig. 22–3). Lasts a few weeks before progressing to...

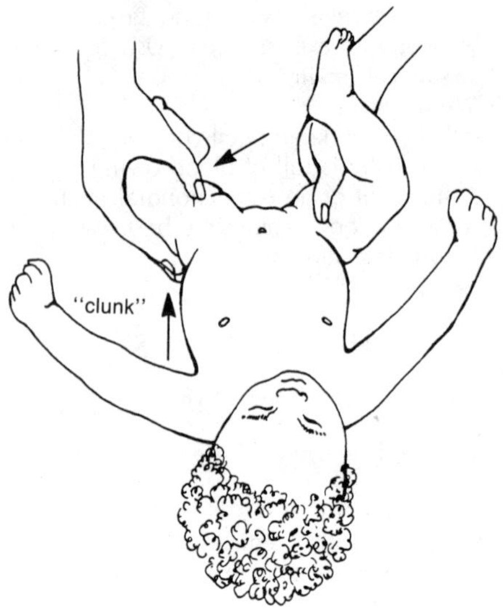

A. Ortolani (reduction) test. With baby relaxed and content on firm surface, the hips and knees are flexed to 90°. Hips are examined one at a time. Examiner grasps baby's thigh with middle finger over greater trochanter, and lifts thigh to bring femoral ead from its dislocated posterior position to opposite the acetabulum. Simultaneously, thigh is gently abdocuted, reducing gently abducted, reducing femoral head into acetabulum. In positive finding, examiner senses reduction by palpable, nearly audible "clunk".

Figure 22–3 Recognition of congenital dislocation of the hip (CDH). (Redrawn after Shelov MD, Mezey AP, Edelmann CM, Jr, Barnett HL. Primary care pediatrics: a symptomatic approach. Norwalk: Appleton-Century-Crofts, 1984:489.)

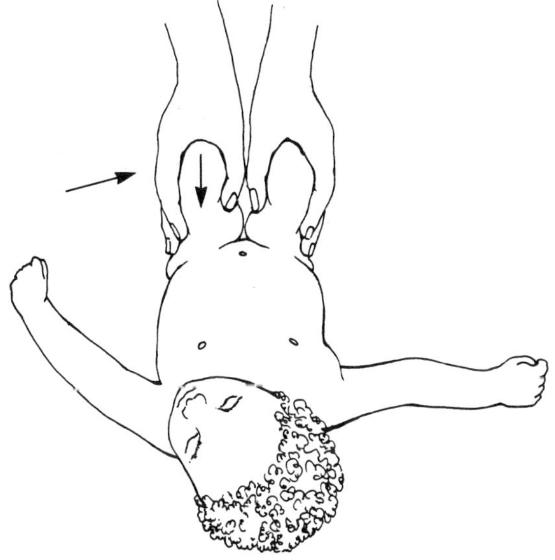

B. Barlow (dislocation) test. Reverse of Ortolani test. If femoral head is in acetabulum at time of examination, the Barlow test is performed to discover any hip instability. Baby's thigh is grasped as above and adducted with gently downward pressure. Dislocation is palpable as femoral head slips out of acetabulum. Diagnosis is confirmed with Ortolani test.

Stage 3. *Fixed dislocation-irreducible*: This is the stage when abduction is limited and thigh looks short (Galeazzi's sign; Fig. 22–4): 3 mo plus.

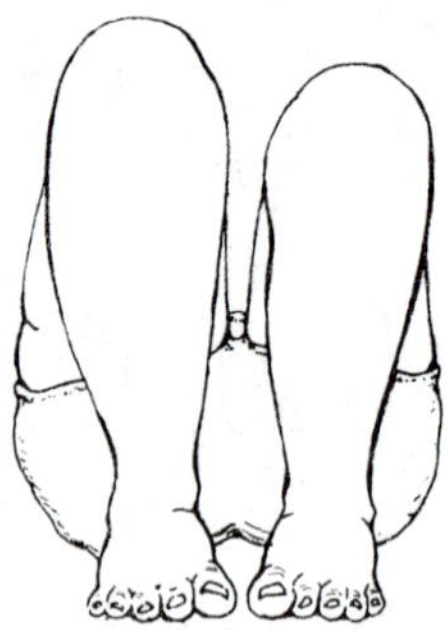

Allis' or Galeazzi's sign: knee is lower on affected side when knees and hips are flexed because femoral head lies posterior to acetabulum in this position.

Figure 22–4   Galeazzi's sign. (Redrawn after Shelov MD, Mezey AP, Edelmann CM Jr, Barnett HL. Primary care pediatrics: symptomatic approach. Norwalk: Appleton-Century-Crofts, 1984:490.)

Differential Diagnosis

- Synovial click: this is a *noise* from the hip like someone "cracking" his knuckles. A positive Ortolani sign is not a noise but the feeling of the femoral head jumping into the joint.
- Congenital adduction contracture in windswept child (i.e., adduction contracture on one hip and abduction contracture on other hip)
- Congenital femoral hypoplasia
- Fixed dislocation in arthrogryposis

Management

- Investigation
  1. Clinical signs best guide for stages 1 and 2
  2. X-ray film or ultrasound for stage 3

- Treatment
  1. Pavlik harness: 0–8 mo
  2. Traction and closed reduction 8–18 mo
  3. Traction, open reduction, innominate osteo-
     tomy, 18–30 mo
  4. Traction, open reduction, innominate osteo-
     tomy, and femoral shortening, 30 mo–5 yr

Legg-Perthes Disease

General Considerations

- Avascular necrosis of femoral head of unknown
  etiology
- Affects primarily children from ages 3–10 yr
  with peak between 5–7 yr
- Boys more frequently affected ($\sim$5:1)
- Child presents with limp, restriction of range of
  movement (ROM), and pain in knee or hip
- Antalgic gait
- Delayed bone age with constitutional delay of
  growth

Management

- Investigation—x-ray (AP and frog leg lateral
  views) may be quite subtle at first
  1. Widening of cartilage space
  2. Widening of epiphyseal line
  3. Femoral head
     - Smaller
     - Dense with subchondral fracture
     - Bone absorption and collapse
     - Repair
  4. Increased width of femoral neck; metaphyseal
     cysts
- Treatment
  1. Child should be referred to orthopaedic
     surgeon
  2. Treatment varies from simple observation to
     bracing or surgery, depending on age of
     child and extent of disease. "Containment" is
     the underlying principle.

Transient Synovitis (Observation Hip)

General Considerations

- Etiology unknown, but often follows viral illness or exertion
- Occurs in age group 2–10 yr
- May be difficult to differentiate from early "septic" hip
- Child usually able to bear some weight on affected hip
- Usually afebrile or low grade fever, and child looks well
- Painful gait
- ↓ ROM with pain at extremes of movement
- Better after a day of rest

Management

- Investigation: WBC, ESR usually normal. X-ray films to exclude Legg-Perthes.
- Treatment
  1. Bed rest (at home in most cases) $\pm$ ASA × 3–5 days
  2. $\pm$ Gentle ROM exercises (springs and slings). Gradual resumption of activity.
  3. Careful observation to rule out early septic arthritis
  4. If recurrent or persistent, need to rule out Legg-Perthes

Septic Hip

General Considerations

- Neonatal: nosocomial infection, often multifocal
- Childhood type usually solitary
- Destroys a hip quickly. The cartilage is dissolved by proteolytic enzymes; the vessels thrombose, leading to avascular necrosis; capsular softening leads to dislocation of hip.

Clinical Features

- Neonatal form may be subtle, e.g., pain on moving hip to change diaper. Swelling follows. Requires high index of suspicion.
- Childhood form: sudden onset of hip pain and diminished range of movement. Fever.

Differential Diagnosis

- Synovitis
- Pelvic osteomyelitis

Management

- Investigation: Aspirate hip under general anesthesia. Blood culture in neonate.
- Treatment
  1. Drain hip surgically
  2. Antibiotics for 3 wk plus

Slipped Femoral Capital Epiphysis (SFCE)

General Considerations

- Serious common condition of obese preadolescents or early adolescence, often with delayed sexual development (ages 9–17 yr)
- 30% bilateral
- Presents either as *acute severe pain* and inability to bear weight following trauma, or more commonly as *insidious ache* in groin or knee—often mistaken for "pulled" muscle
- Tends to lie with leg in some degree of external rotation, with decrease in flexion, internal rotation, and abduction

Management

- Investigations: Frog-leg lateral view of both hips is most useful x-ray view in mild degrees of slip
- Treatment

1. Surgical pinning as emergency
2. Rule out endocrine abnormality if bone age delayed

SPINE

Scoliosis

General Considerations

- Commonest type occurs in adolescent girls—idiopathic or genetic type
- Also seen in neurologic disease—cerebral palsy, Friedreich's ataxia, syringomyelia, and leg length discrepancy
- Mostly progressive until growth is complete. Severe curves progress in adults.
- School screening useful to raise awareness
- Many minimal curves noted in school screening were nonprogressive

Clinical Features

- Forward bend test shows prominence on one side
- Scoliosis usually passes unnoticed when standing vertically

Differential Diagnosis

- Presentation in infancy or early childhood suggests underlying skeletal or neuromuscular disorder

Management

- Investigation: 3 ft *standing* PA x-ray film of spine: a single film is all that is required to confirm and quantify using Cobb angle.
- Treatment
  1. Still growing
     - 10–25 degrees: check every 6 mo using roentgenogram

TABLE 22–2 Clinical Features of Some Common Hip Disorders

	CDH*	Transient Synovitis	Legg-Perthes	SFCE*	Septic Arthritis
Age (yr)	0–4	4–8	3–10	8–15	ANY (0–1)
ROM*	↓ Abduction	↓	↓	↓ Flexion and int. rotation	↓
Pain	None	+ → + +	0 → +	+	+ + + +
X-ray exam	Dislocation	Normal	Abnormal; varies with stage	Abnormal: slip	Frequently normal
Temp.	Normal	Normal	Normal	Normal	↑
ESR*	Normal	Can be ↑	Normal	Normal	↑ Can be normal in early cases
Treatment	External splint early, surgery late	Rest, gentle range of motion exercises	Observation, brace, or surgery depending on age and extent	Surgery	Surgery and antibiotics

* CDH = congenital dislocated hip; SFCE = slipped femoral capital epiphysis; ROM = range of movement; ESR = erythrocyte sedimentation rate.

545

- 25–45 degrees: brace or electrical stimulation
    - 45 degrees +: spinal instrumentation and fusion
2. Growth complete
    - <45 degrees: ignore
    - >45 degrees: spinal instrumentation

Kyphosis

General Considerations

- Round back is common. No solid line separates pathologic from normal. Usually structural.
- When painful, there is usually wedging and osteochondrosis on x-ray film

Management

- Investigation: Standing lateral x-ray film to measure angle of kyphosis between T3 and T12
- Treatment
  1. Still growing
     - <30 degrees: normal
     - 30–45 degrees: mild—watch; stop parents' nagging
     - 45 degrees +: consider Boston brace
  2. Growth complete and 50 degrees +: consider surgical correction

Back Pain

General Considerations

- More likely to be a definite cause in children than in adults

Differential Diagnosis

- Mechanical—spondylolisthesis, Scheuermann's disease, thoracolumbar osteochondritis
- Infection—osteomyelitis
- Tumors and tumor-like conditions—eosinophilic

granuloma, aneurysmal bone cyst, osteoblas-
toma, osteoid osteoma
- Injury

Management

- Investigations: roentgenogram, bone scan, ESR

UPPER LIMB

Pulled Elbow

General Considerations and Clinical Features

- Common in 2–5 yr olds
- Produced by tug on outstretched arm. This
  abolishes normal carrying angle. The radial
  head is "yanked" distally to become trapped in
  the annular ligament.
- Child won't use arm → pseudoparalysis

Differential Diagnosis

- Fracture!

Management

- Investigations: roentgenogram to rule out injury
  (rarely required)
- Treatment
  1. On supination of the forearm, there is a
     "click" felt, which represents the radial head
     escaping from the ligament
  2. Pain disappears immediately!
  3. Occasionally requires a second attempt next
     day

Trigger Thumb

General Considerations and Management

- Infant always holds interphalangeal joint of
  thumb flexed
- Nodule palpable in metacarpophalangeal joint
  crease

- Often noticed suddenly and mistaken for dislocation
- Requires surgical release

NECK

Congenital Muscular Torticollis

General Considerations
- Contracture of sternocleidomastoid muscle
- Breech birth

Clinical Features

- Newborn always turns head to same way
- Pseudotumor at lower end of sternocleido-mastoid
- May be associated with hip dislocation

Management

- Physiotherapy to stretch
- Neglected cases may require surgical release

INJURIES

General Considerations

- Half the deaths in childhood are due to accidents; prevention is a priority
- Sprains are almost unknown in children. They are usually greenstick, buckle, or epiphyseal fractures requiring an x-ray examination to diagnose.
- *Every fracture in a child under 18 mo should be assumed to be due to abuse or neglect until proven otherwise*

Clinical Features

- Metaphyseal-diaphyseal fractures: minor green-stick and buckle fractures produce local pain and tenderness without deformity or swelling
- Growth plate injuries: swelling and tenderness (Fig. 22–5)

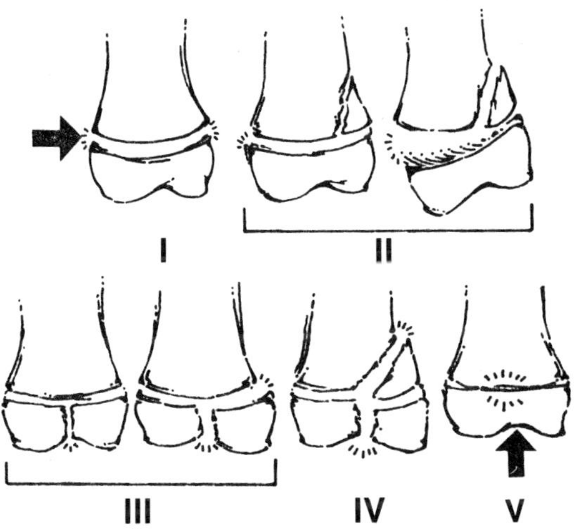

Figure 22–5 Classification of growth plate injuries. Epiphyseal injuries have been classified by Salter and Harris. Types II and III may be seen in displaced or in undisplaced injuries. (From Salter RB, Harris WR. Injuries involving the epiphyseal plate. J Bone Joint Surg 1963; 45A:487.)

Management

- Check circulation and nerve function
- Look for wound. Warn not to eat or drink because anesthesia is often required.
- Splint and x-ray examination. Cover open wounds with sterile dressings.
- Treat
    1. Undisplaced metaphyseal-diaphyseal fractures—immobilize
    2. Displaced metaphyseal-diaphyseal fractures—reduce under anesthesia
    3. Fractures into the joint require open reduction (types 3 and 4)
    4. Open fractures require urgent debridement

Suggested Reading

1. Bobechko WP. Limp affecting the hip and knee in children. Can Fam Physician 1985; 31:1061–1063.
2. Gross RH. Hip problems in children. Postgrad Med 1984; 76:97–105.
3. Yngve DA. Gait problems in children. Postgrad Med 1984; 76:56–64.

23 OTOLARYNGOLOGY

ADENOTONSILLECTOMY

General Considerations

- Absolute and possible indications for adeno-tonsillectomy are very controversial, varying from institution to institution and even among individuals within a division (pediatrics or ENT), since *most* claims of efficacy are based on anecdotal data
- The following is a reasonably acceptable list from each group:
  1. Absolute indications
     - Obstructive sleep apnea, with or without cor pulmonale
     - Dysphagia (tonsillectomy only warranted)
     - Possible malignant disease (unilateral hypertrophy)
     - ± Peritonsillar abscess (quinsy): one episode (as tends to recur)
     - ± Nasal obstruction (hypertrophied adenoids) producing discomfort in breathing, severe speech distortion, or dentofacial maldevelopment
  2. Possible (controversial) indications
     - Chronic or recurrent suppurative otitis media
     - Conductive hearing loss (serous otitis media)
     - Chronic or recurrent tonsillitis: at least three episodes in each of 3 yr, or four in each of 2 yr, or five episodes in 1 yr, associated with fever ($\geq 101°$ F or $38.3°$ C), tonsillar or pharyngeal exudate, cervical lymphadenitis, positive culture for group A β-hemolytic streptococci

- Rheumatic fever in poorly compliant patients
- Mouth breathing, snoring, or halitosis

Complications: Hemorrhage

- Primary—occurring within 24 hr postop
- Secondary—occurring between 5 and 8 days postop—usually secondary to infection
- Giving aspirin in postop period significantly increases risk

Management: Hemorrhage

- Admit patient for at least 1 day for observation in cases of secondary hemorrhage
- Assess fluid status and consider cross matching and starting IV after CBC
- Make a paste of bismuth subgallate in epinephrine (1:1,000) and apply it to pack
- Remove clot and insert pack in nasopharynx or tonsillar fossa for 10 min; postnasal pack may also be required
- Check CBC again at 8 hr after control of hemorrhage
- If bleeding persistent or difficult to control, consider checking PT, PTT, and platelets
- Start antibiotic therapy

FOREIGN BODIES IN EAR

Management

- Visualize with head mirror or headlamp and attempt removal
  1. Soft material: use loop
  2. Hard smooth object: use hook or loop
  3. Insect: kill it before removal by instilling rubbing alcohol
  4. General syringing with warm water is helpful—but do not syringe if FB is vegetable matter, foam, or paper (it may swell)

FOREIGN BODIES IN NOSE

General Considerations and Management

- Foreign body is the commonest cause of unilateral (usually foul smelling) nasal discharge
- Visualize with head mirror or light
- Anesthetize nasal mucosa, and shrink it by inserting cotton packs soaked with cocaine 5% (maximal dose=3 mg/kg)
- Suction off discharge surrounding FB
- Attempt removal with
    1. Forceps: soft material (e.g., paper, cotton)
    2. Hook: solid object

FOREIGN BODIES IN LARYNX, TRACHEOBRONCHIAL TREE, AND ESOPHAGUS

General Considerations

- Not all FBs present as acute problems
- Keep possibility of FB in mind when assessing any child who has enigmatic chronic chest disease or dysphagia
- Remember: "All that wheezes is not asthma, especially if unilateral"
- Diagnosis of FB aspiration established by
    1. History of choking, cyanotic episode
    2. Aphonia + airway distress = laryngeal FB
    3. Examination → stridor or wheeze, unequal expansion of chest, decreased air entry unilaterally; may have normal examination
    4. Radiology: order inspiratory and expiratory chest films—at least two views
        - Collapse suggests complete obstruction
        - Look for FB shadow in trachea
        - Hyperinflation suggests ball valve obstruction
    5. Fluoroscopy: unequal diaphragmatic movement

- Diagnosis of FB in esophagus established by
  1. History of ingestion, dysphagia, regurgitation, vomiting, or drooling
  2. History may be months long
  3. Examination may be normal, or stridor may be present if trachea compressed
  4. Radiology: AP and lateral views reveal position of FB if radio-opaque

Management

- Remove FB endoscopically under general anesthesia
- FB in larynx may cause complete obstruction and require urgent bronchoscopy in emergency department. If bronchoscopist not immediately available, endotracheal intubation may be life-saving.
- Stab tracheotomy is a last resort! Use only for a laryngeal or pharyngeal obstruction

EXTERNAL OTITIS

General Considerations

- Localized infection, usually a furuncle, in the outer third of ear canal
- Diffuse infection occurs following aggressive cleaning of the canal, trauma, or swimming
- *Staphylococcus aureus* commonly causes localized, whereas *Pseudomonas aeruginosa* and *Candida* sp. most commonly cause diffuse infection

Management

- Cleansing the canal is the single most important part of therapy
- Furuncle may require incision and drainage
- Debridement: gently remove infective and epithelial debris from ear canal (by wet swabbing, gentle irrigation, and suctioning)

- Topical antibiotic drops (e.g., those containing polymyxin, neomycin, ± hydrocortisone) for up to 10 days only
- If ear canal occluded by circumferential inflammatory edema, aluminum acetate 1% solution is used. Insert moist cotton wick into ear canal. Keep it wet with the solution until canal has expanded sufficiently to permit debridement after 1–2 days; then use topical antibiotic drops.
- If periauricular swelling, regional adenopathy, and signs of systemic infection are present, systemic antibiotics should be used (e.g., cefuroxime or cloxacillin)
- If difficulty exists in differentiating from furuncle of ear canal or mastoiditis with subperiosteal abscess formation, request ENT consult

EPISTAXIS

General Considerations

- Bleeding is usually from Little's area
- It is more common during acute URIs and in allergic rhinitis

Management

- Mild cases often respond to firm, persistent pressure to nose between fingers for 10 min. Following this, insert cotton plug with petroleum jelly into the nose and leave × 3–4 hr.
- More persistent cases are managed as follows:
    1. May be facilitated by sedation prn (codeine 1 mg/kg IM), visualization (head mirror or light), and suction
    2. Control bleeding with pressure and cotton pledgets moistened with cocaine 5% (maximum 3 mg/kg)
    3. Cauterize with silver nitrate stick behind bleeding point of vessel
    4. Pack nostrils (Oxycel, Gelfoam, petrolatum gauze) only if cautery is ineffective

5. If bleeding persistent, recurrent, or originating posteriorly, request ENT consult. N.B. Persistent bleeding may (rarely) represent a bleeding diathesis.
6. Children with blood dyscrasias should not have cautery with silver nitrate. Control bleeding with Oxycel gauze ± topical thromboplastin and pressure.

FRACTURED NOSE

Management

- Examine nose for septal hematoma or dislocation (causes nasal obstruction and may result in late nasal deformity)
- X-ray may aid in diagnosis but if negative, does not exclude serious pathology
- ENT service should be contacted to reduce deformity early (within 2–3 hr after injury) if no swelling, or late (5–10 days after injury)
- All cases from emergency room with no ENT consultation should be referred to ENT clinic for 3–4 day follow-up to check for late septal hematoma, abscess formation, or deformity (noted after swelling subsides)

CORROSIVE BURNS
OF UPPER GI TRACT

General Considerations

- Esophagus may be damaged by the time the child arrives in the emergency room
- Degree of visible burns in mouth and pharynx may not be indicative of degree of esophageal involvement

Management
(see also Poisoning section)

- Notify ENT service immediately
- Determine nature (acid, alkali, other) and form (solid, liquid) of ingested material if possible
- Do *not* give emetic!
- Do *not* attempt gastric lavage!
- Promote ingestion of appropriate fluids, unless drooling or signs of mediastinal leak (e.g., chest or back pain, dyspnea) present
  1. If alkali ingested, give milk or water
  2. If acid ingested, give milk or water
  3. If bleach ingested, give water or milk
  4. Ages 1–5yrs, give 1–2 cups; >5 yr, give up to 1 L (quart)
- Observe for respiratory distress secondary to laryngeal involvement (hoarseness, stridor, dyspnea)
- Observe for shock. Monitor vital signs carefully!
  1. If shock developing, start IV infusion of fluids (see p 659)
  2. Severe chest and abdominal pain are ominous signs—may be indicative of visceral perforation
- Esophagoscopy is usually performed after oral burns improve (3–5 days), to assess extent of esophageal burn
- Esophageal stricture develops in approximately 15% of cases of caustic ingestion
- The prophylactic use of steroids (prednisone) and antibiotics (ampicillin) following early endoscopy is recommended by some groups

FACIAL NERVE PARALYSIS

General Coinsiderations

- Fairly common in children—may be secondary to Bell's palsy, trauma (also birth), otitis media, aural neoplasm, or intracranial tumor

- Bell's palsy (does not always resolve spontaneously in children) is a diagnosis of exclusion

Management

- Investigations may include
  1. Audiogram
  2. Impedance studies
  3. Nerve conduction tests
  4. Mastoid tomograms, CT
  5. Schirmer's test
  6. Salivary secretion tests
- Therapy
  1. Refer to ENT
  2. Treat underlying condition
  3. Steroids may be useful in Bell's palsy

ACUTE (SUPPURATIVE) OTITIS MEDIA

General Considerations

- An extremely common cause of visits to the
  primary care physician by the young child or
  infant
- Major organisms include *Streptococcus pneumoniae, Haemophilus influenzae, Branhamella
  catarrhalis,* and *Streptococcus pyogenes*
- Symptoms may be vague (irritability, anorexia,
  pulling at the ears) in the infant and young
  child, whereas earache and hearing loss may be
  present in the older child

Management

- (Oral) antibiotic therapy is the mainstay of treatment. Several choices exist
  1. Amoxicillin: probably the most frequently
     prescribed and single most useful drug avail-
     able. Advantages—cheap, effective, easy to
     give ($\uparrow$ compliance), and safe.

2. Trimethoprim-sulfamethoxazole (Bactrim/Septra) is an excellent, effective, cheap alternative to amoxicillin when penicillin sensitivity exists. However, risks of hepatitis and Stevens-Johnson syndrome exist.
3. Erythromycin-sulfisoxazole (Pediazole) covers the same spectrum as cefaclor, but requires qid administration, is expensive, and has sulfa side effects. Useful for ampicillin-resistant *Haemophilus influenzae* and *Branhamella catarrhalis*.
4. Cefaclor, a β-lactamase-resistant drug, is indicated when there is significant risk of infection with these organisms. Associated with rashes and diarrhea, and erythema multiforme and serum sickness in about 1% of recipients. Currently quite expensive.
5. Amoxicillin-clavulanate (Augmentin/Clavulin) is effective against β-lactamase-producing organisms. Expensive; associated with $\sim 15\%$ incidence of diarrhea.
6. Generally one starts with amoxicillin or trimethoprim-sulfamethoxazole and moves to either cefaclor or Augmentin/Clavulin or Pediazole.
7. Treatment is initially for 10 days minimum.
8. In infants <6 wk, early myringotomy may be warranted for culture
9. For perforation with discharge, Garamycin otic drops tid × 10 days is usually recommended.
10. Analgesics and antipyretics as indicated
11. Decongestants or antihistamines are of no proven efficacy
12. Myringotomy indicated for
    - Severe pain—immediately
    - Bulging drum and pain after 48–72 hr of therapy
    - Otitis media with complication (e.g., meningitis, mastoiditis)

- • Residual serous otitis 12 wk after acute otitis despite apparently adequate medical therapy
    - • Immunodepressed (e.g., chemotherapy)
13. If discharge persists after 1 wk of adequate therapy, obtain swabs from deep in external canal for culture and sensitivity studies
14. Mastoid radiographs usually obtained only if disease present for ≥ 3 wk or if acute mastoiditis present (surgery required if air-cell coalescence)
15. If symptoms or discharge persist for >1 wk, check cultures for resistant organism and treat appropriately. Daily microdebridement by ENT may be necessary.

RECURRENT OTITIS MEDIA

Management

- Choice of prophylactic antibiotic (long-term or seasonal) or myringotomy and tympanostomy tube insertion
- Amoxicillin or sulfisoxazole are usual choices for chemoprophylaxis. Failure of this method, despite compliance, is an indication for myringotomy and tympanostomy tube.
- If <6 wk of age, rule out immunodeficiency!

SEROUS OTITIS MEDIA

General Considerations

- Commonest cause of hearing loss in children
- Common accompaniment of adenoidal hypertrophy, atopy, and cleft palate
- If undiagnosed or left untreated, *may* result in delayed onset of speech, learning problems, and chronic ear disease

- Medical
    1. Treat with antibiotics (see acute otitis media) PO × 3–4 wk
    2. Autoinsufflation—Valsalva maneuver
    3. First choice unless
        - Symptoms present for >6 mo at time of diagnosis
        - Bilateral hearing loss >20 db
        - Behavior or speech problem secondary to hearing loss
- Surgical: as above, and if medical therapy fails
    1. Assess each patient individually for required surgical procedure. For example:
        - Adenoidectomy ± tonsillectomy with myringotomy ± insertion of middle ear ventilation tubes have been frequently performed, but are of unclear benefit
        - Insertion of ventilation tube only
    2. Note that these procedures are not free of complications; e.g., tympanostomy tubes may → permanent structural damage to TM and *may* themselves induce cholesteatoma formation

TRAUMATIC PERFORATION OF TYMPANIC MEMBRANE (TM)

Management

- Notify or consult ENT service immediately! Emergency exploration and repair may be required.
- Water to be kept out of the ear

MASTOIDITIS

Management

- Consult ENT service
- If subperiosteal abscess formation—surgical drainage usually required
- If erythema behind ear and no radiographic evidence of coalescence, give cloxacillin 200 mg/kg/day and ampicillin 200 mg/kg/day IV, or cefuroxime
- Wide myringotomy necessary
- N.B. Chronic mastoiditis with chronic otorrhea may be demonstrated by mastoid air cell loss and coalescence on x-ray. Surgery may be necessary to stop otorrhea.

Suggested Reading

1. Bluestone CD. Otitis media in children: to treat or not to treat? N Engl J Med 1982; 306:1399–1404.
2. Eichenwald HE. Otitis media in the child. Hosp Pract 1985; 20:51–61.
3. Moore WR. Caustic ingestions, pathophysiology, diagnosis, and treatment. Clin Pediatr 1986; 25:192.
4. Nelson JD. Current therapy in pediatric infectious disease. Toronto: B.C. Decker, 1986.

24　PLASTIC SURGERY

ABRASIONS

Management

- Cleanse adjacent skin and infiltrate wound with 1% Xylocaine
- Scrub area to remove embedded dirt and prevent tattooing
- If wound is extensive or unable to remove dirt in emergency room, admit patient and scrub wound under general anesthesia
- Tetanus immunization (see p 310)

LACERATIONS

General Considerations

- Hand lacerations
    1. Examine and test flexor and extensor tendons, nerves, intrinsic muscles, joints, bones, vascular supply
    2. If any damage, or diagnosis in doubt, consult plastic surgery
    3. Glass puncture wounds—consult plastic surgery
- Facial lacerations
    1. Of free borders of mouth, nose, eyelids, ears—consult plastic surgery
    2. Involving eye—consult ophthalmology
    3. Use small bites or subcuticular suture to avoid stitch marks

Management

- Cleanse adjacent skin and infiltrate area with 1% Xylocaine (do not use epinephrine in appendages)

- Flush with normal saline only
- Close fascia and deep dermal layers with 4/0 or
  5/0 absorbable sutures (e.g., catgut or Dexon)
- Close mucosa with absorbable sutures
- Close skin using 5/0 or 6/0 nonabsorbable
  sutures (e.g., nylon or polyethylene)
  1. Use 6/0 to close skin on face
  2. Use small bites to avoid large stitch marks
- Tetanus immunization (see p 310)

Follow-Up

- Removal of skin sutures
  1. Face: 5 days
  2. Elsewhere: 7–10 days

NASAL AND FACIAL FRACTURES

Clinical Features and Management

- Examine for
  1. Contour deformity
  2. Pain on deep palpation or chewing
  3. Areas of anesthesia
  4. Crepitus, malocclusion
  5. Subconjunctival hemorrhage, eye movement,
     visual acuity
- Radiograph may be reported as negative. Check
  film. If in doubt, rely on clinical findings or
  suspicions.
- If there is a nasal septal or auricular
  hematoma—consult plastic surgery. It needs to
  be drained, STAT.

CLEFT LIP AND PALATE

Management

- Consult plastic surgery immediately
- Examine child carefully to rule out other mal-
  formations
- Parents need support
- Recognize that there may be feeding problems

Follow-Up

- Lip repair at 3 mo
- Palate repair at approximately 1 yr
- May need a revision of lip or nasal deformity at 5 yr

THERMAL BURNS

- See p 672 for management of smoke inhalation

General Considerations

- Prevent some burns by keeping home water at recommended setting between 49° C (120° F) and 54° C (130° F)
- Cold water immersion of burned area may be helpful within first hour after burning

TABLE 24–1 Duration of Exposure and Water Temperature Producing Third Degree Burns

Temperature		
°C	°F	Duration of Exposure
49	120	More than 5 min
52	125	1.5–2 min
54	130	30 sec
57	135	10 sec
60	140	5 sec
63	145	Less than 3 sec
66	150	1–2 sec
68	155	About 1 sec

TABLE 24–2 Severity of Burn

Degree	Level of Burn	Characteristics
First	Epidermis	Erythema, painful
Second		
Superficial	Superficial dermis	Blisters, painful
Deep	Deep dermis	Eschar, painful
Third	Subcutaneous tissue	Leathery eschar, painless

Clinical Features

- Take careful history of injury; note family setting
- Note degree, locale, and extent of burn
- Beware of child abuse

Management: Outpatient

- Record history of injury; describe burn
- Diagram burn area, noting degree (Fig. 24–1)
- Cool the part; eliminate the agent (copious irrigation with water if a chemical burn)
- Cleanse with saline (use sterile gloves)
- Leave intact blisters alone
- Debride broken blisters and loose debris
- Apply Polysporin and then Sofra-Tulle
- Dress with dry gauze and secure with Kling bandage
- Tetanus immunization (see p 310)
- Analgesics for pain relief if necessary
- Reevaluate in 3–5 days

TABLE 24–3 Criteria for Admission of Patients with Burns to the Hospital

Extent
  Under 2 yr – ≥ 6% of surface area (combination of 2nd and 3rd degree)
  Over 2 yr – ≥ 10% of surface area (combination of 2nd and 3rd degree)
Location: burns of face, neck, hands, feet, perineum
Type: chemical, electrical
Associated injuries: smoke, head injury, fractures, soft tissue trauma
Complicating medical problems: diabetes
Social situation: abuse, self-inflicted, psychologic

Management: Inpatient

- If flame burn and patient confined to smoke filled space
  1. Blood gases, carboxyhemoglobin level, chest x-ray

1st degree erythema ▥ 2nd degree ▤ 3rd degree
not to be included

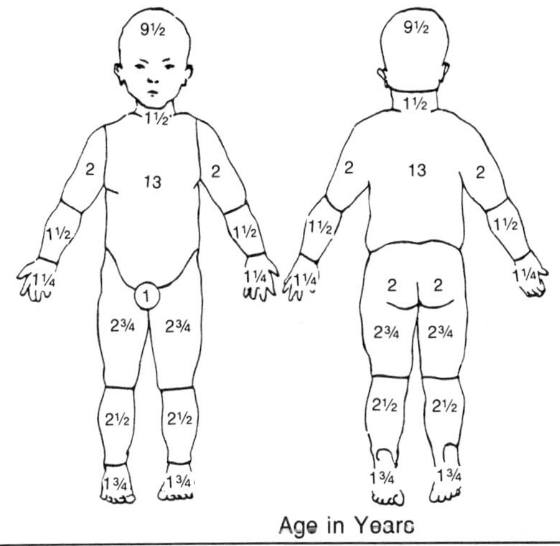

Age in Years

Area	0	1	5	10	15	Adult
Head area	19	17	13	11	9	7
Trunk area	26	26	26	26	26	26
Arm area	7	7	7	7	7	7
Thigh area	5½	6½	8½	8½	9½	9½
Leg area	5	5	5	6	6	7

Total 3rd degree burn_____
Total 2nd degree burn_____

TOTAL BURNS_____

Figure 24–1 Estimation of burn area.

    2. Put child in high FiO_2
    3. See page 672
- Resuscitation
    1. Start large bore IV in unburned area
    2. Take blood for CBC, BUN, electrolytes, protein, and albumin
    3. Insert urinary catheter
    4. Record hourly input and output

5. NPO, nasogastric tube in severe burns, cimetidine 20 mg/kg/day IV divided q6h
6. Give Ringer's lactate
   - 4 ml/kg/% burn over first 24 hr, giving half in first 8 hr post burn (not admission) and half in subsequent 16 hr post burn. Colloids (e.g., plasma) can be used as part of replacement fluid after first 8 hr.
7. In children under 2 yr, give additional maintenance fluid in form of ⅔–⅓ solution at 100 ml/kg evenly distributed over 24 hr
8. Above formula is only a guide and must be reassessed and adjusted according to hourly urine output (Table 24–4), general hydration state, hemoglobin, BUN, serum electrolytes

TABLE 24–4   Hourly Urine Output

Age	0–2 Mo	2–12 Mo	1–5 Yr	5–15 Yr
Optimum	15 ml	20 ml	25 ml	30 ml
Range	5–20 ml	10–30 ml	10–40 ml	15–60 ml

- Upon admission
  1. In depth burn history
  2. Evaluate burn for size (Fig. 24–1), location, and depth
  3. Cleanse in burn bath (lukewarm salt water: ~38° C or 100° F) and debride loose tissue and broken blisters; leave intact blisters alone
  4. Take swabs for culture and sensitivity from nose, throat, and burn
  5. Apply silver sulfadiazine cream to burn areas on body and Polysporin ointment to facial burns
  6. IV penicillin for 3 days is used by some of the consultants at HSC
  7. Tetanus immunization (see p 310)

   8. May require high environmental temperature, e.g., 28–30° C (82–86° F) or higher, to prevent heat loss

   9. Observe for hypothermia with large burns

- Circumferential burns
    1. Loss of capillary integrity leads to massive swelling with resuscitation
    2. Circumferential eschar constriction may compromise distal circulation
    3. Consider immediate escharotomy
- After 24 hours
    1. Adjust IV rate according to clinical status
    2. Continue albumin, plasma, or blood prn
    3. Observe carefully for sepsis
    4. Start feeds (e.g., milk by nasogastric tube) on second postburn day
    5. Beware of ileus

Suggested Reading

1. Demling RH. Burns. N Engl J Med 1985; 313:1389.
2. Grabb WC, Smith JW. Plastic surgery. 3rd ed. Boston: Little, Brown, 1979.
3. McGregor IA. Fundamental techniques of plastic surgery and their surgical applications. 7th ed. New York: Churchill Livingstone, 1980.
4. Wachtel TL, ed. Burns. Crit Care Clin 1985; 1(1), March.

GENERAL MANAGEMENT OF POISONING
Ingested Poison

Dilute Poison

- Dilute nondrug poison by giving water PO
- Do not use milk
- Do not attempt to neutralize poison

Gastric Decontamination

- Induce emesis
  1. Syrup of ipecac: causes vomiting in 80% of children within 15 min
     - Dose
       a. 9–12 mo—10 ml; no repeat
       b. 1–10 yr—15 ml; can repeat once after 20 min
       c. >10 yr—30 ml; can repeat once after 20 min
     - Contraindications
       a. Coma
       b. Convulsions
       c. Caustics
       d. Petroleum distillate hydrocarbons
  2. Gastric lavage
     - Indicated if ipecac is ineffective or patient is comatose
       a. Protect airway if patient is comatose
       b. Suction out stomach contents first
       c. Use large bore orogastric tube
     - Contraindications
       a. Coma—unless an endotracheal tube in place
       b. Caustics

c. Petroleum distillate hydrocarbons (unless containing another toxin, e.g., pesticides)

- Activated charcoal: adsorbs many poisons, making them unavailable for intake by the gut. Give as soon as possible after gastric emptying (patient may vomit after charcoal administration).
  1. Note: Do not give charcoal until ipecac-induced vomiting has subsided
  2. Dose: 1 g/kg; mix appropriate amount in 120–240 ml fluid and give PO or by naso-gastric tube
  3. Contraindications: caustics, hydrocarbons
- Cathartics: cause more rapid transit time, resulting in less absorption
  1. Major indications: delayed-release products, decreased GI motility
  2. Contraindications: caustics, hydrocarbons, diarrhea, abdominal trauma
  3. Dose
     - Sorbitol (70%) 1.5–2.0 ml/kg (maximum 150 ml)
     - Magnesium citrate (5%) 4.0 ml/kg (maximum 200 ml). Magnesium may be absorbed: caution in renal failure patients.

Unknown Poisoning

- Support vital functions
- Proceed as for ingested poison unless poisoning was by another route
- Save vomitus or lavage aliquots and blood and urine samples for toxicology analysis
- Identify symptom complex (if possible) so that specific diagnosis can be made—see Table 25–1

Injected Poison

- If treatment can be started within a few minutes after injection

1. Apply a *venous* tourniquet proximally
2. Do not release tourniquet until patient is in
   an intensive care setting (shock may occur)

Poison by Rectal Route

- Give enema

Inhaled Poison

- Move patient into uncontaminated air
- Maintain clear airway
- Give ventilatory support and oxygen if
  necessary

Poison in Contact with Skin or Eye

- Wash with copious amounts of water for 10–15
  min
- Do not use chemical neutralizers
- If eye contamination, contact ophthalmology
  service for further evaluation and treatment

Toxicology Tests

- Tests can be either qualitative or quantitative
- Substances for which it is reasonable to request
  STAT quantitative values
  1. Acetaminophen   6. Lithium
  2. Carboxyhemoglobin   7. Methanol
  3. Ethanol   8. Methemoglobin
  4. Ethylene glycol   9. Salicylate
  5. Iron   10. Theophylline
- Talk to lab or send clinical information along
  with samples of blood, urine, and gastric fluid
- Toxic screens are notoriously unreliable!
- Rule of thumb: treat the patient, not the level

SPECIFIC POISONS

Salicylate Intoxication

General Considerations

- Toxic dose of ASA: >150 mg/kg
- Note: Oil of wintergreen (methyl salicylate): 1 ml = 1.4 g ASA

Clinical Features

- Hyperventilation, vomiting, pyrexia, tinnitus, lethargy, confusion, dehydration (rare)
- More serious are convulsions, coma, pulmonary edema
- Other complications include hyperglycemia or hypoglycemia and prolonged prothrombin time (clinical bleeding is unusual)
- Chronically intoxicated patients generally are sicker than their serum salicylate level would indicate

Management

- Induce vomiting (p 570) if toxic or unknown dose has been ingested within 4 hr
- Give activated charcoal and a cathartic (p 571) once any lavage or ipecac-induced vomiting has stopped
- Blood for salicylate level (for interpretation of result see nomogram Fig. 25–1). N.B. nomogram *only* for *acute* ingestion
- If patient symptomatic: arterial blood gases, electrolytes, BUN, and blood glucose
  Note: All patients have a mixed acid-base disturbance (metabolic acidosis, respiratory alkalosis). However, infants and young children tend to be acidemic, whereas older children and adults tend to be alkalemic.

- Fluids: give fluids IV
  1. If patient is in shock: give plasma or albumin 10 ml/kg (see p 659)
  2. Parenteral fluid should be given at a rate sufficient to allow for daily maintenance (p 129), to replace the estimated deficit and to correct ongoing losses. Fluid diuresis is not necessary.
  3. Add 40 mmol KCl/L when patient has voided
- Correct metabolic acidosis (p 142)
- Alkalinize urine to pH 8
  1. Give sodium bicarbonate 1–2 mmol/kg over 1 hr and repeat as necessary over the next 8 hr to maintain urinary pH 7.5–8.0
     Note: to prevent paradoxical aciduria, it is essential to give adequate KCl also
     - Alkalinization of urine indicated if
       a. Marked decrease in plasma HCO_3 (respiratory alkalosis is not a contraindication to bicarbonate use)
       b. High serum salicylate level: Done nomogram in toxic range (Fig. 25–1)
       c. Note: Do *not* give sodium bicarbonate if arterial pH >7.5
- Hemodialysis
  1. Renal failure
  2. Aspiration pneumonia or pulmonary edema
  3. Salicylate level >7 mmol/L (100 mg/dl)
  4. Rising or steady salicylate level
  5. Refractory acid-base imbalance
  6. Persistent CNS manifestations

Acetaminophen (Paracetamol) Poisoning

General Considerations

- Toxic dose >150 mg/kg

Clinical Features

- From 2–24 hr after ingestion: nausea, vomiting,

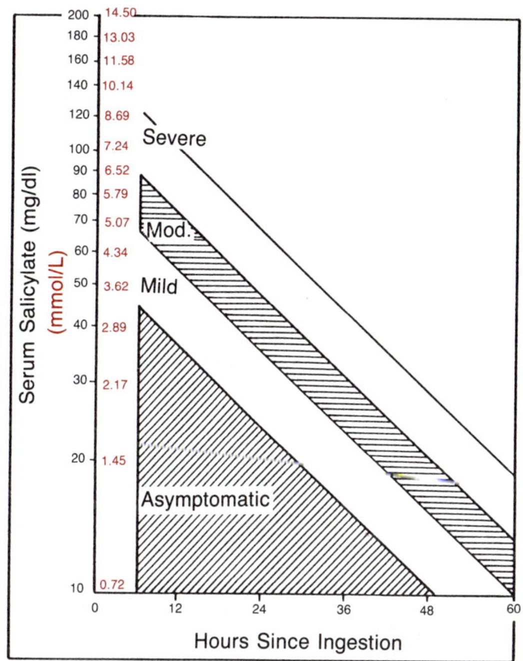

Figure 25–1 Done nomogram for salicylate poisoning. (Adapted from Done AK. Salicylate intoxication. Pediatrics 1960; 26:805).

anorexia, pallor, lethargy. No changes in level of consciousness occur at this stage.

- As initial symptoms decrease, hepatic necrosis develops. Liver becomes enlarged and tender. Liver enzyme levels begin to rise.
- Days 3–6: jaundice, coagulation defects, hypoglycemia, encephalopathy, renal failure

Management

- Induce vomiting using ipecac syrup if patient is

alert
- Activated charcoal not recommended if oral n-acetylcysteine may be used
- N-acetylcysteine
  1. Initiate treatment within 10 hr if possible. Treatment *may* be beneficial if initiated as late as 24 hr following ingestion.
  2. Indications: an acetaminophen plasma level in hepatotoxic range (See Fig. 25–2). If level not available, start treatment if ingested dose is >150 mg/kg
  3. Loading dose = 140 mg/kg PO diluted in 3 volumes of soft drink
  4. Follow with 70 mg/kg q4h PO for 17 doses
  5. If vomiting occurs within an hour after administration, repeat the dose
  6. IV dosing regimen is available; contact poison center for details

Petroleum Distillate Hydrocarbons (PDHs)

General Considerations

- Gasoline, kerosene, charcoal lighter fluid, naphthas, mineral seal oils (furniture polish), and benzine (not benzene)
- PDHs are NOT significantly absorbed through the GI tract. Systemic or pulmonary disease occurs ONLY as a result of aspiration.

Management of Ingestion

- Do NOT induce vomiting or perform gastric lavage (unless hydrocarbon contains another toxin, such as pesticide, in potentially toxic amounts)
- Do NOT give activated charcoal
- Do NOT give oils or cathartics
- Do observe for 2 hr; if no respiratory symptoms, send home

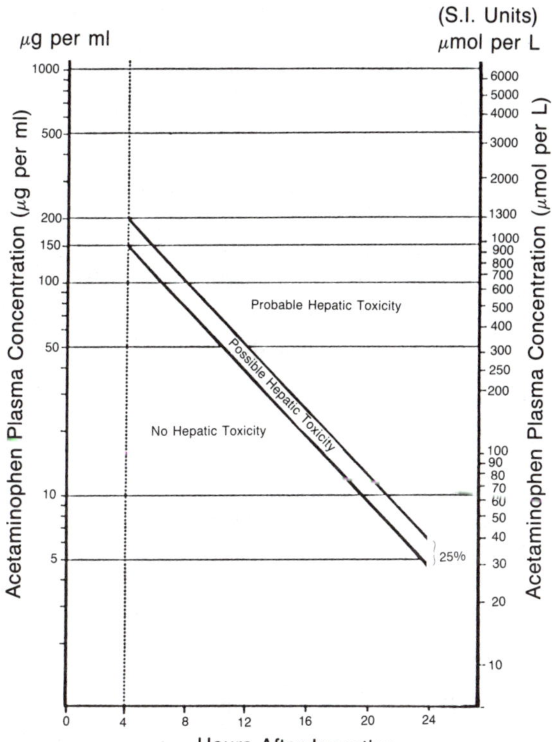

Figure 25–2 Semilogarithmic plot of plasma acetaminophen levels vs time. (Originally adapted from Rumack BH, Matthew H. Acetaminophen poisoning and toxicity. Pediatrics 1975; 55:871–876. The adapted form presented here is used with the permission of Micromedex, Inc., Englewood, CO).

Management of Aspiration

- For patients who are not severely ill but who do have coughing, choking, gagging, or vomiting

1. Take history and do physical examination
2. Observe for 6 hr (repeat respiratory rate and chest examination periodically)
3. Do chest x-ray at end of 6 hr
4. If BOTH exam AND x-ray are normal, send patient home
5. If EITHER exam OR x-ray is abnormal, admit patient for further observation and treatment
6. Symptomatic and supportive care
7. NO prophylactic antibiotics or corticosteroids

Nonpetroleum Distillate Hydrocarbons

General Considerations and Management

- Turpentine, xylene, benzene (not benzine), and toluene are the only four nonpetroleum distillate hydrocarbons
- There is significant GI absorption
- If >1 ml/kg is ingested, it should be removed from stomach using ipecac or lavage (see p 570)
- Treat potential aspiration as for petroleum distillates (p 577)

Barbiturates and Anticonvulsants

Clinical Features

- Drowsiness, ataxia, slurred speech, and nystagmus may occur
- Respiratory depression, hypothermia, aspiration pneumonia, bullous skin lesions, and hypotension may occur in severe cases

Management

- In a conscious patient, induce vomiting with ipecac (see p 570) and follow with activated charcoal and a cathartic
- In a comatose patient, do gastric lavage (with

an endotracheal tube in place)
- Support respiration and circulation
- Alkaline diuresis (see p 574) only for
  phenobarbital intoxication (not effective for
  other barbiturates or anticonvulsants)

Phenothiazines

Clinical Features and Management

- As for barbiturates
- Extrapyramidal reaction: give diphenhydramine
  1–2 mg/kg/dose (maximum 50 mg/dose) IV, IM,
  or PO
- Cardiac arrhythmias: try lidocaine or phenytoin
  (see p 58)

Tricyclic Antidepressants
(e.g., Imipramine, Amitriptyline)

Clinical Features

- Cause central and peripheral anticholinergic
  effects within 6 hr after ingestion
- Anticholinergic effects: fever, mydriasis,
  urinary retention, decreased bowel activity,
  flushed skin
- CNS effects: excitation, muscle twitching, hyperreflexia, delirium, hallucinations, confusion,
  convulsions, and coma
- Cardiovascular effects: tachycardia, conduction
  defects, extrasystoles, and ventricular
  arrhythmia

Management

- Maintain respiration
- IV fluids to maintain adequate blood pressure
- Empty stomach (ipecac or gastric lavage) and
  follow with activated charcoal and a cathartic
  (see p 570)
- Do limb-lead ECG hourly until 6 hr after

ingestion
1. If maximal QRS >0.10 sec = risk of convulsions
2. If maximal QRS >0.16 sec = risk of arrhythmias
- Control seizures with either diazepam or phenytoin (see p 469)
- Cardiac arrhythmia
  1. Try sodium bicarbonate 1–2 mmol/kg IV bolus (may repeat once)
  2. Arrhythmias refractory to sodium bicarbonate: try lidocaine or phenytoin (see p 58)
  3. Cardiac monitor until patient free of arrhythmias for 24 hr

Ethanol

General Considerations

- In small children (<6 yr), 1 ml/kg of absolute ethanol produces a blood concentration of approximately 22 mmol/L (100 mg/dl) 2 hr after ingestion
- Hypoglycemia may result; generally develops within 6 hr after ingestion

Management

- Ipecac within 1–1½ hr after ingestion. If patient is obtunded, significant absorption has occurred and gastric lavage will be nonproductive
- Monitor blood glucose levels
- Avoid CNS-respiratory depressant drugs
- Consider dialysis if ethanol level >110 mmol/L (500 mg/dl)

Iron

General Considerations

- Toxicity is based on the amount of elemental iron ingested

1. Ferrous fumarate = 33% elemental iron
2. Ferrous gluconate = 12% elemental iron
3. Ferrous sulfate = 20% elemental iron

- Toxic dose (elemental iron) >50 mg/kg

Clinical Features

- Early phase (½–6 hr after ingestion): vomiting, bloody diarrhea, lethargy, hypotonia, hypotension, shock, leukocytosis, and hyperglycemia
- Delayed phase (6–48 hr): patient may appear to improve, but in very ill patients this phase may not be evident. Acidosis, hypoglycemia, shock, hepatic failure, pulmonary edema, and coma may occur.

Management

- CBC, electrolytes, blood glucose, and gases
- Serum iron level (STAT)
- Test stool and gastric contents for blood
- Deferoxamine challenge test (useful if serum iron is not available)
  1. An indirect test that detects presence of free circulating iron. Give deferoxamine 25–50 mg/kg (maximum 1 g) IM. If the iron level exceeds the iron binding capacity, the unbound iron is chelated by deferoxamine and excreted in the urine, producing a "vin rose" color.
  2. Note: A serum iron >53μmol/L (300 μg/dl) or a positive deferoxamine test is suggestive of serious poisoning and an indication for deferoxamine therapy
- If a potentially toxic dose has been ingested, use ipecac or gastric lavage. An x-ray examination of abdomen can be used to determine success of gastric emptying.
- Instill 1–2 mmol/kg of 8.4% sodium bicarbonate solution into the stomach. Ferrous carbonate salt results, which is poorly absorbed and less irritating.

- Activated charcoal is ineffective but a cathartic can be used
- Correct electrolyte imbalance and dehydration with appropriate IV fluids. Correct shock with blood products.
- Monitor renal function closely (urine output)
- Deferoxamine: use is determined by serum iron level done within 4–6 hr
  1. <53 μmol/L (<300 μg/dl)—will recover with above supportive measures
  2. 53–90 μmol/L (300–500 μg/dl)—will need brief chelation therapy
  3. >90 μmol/L (>500 μg/dl)—vigorous chelation therapy
  4. Deferoxamine initiated at a continuous IV infusion rate not to exceed 15 mg/kg/hr. Therapeutic regimen is complex; contact poison center for details.
- Hemodialysis or exchange transfusion in patients with serum iron >180 μmol/L (>1,000 μg/dl) or if anuria develops

Theophylline

Clinical Features

- The risk and potential seriousness of theophylline toxicity are directly related to the serum concentration. Patients who are chronically overmedicated may develop severe toxicity with serum levels lower than those causing problems in an acute intoxication.
- GI symptoms: nausea, vomiting, hematemesis
- CNS symptoms: restlessness, irritability, convulsions
- Cardiovascular effects: arrhythmias
- Fever (hypermetabolism)

Management

- Ipecac or gastric lavage (p 570) up to 2 hr following ingestion

- Follow with activated charcoal and a cathartic
  1. N.B. Charcoal in half-doses should be repeated q4h if theophylline levels in toxic range
- Monitor serum theophylline concentrations
- Treat seizures aggressively: use diazepam and barbiturates, not phenytoin
- Treat arrhythmias if they arise
- Hemoperfusion is indicated if
  1. Severe toxicity >440 μmol/L (>80 mg/L) in children. Note: Consider hemoperfusion at lower theophylline levels in situations associated with reduced theophylline clearance (neonates, premature infants, hepatic disease, cardiac failure) or chronic toxicity.
  2. Refractory arrhythmias or convulsions

Alkaline Corrosives

General Considerations and Clinical Features

- Common in drain and oven cleaners
- Esophageal burns can be present without mouth burns
- Presence of two or more symptoms and signs (e.g., dysphagia, oral burns) correlates with esophageal burns

Management

- Emesis and gastric lavage CONTRAINDICATED
- Eye contact: wash eyes thoroughly with water
- Skin contact: wash with running water
- The benefits of prophylactic corticosteroids are questionable
- Contact ENT service if patient symptomatic

Insecticides (Organophosphate Type: e.g., Malathion, Diazinon)

Clinical Features

- Cholinergic signs: vomiting, diarrhea, sweating, salivation, and increased bronchial secretions

- Nicotinic signs: weakness, muscle fasciculations, coma, convulsions, and respiratory insufficiency

Management

- Emesis or lavage if ingested; follow with activated charcoal (see p 570)
- If skin contamination, remove clothes and wash skin with soap and water
- Respiratory problems: treat with suction and assisted ventilation
- If increased bronchial secretions: atropine sulfate, 0.05 mg/kg IV, maximum single dose = 2.0 mg. (N.B. Atropine dose is larger than that used for routine anesthesia.) Repeat every 5 min until secretions dry.
- If respiratory insufficiency, treat supportively and notify poison center
  1. Pralidoxime chloride 25–50 mg/kg up to 2 g IV slowly; repeat in 1 hr if no improvement in muscle activity

Narcotics

General Considerations and Clinical Features

- Heroin, morphine, pethidine-meperidine, methadone, diphenoxylate, propoxyphene, codeine, etc.
- Pinpoint pupils, respiratory depression, coma
- Cyanosis, bradycardia, hypotension

Management

- Maintain ventilation and circulation
- Give naloxone 0.03 mg/kg IV. If no response (and diagnosis is certain), give naloxone 0.1 mg/kg IV. Doses may be repeated as needed to maintain reversal of narcotic signs. Contact poison center or anesthesia department for continuous infusion of naloxone.

SNAKE BITES

General Considerations

- Rattlesnakes are the only poisonous snakes in Canada and one of several in the United States
- Proper identification of snake is important
- Bites are more serious in children than in adults
- The majority of bites are *not* serious!

Clinical Features

- Fang marks
- Local pain (or numbness) and edema are earliest signs and develop within 4 hr after bite
- Local bleeding, ecchymosis
- Lymphangitis
- Severe pain and swelling indicate serious envenomation
- Paresthesias, diaphoresis
- Nausea, vomiting
- Bleeding diathesis, hemolysis, disseminated intravascular coagulation (DIC)
- Arrhythmias
- Renal failure, convulsions

Management

- First aid
  1. Suction (without cutting) over the fang marks within 30 min after bite
  2. Immobilize extremity
  3. Loose superficial venous-lymphatic tourniquet
  4. Transport to hospital
- Wound therapy
  1. Clean and dress wound
  2. Tetanus prophylaxis (see p 310)
  3. Observe for gram negative infection
- Systemic therapy (for severe pain or swelling or systemic symptoms)
  1. Measure and record bite area
  2. IV line

3. CBC, platelets, type and crossmatch
4. PT, PTT, fibrinogen level
5. Electrolytes, Ca, BUN, creatinine, glucose, albumin levels
6. Urinalysis, ECG
7. Antivenin: polyvalent crotalidae antivenin is available; contact poison center for management advice

TABLE 25–1   Common Signs and Causes of Poisoning

System	Sign	Causes
Cardiovascular	Bradycardia	Digitalis compounds
		Beta-blocking agents
	Tachycardia	Sympathomimetics
		Anticholinergic agents
		Theophylline
	Hypertension	Sympathomimetics
		Phencyclidine
	Hypotension	Hypnotic-sedatives
		Narcotic analgesics
	Arrhythmias	Theophylline
		Digitalis compounds
		Tricyclic antidepressants
Respiratory	Bradypnea	Narcotics
		Ethanol
		Hypnotic-sedatives
	Tachypnea	Salicylates
		Carbon monoxide
		Methanol
Temperature	Hyperthermia	Salicylates
		Anticholinergic agents
		Theophylline
	Hypothermia	Ethanol
		Phenothiazines
Neurologic	Ataxia	Ethanol
		Barbiturates
		Phenytoin
	Miosis	Narcotics
		Barbiturates
		Phenothiazines
		Clonidine
		Benzodiazepines
	Mydriasis	Sympathomimetics
		Anticholinergic agents

TABLE 25–1 Common Signs and Causes of Poisoning *(Continued)*

System	Sign	Causes
	Nystagmus	Phenytoin
	Convulsions	Sympathomimetics
		Anticholinergic agents
		Camphorated oil
		Lindane (γ-benzene hexachloride)
		Strychnine
		Theophylline
	Coma	CNS depressants
		Anticholinergic agents
		Narcotics
		Asphyxiant gases
		Salicylates
	Psychosis	Anticholinergic agents
		Sympathomimetics
		Hallucinogens
		Salicylates
Oral cavity	Dryness	Sympathomimetics
		Anticholinergic agents
		Narcotics
	Acetone smell	Acetone
		Methanol
		Isopropyl alcohol
		Phenol
		Salicylates
	Alcohol smell	Ethanol
	Almond smell	Cyanide
	Garlic smell	Arsenic
		Phosphorus
		Organophosphate insecticides
		Thallium
	Wintergreen smell	Methylsalicylate
	Petroleum smell	Hydrocarbons
Skin	Cyanosis	Methemoglobinemia
Gastrointestinal	Emesis, hematemesis	Iron
		Arsenic
		Colchicine
		Salicylates
		Theophylline

SPIDERS

Black Widow

- Mild–moderate pain on envenomation
- Muscle spasms within 2 hr
- May cause abdominal pain and rigidity
- Symptomatic supportive care
- Tetanus prophylaxis (see p 310)
- Antivenin is available; contact poison center for management advice

Brown Recluse

- May be no pain on envenomation
- Local vesicles may progress to ulcerations
- Hematologic, cardiovascular, and renal effects may occur
- No antivenin is available
- Many treatment regimens have been proposed, some of which need to be started early after bite; contact poison center for recommendations

Suggested Reading

1. Blumer JL, Reed MD. Pediatric toxicology. Pediatr Clin North Am 1986; 33:245–450.
2. Goldfrank LR, et al. Toxicologic emergencies: a handbook in problem solving. 3rd ed. Norwalk: Appleton-Century-Crofts, 1986.
3. Haddad LM, Winchester JF. Clinical management of poisoning and drug overdose. Philadelphia: W.B. Saunders, 1983.

26 RESPIROLOGY

NORMAL ANATOMY OF LUNGS

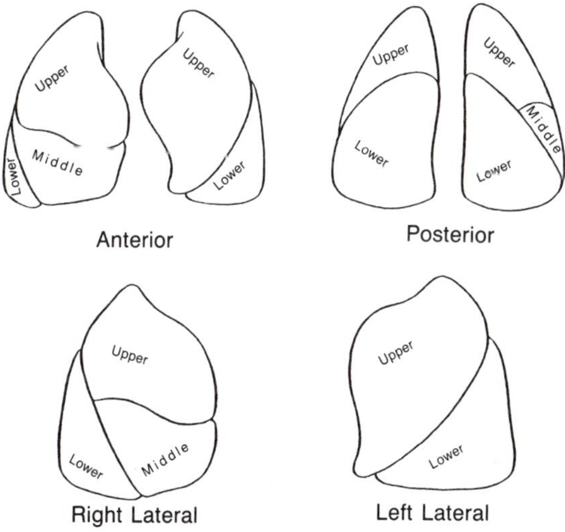

Figure 26–1 Division of lungs into lobes. Minor variations in fissures may occur, producing somewhat different lobar proportions, incompletely separated lobes, or supernumerary lobes. These patterns are the most common, however. (From Kendig EL, Chernick V. Disorders of the respiratory tract in children. 14th ed. Philadelphia: W.B. Saunders, 1983:73.)

BACKGROUND PHYSIOLOGY

The Alveolar Gas Equation

- Alveolar oxygenation can be estimated as follows:

$$P_AO_2 = P_IO_2 - \frac{PaCO_2}{R}$$

  where A=alveolar; a=arterial; P=pressure; P_IO_2=partial pressure of O_2 in inspired air; R=respiratory exchange quotient= 0.8. For example, in room air at sea level:

$$P_AO_2 = \% \text{ inspired } O_2 \text{ (as fraction)} \times \text{(P barometric} - \text{vapor pressure mm Hg)} - \frac{PaCO_2}{R}$$

$$= \frac{21}{100} \times (760 - 47) - \frac{40}{0.8}$$

$$= 150 - \frac{40}{0.8} = 100 \text{ mm Hg}$$

  A − a gradient ($P_AO_2 - PaO_2$) should be ≤ 16 mm Hg
- If patient hypoxemic and retaining CO_2, relative contribution of hypoventilation versus impaired gas exchange can be determined knowing A − a gradient
- If A − a gradient normal, may correct hypoxemia by ensuring adequate ventilation
- A − a gradient increased in all causes of hypoxemia except hypoventilation

Causes of Hypoxemia

- Ventilation/perfusion ($\dot{V}/\dot{Q}$) mismatch
- Right to left shunt
- Hypoventilation
- Impedance to gas diffusion

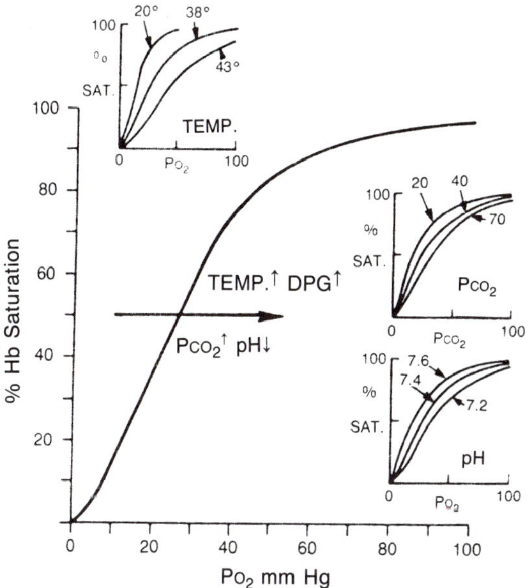

Figure 26–2 Oxyhemoglobin dissociation curve. Shift of the oxygen dissociation curve by pH, PCO₂, and temperature. As curve shifts to the right, oxygen unloading to tissues is enhanced. (Modified from West JB. Respiratory physiology: the essentials. 2nd ed. Baltimore: Williams & Wilkins, 1979:73.)

Review of Blood Gas Analysis

- Obtain sample by arterial puncture (see p 716) or arterialized capillary blood sampling
- Interpret results with clinical setting in mind
- Inspired O_2 concentration must be known
- For interpretation of acid-base abnormalities see p 141

PULMONARY FUNCTION TESTING

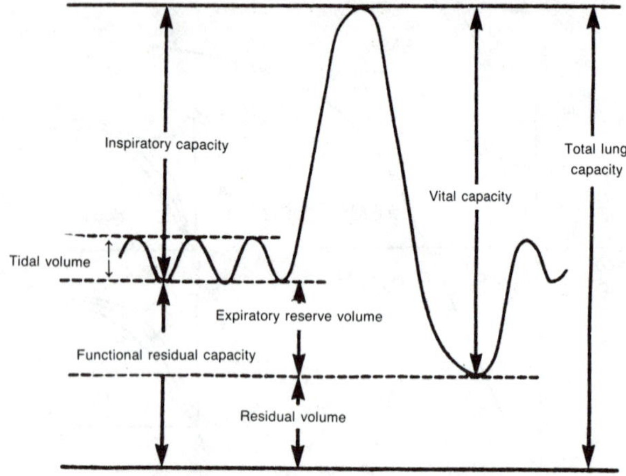

Figure 26–3   Lung volume subdivisions.

Patterns of PFTs Observed

- See Table 26–1 for normal values of FVC, FEV$_1$, and PEFR

Obstructive

- Forced vital capacity (FVC) normal or decreased
- Forced expiratory volume in 1 sec (FEV$_1$) decreased
- Forced expiratory flow at 75 to 25% lung volume (FEF 25–75) decreased
- Ratio of FEV$_1$/FVC <80% (normal: >80%)
- Total lung capacity (TLC) normal or increased
- Functional residual capacity (FRC) normal or increased
- Residual volume (RV) normal or increased
- RV/TLC normal or increased (normal is 20%)

Restrictive

- FVC decreased
- FEV_1 decreased
- $FEV_1/FVC \geq 80\%$
- TLC decreased
- RV normal or decreased (RV may be slightly increased in some neuromuscular disorders.)
- FRC normal or decreased

UPPER AIRWAY OBSTRUCTION

Respiratory Distress (see p 668)

Choking (see p 655)

Epiglottitis (see p 595)

General Considerations

- Various clinical situations can result from upper airway obstruction, ranging from mild respiratory distress with stridor to acute complete airway obstruction requiring urgent emergency care. The upper respiratory tract includes the airway from the nares and mouth to the carina.

Clinical Features

- Inspiratory phase of respiration prolonged
- Subcostal, suprasternal, and supraclavicular retractions
- Increased respiratory rate
- Stridor
- Barking cough is suggestive of subglottic or tracheal obstruction

Management

- Depends on etiology of obstruction (N.B. Epiglottitis: see below.)

TABLE 26–1   Normal Values for Peak Flow, FVC, and FEV_1*

Height (cm)	Male			Female		
	FVC(L)[†]	FEV_1(L)[†]	PEFR(L/min)[†]	FVC(L)	FEV_1(L)	PEFR(L/min)
110				1.146	0.976	145
115	1.311	1.134	160	1.268	1.078	157
120	1.452	1.250	175	1.403	1.191	170
125	1.609	1.378	191	1.552	1.316	184
130	1.782	1.519	208	1.718	1.454	199
135	1.975	1.674	226	1.901	1.606	216
140	2.188	1.845	247	2.104	1.774	234
145	2.424	2.034	269	2.328	1.960	253
150	2.685	2.241	293	2.576	2.165	274
155	2.975	2.470	319	2.851	2.392	296
160	3.296	2.723	348	3.155	2.642	321
165	3.652	3.001	379	3.491	2.919	347
170	4.046	3.308	414	3.864	3.225	376
175	4.482	3.645	451	4.276	3.562	407
180	4.966	4.018	491	4.732	3.936	441
185	5.502	4.428	536	5.236	4.348	477
190	6.095	4.881	584	5.794	4.803	517

* Values obtained with Roxon portable battery-operated turbine spirometer at the Hospital for Sick Children.
† FVC, forced vital capacity.
FEV$_1$, forced expiratory volume in 1 sec.
PEFR, peak expiratory flow rate.

- Investigations may include AP and lateral soft tissue x-ray views of neck and chest. Obtaining radiologic investigations should NEVER delay the establishment of an artificial airway in severe airway obstruction, and should be performed ONLY if the highest level of supervision in the radiology suite is available.
- Barium swallow useful in detecting vascular compression
- Laryngoscopy and bronchoscopy very helpful
- CT scan occasionally needed

Epiglottitis

Clinical Features and Differential Diagnosis

- See Table 26–2

Management

- Truly a pediatric emergency: must be diagnosed and treated promptly if survival is to be assured
- Diagnose on clinical gounds—"the four Ds," i.e., dysphagia, dysphonia, drooling, and distress
- DO NOT OBTAIN X-RAYS OR BLOOD WORK (child may deteriorate while procedures are being done)
- DO NOT TRY TO EXAMINE THROAT OR LOOK FOR EPIGLOTTIS
- DO NOT AGITATE CHILD. Keep NPO.
- CALL ENT AND ANESTHESIA PERSONNEL STAT—intubation done in OR; tracheotomy rarely necessary today
- Once child is intubated: IV fluids and antibiotics appropriate for coverage against *H. influenzae* (ampicillin and chloramphenicol together or cefuroxime by itself)
- Give IV antibiotics until over acute phase; then continue with oral antibiotics for 7 to 10 days total coverage
- Rifampin prophylaxis recommended for patients and family (see p 300)
- Other *H. influenzae* infections may coexist, e.g.,

TABLE 26–2 Epiglottitis and Croup

Factor	Epiglottitis	Croup	Bacterial Tracheitis
Age	Usually older (2–6 yr)	Usually younger (6 mo–4 yr)	Any age
Sex	M = F	M > F	M = F
Agents	Bacterial: *H. influenzae* type b(+ + +), β-hemolytic strep (+)	Viral: parainfluenza 1(+ + +), RSV, parainfluenza 2,3 (+), influenza	Bacterial: *S. aureus*, pneumococcus, *H. influenzae*
Seasons	Year round	Late spring, late fall	Any time
Recurrence	Rare	Fairly common	Rare
Clinical	Toxic	Nontoxic	Toxic
	Severe airway obstruction		Croup-like cough
	Drooling, sitting	Not drooling	
	Stridor	Stridor common	Stridor
	Sternal recession	Sternal recession common	
Progression	Rapid	Usually slow	Moderately rapid

septic arthritis and meningitis, and should be
considered

Croup (Acute Laryngotracheobronchitis)

Clinical Features

- See Table 26-2
- History of barking cough, hoarseness and
  coryza
- Child may be distressed, restless, and cyanotic
- Differential diagnosis includes epiglottitis,
  bacterial tracheitis, foreign body aspiration, and
  diphtheria

Management

- Avoid agitation as much as possible; parent at
  bedside reduces anxiety
- Mild croup may be managed at home with PO
  fluids and humidity
- Warn parents that croup may be worse at night.
  May clear in cold air outside.
- Stridor at rest, moderate chest wall retractions,
  decreased air entry, and an anxious restless
  child are all indicators of moderate to severe
  disease and signal the need for hospitalization
- A rising respiratory rate correlates well with a
  falling PaO_2. Hypercapnia occurs late in upper
  airway obstruction and is a sign of increasing
  respiratory failure.
- If concerned about degree of respiratory failure,
  arterial blood gases are indicated to measure
  hypoxemia, hypercapnia, and acid-base status
- Nurse in O_2 (30–40%) and humidity (croupette)
- Racemic epinephrine 0.5 ml of 2.25% solution
  in 3 ml normal saline by mask may provide
  relief. Effect may last 30–60 min. May repeat
  q1–2h if necessary. A child who has received
  racemic epinephrine must be admitted for
  observation.

- If not responding to racemic epinephrine, should be observed in ICU setting and may require intubation
- Use of steroids in severe croup is controversial

Foreign Body Aspiration

General Considerations

- Aspiration of a foreign body may present as acute upper or lower airway obstruction or as a chronic respiratory problem
- Esophageal foreign body may also cause respiratory distress

Clinical Features

- Most important to take careful history for possible aspiration, e.g., history of choking while eating peanuts
- Often a history of wheezing, stridor, cough, and recurrent pneumonias
- Physical examination may reveal tachypnea, cough, wheeze, stridor, mediastinal shift, and evidence of hyperinflation

Differential Diagnosis

- If onset of symptoms is not acute, diagnosis is more difficult
- Infectious causes of upper and lower respiratory tract obstruction, such as croup, epiglottitis, bronchiolitis, and pneumonia, may need to be considered
- Asthma should be considered if cough and wheeze are the features of presentation

Management

- For treatment of choking person see p 655
- *If* the patient is *stable,* obtain inspiratory and expiratory films (useful to determine whether

there is unilateral air trapping)
- Make sure x-ray shows region from mouth
  to below diaphragm
- Opaque foreign bodies or a lucent outline of
  nonradiopaque foreign bodies may be visible
- Look for hyperinflation with contralateral mediastinal shift, paradoxical diaphragmatic movement on sequential films or fluoroscopy
- Esophageal foreign body such as a coin is seen
  head on in PA view as opposed to a tracheal
  foreign body, which is seen head on in lateral
  view
- Appropriate method of further investigation and
  treatment is bronchoscopy

LOWER AIRWAY DISEASE

Bronchiolitis

General Considerations

- Common age less than 1 yr with peak less than
  6 mo
- Etiology usually RSV, but can be any respiratory
  virus

Clinical Features

- Prodromal signs include upper respiratory tract
  infection ± fever, poor feeding, and irritability
- Physical signs include fever, dehydration,
  wheezing, dyspnea, tachypnea (rate 50 to
  80/min), intercostal indrawing with use of accessory muscles, and tachycardia. Rhonchi ±
  diffuse crepitations on auscultation.
- May see hyperinflation with increased AP
  diameter and hyperresonance

Differential Diagnosis

- May be hard to differentiate from asthma
- Pneumonia and aspiration should be considered

Management

- Chest x-ray PA and lateral. (Usually have hyperinflation, ↑ linear markings, and areas of atelectasis.)
- Arterial blood gases (hypoxemia initially, then hypoxemia and hypercapnia in more severe cases)
- Nasal swab for rapid detection of RSV antigen (e.g., fluorescent antibody technique)
- Humidified O_2 (30–40%) appropriate
- Ensure adequate hydration (IV if oral intake poor and dehydration present)
- Salbutamol (0.5% solution) 0.01 to 0.03 ml/kg in 3 ml normal saline by inhalation is worth a trial
- Intubation and ventilation are rarely required
- Ribavirin guidelines
  1. Ribavirin is an antiviral drug recently approved in aerosolized form for therapy of hospitalized children with RSV infection. It is recommended for the treatment of children with severe RSV infections. The severity of infection should be assessed clinically (apnea, severe retractions, tachycardia or bradycardia, tachypnea, cyanosis) and by arterial blood gases (falling PaO_2, rising $PaCO_2$).
  2. Infants with congenital heart disease, BPD, chronic lung disease, or who are immuno-suppressed, immunodeficient, or less than 8 wk old are at increased risk for severe RSV infection and should be considered for Ribavirin therapy.
  3. Therapy requires special small particle aerosol generator (SPAG–2) and will most likely be used in an ICU setting

Follow-Up

- Mortality <1%. Thirty percent of patients may have subsequent recurrent wheezing episodes. Recurrent wheeze likely due to asthma.

Pneumonia

General Considerations

- Annual attack rates for pneumonia in preschool-
  ers average 40 per thousand and gradually drop
  to 9 per thousand in the adolescent years
- Incidence greatest in first year of life
- Overall, viruses are the most common etiologic
  agents (see Tables 26–3, 26–4)

Clinical Features

- See Tables 26–5, 26–6

Management

- Investigation
  1. CBC, differential count
  2. Blood culture
  3. Sputum culture (nasopharyngeal cultures are
     not representative of pneumonia's etiology)
  4. Arterial blood gases if patient in respira-
     tory distress
  5. Chest x-ray PA and lateral
  6. Tuberculin skin test
  7. Cold agglutinin titer
  8. Diagnostic thoracentesis if significant pleural
     fluid is present
- Treatment

  1. General supportive care needed including
     IV or PO fluids
  2. O_2 30 to 40% by mask
  3. IV or PO antibiotics appropriate for most
     likely etiologic organism or organism
     cultured (Table 26–7)
  4. Hospital admission based on clinical status
     of patient
  5. Empyema requires chest tube drainage
  6. In compromised patients may use ceftazidime
     alone or tobramycin plus ticarcillin/
     piperacillin. In addition, consider anaerobic

TABLE 26–3 Relative Causes of Acute Lower Respiratory Infection in Normal Children According to Age

	<2 wk	2 wk–3mo	4 mo–5 yr	6–18 yr
Bacteria	+ + + +	+ +	+ +	+
Virus	+ +	+ + + +	+ + + +	+ +
Mycoplasma	– –	– –	+	+ + + +
Chlamydia	– –	+ + +	– –	– –
Pneumocystis, tuberculosis, and fungus are rare causes of pneumonia at any age.				

Modified from Long SS. Treatment of acute pneumonia in infants and children. Pediatr Clin North Am 1983; 30:298.

TABLE 26–4   Epidemiology of Viral and Mycoplasma Pneumonias

Agent	Season	Age (Yr)		
		<1	1–5	>6
RSV	Winter to early spring	+ + + +	+	– –
Parainfluenza virus, type 3	Fall to spring	+	+ + +	+ +
Parainfluenza virus, type 1	Fall to spring	+	+ +	+ + +
Mycoplasma	Year-round	– –	+ +	+ + + +
Influenza	Fall and winter	+ +	+ + +	+ +

Modified from Nussbaum E, Galant S. Pediatric respiratory disorders: clinical approaches. Orlando: Grune & Stratton, 1984:138.

TABLE 26–5 Etiologic Agents for Acute Bacterial Pneumonia According to Age and Syndrome

Agents	Uncomplicated Pneumonia			Complicated Pneumonia		Hospital Associated Pneumonia
	<3 mo	3 mo–5 yr	5–19 yr	Pleural Fluid	Lung Abscess	
S. pneumoniae	+ + +	+ + + +	+ + + +	+ +	+	+ +
H. influenzae	+	+ + +	+	+ + +	+	+
Group A strep.	–	+	+	+ +	–	–
Mouth flora	–	–	–	+ + +	+ + + +	+ + +
S. aureus	+ +	+	+	+ +	+ +	+ +
Group B & D strep.	+ + +	–	–	–	–	–
Enteric bacilli	+ + +	–	–	+	+ +	+ +
Tuberculosis	–	±	±	+	+	–

Modified from Long SS. Treatment of acute pneumonia in infants and children. Pediatr Clin North Am 1983; 30:304.

TABLE 26–6 Epidemiologic, Clinical, and Laboratory Features of Acute Pneumonia in Normal Infants and Children According to Etiologic Agents

	Bacteria	*Virus*	*Mycoplasma*
History and Physical			
Temperature	Majority $\geq$39° C	Majority <39°C	Majority <38° C
Onset	Abrupt, may follow URI	Gradually worsening URI	Gradually worsening cough
Others in home ill	Infrequent	Frequent. concurrent	Frequent, weeks apart
Associated signs, symptoms	Respiratory distress common; meningitis and septic arthritis occasionally coexist; pleuritic chest pain common	Frequent—myalgia, rash, conjunctivitis, pharyngitis, mouth ulcers, diarrhea	Frequent—headache, sore throat, myalgia; Occasional—rash, conjunctivitis, myringitis, enanthem; Hacking paroxysmal cough—sometimes productive
Toxicity	+ + +	+	+
Laboratory Findings			
X-ray	Usually infiltrate in distribution of lobe or subsegment of lobe	Interstitial pattern—may be diffuse	May be lobar or diffuse
Pleural fluid	May occur; may be large	Infrequent, majority small	Infrequent, majority small
Peripheral WBC	Majority >15 × 10^9/L granulocytes predominant	Majority <15 × 10^9/L lymphocytes predominant	Majority normal or <15 × 10^9/L
↑C-reactive protein	Majority	Elevated in adenovirus; otherwise variable	Infrequent

Modified from Long SS. Treatment of acute pneumonia in infants and children. Pediatr Clin North Am 1983; 30:299.

coverage and staphylococcal coverage as
each case dictates.

7. Open lung biopsy may be needed for diagnosis in immunosuppressed patients or those
with deteriorating courses despite rigorous
therapy

Follow-Up

- Prognosis ultimately depends on seriousness of
initial infection
- Staphylococcal pneumonia usually requires 3
wk therapy, minimum
- Follow patient with chest x-ray at 4–6 wk to
document resolution of radiographic changes

TABLE 26–7 Antibiotics to Use for Pneumonias

Antibiotics in Uncomplicated Pneumonia

Age	Inpatient	Outpatient
<6 wk	IV ampicillin and gentamicin	--
6–12 wk*	IV cefuroxime	--
3 mo–5 yr	IV cefuroxime	Amoxicillin
5–19 yr	Penicillin G or erythromycin	Penicillin V or erythromycin

Antibiotics in Complicated Pneumonia

Pleural Effusion	Lung Abscess
Cefuroxime	Cloxacillin ± Clindamycin

* Add erythromycin if *Chlamydia* is a concern.

Asthma (Acute)

General Considerations

- Asthma affects 5 to 10% of children
- Mucosal inflammation, increased airway smooth

muscle tone, and mucus plugging result in
increased airway resistance
- Hyperinflation and increased airway resistance
lead to increased work of breathing
- Nonuniform changes result in V/Q mismatch
and hypoxemia
- Spectrum of acute illness from mild, easily
reversible obstruction to life threatening situation with severe airway obstruction

Clinical Features

- Obtain history of duration and course of attack.
Triggering factors may include viral respiratory
tract infections, cold air, exercise, chemical irritants, tobacco smoke, stress, and allergens
- Determine number of hospital admissions, dependency on steroids, and history of ICU ad-
missions
- Medication and adverse reaction history need
to be checked
- Assess for evidence of fatigue and restlessness
- Assess for altered mental status and inability to
speak
- Beware respiratory rate >30/min, heart rate
>110/min in older child
- Look for use of accessory muscles of respiration, asymmetry of air entry, evidence of sub-
cutaneous emphysema, pneumothorax, or
pneumomediastinum
- Assess for evidence of cyanosis
- Assess for pulsus paradoxus. Beware if >15 mm
Hg

Differential Diagnosis

- Bronchiolitis in infant may be hard to
distinguish from asthma
- Foreign body aspiration and gastroesophageal
reflux can masquerade as asthma

Management

- Investigation
  1. Arterial blood gases in moderate or severe cases—beware of the patient with a normal, rising, or elevated $PaCO_2$
  2. Chest x-ray (if clinically indicated) may show hyperinflation, increased peribronchial markings, atelectasis, evidence of pneumothorax, or pneumomediastinum
  3. Pulmonary function testing with portable spirometric device can give objective assessment of degree of obstruction. In severe asthma, peak flow rates ≤ 20 to 30% predicted value
- General treatment
  1. Humidified oxygen 30 to 40% by mask or nasal prongs
  2. Follow status with arterial blood gas measurements as clinically dictated
  3. Correct fluid deficits if dehydration present and provide maintenance IV fluids and electrolytes
  4. Avoid fluid overload
- Specific treatment
  1. Sympathomimetic drugs
     - Treatment of choice salbutamol (0.5% solution) 0.01 to 0.03 ml/kg (maximum 1 ml) in 3 ml normal saline by mask hourly. In mild cases give masks q3–4h.
     - Alternatively, in moderate to severe asthma may give initial dose of 0.03 ml/kg (maximum 1 ml) followed by 0.01 ml/kg (maximum 0.33 ml) in 3 ml normal saline q20 min by mask
  2. Theophylline
     - IV drug may be aminophylline (80% theophylline) or theophylline
     - Obtain theophylline level if child is on oral theophylline
     - Effect is dose related; therefore a level in

the upper limit of the therapeutic range is
best
- If no theophylline on board, give IV loading dose of 6.0 mg/kg theophylline over 20
  min
- If child received oral theophylline within
  12 hr prior to admission, a serum theophylline concentration should be measured. As
  a rule of thumb, each 1.0 mg/kg of theophylline raises the serum levels by 10
  μmol/L (1.8 mg/L)
  Alternatively, if unable to obtain stat theophylline levels, give loading dose of theophylline of 3.0 mg/kg
- Following loading dose, start on maintenance theophylline as intermittent
  bolus or by continuous drip (see p 849
  for doses)
- Theophylline metabolism decreased by
  liver disease, congestive heart failure, viral
  disease, and concurrent erythromycin or
  cimetidine administration. Beware of toxic
  levels.
- Phenobarbital and cigarette smoking increase theophylline metabolism. Beware
  subtherapeutic levels.
3. Corticosteroids
   - Results from clinical trials of steroids in
     acute asthma are conflicting. Most physi-
     cians administer steroids in moderate to
     severe cases.
   - IV steroids are indicated if child is on
     maintenance oral or inhaled steroids or if
     child has needed IV steroids in the last 6
     mo
   - Steroids should be used in addition to
     aggressive bronchodilator therapy
   - Give IV hydrocortisone bolus 4 to 6 mg/kg,
     then same amount q4 to 6h
   - Alternatively, IV methylprednisolone 0.5–1
     mg/kg/dose q6h
   - If patient improves, convert to oral steroids

in 48 hr; taper over following week
4. Anticholinergic drugs
    - Clinical trials show nebulized ipratropium bromide (Atrovent) useful in treatment of acute asthma when combined with β_2 agents (e.g., salbutamol)
    - May give 250 μg ipratropium bromide every 4 hr with salbutamol mask
5. Antibiotics
    - Antibiotics have no role in treatment unless bacterial infection is documented
- Warning
  1. Remember: respiratory failure and fatigue may develop despite optimal therapy
  2. ICU care essential for trial of IV salbutamol or possible intubation and ventilation

Chronic Asthma

General Considerations

- Asthma is a chronic respiratory disease. Treatment plans should address social, psychological, and medical needs
- Regular follow-up and PFTs valuable to determine response to therapy

Management

- Environmental control
  1. History of specific allergic or irritant factors should be obtained
  2. Smoking in home to be discouraged
  3. Antidust programs may be tried but can be difficult to comply with
- Immunotherapy
  1. Not generally useful in asthma
  2. Should be considered only if attacks are triggered by specific unavoidable allergens
- Exercise programs
  1. Exercise is to be encouraged. Swimming often is well tolerated even in patients whose

asthma is triggered by exercise.
  2. Inhalation of β_2 drugs or sodium cromogly-
     cate prior to activity is often beneficial (see
     below)
- Pharmacotherapy
  1. May require one or more of following
     categories of drugs
     - Sympathomimetic drugs
       a. Preferably given by inhalation but also
          can be given orally
       b. Side effects include tachycardia and
          tremor
       c. Inhaled β_2 drugs may be given by com-
          pressor, metered dose inhaler, or
          Rotahaler
       d. By compressor, may put salbutamol in 3
          ml normal saline or in 2 ml of 1%
          sodium cromoglycate
       e. Doses of salbutamol: 0.01–0.03 ml/kg
          (maximum 1 ml) of 0.5% solution in 3
          ml normal saline by mask q4–6h. Alter-
          natively, may use metered dose inhaler
          salbutamol: 100–200 μg (1–2 puffs) qid.
       f. For children aged 4–7 yr, spacer attach-
          ment useful or may try dry powder inhal-
          er (Rotahaler)
       g. Oral β_2 drugs used in those too young
          for metered dose inhaler and no access
          to compressor
       h. Salbutamol PO 0.3 mg/kg/day ÷ tid or
          orciprenaline (Alupent) PO 2 mg/kg/day
          ÷ tid (maximum 20 mg/dose)
     - Theophylline
       a. Sustained release oral preparations given
          q12h best (e.g., Theo-Dur,
          Somophyllin-12); see p 849 for doses
       b. Occasionally may benefit from use of
          small 1600 hr dose in addition to doses
          given morning and night
       c. Adverse GI side effects avoided by start-
          ing patient on 50% dose and increasing

gradually
  d. Follow patient for side effects and moni-
     tor level: therapeutic range is 55 to 110
     μmol/L (10 to 20 mg/L)
- Sodium cromoglycate (cromolyn sodium)
  a. Solely a prophylactic agent
  b. Often useful before exposure to cold or
     in exercise induced bronchospasm
  c. Trial of 2 mo warranted in patients need-
     ing daily medications
  d. No role in acute asthma attack
  e. Usually delivered as dry powder—1 spin-
     cap qid
  f. Metered dose inhaler delivering 1 mg/puff
     available, with appropriate dose being 2
     mg (2 puffs) qid
  g. When using salbutamol by compressor,
     may use 2 ml of 1% sodium cromogly-
     cate in place of saline
- .Corticosteroids
  a. Chronic or intermittent therapy added for
     patients inadequately controlled with
     above medications
  b. Majority of patients with moderate to
     severe asthma controlled with inhaled
     steroid, such as beclomethasone 300 to
     400 μg/day (2 puffs 3 to 4 times/day)
  c. Use of high dose beclomethasone inhala-
     tion (1600 μg/day) shown successful in
     some adult studies
  d. Adrenal suppression possible with high
     dose inhalation
  e. Low dose side effects include hoarseness
     and oral candidiasis
  f. Severe asthma may need oral steroids for
     adequate control
  g. Steroid side effects minimized with alter-
     nate day, single morning dose regimen
  h. Daily oral steroids occasionally required
- Anticholinergic drugs
  a. Ipratropium bromide (Atrovent) available

in metered dose inhaler
b. Dose 20 μg/puff, 2 puffs qid
c. Slower but more prolonged bronchodilation compared to β_2 drugs
d. Role in acute and chronic asthma still evolving

CYSTIC FIBROSIS

General Considerations

- Incidence of CF in North American Caucasian population between 1:1,900 and 1:3,700 live births; 1:17,000 in American blacks; 1:90,000 in Orientals
- Autosomal recessive inheritance pattern with carrier rate approximately 1:20 in Caucasians

Clinical Features

- See Table 26–8

Diagnosis

- Quantitative analysis of sodium chloride content in sweat using urecholine or pilocarpine iontophoresis most reliable method of diagnosis
- Minimum of 100 mg sweat should be collected
- May be difficult to obtain enough sweat in first weeks of life
- Sweat chloride >60 mmol/L in 98% of cases of CF
- False positive results seen with poor lab technique, nephrotic syndrome, Addison's disease, malnutrition, nephrogenic diabetes insipidus, G–6–PD deficiency, glycogen storage disease, ectodermal dysplasia, and hypothyroidism
- Pancreatic dysfunction determined by use of 3 to 5 day fecal fat collection

**TABLE 26–8 Clinical Features Present
at Diagnosis of CF**

Age and Clinical Feature	Approximate Incidence, %
0–2 yr	
Meconium ileus	10
Obstructive jaundice	
Heat prostration/hyponatremia	
Hypoproteinemia/anemia	
Bleeding diathesis	
Failure to thrive	
Steatorrhea	
Bronchitis/bronchiolitis	
Staphylococcal pneumonia	
Rectal prolapse	20
2–12 yr	
Recurrent pneumonia/bronchitis	60
Malabsorption	85
Nasal polyps	
Intussusception	1–5
13 yr +	
Chronic pulmonary disease	70
Clubbing	
Abnormal glucose tolerance	20–30
Chronic intestinal obstruction	10–20
Recurrent pancreatitis	
Focal biliary cirrhosis	15–25
Portal hypertension	2–5
Gallstones	4–12
Diabetes mellitus	1
Aspermia	98

From MacLusky I, McLaughlin FJ, Levison H. Cystic fibrosis. Part
I. Curr Prob Pediatr 1985; 15(6):13.

Management

- Nutritional Management (Table 26–9)
- Respiratory Management
    1. Frequent sputum for culture and sensitivity
    2. Physiotherapy—most patients practice postural
       drainage bid to tid in conjunction with bron-
       chodilator therapy
    3. Inhalation therapy—mist alone no longer
       practiced

TABLE 26–9 Nutritional Management

Calories	120 to 150%
Protein	RDA*
Essential fatty acids	3 to 5% total calories
Vitamin A	5,000 to 10,000 IU/day
Vitamin D	400 to 800 IU/day
Vitamin E	100 to 300 IU/day (water soluble form)
Vitamin K	5 mg twice weekly for infants 5 mg daily for children and older
Vitamin B's	RDA × 2
Vitamin C	RDA × 2

Pancreatic enzymes:

Infants: Add one regular cotazym capsule or ⅓ tsp. powder to 4 oz. of formula (8,000 units lipase/120 ml formula)

Children and Adults: Regular capsules = 6/meal (48,000 units lipase/meal); 2/snack (16,000 units lipase/snack) Enteric-coated microspheres (cotazym ECS) = 3/meal (24,000 units lipase/meal); 1/snack (8,000 units lipase/snack)

N.B. Enteric-coated capsules are not to be used in children who cannot swallow capsules whole, as mucosal ulceration may develop.

* Recommended daily allowance.
Modified from MacLusky I, McLaughlin FJ, Levison H. Cystic fibrosis. Part II. Curr Prob Pediatr 1985; 15(7):11.

4. Bronchodilators often helpful, as high percentage of CF population have component of hyperreactive airway disease
5. Salbutamol (0.5% solution) 0.01 to 0.03 ml/kg (maximum 1 ml) in 3 ml normal saline bid to tid before physiotherapy is useful
6. Mucolytic therapy with 2 ml of 20% acetylcysteine occasionally needed to reduce sputum viscosity
7. Inhalational antibiotics not routinely used at this time
8. At HSC, long term daily oral antibiotics tailored to sputum C+S results are prescribed, e.g., cloxacillin, co-trimoxazole, or oral cephalosporins

- Management of Acute Chest Exacerbation
    1. CF characterized by recurrent acute chest exacerbations manifested by fevers, increased cough, shortness of breath, sputum production, anorexia, and weight loss
    2. With exacerbations, an increased WBC and ESR may be seen, especially with *Pseudomonas cepacia* infection
    3. Check for deterioration in PFTs, ABGs, and chest x-ray
    4. Requires hospitalization
    5. IV antibiotics appropriate for sputum C+S
    6. Regular physiotherapy with inhalational treatments
    7. Nutritional support
    8. O_2 if necessary

PLEURAL EFFUSION

General Considerations

- Defined as excess accumulation of fluid in pleural cavity
- Usually secondary to an underlying disorder
- Fluid analysis needed to distinguish transudate, exudate, chyle, or blood

Investigation and Management

- In adult, x-ray changes on upright film not usually present until 400 ml fluid accumulated. Lateral decubitus films can detect smaller quantities.
- Other radiologic features include uniform fluid density, widened intercostal interspaces on affected side, and possible tracheal and mediastinal shift contralaterally
- An exudate meets at least one of the following criteria, whereas a transudate meets none of these criteria:

   1. Pleural LDH $>\frac{2}{3}$ upper limit of normal for
      serum LDH
   2. Protein: Pleural/serum >0.5
   3. LDH: Pleural/serum >0.6
- Send fluid for cytology (cell differential, RBC, WBC, and malignant cells), biochemistry (protein, glucose, pH, LDH, fat content if chylous), microbiology (Gram stain, C+S, acid-fast staining, virology), and immunologic investigations when appropriate (e.g., complement studies)
- Transudates associated with congestive heart failure, nephrotic syndrome, acute glomerulonephritis, cirrhosis, myxedema, sarcoidosis, and Meigs' syndrome
- Exudates commonly caused by infection (bacterial, viral, mycoplasma, mycobacterial, fungal). Can also be caused by collagen vascular diseases, malignant disease, pancreatitis, and subdiaphragmatic abscess

Management of Parapneumonic Effusions

- Obtain chest x-ray PA and lateral
- If diaphragm is obscured or there is blunting of posterior costophrenic angle, obtain decubitus films
- Obtain ultrasound if films suggest loculated fluid
- If >10 mm fluid thickness on decubitus film or loculation present, perform thoracentesis
- Chest tube if thick pus, positive Gram stain, pH <7.0, glucose <3.3 mmol/L (<60 mg/dl), or severe respiratory distress
- If $7.0 <$ pH < 7.2 or LDH $>1,000$, consider chest tube drainage or serial thoracentesis. Generally, serial thoracentesis inappropriate in children.
- Treatment appropriate for suspected organisms or culture results

PNEUMOTHORAX

General Considerations

- Pneumothorax defined as presence of gas in pleural space
- Causes include
  1. Pressures developed during first breath
  2. Iatrogenic (e.g., procedures)
  3. Hyaline membrane disease
  4. Aspiration syndromes
  5. Cystic fibrosis
  6. Asthma
  7. Infection
  8. Malignant disease
  9. Blunt or penetrating trauma
  10. Spontaneous
- Incidence of spontaneous pneumothorax is highest in tall, thin, young adult males (approximately 1:10,000). Usually due to rupture of apical pleural blebs.

Clinical Features

- Dyspnea, chest pain, or shoulder tip pain
- On physical may see marked respiratory distress and cyanosis
- Chest wall movement decreased on affected side
- Percussion note on affected side tympanitic
- Larynx, trachea, and mediastinum may be shifted contralaterally
- Cardiac function may be compromised if pneumothorax is under tension

Management

- Radiologic evidence includes spectrum of obvious air in pleural cavity to thin lucent rim devoid of lung markings
- Small pneumothorax ($< 5\%$) requires only observation, with spontaneous resolution within

1 wk usual
- Small pneumothoraces resolve more quickly with 100% O_2, which will increase N_2 gradient between pleural gas and blood. Beware CO_2 retainer depending on hypoxic drive. Avoid hyperoxia in premature infants.
- Larger pneumothoraces require chest tube drainage to underwater seal
- To prevent recurrences in patients at risk for recurrent pneumothoraces, consider chemical pleurodesis (e.g., quinacrine)
- Recurrent pneumothoraces may need open thoracotomy and pleural bleb excision/plication and stripping of apical pleura

Suggested Reading

1. Kendig EL, Chernick V. Disorders of the respiratory tract in children. Philadelphia: W.B. Saunders, 1983.
2. West JB. Respiratory physiology—the essentials. 2nd ed. Baltimore: Williams & Wilkins, 1979.

General Considerations

- For causes of arthritis in childhood (see Table 27–1)
- Table 27–2 contains normal values for range of motion of joints
- Table 27–3 contains values for synovial fluid in various conditions
- See Table 27–4 for an approach to the investigation of suspected rheumatic disorder

JUVENILE RHEUMATOID ARTHRITIS (JRA)

General Considerations

- Diagnostic criteria for JRA
  1. Arthritis in one or more joints for at least 6 wk
  2. Onset < 16 yr
  3. Exclusion of other rheumatic diseases
  4. See Table 27–5 for the classification of JRA

Clinical Features

- See Table 27–6

Differential Diagnosis of Arthritis in Childhood

Condition	Monarticular	Polyarticular
Trauma	+	
Infection		
Septic arthritis		
S. aureus, Haemophilus influenzae	+	
Meningococcus, gonococcus	±	+
Mycobacteria	+	
Virus related		
Rubella, hepatitis		+
Osteomyelitis	+	
Childhood malignant disease		
Leukemia, neuroblastoma	+	+
Hematologic disorder		
Hemophilia	+	+
Sickle cell disease	+	+
Rheumatic disease		
Juvenile rheumatoid arthritis	+	+
Spondyloarthropathies		
Juvenile ankylosing spondylitis	+	+
Arthritis with inflammatory bowel disease	+	+
Reactive arthritis		
Reiter's syndrome	+	+
Postinfectious (*Salmonella, Shigella, Yersina*)	+	+

TABLE 27–1 Differential Diagnosis of Arthritis in Childhood (Continued)

Condition	Monarticular	Polyarticular
Psoriatic arthritis	+	+
Systemic lupus erythematosus		+
Dermatomyositis		+
Scleroderma		+
Mixed connective tissue disease		+
Vasculitis syndromes		
Henoch-Schönlein purpura		+
Kawasaki disease		+
Polyarteritis nodosa		+
Behçet's syndrome		+
Rheumatic fever		+
Miscellaneous conditions		
Transient synovitis	+	
Orthopaedic conditions		
Slipped capital upper femoral epiphysis	+	
Perthes disease	+	
Osteoid osteoma	+	
Osteochondritis syndromes	+	
Chondromalacia patellae	+	
Serum sickness		+
Noninflammatory conditions		
Limb pains ("growing pains")	+	+
Psychogenic	±	+
Lyme arthritis	+	±

TABLE 27–2 Normal Range of Motion of Various Joints in Children

	Flexion	Extension	Internal Rotation	External Rotation	Abduction	Adduction
Hip	120°	30°	35°	45°	45–50°	20–30°
Knee	135°	2–10°	10°	10°	0	0
Ankle	50°	20°				
Subtalar-midtarsal	--	--	5° inversion	5° eversion	10° forefoot	20°
First MTP	45°	70–90°				
Wrist	80°	70°			20° radial deviation	30° ulnar deviation
Elbow	135°	0–5°	90° supination	90° pronation		
Shoulder	90°	45°	55°	40–45°	180°	45°
MCPs	90°	30–45°			20°	0
Thumb	70° palmar	0				
Neck	45°	50°	80° right	80° left	40° lateral bend	40° lateral bend

From Jacobs CJ. Pediatric rheumatology for the practitioner. New York: Springer-Verlag, 1982:8.

TABLE 27–3 Synovial Fluid Analysis

	Normal	Inflammatory	Infectious
Color	Colorless to straw	Yellow	Variable
Turbidity	Clear	Clear to turbid	Turbid
White cell count	$<0.2 \times 10^9$/L (<200/mm^3)	2.0–75.0×10^9/L ($2{,}000$–$75{,}000$/mm^3)	Often $>100.0 \times 10^9$/L ($>100{,}000$/mm^3)
Neutrophils (%)	<25	>50	>75
Glucose	Nearly equal to blood glucose	<2.8 mmol/L (50 mg/dl) *below* blood glucose	>2.8 mmol/L (50 mg/dl) *below* blood glucose
Culture	Negative	Negative	Often positive

Modified from Kelley WN, Harris ED, Ruddy S, Sledge CB. Textbook of rheumatology. Vol. 1. 2nd ed. Philadelphia: W.B. Saunders, 1985:562.

TABLE 27–4   Investigation of Suspected Rheumatic Disorder

Blood tests
    Complete blood count and differential
    ESR
    Urea, creatinine
    AST (SGOT), alkaline phosphatase, bilirubin
    Immunoglobulins
    LE cell preparation (rapid return—not sensitive or specific)
    ANA (antinuclear antibody)
    RF (rheumatoid factor)
    C3, C4 if SLE suspected
Urine
    Urinalysis
    Urine microscopy
X-ray of joints as indicated clinically

TABLE 27–5   Classification of Juvenile Rheumatoid Arthritis*

Systemic	Fever, rash, hepatosplenomegaly, lympha-denopathy, serositis, leukocytosis, anemia
Polyarticular	Five or more joints
Pauciarticular	Four or fewer joints

* Classification based on clinical presentation within first 6 mo after onset of disease.

TABLE 27–6 Subgroups of JRA

	Pauciarticular Type I	Pauciarticular Type II	Polyarticular RF-Negative	Polyarticular RF-Positive	Systemic Onset
% of JRA patients	30	15	25	10	20
Sex	80% girls	90% boys	90% girls	80% girls	Male = female
Age at onset	Early childhood	Late childhood	Throughout childhood	Late childhood	Throughout childhood
Joints	Large joints—knee, ankle, elbow	Large joints—hip girdle	Symmetric—any joints	Symmetric—any joints	Usually polyarticular—any joints
Sacroiliitis	No	Common (late)	No	Rare	No
Iridocyclitis	30–50% chronic iridocyclitis	10–20% acute iridocyclitis	Rare	No	No
RF	Negative	Negative	Negative	100%	Negative
ANA	60%	Negative	25%	75%	Negative
Association with HLA-B27	No	Yes	No	No	No
Ultimate morbidity	Ocular damage 10%	Subsequent spondyloarthropathy ?%	Severe arthritis 10–15%	Severe arthritis >50%	Severe arthritis 25%

RF = rheumatoid factor.
ANA = antinuclear antibodies.
Modified from Schaller JG. Chronic arthritis in children. Clin Orthop 1984; 182:79–87.

Management

- Education of patient and family
- Drug therapy
  1. First line
     - Salicylates
       a. ASA 60–100 mg/kg/day in 4 divided doses, with meals
       b. Monitor levels; observe for side effects and toxicity
     - Nonsteroid anti-inflammatory drugs, e.g., naproxen (Naprosyn), tolmetin sodium (Tolectin), indomethacin (Indocid)
  2. Second line
     - Hydroxychloroquine
     - Gold salts
     - D-Penicillamine
  3. Corticosteroids—specific indications
     - Local—eyes (for uveitis); intra-articular
     - Systemic—indicated for
       a. Systemic JRA with life-threatening complications or fever unresponsive to nonsteroidal anti-inflammatory drugs
       b. Chronic uveitis unresponsive to topical therapy
       c. Severe polyarticular JRA
  4. Immunosuppressive agents
- Physical and occupational therapy
  1. Exercise to maintain range of motion of joints and muscle strength
  2. Encourage activities such as swimming and bicycle riding
  3. Splints help to prevent deformity
- Heat (e.g., warm bath)—helps to relieve pain and stiffness, may be useful in early morning
- Rest—no place for prolonged bed rest. Ensure adequate rest period at night; may require rest period during the day.

- Consultations
    1. Ophthalmologist—mandatory
    2. Multidisciplinary approach best—
       physiotherapy, occupational therapy, social
       worker, involvement of school, orthopaedic
       surgeon
    3. Pediatric rheumatologist—if there is poor
       response to first line drug therapy

SPONDYLOARTHROPATHIES

General Considerations

- No accepted diagnostic criteria in children
- Prototype—juvenile ankylosing spondylitis (JAS)
- May be associated with inflammatory bowel
  disease or psoriasis or may follow gastrointestinal or genitourinary infection

Clinical Features

- Cassidy (1982, p 285) indicates the following:
    1. Age—late childhood, early adolescence
    2. Male:female $= >6:1$
    3. Family history of related disease
    4. Peripheral arthritis—pauciarticular, asym-
       metric, lower extremities most commonly
       involved
    5. Axial arthritis—often occurs late; sacroiliac or
       lumbosacral spinal symptoms only in 20% at
       onset
    6. Enthesitis—tenderness at sites of insertion of
       tendons and ligaments to bone, e.g., heel
       pain at Achilles tendon insertion
    7. Absence of antinuclear antibodies (ANA) and
       rheumatoid factor (RF)
    8. HLA-B27 in 90%
    9. N.B. Early stages of JAS may be indistinguish-
       able from pauciarticular JRA

SYSTEMIC LUPUS ERYTHEMATOSUS

- Criteria for diagnosis—see Table 27–7
- Autoantibody patterns—see Table 27–8

TABLE 27–7   1982 Revised Criteria for Classification of Systemic Lupus Erythematosus (SLE)

Malar rash
Discoid rash
Photosensitivity
Oral or nasopharyngeal ulcers
Arthritis—involving two or more peripheral joints
Serositis
    a. Pleuritis *or*
    b. Pericarditis
Renal disorder
    a. Persistent proteinuria (>0.5 g/day or $>3+$) *or*
    b. Cellular casts
Neurologic disorder
    a. Seizures *or* ⎱ in absence of offending drugs or
    b. Psychosis ⎰ metabolic abnormalities
Hematologic disorder
    a. Hemolytic anemia *or*
    b. Leukopenia—$<4.0 \times 10^9$/L ($<4,000$/mm^3) *or*
    c. Lymphopenia—$<1.5 \times 10^9$/L ($<1,500$/mm^3) *or*
    d. Thrombocytopenia—$<100 \times 10^9$/L ($<100,000$/mm^3)
       in absence of offending drugs
Immunologic disorder
    a. Positive LE cell preparation *or*
    b. Anti-nDNA antibody *or*
    c. Anti-Sm antibody *or*
    d. False positive serologic test for syphilis
ANA—in absence of drugs associated with "drug-induced lupus syndrome"

- **Diagnosis—requires four or more of these 11 criteria, serially or simultaneously**
- Additional features to be considered in diagnosis of SLE:
  - Raynaud's phenomenon
  - Alopecia
  - Constitutional symptoms—fever, lymphadenopathy, hepatosplenomegaly

TABLE 27–8 Autoantibodies in SLE

Antibody	Prevalence in SLE	Fluorescent Staining Patterns	Other Disease Associations	Clinical Associations
Anti-nDNA (Anti-double stranded DNA)	40–60%	Peripheral or rim	Specific for SLE	Renal disease Hypocomplementemia Worse prognosis
Anti-Sm	25–30%	Speckled	Specific for SLE	Better prognosis if anti-nDNA absent
Anti-nRNP	30–35%	Speckled	Not specific for SLE 100% in MCTD	Arthritis, Raynaud's phenomenon, sclerodactyly, serositis, myositis, ↓ prevalence of renal disease Better prognosis
Antihistones	60%	Homogeneous	Drug-induced lupus	
Anti-Ro (= anti-SSA)	25–40%		Sjögren's syndrome ANA negative lupus Neonatal lupus SLE with homozygous C2 and C4 deficiency	Photosensitivity Subacute cutaneous lupus
Anti-La (= anti-SSB)	10–15%		Sjögren's syndrome Neonatal lupus	Almost always associated with anti-Ro

DERMATOMYOSITIS

General Considerations

- Diagnostic criteria of dermatomyositis
  1. Symmetric, progressive proximal muscle weakness
  2. Classic dermatomyositis rash
     - Swelling and heliotrope hue of upper eyelids
     - Erythematous or violaceous eruption over extensor surfaces, particularly interphalangeal joints, elbows, and knees
  3. Serum muscle enzyme elevation—creatine kinase, aldolase, AST(SGOT), and LDH
  4. EMG evidence of myositis
  5. Muscle biopsy findings typical of dermatomyositis

MIXED CONNECTIVE TISSUE DISEASE (MCTD)

General Considerations

- Comprises a syndrome of a combination of features of
  1. Systemic lupus erythematosus
  2. Scleroderma (high incidence of Raynaud's phenomenon, abnormal esophageal motility, sclerodactyly, and lung disease)
  3. Dermatomyositis or polymyositis
  4. Arthritis is prominent
- ANA profile
  1. High titer antibody to RNP (= ribonuclease sensitive component of extractable nuclear antigen, ENA)
  2. Absence of other ANAs

HENOCH-SCHÖNLEIN PURPURA

Clinical Features

- Skin lesions (100%)
  1. Nonthrombocytopenic purpura, particularly over buttocks and lower limbs: necessary for diagnosis
  2. Angioedema
- Arthritis-arthralgia (in ~ ⅔ of cases)
  1. Involves large joints, especially knees and ankles
  2. Frequently periarticular swelling present
  3. Transient
- Gastrointestinal involvement (in ~ ⅔ of cases)
  1. Colicky abdominal pain—may precede arthritis and purpura
  2. Intussusception and significant hemorrhage (in <5% of cases)
- Renal involvement (in ~ 40% of cases)
  1. Nephritis with hematuria or proteinuria
  2. Progressive renal failure (in <5% of cases)
- Central nervous system involvement
- Acute scrotal swelling

Management

- Supportive
- Prednisone may be indicated for
  1. Severe gastrointestinal involvement
  2. Severe central nervous system involvement
  3. Severe renal involvement
  4. Severely painful soft tissue swelling
  5. Scrotal or testicular involvement

Suggested Reading

1. Ansell BM. Chronic arthritis in childhood. Ann Rheumat Dis 1978; 37:107–120.
2. Cassidy JT. Textbook of pediatric rheumatology. New York: John Wiley, 1982.
3. Jacobs JC. Pediatric rheumatology for the practitioner. New York: Springer-Verlag, 1982.
4. Schaller JG. Chronic arthritis in children. Clin Orthop 1984; 182:79–87.

28 SURGERY

NEONATAL ABDOMINAL EMERGENCIES

General Principles

- History of vomiting bile-stained fluid in the first few days of life indicates intestinal obstruction until proven otherwise
- Sepsis is the major medical consideration in the differential
- A careful history must be sought, paying particular attention to
  1. History of polyhydramnios
  2. Excessive salivation ("mucousy"), cyanosis, and choking with feeds
  3. Abdominal distention
  4. Delayed passage of meconium, more than 24 hr after birth (meconium may be passed from bowel distal to an obstruction)
  5. Large gastric aspirate in the delivery room
- A careful physical examination must be carried out to rule out congenital abnormalities *other than* those responsible for the presenting symptoms

Basic Management

- Cross match ~ 100 cc of packed red cells at admission
- Avoid hypothermia
- Correct electrolyte abnormalities, fluid deficits, acid-base derangements
- Chest and abdominal x-rays should be obtained
- A No. 10 nasogastric tube should be passed in all cases of suspected intestinal obstruction in newborns >2,000 g, or No. 8 if <2,000 g

- A radiocontrast enema is often helpful in establishing the diagnosis in cases of intestinal obstruction

SPECIFIC SURGICAL EMERGENCIES

Esophageal Atresia

General Considerations and Clinical Features

- Commonly associated with a distal tracheoesophageal fistula (TEF)
- Presents with history of polyhydramnios, excess salivation, choking with feeds $\pm$ cyanotic spells

Investigations

- Diagnosis made by inability to pass a No. 10 nasogastric tube into the stomach, and demonstration of its tip in air-filled dilated proximal esophagus (usually T3-T5) radiologically
- An air-contrast outline of the pouch can be obtained by taking a chest x-ray while insufflating the pouch with air through the tube
- If doubt exists about the diagnosis, 0.5 cc of bronchography contrast medium can be instilled into pouch through a catheter under fluoroscopic control

Treatment

- Operation to correct atresia with fistula usually done within 24 hr after diagnosis. Reasons for further delay most commonly include
  1. Pneumonitis from aspiration of gastric contents
  2. Severe associated cardiac (or other) anomalies
- While awaiting surgery, the infant should be kept in Fowler's position with a suction tube in the proximal pouch

Duodenal Atresia or Stenosis

General Considerations and Clinical Features

- Common in Down syndrome
- Presents with
    1. Bile-stained vomiting in first 1–3 days of life (depending on degree of obstruction). If obstruction proximal to ampulla of Vater, vomitus is *not* bile stained (less than 10% of cases)
    2. Abdomen not distended
    3. ± Jaundice

Investigations

- Abdominal x-rays → "double bubble" pattern classically
- Acid-base and electrolyte status
- Urgent radiocontrast enema indicated to rule out malrotation, volvulus, and colonic atresias, especially if surgery is not undertaken immediately

Treatment

- See under General Principles (p 634)
- Early surgery

Small Intestinal Atresia

General Considerations and Clinical Features

- May be associated with cystic fibrosis
- Presents with
    1. Abdominal distention
    2. Bilious vomiting
    3. Failure to pass meconium (occasionally some meconium may be passed)
    4. Palpable distended loops of bowel often present

Investigations

- Plain abdominal films show intestinal distention and multiple air-fluid levels
- Radiocontrast enema: helpful in defining level and cause of obstruction and ruling out a more distal second obstruction

Treatment

- As for duodenal atresia

Malrotation with Midgut Volvulus

Clinical Features

- Presents with
  1. Bilious vomiting
  2. Abdominal distention
  3. ± Blood in stool (hematochezia)
  4. In a neonate, presentation may be similar to that seen with necrotizing enterocolitis (NEC)
  5. Peritoneal signs may be present

Investigations

- Abdominal plain film may show multiple air-fluid levels, or a relatively gasless abdomen. Occasionally the film is compatible with duodenal obstruction
- Urgent radiocontrast enema or upper GI study is necessary to confirm the presence of malrotation or duodenal obstruction

Treatment

- Resuscitation, correction of electrolyte and acid-base abnormalities, and passage of nasogastric tube for suction are important precursors of surgical therapy
- Delay in treatment can be catastrophic, with high morbidity and mortality!

Meconium Ileus

General Considerations and Clinical Features

- Almost always (>95%) associated with cystic fibrosis (CF); therefore FAMILY HISTORY IMPORTANT
- Symptoms usually those of bowel obstruction and resemble those of intestinal atresia
- Complicated meconium ileus may present with signs of peritonitis ($\pm$ intra-abdominal calcifications) as a result of intrauterine volvulus or perforation of the gut

Investigations and Treatment

- Abdominal plain films: similar to those of intestinal atresia, except distended bowel may have "ground glass" appearance and air-fluid levels may be absent, $\pm$ intra-abdominal calcifications
- In uncomplicated meconium ileus, gastrograffin or Hypaque Muco-myst enema is used to relieve the obstruction in an attempt to avoid surgery. Repeated attempts are often necessary to produce complete resolution
- Surgery is required in ~ 50% of patients
- N.B. ALL PATIENTS SHOULD HAVE A SWEAT CHLORIDE DONE TO RULE OUT CF

Hirschsprung's Disease

General Considerations and Clinical Features

- Early diagnosis is crucial in order to decrease risk of enterocolitis
- Clinical features may include
  1. A delay in passage of meconium (>24 hr)
  2. Intestinal obstructive signs and symptoms with no mechanical explanation
  3. Failure to thrive with irregular bowel movements (late presentation)

4. Rectal examination often results in explosive egress of liquefied meconium and air in previously obstructed infant
5. Meconium plug syndrome and L colon syndrome may present in identical fashion

Investigations

- Barium enema may not be diagnostic in the first few days of life but *is* useful in excluding other causes of bowel obstruction. Barium is not cleared in a delayed film 24 hr later in Hirschsprung's disease.
- Rectal biopsy necessary to confirm absence of ganglion cells

Treatment

- A decompressing colostomy is usually necessary, pending later definitive pull-through surgery

Necrotizing Enterocolitis

General Considerations and Clinical Features

- Most common in stressed, premature, ± hypoxic babies
- Common cause of
  1. Abdominal distention
  2. Feeding intolerance   } in the appropriate clinical setting
  3. Bloody stools

Investigations

- In the acute stages, frequent assessments including abdominal x-rays are necessary to exclude pneumoperitoneum
- The x-ray appearance may be quite variable, ranging from thickened bowel loops and free peritoneal fluid to pneumatosis intestinalis or gas in the portal vein

- CBC, differential, and platelet count may indicate a septic process with neutropenia ± thrombocytopenia
- Full septic screen including lumbar puncture, blood and stool cultures
- Barium enema contraindicated during acute episode, unless diagnosis is in doubt

Treatment

- Supportive medical therapy
  1. IV fluids (*may* need colloids initially)
  2. IV antibiotics (e.g., ampicillin, gentamicin, and clindamycin) × 7–10 days
  3. Nasogastric suction + NPO
  4. May need ventilatory support
- Indications for surgical intervention include
  1. Free perforation
  2. Increasing abdominal wall erythema
  3. Failure of medical therapy

Complications

- Late strictures (3–4 wk after the acute episode) may produce symptoms of bowel obstruction
- ''Short gut'' syndrome with malabsorption

Diaphragmatic Hernia (Bochdalek)

General Considerations and Clinical Features

- Presents with ± respiratory distress (earlier onset → poorer prognosis), ± scaphoid abdomen
- More commonly L sided

Investigations

- CXR—diagnostic (e.g., bowel loop in thoracic cavity)
- Monitor preductal and postductal arterial gas levels

Treatment

- Pass nasogastric tube
- Resuscitate with ETT, ventilation, $\pm$ paralysis
- Transfer to tertiary center ASAP
- Poor prognostic signs
  1. Respiratory distress in first 12 hr of life
  2. Hypoplastic lungs, persistent pulmonary hypertension, and "high" ventilatory requirements
- N.B. Surgical repair of defect delayed until infant fully resuscitated and in stable condition

Gastrointestinal Bleeding

General Considerations

- The age of onset of GI hemorrhage can often be a useful guide to probable etiology (Table 28–1)

TABLE 28–1 Common Causes of Gastrointestinal Bleeding (According to Age)

Neonate (0–30 days)	Infant (30days–1 yr)
1. Swallowed maternal blood	1. Meckel's diverticulum
2. Gastric erosions or peptic ulceration	2. Enteric duplications
3. Necrotizing enterocolitis (NEC)	3. Gastroenteritis
4. Midgut volvulus	4. Reflex esophagitis
5. Anal fissures	5. Intussusception
	6. Anorectal fissures
	7. Peptic ulceration
Child (1–12 yr)	**Older Child (>12 yr)**
1. Juvenile polyps	1. Juvenile polyps
2. Esophageal varices	2. Esophageal varices
3. Peptic ulcer disease	3. Peptic ulcer disease
4. Meckel's diverticulum	4. Inflammatory bowel disease
5. Gastroenteritis	5. Anorectal fissures
6. Anorectal fissures	
7. Inflammatory bowel disease	

Management

- Determine level of bleeding
  1. Hematemesis or "coffee ground" vomiting or melena *usually* means bleeding above the ligament of Treitz
  2. Dark or bright red rectal bleeding *usually* means bleeding from small bowel or colon
  3. Massive upper GI bleeding can cause hematochezia
- Insert nasogastric tube to help determine level of bleeding
- Insert large-bore peripheral IV
- Commence iced saline lavage of stomach if blood is coming from nasogastric tube (controversial)
- Cross match 20–40 cc of whole blood or packed cells per kg of body weight
- Monitor vital signs and urine output (Foley catheter)
- Admission to ICU is necessary if bleeding requires transfusion
- Gastrointestinal bleeding usually self-limited in children

Diagnostic Procedures

- Endoscopy: for localization of acute, ongoing bleeding for both upper GI and colonic bleeding
- Angiography: for severe, ongoing bleeding below ligament of Treitz
- Air contrast barium studies: excellent in detecting esophageal varices, peptic ulceration, colonic polyps, and inflammatory bowel disease after the acute bleeding has been controlled
- Meckel's scan: for diagnosis of ectopic gastric mucosa within a Meckel's diverticulum or intestinal duplication
- Technetium-labeled red cell scan: for localization of persistent or intermittent gastrointestinal bleeding

Intussusception

General Considerations and Clinical Features

- Most commonly occurs between the ages of 3 mo and 2 yr
- May follow or accompany an upper respiratory tract infection or gastroenteritis
- The classic presentation of colicky abdominal pain, currant jelly stools, and palpable abdominal mass is not often seen
- Intussusception must be suspected in all infants with intermittent crying from presumed abdominal pain or with symptoms of bowel obstruction. May present, however, with no obvious significant colicky pain.

Management

- Barium enema confirms diagnosis and can be used to reduce intussusceptions in ~75% of cases. (Air contrast enemas also used.)
- Prior to enema, the child should have an IV started
- After successful hydrostatic reduction, there is ~10% incidence of recurrence
- If enema unsuccessful, operative reduction should follow immediately after rapid rehydration
- Hydrostatic reduction of an intussusception *should not* be attempted in cases with clinical evidence of peritonitis, or in those acutely ill with far advanced intestinal obstruction, because of the danger of perforation

Appendicitis

General Considerations and Clinical Features

- The clinical presentation of appendicitis may be quite variable

- In general, periumbilical pain is the first symptom, followed by a low grade fever, anorexia, and localization of the pain to the right lower quadrant. Vomiting usually follows the onset of pain.
- May present with fever and diarrhea with little, if any, abdominal pain, leading to an incorrect diagnosis of gastroenteritis
- Appendicitis should be considered in any child in whom treatment for suspected gastroenteritis does not bring about the anticipated amelioration in symptoms of diarrhea, abdominal pain, and fever within 24 hr
- Gastroenteritis may precede or coexist with appendicitis
- The most reliable clinical finding is tenderness and guarding over McBurney's point
- Leukocytosis and fever are not always present
- Rectal examination is often helpful to assess pelvic inflammation
- In children < 5 years of age, the incidence of ruptured appendicitis is very high

Management

- Intravenous rehydration is started
- Antibiotics (usually ampicillin, gentamicin, and clindamycin) are used for all cases of ruptured appendicitis and continued for 5–7 days
- A dose of an antibiotic, usually cefoxitin, is given preoperatively for prophylaxis in unruptured appendicitis
- When the diagnosis is not certain, children are often admitted for observation

Hypertrophic Pyloric Stenosis

General Considerations and Clinical Features

- Usually occurs in infants between 3 and 6 wk of age, but may occur sooner

- The patients are usually males, and often there is a family history of pyloric stenosis
- The symptoms include forceful vomiting of previously ingested food, and the baby is often very hungry immediately afterward
- Jaundice and constipation are frequent accompanying features
- The diagnosis is made by palpating the pyloric "tumor." This is extremely difficult to do unless the baby is relaxed and not crying, and hard to do if the stomach is full. Hence the following method is recommended:
  1. Insert No. 10 nasogastric tube and connect to suction
  2. Allow the baby to drink a solution of dextrose water
  3. As the baby relaxes, the hypertrophied pylorus is felt midway between the xiphisternum and the umbilicus in the middle position of the upper abdomen
  4. Structures that can be mistaken for the pylorus include L lobe of liver and R kidney
- Observe for a gastric wave
- If a hypertrophied pylorus can be felt, no further diagnostic procedures are needed

Management

- If the diagnosis is in doubt, an upper GI series or ultrasound can be used to determine its presence
- Metabolic alkalosis with hypochloremia and hypokalemia are frequent metabolic derangements
- Mild to moderate dehydration is present in most cases, but it can be severe if the diagnosis is made late
- With the above in mind, therapy is approached as follows:
  1. Correct fluid and electrolyte status prior to operative intervention. This is achieved with

a solution containing 0.45% saline with 20
mEq (mmol)/L of KCl at 150 ml/kg/day.
2. Blood pH and electrolyte levels are used to
monitor infant's progress

Differential Diagnosis

- Gastroesophageal reflux can present with similar symptoms
- Congenital adrenal hyperplasia: consider if K^+ is high and Na^+ low, especially with associated ambiguous genitalia

Ingested Foreign Body (FB)

General Considerations and Management

- Most swallowed FBs pass spontaneously
- Plain films (x-rays) of the neck, chest, and abdomen localize radio-opaque foreign bodies
- Endoscopy is used in removing all foreign bodies held up in the esophagus or present in the tracheobronchal tree
- Long, sharp objects in the stomach may be removed endoscopically or with a magnetic probe under fluoroscopy. Once past the pylorus, they may be allowed to advance spontaneously unless symptoms of persistent abdominal pain develop, or if impaction of the object against the intestinal wall results in arrest of distal migration. Laparotomy is then indicated.
- Enemas or cathartics *should not* be used to hasten the evacuation of most foreign bodies. An exception to this rule is ingestion of microbatteries used for cameras and calculators. After 48 hr, leakage of corrosive fluids contained within the battery can result in bowel perforation. Enemas can be used to help evacuate such batteries.

OTHER COMMON SURGICAL CONDITIONS

Inguinal Hernias

General Considerations

- Can occur at any age, and generally should be repaired shortly after diagnosis. When incarcerated hernia cannot be reduced, emergency surgery is necessary.
- High incidence of incarceration below age 1 yr, with danger of testicular artery thrombosis, as well as intestinal obstruction
- In premature infants, repair usually delayed until a weight of 2,500 g is attained

Hydrocele

General Considerations

- Communicating hydrocele (fluid hernia) should be treated as an inguinal hernia. In these cases the scrotal or inguinal mass will change in size.
- Hydroceles which are present shortly after birth usually do not freely communicate with the peritoneal cavity and often resolve spontaneously
- In the absence of a clinical hernia, repair of a noncommunicating hydrocele is not indicated unless it persists beyond 1 yr

Undescended Testis (Cryptorchidism)

General Considerations

- Testes often retract into the inguinal canal in young males; if a testis can be brought into the scrotum with gentle traction, it is not truly undescended

- Orchidopexy is not recommended before the age of 2 yr unless a symptomatic inguinal hernia is also present
- Hormonal therapy is not usually successful in altering the position of the undescended testes but may increase their size and make operation easier
- Hypospadias and cryptorchidism either alone or together may be an expression of intersexuality, as well as indicative of other major genito-urinary malformations

Testicular Pain

General Considerations and Management

- It is often difficult to differentiate between epididymo-orchitis, testicular torsion, and torsion of the appendix testis
- If the scrotum is swollen but only moderately tender and the onset of pain has been gradual, torsion is unlikely
- If torsion of the testis cannot be excluded on clinical grounds, immediate exploration is indicated
- Radionuclide imaging of the testis and Doppler flow study of the testicular artery may not be reliable diagnostic tests

Biliary Atresia

General Considerations and Management

- Usually presents with progressive conjugated hyperbilirubinemia in the first month of life
- Associated developmental anomalies may coexist: situs inversus, dextrocardia, polysplenia
- Differential diagnosis usually includes neonatal hepatitis or metabolic diseases resulting in hepatic dysfunction

- Liver biopsy and liver scan (e.g., HIDA) are most useful tests discriminating between neonatal hepatitis and biliary atresia
- Portoenterostomy (Kasai procedure) is most successful in relieving jaundice if done before the age of 3 mo
- Liver transplantation is currently becoming a realistic hope for "cure" in eligible candidates

Umbilical Problems

General Considerations and Management

- Hernia: this type of hernia (common in blacks) rarely incarcerates and usually closes spontaneously. If present to age 2 yr, requires surgical repair
- Granuloma
  1. Results from chronic infection at site of umbilical cord separation
  2. Cautery with silver nitrate sticks can remedy the problem
  3. Must be differentiated from omphalomesenteric duct remnants, which may require excision and abdominal exploration

Cervical Masses

General Considerations and Management

- Torticollis: managed with physiotherapy unless there is restriction in range of motion after suitable trial of conservative therapy, or if facial asymmetry develops
- Branchial cleft malformation: can be a cyst or sinus and may be bilateral and is located along anterior border of sternocleidomastoid. Resection is usually necessary.
- Thyroglossal duct cyst: mass close to midline overlying the hyoid bone. It can become infected and present as an abscess. It requires resection.

- Cervical abscess: usually originates in a submandibular or posterior cervical lymph node and is caused by staphylococcus or streptococcus. Antibiotic therapy limits extent of cellulitis until abscess is fully fluctuant and ready to drain.

Suggested Reading

1. Filston H, Izant RJ. Congenital anomalies presenting with obstructive gastrointestinal symptoms. In: Klaus MH, Fanoroff AA, eds. Care of the high-risk neonate. Philadelphia: W.B. Saunders, 1986.
2. Schwartz MA, Lobe TE. Pediatric surgery (entire issue). Pediatr Clin North Am 1985; 32(5).
3. Welch KJ, Randolph JG, Ravitch MM, O'Neill JA Jr, Rowe MI, eds. Pediatric surgery. 4th ed. Chicago: Year Book, 1986.

III

EMERGENCIES

EMERGENCIES

ABBREVIATIONS

BP	Blood pressure
BUN	Blood urea nitrogen
CBC	Complete blood count
CPAP	Continuous positive airway pressure
Cr	Creatinine
CXR	Chest x-ray
DIC	Disseminated intravascular coagulation
ECG	Electrocardiogram
IM	Intramuscular
IPPV	Intermittent positive pressure ventilation
IV	Intravenous
$PaCO_2$	Partial pressure of carbon dioxide in arterial blood
PaO_2	Partial pressure of oxygen in arterial blood
WBC	White blood cell count
Hb	Hemoglobin
X-match	Cross match
FiO_2	Fractional concentration of oxygen in inspired air
COHb	Carboxyhemoglobin

CARDIOPULMONARY RESUSCITATION

- A quick guide to resuscitation drugs is inside the front cover.

Pediatric Basic Life Support

General Considerations

- Unlike arrest in adults, the precipitating factor in the majority of pediatric cardiac arrests is not a cardiac event
- Major causes of a pediatric cardiac arrest are

hypoxia and hypovolemia, and resuscitation should be directed at reversing these two disorders.

Management

- Determine unresponsiveness
- Call for help
- Open the airway
  1. Head extension
  2. Chin lift
  3. Jaw thrust
- Check breathing
  1. Look, listen, and feel
  2. If patient is breathing, check for cause of coma
- Ventilate
  1. Mouth to mouth or
  2. Mouth to nose
- If chest not moving, see p 658
- Check pulse: carotid, brachial, or precordial
- If pulse absent or inadequate, then cardiac compression
  1. Infant: on sternum just below intermammary line, 100/min, 1.5 to 2.5 cm, using two or three fingers
  2. Child: lower sternum, 80–100/min, 2.5 to 4 cm, using heel of hand

Pediatric Advanced Life Support

- Oxygen:
  1. The provision of 100% oxygen as soon as possible should be a priority
  2. Have self-inflating bag and masks available
- Endotracheal intubation (see p 674)
- Establish IV access
  1. Cut-down on long saphenous vein, ante-cubital fossa, or femoral vein. In abdominal trauma, sites on upper body are preferred.
  2. Transcutaneous access to central veins if experienced personnel are available

- If IV access is not established early, endo-tracheal route can be used for epinephrine, atropine, isoproterenol, or lidocaine (same doses as IV)
- Intracardiac injections pose significant hazards and should be reserved for experienced personnel who fail to establish any other route. Subxiphoid route is recommended. (May be used for epinephrine and bicarbonate.)

TABLE 1 Drug Therapy

Diagnosis	First Line Therapy	Secondary
Asystole, bradycardia or normal rate with no pulse	Oxygen, bicarbonate, and epinephrine	Atropine, isoproterenol, ± calcium
Ventricular fibrillation	Defibrillation and oxygen	Lidocaine Epinephrine Bicarbonate
Tachycardia	Oxygen Expand intravascular volume	

- IV fluids
    1. Intravascular volume expansion is frequently required during resuscitation
    2. Fluids used include Ringer's lactate, normal saline, and plasma. However, the type of solution is not as critical as the volume administered.
    3. In the absence of central venous pressure measurements, use 20 ml/kg as an initial bolus and 10–20 ml/kg during the subsequent hour, based on the response to this volume as observed by blood pressure and peripheral perfusion
- Defibrillation
    1. For ventricular fibrillation
        - Initially 2 joules/kg (2 watt-sec/kg)
        - If unsuccessful, then 4 joules/kg

(4 watt-sec/kg)
- • Repeat once, if necessary, 4 joules/kg (4 watt-sec/kg)
2. If still in ventricular fibrillation, correct hypoxemia and acidosis; administer epinephrine and repeat defibrillation at 4 joules/kg (4 watt-sec/kg) as necessary

- Emergency drug doses—see Table 2

Continuing Support

- Monitor arterial blood gases and electrolytes, and correct any abnormality as necessary
- Continue with elective hyperventilation even if spontaneous respiratory effort returns. Posthypoxic encephalopathy can be minimized by maintaining effective cerebral perfusion and oxygenation in the postarrest period.
- Maintain normothermia. Hypothermia is common during resuscitation.
- Continue to keep parents and family informed

CHOKING

General Considerations

- Aspiration of foreign material or a foreign body should be suspected in witnessed cases of sudden airway obstruction in previously healthy children, and in the unconscious child whose airway remains obstructed during the normal resuscitation maneuvers

Management

- If GOOD AIR EXCHANGE (forceful cough, wheezing inspiration, and loud cry), ALLOW CHILD TO CONTINUE WITH SPONTANEOUS EFFORTS TO CLEAR THE AIRWAY
- If POOR AIR EXCHANGE (very weak or nonexistent cough, no cry) OR TOTAL AIRWAY OBSTRUCTION, then for the:

TABLE 2 Emergency Drug Doses[*]

Drug	Concentration	Dose	Maximum Individual Dose
Sodium bicarbonate[1]	8.4% = 1 mmol/ml	2–3 ml/kg initially (2–3 mmol/kg) then 1–2 ml/kg (1–2 mmol/kg) q10–20 min of arrest time	
Epinephrine[3]	1:10,000 = 0.1 mg/ml (prefilled syringe) Infusion:	0.1 ml/kg MINIMUM 1 ml (0.01 mg/kg minimum 0.1 mg) 0.1–1 μg/kg/min	10 ml
Atropine[3]	0.1 mg/ml (prefilled syringe)	0.2 ml/kg MINIMUM 1 ml (0.02 mg/kg minimum 0.1 mg) May give q20 min	10 ml
Isoproterenol[3]	Supplied as 0.2 mg/ml: DILUTE 0.2 mg to 20 ml = 10 μg/ml Infusion:	0.3 ml/kg (3 μg/kg) 0.05–1.0 μg/kg/min	10 ml (of the diluted solution)
Calcium chloride	10% = 100 mg/ml	0.1 ml/kg (10 mg/kg) May repeat q10–20 min	10 ml

Calcium gluconate	10% = 100 mg/ml	0.3 ml/kg (30 mg/kg) May repeat q10–20 min	20 ml
Lidocaine[3]	2% = 20 mg/ml Infusion:	0.05 ml/kg (1 mg/kg) 20–50 μg/kg/min	5 ml
Dextrose[2]	50% = 0.5 g/ml	1–2 ml/kg (0.5–1 g/kg)	
Dopamine	Infusion:	5–20 μg/kg/min	25 μg/kg/min

* See also quick guide to resuscitation drugs inside front cover.
1. For use in prematures and newborns, dilute 1:1 with sterile water and give twice the volume (i.e., same dose).
2. In young children, dilute 1:1 with sterile water (to a 25% solution) to avoid damage to soft tissues.
3. May be given by ETT if no IV access is available (same doses).

FOR QUICK CALCULATION OF DRUG INFUSIONS USING SYRINGE PUMP: Wt(kg) × 3 × starting dose required (μg/kg/min) = amount of drug (mg) to be added to a 50 ml syringe. Then run at 1 ml/hr. Alternatively one may use drug infusion table (see p 682).

1. Older child (>1 yr)
   - Six to 10 abdominal thrusts (Heimlich maneuver). These thrusts may be administered in the standing position in the older conscious child, or the heel of one hand can be placed on the abdomen between the umbilicus and the rib cage with the child in a recumbent position. The thrusts should be directed inward and upward.
   - If the above maneuvers are unsuccessful, head extension and tongue-jaw lifts (anterior displacement of the mandible, using fingers behind the mandibular ramus or by gripping the mandible anteriorly and lifting forward) may help relieve the obstruction. If the foreign body is visualized, finger sweeps may be used to remove it. Blind finger sweeps may further impact the foreign body and should be discouraged.
   - When the child is unconscious, continue with basic CPR (p 653) and attempts at ventilation, because air exchange may well be possible. If ventilation is not possible, repeat above maneuvers.
2. Infant
   - In the choking infant, abdominal thrusts may be traumatic, and they should be avoided if other means are effective
   - Place the infant, 60 degree head down, lying on the rescuer's forearm
   - Administer four back blows between the shoulder blades with the heel of the rescuer's hand
   - If unsuccessful, turn the infant over and administer four chest thrusts (as with cardiac compression)
   - Attempt to visualize foreign body in mouth—if seen, remove with finger sweeps
   - Open airway with tongue-jaw lift technique
   - Attempt to ventilate

- Repeat the above maneuvers until ventilation is possible
- If unsuccessful, abdominal thrusts may be attempted

SHOCK

General Considerations

- Traditionally shock is categorized into
  1. Hypovolemic
  2. Septic
  3. Cardiogenic
  4. Anaphylactic
  5. Neurogenic

  Different forms of shock may merge in a pathophysiologic sense

Clinical Features

- Recognize some of the following:
  1. Sick looking
  2. Pallor
  3. Cyanosis (if Hb adequate), central or peripheral
  4. CNS disturbance (agitation to depression)
  5. Tachypnea
  6. Tachycardia, hypotension
  7. Poor capillary refill
  8. Acidemia (metabolic or mixed acidosis)
  9. Oliguria

Management

- Immediate treatment
  1. Improve oxygen delivery to tissues
     - Oxygen: by mask, nasal cannula or hood. Consider intubation if severely hypoxic.
     - Artificial ventilation: if there is respiratory failure, severe respiratory distress, or marked acidemia. Artificial ventilation reduces work of breathing and cardiac demands, especially in cardiogenic and septic shock.
  2. Improve cardiac performance
     - If hypovolemic, restore circulating blood

volume with normal saline, plasma, albumin, or blood. Start with 20 ml/kg and
reassess. (Remember: BP may be well
maintained by tachycardia and peripheral
vasoconstriction even in the presence of
severe hypovolemia.)
- In all other patients, give volume challenge
  with 10 ml/kg normal saline to augment
  stroke volume by increasing ventricular
  preload
- Increase contractility
  a. Correct pH
     - Ventilation
     - $NaHCO_3$ if pH still <7.25 once $PaCO_2$
       <40 (give weight [kg] $\times$ base deficit $\times$
       0.15 mmol).
     - Repeat if necessary
  b. Inotrope infusion
     - Dopamine 5–20 μg/kg/min. N.B.
       Dopamine should always be ad-
       ministered through a central line when
       possible because of the risk of tissue
       necrosis, although in an emergency
       setting the drug may be administered
       peripherally for a short period, prefer-
       ably through a separate line.
     - Epinephrine 0.1–1 μg/kg/min (rarely
       needed except in severe shock)
     - See drug infusion table (p 682)
- Investigations
  1. Arterial blood for
     - Hb, WBC with differential, platelets, coagu-
       lation screen
     - Blood gas and acid-base levels
     - Electrolytes, BUN, creatinine
     - Culture if appropriate
     - X-match if appropriate
  2. Chest x-ray
  3. Sepsis work-up if appropriate
- Further management
  1. Detailed history, best obtained by another
     MD during initial resuscitation

2. Detailed physical examination
   - Assess neck veins, fontanelle, mucous membranes, skin turgor for signs of hypovolemia. N.B. *Full neck veins and shock: beware of pneumothorax and cardiac tamponade.*
   - Fever, focal signs of infection (may be minimal); beware of rash consistent with meningococcemia
   - Signs of heart failure, especially gallop rhythm, cardiomegaly, pulse differential, lung crackles, hepatomegaly
   - Urticaria, mucosal edema, bronchospasm
3. Nasogastric tube and empty stomach to decrease risk of aspiration
4. Urethral catheter for initial urine volume
5. Further management based on diagnostic clues and response to initial therapy (for further management of septic shock, see p 340)

ANAPHYLAXIS

General Considerations

- Anaphylaxis is an immediate (type I) hypersensitivity reaction that can lead to life-threatening cardiorespiratory decompensation brought about by the release of vasoactive amines
- Hypotensive shock may occur and may be accompanied by laryngeal or bronchial obstruction and cutaneous reaction
- Treat patient at first sign of anaphylaxis. Do not wait for symptoms and signs to evolve.

Management

- Assess airway patency and cardiovascular status (CPR if necessary)
- Discontinue any ongoing parenteral medications or blood products being given at time of reaction
- O_2 by mask

- Medications
  1. Epinephrine (1:1,000) 0.01 ml/kg (minimum
     0.1 ml/dose, maximum 1.0 ml) SC *or*
     Epinephrine (1:10,000) 0.1 ml/kg (minimum
     1 ml/dose, maximum 10 ml) IV
     May repeat once in 5 min *and*
  2. Diphenhydramine (Benadryl) 1–2 mg/kg
     (maximum 50 mg) IM/IV *and*
  3. If severe reaction, use hydrocortisone (Solu-
     Cortef)
     - 5–10 mg/kg IV
     - Can add same amount to IV fluids over
       next 8 hr
- If BP falling, treat as shock (see p 659)
- If bronchospasm present, treat as in asthma (see
  p 608)
- Observe patient for recurrence of symptoms,
  which may occur over the next 24 hr. This "late
  reaction" can be life threatening.
- See p 22 for management of anaphylaxis once
  acute episode is resolved

TRIAGE OF THE MAJOR TRAUMA PATIENT

General Considerations

- The pediatric victim of multiple trauma
  deserves the highest level of medical attention
  available
- The history of the mechanism and force of the
  trauma is invaluable as a guide to being suspicious of injury. For example, a child who has
  fallen from a three-story balcony deserves
  thorough assessment and observation even if
  initially there appear to be only minor injuries.
- Common life threatening problems in the immediate period after the traumatic event include
  acute respiratory failure (e.g., airway obstruction
  or apnea) and hemorrhagic hypovolemia

Management

- Immediate management
  1. The initial attention of medical staff should be directed toward basic resuscitation, with maintenance of the airway, breathing, and circulation (see p 652)
  2. Additional experienced staff should be alerted
  3. Consider transfer to a pediatric trauma center *after*
     - Organizing the transfer through direct physician-to-physician contact
     - Stabilization
- Stabilization involves
  1. Securing a patent airway
     - Assume that the patient has a fractured cervical spine
     - Clear the pharynx; position the chin and jaw as for CPR
     - Intubate the trachea if
       a. Simpler measures of clearing airway fail
       b. The patient has a Glasgow coma score of 7 or less (see p 481)
       c. There is an airway burn
  2. Assisting ventilation if there is
     - Apnea
     - Inefficient ventilation due to chest trauma
     - A Glasgow coma score of 7 or less (see p 481)
  3. Securing intravenous access preferably with two wide bore cannulas
  4. Securing reasonable hemostasis and treating hypovolemic shock
     - Even in the presence of head injury, 10–20 ml/kg of Ringer's lactate or 10 ml/kg of a colloidal solution is a reasonable volume of fluid to infuse rapidly into a patient with signs of hypovolemic shock after trauma
     - Have sufficient fluid available to continue resuscitation during transport of the patient

- Give blood if more than 10% of the child's blood volume has been lost (blood volume in a child is 80 ml/kg)
  - Antishock trousers may be helpful if available in pediatric size (do not inflate the abdominal component if there is suspicion of diaphragmatic rupture)
5. Examination of the patient "top to toe" for significant injury (see assessment below)
6. Passage of a nasogastric or orogastric tube (consider the latter in the presence of facial or basal skull fractures)
7. Administration of oxygen to all patients
8. In hospitals with medium level trauma care facilities, baseline investigations should be performed before transport to a pediatric trauma center: blood gases, hemoglobin, X-match, electrolytes, and chest x-ray
9. Insertion of chest drains into all ventilated patients with documented pneumothorax or hemothorax
10. Measures to avoid hypothermia to which children are more prone than adults (see p 676)

- Further assessment: Examine the following for the presence of:
  1. Head
     - Laceration, bruising, swelling $\pm$ fracture
     - Hemorrhage from nose, mouth, or ears or clear fluid from nose or ears
  2. Neck
     - Tenderness
     - Laryngeal or tracheal injury (abnormal cry, stridor, subcutaneous emphysema)
     - Assume there is cervical spine fracture
  3. Chest
     - Flail segment or penetrating wounds
     - Signs of pneumothorax or hemothorax (tracheal deviation, auscultation for reduced air entry, chest expansion)
     - Rib fractures, bruising over precordium

4. Abdomen
    - Penetrating wounds
    - Bowel sounds
    - Guarding
    - Peritoneal lavage should not be performed unless discussed with a pediatric surgeon
5. Pelvis
    - Instability or pain on compression
    - Perineal injury
6. Extremities
    - Fractures-dislocations (remove clothing!)
    - Pulses, perfusion
7. Back
    - Tenderness of spine
    - Bruising of flanks

TRANSPORT OF THE TRAUMATIZED CHILD

General Considerations

Aim: To avoid deterioration in transport in order to arrive with a stable patient

Caution: Monitoring during transport is difficult, and the performance of medical tasks is much harder. The key to a successful transport is the stabilization of the patient and adequate fixation of all lines, drains, and tubes!

Discuss the transport with receiving physician—either:
1. Trauma team leader: usually the general surgeon on call
2. ICU physician: an intensivist often experienced in transport
3. Emergency room physician: experienced in medical emergencies

Consider asking the receiving hospital to transport the patient if they have transport capability

Management

- Land vs. helicopter vs. fixed wing

1. Land
   - Quicker to arrange
   - Can be stopped en route to perform tasks or diverted to another hospital if patient suddenly deteriorates
   - Slower for long journeys
   - Requires more fluids, drugs, oxygen for the trip
   - Paramedic assistance may not be available
2. Helicopter
   - Not always available (already in use, bad weather)
   - May require land transport to heliport
   - Fast for medium distance transport
   - Usually well equipped
   - Paramedic support usually provided
3. Fixed wing
   - Slow to arrange
   - May not have equipment or personnel provided
   - Requires land transport at each end
   - Useful for long distance transport to a major facility once patient is stabilized

In addition, transport by helicopter or fixed wing aircraft involves transport at altitude. The extra problems include

- Increased gas volume during ascent, e.g., expansion of pneumothorax, air in stomach, air in inflated cuff of endotracheal tube, air above fluid level in drip chamber of intravenous line
- Fall in the partial pressure of oxygen; worse in unpressurized craft
- Often increased background noise levels, making auscultation difficult
- Vibration of concern in new spine fractures (though road transport may be as bad)
- Confined space, with difficult access to the patient, especially if the aircraft interior is not designed for regular patient transport

- Prior to transport
  1. Check equipment
     - Intubation equipment
     - Adequate oxygen supply
     - Sufficient fluids for maintenance and resuscitation
     - Drugs available, drawn up, and at hand (e.g., anticonvulsants)
     - Suction equipment
     - Humidification, e.g., small condenser humidifier on endotracheal tube
     - ECG monitor
     - BP cuff or Doppler monitor
     - Oxygen saturation monitor if available
     - Precordial or esophageal stethoscope
  2. Ensure that appropriate personnel accompany the child, e.g., MD, transport trained RN, or paramedic
- Respiration
  1. Secure the airway: endotracheal Intubation is usually necessary—a well-taped nasal tube is preferable to an oral tube. Use a bite block in orally intubated patients.
  2. Ensure adequate ventilation: head injury patients with Glasgow coma scores (see p 481) of 7 or less should be mildly hyper-ventilated and paralyzed for transport
  3. Use excess oxygen rather than too little
  4. Insert chest drainage tubes if there is pneu-mothorax and attach to Heimlich valves to avoid clamping chest drains
  5. Use a condenser humidifier (i.e., Swedish nose)
- Cardiovascular
  1. Stabilize the blood pressure and pulse rate before transport
  2. Antishock trousers may be helpful. Do not use the abdominal section if diaphragmatic rupture is suspected.
  3. Two intravenous cannulas are advisable. Port-

able syringe drivers are preferable to hanging fluid bags because of limited head room.
4. Remember: BP may be well maintained by tachycardia and peripheral vasoconstriction even in the presence of severe hypovolemia
- Also:
  1. Nasogastric tube to open drainage
  2. Remember possibility of cervical spine fracture
  3. Immobilize limb fractures
  4. Insert urinary catheter unless urethral injury is suspected
  5. Aim to maintain normothermia
  6. Consider taking finger-prick blood sugar estimation strip for at-risk patients (neonates, fasting, liver failure)
  7. Keep record of observations during transport

RESPIRATORY FAILURE

Asthma: see p 606

Choking: see p 655

Epiglottitis: see p 595

Respiratory Arrest: see p 652

General Considerations

Definition: Respiratory failure is the inability of the respiratory system to meet the body's demand for oxygen delivery and carbon dioxide elimination. It need not be due only to lung disease—a multitude of conditions including neurologic, cardiac, and multisystem disorders may result in inadequate gas exchange.

Common Clinical Features in Respiratory Failure

- Decreased or absent breath sounds
- Tachypnea or bradypnea-apnea

- Severe retractions and use of accessory muscles
- Cyanosis
- Restlessness or stupor, hypotonia, weak gag
- Grunting
- In obstructive failure—drooling, stridor, wheeze (depending on level of obstruction)
- $PaO_2 < 60$
- $PaCO_2$
  1. Low, normal: seen in failure usually due to ventilation-perfusion mismatch (e.g., pneumonia, sepsis, asthma). Called type I failure.
  2. High: seen in hypoventilation (e.g., coma, paresis, obstruction, or terminal stages of type I failure when fatigue develops). Called type II failure.

Management

- Immediate management
  1. Significant apnea (i.e., respiratory arrest) warrants initiation of an arrest protocol (see p 652)
  2. If patient is alert with respiratory distress, manage *gently* but not slowly
  3. If patient is stuporous or weak, consider first improving the airway with correct positioning and insertion of oropharyngeal airway
  4. Provide humidified oxygen to all patients. Note:
     - In upper airway obstruction, although hypoxia may be relieved by oxygen administration, once hypoxia develops it is imperative that the obstruction be relieved immediately. Certain children may be made more restless by the method of oxygen delivery; hence many hospitals do not routinely administer oxygen to this group.
     - Retinopathy of prematurity and chronic obstructive airway disease should never be excuses to avoid oxygen in respiratory distress; they are merely indications to

monitor that therapy more closely
5. Minimal handling, but monitor vital signs
   closely, since deterioration can be precipitous
   and hypoxia is the commonest cause of
   cardiac arrest in children
6. Establish IV if patient is unable to feed because of distress, is likely to be intubated, or
   requires IV medications and rehydration.
   Note: In children with upper airway obstruction, the anxiety produced by insertion of an
   intravenous cannula may exacerbate the
   respiratory distress. For example, in most
   pediatric hospitals, children with epiglottitis
   WOULD NOT receive an intravenous cannula until induction of anesthesia for
   intubation.
7. Consider pneumothorax-effusion as cause of
   distress
- Investigations
  1. Blood gases (but be careful in upper
     airway obstruction: clinical assessment is
     usually just as helpful in determining therapy,
     whereas the distress associated with drawing
     the sample may precipitate complete
     obstruction)
  2. Chest x-ray (often more helpful than clinical
     examination)
  3. Obtaining a lateral neck x-ray or chest x-ray
     should NEVER delay the establishment of an
     artificial airway in severe airway obstruction,
     and should be performed ONLY if the
     highest level of supervision in the radiology
     suite is available
- Other management
  1. Aerosols: consider salbutamol 0.03 ml/kg
     (maximum 1 ml) of 0.5% solution in 3 ml
     normal saline by mask (as in asthma, p 608)
     when bronchoconstriction is a component.
     Consider racemic epinephrine (2.25% solu-
     tion) 0.5 ml in 3 ml normal saline for sub-
     glottic edema.

2. Pharyngeal suctioning—avoid in upper airway obstruction
3. Fluids: adequate hydration is necessary to ensure that secretions do not become inspissated. Nevertheless humidification of inspired gases reduces respiratory fluid losses so that usual maintenance fluid volumes may represent overhydration and risk interstitial edema in these patients.
4. Intubation
   - Provides a means of guaranteeing a high inspired oxygen concentration
   - Protects and secures the airway
   - Facilitates tracheobronchial toilet
   - Permits CPAP/IPPV
   - The indication for intubation depends on current trend of the illness and the severity of distress. Remember: when intubation is indicated, oxygen delivery with IPPV should always be attempted with bag and mask until expert assistance with intubation arrives.
5. IPPV is often required in type II failure, whereas CPAP with supplemental oxygen may be adequate in some cases of type I failure
6. Physiotherapy may be of value for conditions in which secretions block major bronchi
7. Specific therapy for underlying etiology of respiratory failure, e.g., antibiotics after culturing blood and secretions in pneumonia, antifailure therapy in heart disease

NEAR DROWNING

General Considerations

- Immediate and continuous resuscitation is of paramount importance in the prehospital and early hospital care
- Hypothermia may be present, making cardiac

resuscitation difficult, although the prognosis
may be improved (see p 676)

Management

- If respiratory or cardiac arrest is present, see
  p 652
- If comatose, in order to prevent secondary brain
  insult, begin intensive therapy with controlled
  ventilation, circulatory support, and measures to
  reduce raised intracranial pressure. Monitor in
  an intensive care unit (see p 478).
- Insert a nasogastric tube. Near drowning victims
  frequently swallow large volumes of water and
  risk pulmonary aspiration if consciousness is
  impaired.
- If conscious state is normal or minimally impaired, remain in hospital for close observation
  for 24 hr
- Acute respiratory failure may occur, usually
  secondary to pulmonary aspiration (see p 668)

SMOKE INHALATION

General Considerations

- Give 100% oxygen from time of rescue until
  proven unnecessary
- Mechanism of injury
    1. Thermal injury—mainly affects the upper air-
       way with edema and obstruction, which can
       worsen over the first hours after injury
    2. Particulate material—results in tracheo-
       bronchitis
    3. Toxic fumes—may reach the distal airways
       and cause alveolitis
    4. Carbon monoxide and cyanide can enter the
       blood and poison cellular respiration

Clinical Features

- Consider the possibility of severe smoke inhalation in all fire victims, but especially those with

1. History of exposure in a confined space
2. Facial burns, singed nasal hairs, hoarse voice
3. Carbonaceous sputum

Management

- Investigations
  1. Arterial blood gas analysis
     - Frequently shows metabolic acidosis
     - PaO_2 does NOT reflect available oxygen in the presence of carboxyhemoglobin
  2. Carboxyhemoglobin level: elevated levels require treating with 100% oxygen; reduces half-life to ~60 min
  3. Chest x-ray: essential as baseline but may be normal in the first 24 hr in up to 40% of patients
- Treatment
  1. Airway patency
     - A secure airway, with an endotracheal tube if necessary, is essential for adequate respiratory exchange
     - The development of upper airway edema may make late intervention difficult or impossible. Endotracheal intubation also makes possible the application of IPPV/ PEEP or CPAP and aids oxygen therapy, humidification, and tracheobronchial hygiene.
     - Relatively high ventilation pressures and PEEP may be required because of the alveolar capillary leak, reduced compliance, and possible pulmonary edema
  2. Supplemental oxygen: high FIO_2 (100% if possible) until COHb levels are <0.05 (5%) or 5–6 hr of therapy
  3. Bronchial hygiene
     - Adequate humidification, physiotherapy, and tracheal suction are essential
     - Bronchoscopy in rare circumstances may

be necessary to remove tracheal debris
4. Fluids
- As with all burn patients, adequacy of urine output is a good yardstick of adequacy of rehydration: aim for 1 ml/kg/hr
- Patients with smoke inhalation are at risk of adult respiratory distress syndrome (ARDS). Thus more careful monitoring of fluid balance and circulating blood volume is required.
5. Antibiotics: not recommended prophylactically
6. Steroids: no evidence to support their use is currently available

INTUBATION

Indications

- To secure the airway
  1. Severe airway obstruction
  2. Unprotected airway (e.g., coma or prolonged seizures)
- Deliver high oxygen concentration when adequate arterial oxygenation cannot be delivered by simple means, e.g., O_2 mask or hood
- Deliver positive pressure ventilation, e.g., in respiratory failure with CO_2 retention or exhaustion that does not respond to other therapy

General Considerations

- Intubation should NOT be attempted by the inexperienced if more skilled personnel are available
- In the apneic patient, positive pressure ventilation by bag and mask technique with oxygen MUST be administered before attempts at laryngoscopy
- N.B. Airway obstruction that may appear complete often can be partially overcome by bag and mask technique, allowing correction of

hypoxemia and preparation for intubation
- Suctioning equipment should be available when bagging, as well as prior to intubation
- Preoxygenation and a rapid sequence induction with cricoid pressure should be used in any elective intubation in the emergency department, unless there is anatomic airway obstruction
- Muscle relaxant and sedating drugs SHOULD NOT be used in patients with anatomic airway obstruction. Intubation in these patients must NEVER be attempted by the inexpert unless a dire emergency exists.
- Nasal intubation should be attempted only after oral intubation is established and the patient is stable. It should not be performed if a basal skull fracture or severe facial injury is suspected.
- The technique of intubation should be learned under controlled circumstances, e.g., in the operating room

Endotracheal Tubes

- Size
  1. The correct size endotracheal tube (ETT) is a compromise between the risks of pulmonary aspiration and laryngeal mucosal ischemia
  2. The appropriate ETT is the largest one that allows a leak of air around the tube when 25–30 cm H_2O positive pressure is applied
     - See chart giving tube size for age and weight—inside front cover
     - A rough guide to ETT size (internal diameter) in children older than 1 yr is:

       $$\frac{\text{age (yr)}}{4} + 4 \text{ mm}$$

  3. Expect to use a smaller ETT if
     - Down syndrome
     - History of airway obstruction
  4. For patients with croup, select 3.0 mm for

<6 mo, 3.5 mm for 6–24 mo, and $\frac{age\ (yr)}{4}$ + 3 mm for older patients

- Position
  1. Correct position is with the ETT tip at mid-tracheal level, confirmed by x-ray; check for equal chest movement and breath sounds
  2. A rough guide for distance to insert to mid-trachea
     - Oral ETT: (tube size × 2) + 4 cm
     - Nasal ETT
       a. ≤4 kg: (1.5 × weight [kg]) + 6 cm
       b. >6 mo (<1 yr): 12–13 cm
       c. ≥1 yr: age (yr) + 13 cm
- Further care
  1. Securely fix endotracheal tube
  2. Restrain arms and legs to prevent self-extubation
  3. Transfer to appropriate area where facilities for continuous nursing and medical care are available
  4. Ascribe further breathing difficulty to ETT blockage until disproven

EMERGENCY MANAGEMENT OF HYPOTHERMIA

General Considerations

- Definition: hypothermia is a core temperature less than 35° C
- Patients at risk are
  1. Neonates, especially prematures
  2. Victims of immersion or exposure to cold
  3. Those in coma or paralyzed
  4. Those with endocrine diseases such as hypothyroidism or hypoadrenalism
- For hospitalized patients the best treatment is prevention
  1. By avoiding prolonged exposure during procedures and transport
  2. Nursing in the thermoneutral range

3. When patients need large fluid volumes, heating the infusions
4. Regularly noting the temperature of acutely ill children

Clinical Features

- Cardiovascular system
  1. Initially there is a sympathetic stimulation with later depression of BP and cardiac output as the core temperature falls
  2. ECG shows prolongation of all phases of the cardiac cycle, and a J wave (elevation of the ST segment) may be seen at 32–33° C
  3. Supraventricular arrhythmias are common below 33° C and ventricular below 30° C
- Nervous system: rigidity and pupillary dilation occur at 30–33° C, with coma under 28–30° C and no pupillary light reflex under 25° C
- Respiratory system: in older children apnea occurs below 26° C. However, apneic episodes are a common feature of mild hypothermia in premature neonates.
- Renal: "cold diuresis" occurs; hypokalemia or hyperkalemia may occur

The major risks of hypothermia and rewarming are hypovolemia, acidosis, hypokalemia, and hypoglycemia

Diagnosis

- Be suspicious for the diagnosis
- A low temperature reading rectal thermometer is necessary
- In profound hypothermia the differential diagnosis is death: if hypothermia is the primary disorder (rather than merely secondary to death from other causes), resuscitation should be continued until the core temperature is over 33° C.

Management

- Investigations
  1. CBC, electrolytes, Cr/BUN, glucose (especially in neonates), amylase, blood gases, drug screen, coagulation screen, and thyroid function
  2. Chest x-ray and ECG
  3. Monitor ECG, core temperature, urine output, and temperature of inspired gases
- Treatment
  1. Over 32° C
     - Remove from cold stress
     - Remove wet clothing
     - Cover
     - Heat IV fluid to 37° C using "blood warmer" devices
     - Note: there is some controversy regarding active rewarming with warming blankets, since there is a risk of burns and acidemic-hyperkalemic blood returning from the cold extremities
  2. Under 32° C
     - If arrested, resuscitate (see p 652)
     - Note: arrhythmias may be resistant to cardioversion until rewarming occurs
     - Ventilate with oxygen (avoid hyperventilation)
     - Treat metabolic acidosis
     - Other simple measures include warming IV solutions, warm gastric or rectal lavage, and radiant heater lamps
     - Peritoneal lavage with 37–43° C dialysate solution can be used in severe cases; heart-lung bypass, although ideal, is usually impractical
  3. In all cases, a useful adjunct to rewarming is inhalation of heated gases (in severe cases by endotracheal tube with heated humidified gases at 37° C, or in milder cases by mask with inspired gas at 42–46° C)

Frostbite

- Cold-induced tissue injury may accompany hypothermia or may occur independently
- Usually restricted to head and extremities: the frozen part is white and firm
- AFTER the core temperature has returned to normal, immerse the injured extremity for about 20 min into water kept between 37 and 40° C (do not start to thaw an extremity if there is any chance of the patient being reexposed to the cold)
- Refer patient to plastic surgery

EMERGENCY MANAGEMENT OF HYPERTHERMIA

General Considerations

- Fever is a core temperature over 38° C. Abnormally high core temperature occurs when
    1. Metabolic-environmental heat exceeds the body's thermoregulatory capacity for dissipation, e.g., in young athletes exercising in warm environments (made worse by dehydration or incidental fever) and in children overheated in cars, or neonates under overhead heaters
    2. The hypothalamic set point for temperature control is raised by
        - Pyrogens in sepsis, toxemia
        - Injury to the hypothalamus
- Over 40° C there may be failure of mechanisms for temperature control

Clinical Features

- Milder forms of environmental overheating (e.g., ''heat exhaustion'') are characterized by water depletion, with
    1. Lethargy
    2. Thirst
    3. Headache

    4. Vomiting
    5. Tachycardia and hypotension
    6. Hemoconcentration
    7. Hypernatremia
- Severe hyperthermia (e.g., "heat stroke" with core temperature over 41° C) is characterized by
  1. More severe neurologic dysfunction (combativeness, delirium, convulsions, and when temperature >43° C—coma)
  2. Vomiting and diarrhea
  3. Sweating (may stop when temperature >41.6° C)
  4. Risk of rhabdomyolysis, acute tubular necrosis, and DIC
- If there is no history consistent with environmental overheating, look for signs of sepsis. Beware: infants with infection, including meningitis, may lack features pointing to the site of infection early in the illness.

Management

- Investigations and monitoring
  1. Monitor for hypoglycemia
  2. Record urine output and vital signs
  3. Search for sepsis. The thoroughness of a search for sepsis is influenced by the history, child's age (be more suspicious in small infants), general appearance, and clinical signs of infection.
- Treatment
  1. Mild hyperthermia can be treated by
     - Removal of the heat source
     - Antipyretics (acetaminophen 40–60 mg/kg/day PO/PR ÷ q4–6h)
     - Fluid replacement
     - Cooling with ice packs to head and trunk
  2. More severe hyperthermia requires in addition
     - Rapid cooling; consider immersion of the trunk in cold water

- Cardiovascular support (see shock, p 659)
- Oxygen
- Chlorpromazine (0.5 mg/kg/dose IM) to reduce shivering, if the cardiovascular status is stable

TABLE FOR CALCULATION OF DRUG INFUSION DILUTION

- See Fig. 1 (p 682)

Suggested Reading

1. Fleisher G, Ludwig S, eds. Textbook of pediatric emergency medicine. Baltimore: Williams & Wilkins, 1983.
2. Levin DL, Morriss FC, Moore GC. A practical guide to pediatric intensive care. 2nd ed. St. Louis: C.V. Mosby, 1984.
3. Tintinalli JE, ed. Symposium on resuscitation. Emerg Med Clin North Am 1983:1(3).
4. Wilkins EW, ed. MGH textbook of emergency medicine. Baltimore: Williams & Wilkins, 1983.

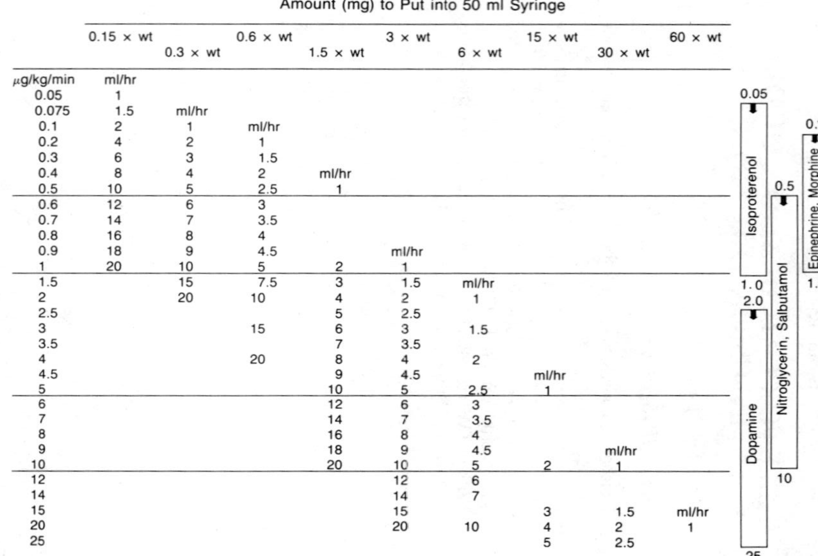

Amount (mg) to Put into 50 ml Syringe

μg/kg/min	0.15 × wt	0.3 × wt	0.6 × wt	1.5 × wt	3 × wt	6 × wt	15 × wt	30 × wt	60 × wt
	ml/hr								
0.05	1								
0.075	1.5	ml/hr							
0.1	2	1	ml/hr						
0.2	4	2	1						
0.3	6	3	1.5						
0.4	8	4	2	ml/hr					
0.5	10	5	2.5	1					
0.6	12	6	3						
0.7	14	7	3.5						
0.8	16	8	4						
0.9	18	9	4.5		ml/hr				
1	20	10	5	2	1				
1.5		15	7.5	3	1.5	ml/hr			
2		20	10	4	2	1			
2.5				5	2.5				
3			15	6	3	1.5			
3.5				7	3.5				
4			20	8	4	2			
4.5				9	4.5		ml/hr		
5				10	5	2.5	1		
6				12	6	3			
7				14	7	3.5			
8				16	8	4			
9				18	9	4.5		ml/hr	
10				20	10	5	2	1	
12					12	6			
14					14	7			
15					15		3	1.5	ml/hr
20					20	10	4	2	1
25							5	2.5	

30	15	6	3	1.5
40	20	8	4	2
50		10	5	2.5
100		20	10	5
150			15	7.5
200			20	10

Figure 1 Table for calculation of drug infusion dilution (can also use calculations at the bottom of table on p 657)

(1) Select desired drug dosage to be delivered in μg/kg/min (see named bars to right of chart—start at lower end of the dose range and adjust according to response). (2) Select infusion rate of syringe pump in ml/hr from table. (3) Calculate number of milligrams of drug to be mixed in 50 ml syringe: wt = patient's weight (kg). If 250 ml bag is used, add same mass of drug, but run at 5 × rate quoted in table.

For example, a 7 kg infant requires dopamine: from the bars on the right of the chart, the range of dosages for dopamine is 2 to 25 μg/kg/min; start with 2 μg/kg/min. We will opt for a rate of fluid infusion of 1 ml/hr. For 1 ml/hr to give 2 μg/kg/min, we need to put 6 × weight, i.e., 42 mg into 50 ml of solution.
(Modified from Shann F. Continuous drug infusion in children: a table for simplifying calculation. Crit Care Med 1983; 11:462-463.)

IV

PROCEDURES

PROCEDURES

BLOOD COLLECTION AND INTRAVENOUS INFUSION

Venipuncture

Sites

- Antecubital veins (e.g., median and cephalic veins)—route of choice in all age groups
- Veins at dorsum of hand (e.g., dorsal venous arch)
- Scalp veins—a useful alternative for newborns and infants, but moreso for infusions than for phlebotomy
- External jugular vein—easy accessibility in patients with otherwise difficult venous access
- Internal jugular vein
- Femoral vein
- N.B. Any available vein may be used in critical situations

Technique

- For venipuncture of lower arms, lower legs, hands, and feet
  1. The child or infant is immobilized and the site prepared with an appropriate antiseptic, e.g., alcohol or Betadine
  2. Apply a tourniquet proximal to desired site for venipuncture, to distend veins distally
  3. A 20–25 gauge needle or "butterfly" scalp vein infusion needle, with syringe attached, can be used
  4. The skin is pierced with the needle, bevel up, just distal to the intended site of venipuncture

5. The needle is gently but forcibly introduced into the vein with a sharp jab (while maintaining some traction on overlying skin)
6. Gentle suction is applied with the syringe to withdraw blood from the vein without collapsing it. The flow of blood may be facilitated by gently "pumping" circumferentially with the fingers, proximal to the site of phlebotomy
7. When blood is withdrawn, release the tourniquet and apply pressure to the puncture site for 1–2 min

- For scalp veins, proceed as above with the following exceptions and additions:
  1. The scalp may have to be shaved prior to insertion of the needle
  2. The tourniquet is applied circumferentially around the head from the forehead to the occiput (preferably using a rubber band)
  3. For this location a butterfly needle with an attached catheter is preferable
- External jugular venipuncture
  1. Position child on table, with head rotated to one side, ~ 90 degrees
  2. Child should be restrained, preferably using "mummying" technique, with sheet or blanket
  3. Extend head over edge of table (or place towel roll beneath shoulders), 45 degrees toward the floor
  4. Assistant should hold patient's head in position
  5. Make infant cry (if not already doing so!) to distend vein
  6. Using 20–22 gauge needle, 2–4 cm long, attached to syringe; penetrate skin in caudal direction where vein crosses sternocleidomastoid muscle
  7. Exert negative pressure on syringe and penetrate distended vein with sharp jab. Blood will flow freely into syringe once vein is entered.

8. Apply firm pressure over puncture site once needle is withdrawn
- Internal jugular venipuncture
THIS IS A POTENTIALLY DANGEROUS PRO-CEDURE; MAY → hematoma, subcutaneous emphysema; proceed with care! This location should be a last resort only!
1. Adequate restraining is absolutely required, using mummying plus help from assistants
2. Child is positioned as described above for external jugular puncture
3. Select a point on posterior border of sternocleidomastoid at junction of upper ⅓ and lower ⅔
4. Place a finger in sternal notch. Insert needle (22 gauge, 4 cm) at selected site, parallel to floor and aimed at finger 2 cm above sternal notch.
5. Transfix vein while exerting negative pressure on syringe. Blood is often obtained while needle is being withdrawn.
6. At completion, sit child upright, while applying firm pressure over puncture site for 2–5 min
- Femoral venipuncture
1. Not a desirable site, as may → septic arthritis of hip joint. Use only in emergency situations.
2. Place child in frog-leg position
3. Assistant should be available to hold legs in proper position
4. Identify femoral pulse (artery)
5. After preparing site carefully with antiseptic agent(s), insert needle just medial to femoral pulse, 1–2 cm distal to flexion crease of groin, aiming vertically, slightly cephalad, and slightly laterally, to transfix vein
6. Withdraw needle slowly, exerting traction on plunger
7. When blood appears in syringe, stop with-

drawing needle and remove appropriate
quantity of blood

8. At completion, maintain pressure on puncture site for 2–3 min

Notes About IV Infusions

- Many of the sites noted above, especially ante-
cubital, dorsum of hands, scalp, and dorsum of
feet, can be used for IV infusions
- Proceed as for venipuncture, except for following points:
  1. Extra care should be taken in preparing site
  aseptically
  2. A "butterfly" or intravenous catheter (e.g.,
  Angiocath) is used, the system flushed
  through with normal saline prior to insertion
  into vein, and attached to a syringe filled
  with same. The nondominant limb should be
  selected if at all possible.
  3. Following intravenous insertion of needle or
  catheter, the system is again slowly flushed to
  rule out extravasation
  4. The system is connected to infusion fluid,
  after the needle or catheter has been securely taped (with sterile tapes), and an armboard
  applied if appropriate
  5. IV catheters or "butterflies" should not remain in situ for >48–72 hr, to decrease risk
  of thrombophlebitis and its sequelae
  6. For intra-abdominal trauma, avoid using lower limb veins.

DERMATOLOGIC PROCEDURES

Skin Biopsy

- A punch biopsy technique is most efficient. Occasionally an elliptical excision is preferable
when the disease is deep seated or the whole
lesion is to be removed

Technique for Punch Biopsy

- Obtain consent for procedure. Advise that there will be a small scar.
- Assemble skin biopsy tray (contains forceps, needle driver, iris scissors), 3 or 4 mm punch, Xylocaine, syringe and needles, suture material, povidone-iodine and alcohol preps, sterile gloves, and specimen bottle (10% formalin)
- Select site. If eruption is widespread, select a well-developed representative lesion in least conspicuous site. If eruption is vesicular, or suspected vasculitis, select the newest lesion.
- Cleanse site with povidone-iodine and alcohol. Inject local anesthetic.
- Gently stretch skin surrounding lesion perpendicular to the natural skin creases (so that the round punch defect becomes elliptical and closes better). Hold punch at right angles to skin and push down firmly 3–4 mm, rotating punch slightly for a clean cut.
- Carefully withdraw punch. To remove specimen from site, spear it with a needle, elevate it above skin surface, and snip base with iris scissors (do not squeeze with forceps as this will distort the histopathology).
- Suture if necessary

Wood's Lamp Examination

- Emits light in ultraviolet A spectrum (360 mm). It is useful in the following circumstances:

Detection of Fluorescent Organisms

- Tinea capitis caused by the *Microsporum* species shows a green fluorescence. A negative examination does not exclude a fungal infection, however, as other fungal species causing scalp ringworm do not fluoresce.
- The bacteria causing erythrasma (*Corynebacterium minutissimum*) show coral red fluorescence

Delineation of Pigmentary Disorders

- Depigmented lesions (vitiligo) show accentuated contrast with normal skin. Hypopigmented lesions do also, but to a lesser extent.
- Hyperpigmentation caused by increased epidermal melanin such as freckles are more prominent under Wood's lamp, whereas dermal melanin is not accentuated

Miscellaneous

- Porphyrins fluoresce (e.g., in urine)
- Tetracycline in teeth fluoresce

SURGICAL PROCEDURES

- N.B. The following guide is intended to help physicians who are faced with a clinical situation that requires the immediate implementation of one of the following simple surgical procedures. It is not designed to serve as a substitute for learning the techniques from an experienced teacher. Help from such an individual should be sought whenever possible.

Intravenous Cutdown

Indications

- Any situation in an infant or child that requires urgent venous access, but when such access is difficult to obtain in the usual way, e.g., severe dehydration or shock from any cause, during cardiopulmonary resuscitation, or following multiple injuries or trauma
- In patients on long-term intravenous therapy, when percutaneous IV cannulation is impossible, and operative insertion of a central venous catheter is not feasible

Technique

- Equipment needed: a No. 15 blade scalpel, 4–0

silk ligatures, 4–0 nylon silk stitch, a fine hemostat, fine scissors, No. 5 umbilical artery (UA) catheter or 22 gauge intravenous catheter, 1% Xylocaine without epinephrine, gauze sponges, disinfectant solution, surgical gloves, sterile towels, good lighting, tourniquet
- An assistant who can help with immobilizing the child is helpful
- It is easiest to cut down on the long saphenous vein at the ankle, ~ 1 cm above and ~ 1 cm medial to the medial malleolus
- Infiltrate the skin over the vein with 1% Xylocaine
- A 1 cm transverse incision is made, and the subcutaneous fat is gently spread using the hemostat in a direction parallel to the vein. (The vein may be visible as a bluish tubular structure.)
- If not, the tips of the hemostat are pushed to the deep fascia overlying the bone and used to lift all the more superficial soft tissues
- The tips of the hemostat are then opened. Fat and other soft tissues will separate, leaving the vein visible as a white cordlike structure if it is empty of blood.
- Two 4–0 silk ties are passed around the vein. The distal tie is ligated and used to apply downward traction on the vein.
- A small nick is made on the surface of the vein and used to insert the UA catheter
- The catheter is advanced, preferably until blood can be freely drawn back
- Alternatively, an ordinary No. 22 or 20 IV catheter can be used to cannulate the vein under direct vision
- The proximal 4–0 tie is used to secure the vein to the catheter
- A 4–0 nylon stitch is used to close the incision and secure the hub of the catheter to the skin
- The antecubital fossa provides another access site, although the size of the veins here is

smaller than in the ankle, and their distribution is more variable
- In most cases of abdominal trauma, it is safer to start a cutdown in the upper extremities

Chest Tube Insertion

Indications

- Proven or suspected tension pneumothorax after trauma
- Symptomatic pneumothorax
- Hemothorax
- Empyema
- Symptomatic pleural effusion
- Any size pneumothorax in patient on ventilator

Technique

- Equipment needed: 1% Xylocaine, chest tube (No. 12 for newborn, No. 16 for infant, No. 22 for child less than 40 kg, No. 24 for child over 20 kg or adult), scalpel with No. 15 blade, hemostat, Kelly forceps, 2–0 nylon skin suture, Pleurovac or bottle with underwater seal drain (or Heimlich valve if available), tubing for Pleurovac
- The sixth intercostal space at the midaxillary line can be used to insert chest tubes for all indications
- In cases of suspected tension pneumothorax, a 20 gauge Intracath connected to IV tubing with the other end placed under water in a small cup can be inserted into the second interspace in the midclavicular line
- After the catheter is inserted, the needle is withdrawn and air allowed to drain, relieving the tension in the pleural cavity and allowing for a more controlled insertion of the chest tube
- After the skin overlying the chosen insertion point is infiltrated with Xylocaine (if the clinical situation permits), a skin incision is made, and

Kelly forceps are advanced through the chest wall between the fifth and sixth ribs. The tips are spread once inside the pleural cavity, creating a tunnel.

- The Kelly forceps are then used to grasp the tip of the chest tube and to push it through the previously made tunnel into the pleural cavity. Considerable force may be necessary to do this, particularly in larger children.
- Alternatively, a chest tube may be inserted using a trocar. After a skin incision is made, the tube and trocar are advanced by pushing perpendicular to the chest wall into the pleural cavity. *Great care must be used to control the penetration of the trocar into the pleural cavity in order to prevent injury to underlying vital structures.* The chest tube is carefully advanced over the trocar into the pleural cavity. The trocar is then withdrawn.
- The chest tube must remain clamped with a Kelly forceps while it is being inserted before being connected to the tubing, thus preventing the inspiration of air into the pleural cavity
- After the tube is advanced a few centimeters, it is fixed to the skin with the nylon suture. It is connected to the Pleurovac and the underwater seal.
- The suction chamber should be filled with water to a height of 15–20 cm before insertion of the tube so that the tube can be unclamped quickly
- A chest x-ray should be obtained if possible to confirm the position of the tube, and to assess its effects

Tracheotomy

Indications

- Upper airway obstruction after trauma to the face and oral cavity when endotracheal intubation is not possible

- Any case of severe upper airway obstruction with impending cardiac arrest when endotracheal intubation is not possible

Technique

- Equipment needed: scalpel, antiseptic agent
- With the patient supine, the area below the thyroid cartilage but superior to the cricoid is palpated. This is the cricothyroid membrane. The area is prepared with appropriate antiseptic agent.
- The skin is incised transversely over the membrane. The scalpel is quickly pushed through the overlying tissues and through the membrane.
- Without removing the scalpel from the lumen of the trachea, turn it through 90 degrees so that a longitudinal incision in the trachea can also be made
- The resulting cruciate incision can be dilated with any available blunt instrument to allow air to enter
- If possible, a suction catheter should be forced down the trachea to clear any blood or secretions

Incision and Drainage of Abscess

Indications

- The most frequent site of suppurative lymphadenopathy in infants is in the cervical lymph nodes. An area of redness and induration will grow in size, and the induration will soften in a central area. Systemic antibiotics should be used if there is surrounding cellulitis.

Technique

- Equipment needed: 1% Xylocaine, scalpel with No. 15 blade, hemostat, Betadine soaked 1/4" gauze

- The skin overlying the softest area of the lump is infiltrated with Xylocaine. A small incision is made in the skin and deepened until the abscess cavity is entered. The pus is squeezed out. Gentle probing with a hemostat may help to evacuate loculated pockets of pus.
- After most of the pus is evacuated, a small length of gauze soaked in Betadine is packed into the abscess cavity. A clean dressing is applied. The packing may be removed 48 hr later; the surrounding swelling will gradually resolve.
- The above procedure can be done under local anesthesia in easily restrained babies, but in older children a general anesthetic may be required

NEONATAL PROCEDURES

Umbilical Vein Catheterization

Indications

- Emergencies, e.g., delivery room resuscitation when immediate venous access is required. Cardioactive and vasoactive drugs may be given via this route.
- Exchange transfusion, e.g., for Rh isoimmunization
- To monitor central venous pressure (CVP) in critically ill infants.
  N.B. For CVP monitoring, the catheter should be advanced into the inferior vena cava (IVC) via the ductus venosus. (For complications, see section under Exchange Transfusions, p 419.)

Technique

- Infant is kept warm in incubator or under radiant heater during procedure
- The shoulder-umbilicus length should be measured, and the appropriate calculation made

(from graph—Fig. 2) to determine catheter insertion length
- Umbilical tape is loosely tied at the base of the stump in the event of bleeding
- The umbilicus is "prepped" with antiseptic solution (e.g., Betadine) and draped. Then it is cut with scalpel to within 1.0–1.5 cm of the abdominal wall.
- Identify exposed vessels (two arteries, thick walled, and one vein, thin walled and larger)
- Insert catheter (size No. 5 or 8), which is connected to syringe via three-way stopcock ± blunt-ended needle (system filled with heparinized saline solution: 0.5–1 unit heparin/ml of normal saline), while maintaining gentle traction on cord stump
- The catheter is secured with a "pursestring" suture around the stump, followed by a "bridge tape" support (see Fig. 1)
- Confirm position of catheter with x-ray
- Following emergency procedure, the UVL should be removed and replaced with an umbilical artery line (UAL) or peripheral venous line as soon as possible

Umbilical Artery Catheterization

Indications

- To monitor mean arterial pressure (MAP) and arterial blood gas levels (ABGs) in the very sick infant
- Dextrose-containing solutions can also be infused via this route

Technique (See Fig. 1)

- Steps 1–5 as per UVL insertion
- After identifying the arteries, the closed tip of an iris forceps (or probe) should be gently inserted into the vessel lumen and then slowly released (or removed) to open the lumen. The

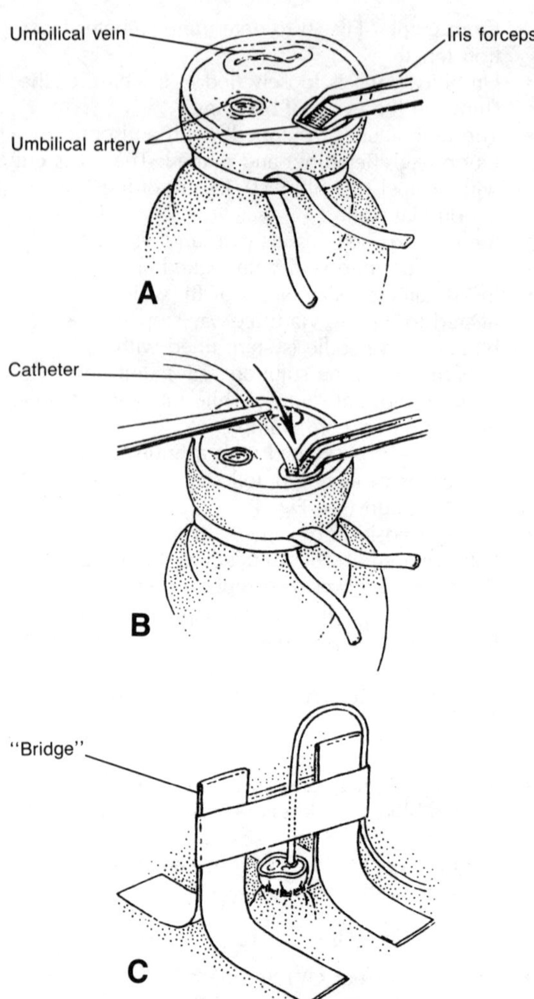

Figure 1 Umbilical artery catheterization. (Adapted from Klaus MH, Fanaroff AA, eds. Care of the high risk neonate. 3rd ed. Philadelphia: W.B. Saunders, 1986:431.)

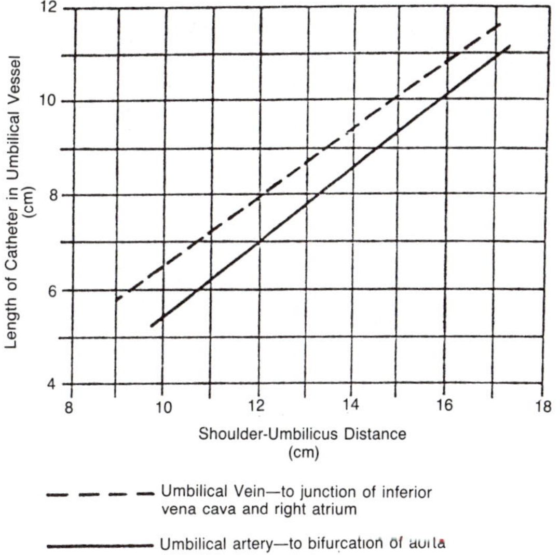

Figure 2 Determination of length of catheter to be inserted for appropriate arterial or venous placement. Determination of length of catheter to be inserted for appropriate arterial or venous placement. The length of the catheter read from the diagram is to the umbilical ring; the length of the umbilical cord stump present must be added. The shoulder-umbilicus distance is the perpendicular distance between parallel lines at the level of the umbilicus and through the distal ends of the clavicles. (From Klaus MH, Fanaroff AA, eds. Care of the high risk neonate. Philadelphia: W.B. Saunders, 1986:430.)

lumen should be maintained open for 45–60 sec at least.

- A sterile catheter of appropriate size (3.5 F for infants <1,500 g, and 5.0 F for infants >1,500 g) connected to syringe via three-way stopcock and blunt-ended needle (system filled with heparin in normal saline or dextrose-containing solution [1 unit heparin/ml])

- The catheter is slowly but firmly threaded into the artery (with traction on stump) to the desired length. Confirm its position (L3–L4 preferably) with x-ray. Secure line as for UVL (see Fig. 1).

Complications

- Blanching of toes, legs, or buttocks—possibly secondary to vasospasm—requires removal of the catheter in most cases. (Warming of the contralateral leg may help in some cases.)
- Hypertension secondary to high umbilical artery catheters has been described (although it also occurs with low catheters)
- Hemorrhage from loose connections or careless use of stopcocks is a major complication

Neonatal Endotracheal Intubation

Indications

- To facilitate ventilation in infants unable to do so adequately on their own or with non-ETT CPAP, e.g., apnea resistant to drug therapy
- To aspirate meconium from trachea of infant at birth
- For (routine) surgical procedures on infants, e.g., PDA ligation

Technique (See Fig. 3)

- In emergency situations, oral intubation may be preferred, followed by elective nasotracheal intubation, depending on the preference of your unit
- Intubation is best performed with the help of an assistant who can stabilize the infant's head and assist with taping of the ETT in situ
- Prior to intubation, the infant should be ventilated with bag and mask in 100% O_2 until heart rate and central color are satisfactory. This

should be repeated between reattempts at intubation, allowing the infant to recover.

- Tube size should be selected appropriately (Table 1), but one size above and below should also be available
- Intubation should be performed under sterile conditions under radiant heater or in incubator
- Use laryngoscope with Miller 0 (premature) or 1 (>2,500 g infant) blade
- The baby's head should be extended (*not* hyperextended) and held in position by the assistant or by fourth and fifth fingers of L hand of person intubating
- Cricoid pressure may assist visualization of vocal cords
- The laryngoscope blade is passed into the right side of the infant's mouth and then swept gently to the midline, to move the tongue out of the way (see Fig. 3). It is then advanced until the cords are visualized.
- The ETT is then inserted between the cords to about 2 cm below the glottis. (An obturator may be required for oral intubation; a Magill forceps is useful for nasal intubation.) The ETT should be secured with tape after application of tincture of benzoin.
- The approximate distance on insertion of the ETT can be calculated from the graph in Figure 4
- The tube position can be checked clinically by auscultating for equal air entry on both sides of the chest, but should be confirmed with a chest x-ray

Complications

- Traumatizing the gums with the blade during intubation
- Intubation of R main stem bronchus with collapse of contralateral side
- Failure to respond to cardiac monitor (bradycardia) during procedure, thereby unnecessarily stressing the infant

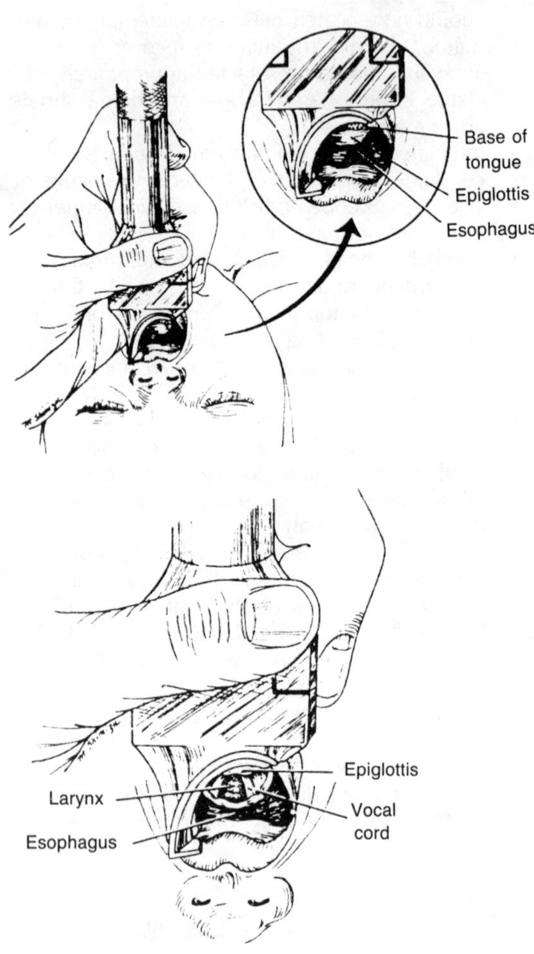

Figure 3 Neonatal endotracheal intubation. (From Klaus MH, Fanaroff AA, eds. Care of the high risk neonate. Philadelphia: W.B. Saunders, 1986:40.)

702

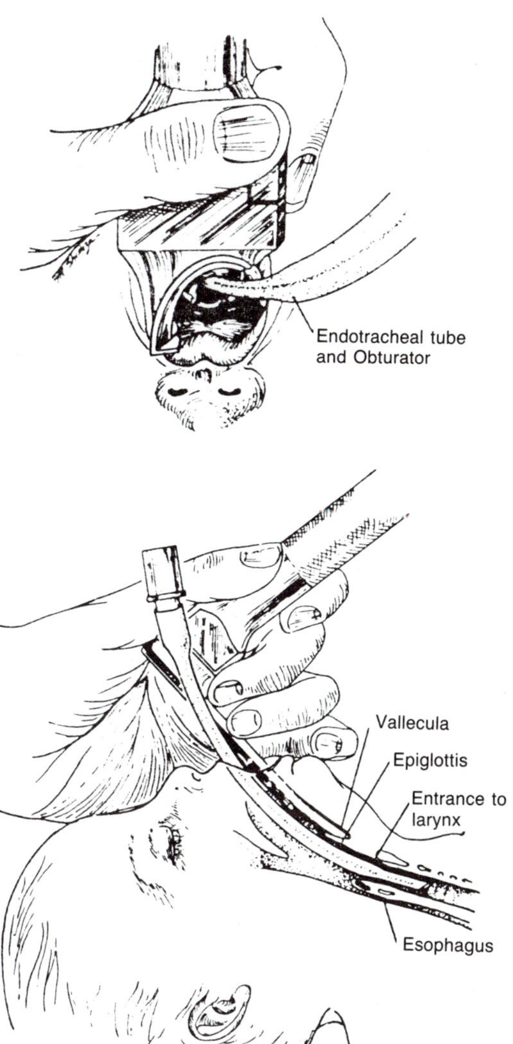
Endotracheal tube
and Obturator
Vallecula
Epiglottis
Entrance to
larynx
Esophagus

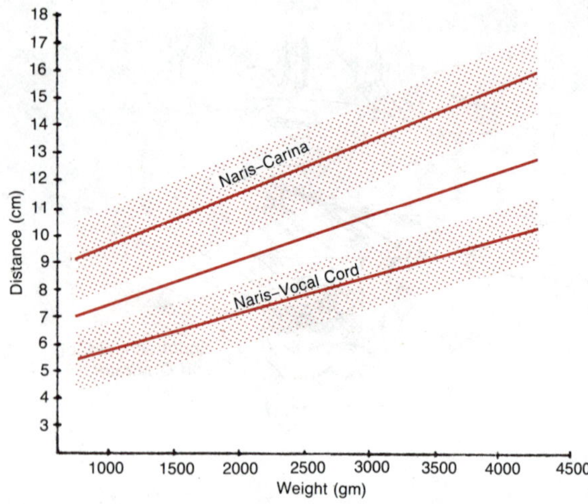

Figure 4 Estimation of ETT length for intubation. (Adapted from Coldiron J. Estimation of nasotracheal length in neonates. Pediatr 1968; 41:823.)

TABLE 1   ETT Sizes (Internal Diameters)

Tube Size (mm, Inside Diameter)	Infant Weight (g)	Suction Catheter Size
2.5	<1,000	5F
3.0	1,000–2,000	6F
3.5	2,000–3,000	8F
4.0	>3,000	8F

Needle Aspiration in Pneumothorax

Indications

- Therapeutic and diagnostic procedure for suspected tension pneumothorax in critically ill patients with respiratory or hemodynamic compromise

Technique

- A 23 or 25 gauge scalp needle attached to a three-way stopcock and a 20 ml syringe (sterile) is prepared
- The skin is cleansed with appropriate antiseptic solution, e.g., Betadine
- The needle is inserted into the third or fourth intercostal space at the midclavicular line, or the fourth intercostal space at the anterior axillary line, at an angle of 60 degrees directed cephalad (see Fig. 5)
- Air is removed until the clinical condition improves; then a chest tube should be inserted semielectively and a CXR done

Complications

- A bronchopleural fistula may rarely develop

Chest Tube Placement

Indications

- Infants with continuing air leak, associated with hemodynamic or respiratory compromise. Asymptomatic (usually small) pneumothoraces rarely require tube placement, but should be closely monitored.

Technique

- A No. 8 or 10–12 F is generally satisfactory for preterm and full-term infants, respectively, depending on the size of the pneumothorax. Often more than one tube is required.
- The chest wall is prepped with appropriate antiseptic (e.g., Betadine)

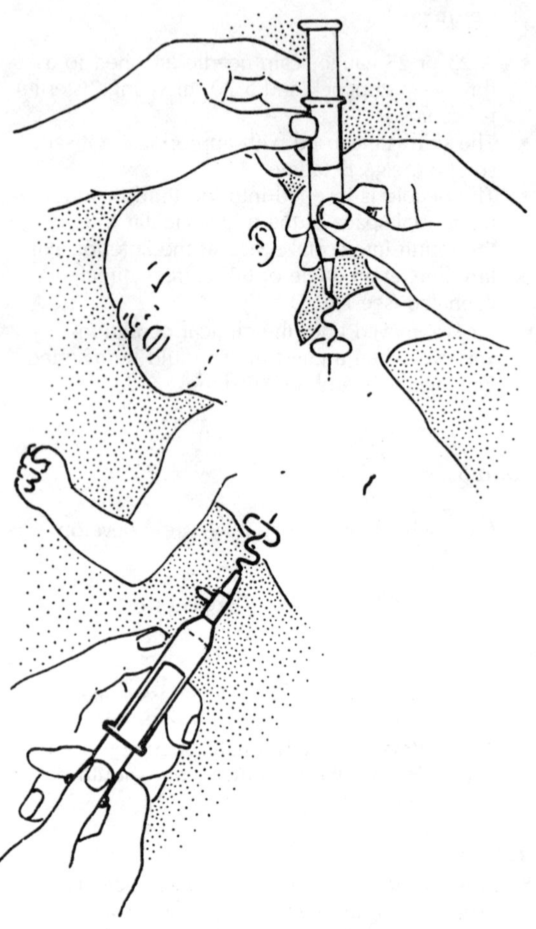

Figure 5 Positions for needling chest for tension pneumothorax and for chest tube positioning. For small infants the lateral position is preferred. (Adapted from Brady JP, Lewis K. Newborn emergencies. In Pasco DJ, Grossman M, eds. Quick reference to pediatric emergencies. 3rd ed. Philadelphia: J.B. Lippincott, 1984.)

- The infant should be positioned with the side of the chest with the pneumothorax elevated to a near vertical position
- The chest is draped, with a small aperture at the site for insertion
- A small (1.0–1.5 cm) incision is made with a scalpel in the fourth or fifth interspace (e.g., approximately in the nipple line) in the midaxillary line or anterior axillary line
- A hemostat is used to open the incision to the intercostal muscle, and then the hemostat is closed and used to penetrate through the pleura. A "pop" should be felt.
- The catheter is then grasped by the hemostat and directed into the pleural space to a predetermined distance
- "Humid air" will form in the catheter, confirming its entry into the pleural space
- The catheter should then be secured with a suture to the chest wall and antibiotic ointment applied (optional). A small sterile dressing is then placed over the chest tube at the distal end.
- A CXR is done after the procedure to confirm its location and efficacy
- The tube should be connected to an underwater seal or Pleurovac that is placed to suction of ~10–20 cm water
- The chest tube can usually be removed after 72 hr if there has been no reaccumulation of air with suction turned off or tube clamped for 24 hr. A postremoval CXR should always be done.

Complications

- Bronchopleural fistula formation, especially with use of a trocar for insertion
- Infection
- Scar or keloid formation at site of insertion

NEPHROLOGIC AND UROLOGIC PROCEDURES

Insertion of Acute Peritoneal Dialysis (PD) Catheter

Indications

- Signs of uremia, e.g., CNS disturbance, uremic pericarditis, bleeding
- Failure of medical therapy of fluid overload
- Symptomatic or potentially life-threatening electrolyte disturbance that cannot be corrected otherwise
- Severe metabolic disorders
- Presence of a dialyzable toxin

Technique

- If previous abdominal surgery, coagulopathy, or anticipate a long period of dialysis—surgeon should insert
- Sedate properly
- Empty bladder by catheterization if necessary
- Anesthetize—1% Xylocaine without epinephrine
- Prepare appropriate site aseptically with antiseptic, e.g., Betadine/alcohol
- Site
  1. Below the umbilicus, one-third of the distance between symphysis and umbilicus, or
  2. Just lateral to rectus muscle, at or just above the level of the umbilicus or
  3. At McBurney's point
- Insert 16 gauge IV catheter into peritoneal cavity
- Run 10 cc/kg IV fluid into peritoneal cavity
- Remove catheter
- Make small skin incision
- Introduce PD catheter—firm steady pressure— sensation of "pop" when peritoneum entered; remove stylet
- Direct tip into pelvic fossa
- Fix with pursestring suture

Solution

- Start with 10–20 ml/kg—1.5% (2.5% or 4.25% if severe fluid overload) dianeal
- Add heparin 500 units/L for first few exchanges until fibrin clots disappear (usually 24 hr)
- Run in over 10–15 min; dwell for 20–30 min; then run out over 10–15 min
- Increase dwell time or volume of solution as condition allows

Complications

- Bowel perforation if coexistent bowel distention
- Bladder perforation
- Infection, especially if left in for long periods

Bladder Catheterization

Indications

- To obtain sterile urine sample from child unable to produce midstream clean-catch specimen
- Relief of bladder outlet obstruction
- Indwelling—for accurate monitoring of urine output

TABLE 2   Catheter Sizes

	Intermittent Catheterization	Indwelling Catheters
0–5 yr	3½–5 F feeding tube	3½–5 F feeding tube
5–7 yr	5 F feeding tube	5 F feeding tube
7–10 yr	8–10 F disposable urinary catheter	8–10 F Foley (Sialastic)
10–14 yr	10 F disposable urinary catheter	10 F Foley (Sialastic)
>14 yr	12–14 F disposable urinary catheter	10–14 F Foley (Sialastic) (N.B. Foleys >14 F are latex)

Technique

<table>
<tr><td align="center">Male</td><td align="center">Female</td></tr>
<tr><td>

- Retract prepuce if uncircumcised
- Swab penis to base with appropriate antiseptic (e.g., Betadine)

</td><td>

- Separate labia and swab periurethral area with antiseptic

</td></tr>
</table>

- Drape sterile towel above and below urethra

- Lubricate catheter

<table>
<tr><td>

- Apply caudal traction to penis

</td><td>

- Separate labia

</td></tr>
</table>

- Introduce catheter into urethral meatus
- Advance with gentle forward pressure until urine is obtained
- Return prepuce to its normal position if necessary
- If Foley catheter used, inflate balloon with sterile saline or water
- Attach outlet end aseptically to closed drainage system

Suprapubic Bladder Aspiration

Indications

- To obtain urine in infant or neonate who cannot void on command
- To confirm suspected infection (UTI) in infant or neonate with equivocal results or several colony counts. Any bacteria grown from urine obtained by this method are significant.

Technique (Fig. 6)

- Ensure full bladder (palpable bladder; dry diaper >60 min)
- Immobilize infant in supine position (frog-leg posture)
- Prepare lower abdomen with appropriate antiseptic (e.g., Betadine-alcohol)
- Some recommend compressing urethra by pressure through the rectum in the female or by gentle penile pressure in the male, to prevent spontaneous voiding, but this is rarely necessary
- Aspiration site: 1–2 cm above symphysis pubis in midline. (Often a transverse lower abdominal crease just above the symphysis provides an excellent landmark.)
- Advance needle (22 gauge, 2–3 cm) at angle of 10–20 degrees from perpendicular to abdominal wall; aspirate while advancing cephalad
- If no urine obtained after entering 2–2.5 cm, change angle slightly and try again once
- Once urine obtained, needle is quickly withdrawn with swift motion

Complications

- Transient hematuria
- Bowel penetration (usually benign)

PROCEDURES

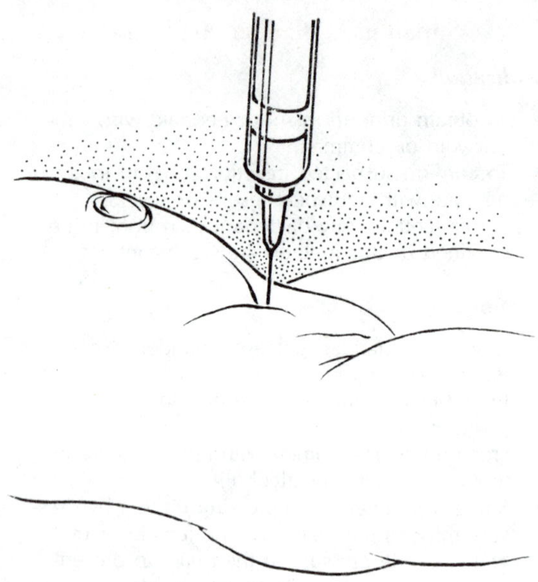

Figure 6 Suprapubic bladder aspiration.

"NEUROSURGICAL" PROCEDURES

Subdural Tap

Indications

- To diagnose acute subdural collections, in any infant whose coronal sutures are sufficiently open to allow passage of a needle
- To sample subdural collection for hematologic, microbiologic, and biochemical studies in above infants
- To drain subdural collection to reduce intracranial pressure when possible

Procedure (Fig. 7)

- Preferably performed by a neurosurgeon when possible
- Patient should be restrained or sedated if desirable or necessary during this procedure
- Identify the junction of the coronal suture and anterior fontanelle (see arrow—Fig. 7)
- Prepare site with Betadine and alcohol (shaded area). Drape with sterile towels.
- Using a sharp but short beveled subdural needle (19–23 gauge), insert it at right angle to the skull surface

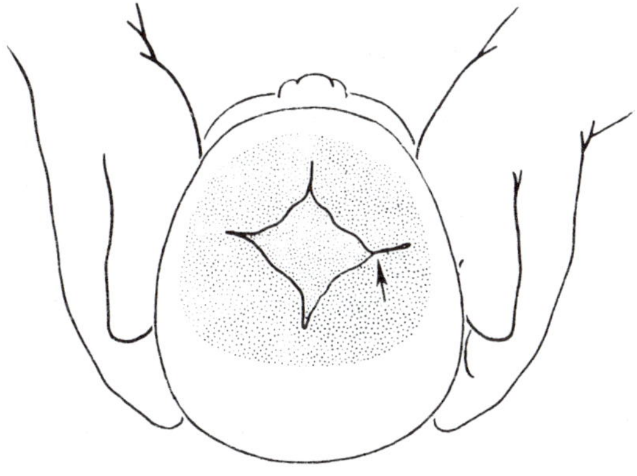

Figure 7   Subdural tap. Arrow indicates the insertion site of the needle (junction of the coronal suture and anterior fontanelle). (Adapted from Fletcher MA, MacDonald MG, Avery GB. Atlas of procedures in neonatology. Philadelphia: J.B. Lippincott, 1983:83.)

- Just after the needle passes through the dura, a resistance ("pop") will be felt. Remove stylet.
- Do not insert needle more than 0.5 cm
- Wait for fluid to emerge spontaneously into sterile tubes (DO NOT aspirate)
- Remove needle, and apply firm pressure to puncture site
- The puncture hole should be closed with a single silk suture through the puncture site. Apply sterile collodion dressing and place patient in supine position, with head elevated 10–15 degrees.

Complications

- Subdural bleeding
- Infection
- Trauma to underlying cortex

Ventricular Tap

Indications

- Performed in an emergency in a baby who has a noncommunicating hydrocephalus. If at all possible, consult neurosurgical service first, but if medullary signs are present, the tap is urgently necessary.

Technique

- Proceed as for a subdural tap. Aim the needle in the coronal plane to the inner canthus of the ipsilateral eye and in the sagittal plane to the front on the ear. When ventricle is struck, decompress *slowly* by leaving stylet partially in situ. Allow CSF to drain spontaneously.
- Submit CSF for usual bacteriologic and biochemical determinations. If search for tumor cells is to be made, the CSF must be sent immediately to the pathology laboratory.
- The puncture hole is closed as described above

Complications

- As for subdural tap

Lumbar Puncture (LP)

Indications

- Any condition requiring biochemical or cyto-
  logic assessment of CSF (e.g., meningitis,
  Guillain-Barré syndrome, leukemia, metabolic
  disorders)
- Instillation of intrathecal chemotherapy (Table 3)
- Contraindicated in bleeding diathesis, infection
  over skin or along needle insertion site, or ↑
  ICP (see below)

TABLE 3   Total Volume for Intrathecal Administration

Child's Age	Total Volume for IT Injection*
Up to 1 yr	6 ml
1–2 yr	8 ml
2–3 yr	10 ml
>3 yr	12 ml

* Drug solution plus 0.9% sodium chloride for dilution.

Technique

- *Be sure to exclude ↑ ICP* (by examining fundus
  or using CT scan) *prior to performing LP*. Consult neurosurgery if this is suspected.
- Proper positioning and adequate restraint of
  patient are absolutely essential to a successful
  tap
- Place patient with back fully flexed and either
  sitting up or lying on one side with hips, knees,
  and neck flexed
- Patients with cardiorespiratory compromise
  need close monitoring during the procedure, or

may need it deferred until more stable
- An imaginary line is drawn between the two iliac crests, and the intervertebral space (L3–L4) at, below, or above this line located. Avoid L2–L3 space in infant.
- Skin is prepared with appropriate antiseptic (e.g., Betadine) and draped with sterile towels
- In infants and older children (not neonates) infiltrate skin and subcutaneous tissue with 1% Xylocaine
- An appropriate needle is selected (21–23 gauge short needle with stylet for infants, and 20–21 gauge long needle with stylet for older children) and inserted in the midline, just below the spinous process, angled toward the umbilicus, and slowly advanced until a "pop" is felt (except in infant) as the dura is penetrated
- When fluid appears, a three-way stopcock and manometer may be attached and the opening pressure measured (useless in crying child). DO NOT ASPIRATE FLUID.
- Fluid is collected in appropriate tubes and sent for biochemical (glucose, lactate, protein), bacteriologic (culture, Gram stain, cell count, antigen detection tests, e.g., CIE or latex agglutination), and cytospin, as appropriate
- An extra specimen may be left refrigerated for later testing, e.g., metabolic tests

"RESPIRATORY" PROCEDURES

Arterial Blood Gas Sampling

Indications

- Necessary for proper determination of blood oxygen and carbon dioxide content as well as analysis of acid-base status

Technique

- Preferred sites for arterial puncture in older

children are radial and brachial arteries

- In infants, may use radial, brachial, dorsalis pedis, and posterior tibial arteries
- Avoid femoral artery puncture as may produce septic arthritis of hip
- Use 25 gauge needle and heparinized syringe
- Palpate artery; cleanse puncture site with antiseptic, e.g., Betadine-alcohol, and insert needle at 60 degree angle with bevel up
- Slowly withdraw needle until blood enters needle; then hold steady while gradually pulling plunger up barrel
- After 1–2 cc withdrawn, remove needle from artery and apply pressure firmly for $\sim$ 5 min
- Remove air from syringe; cap and transport to lab on ice

Complications

- Hemorrhage $\pm$ hematoma formation
- Arterial spasm—especially risky in brachial and femoral arteries because of inadequate collateral circulation
- Septic arthritis from femoral "stab" (area often contaminated)

Arterial Line Insertion

Indications

- Accurate, frequent monitoring of arterial blood gas status and mean arterial pressure (MAP) in intensive care setting
- Not to be used for drug administration or infusion of large fluid volumes ($>$2–3 ml/hr)

Technique

- The posterior tibial or radial arteries are the most frequently selected sites (usually good collateral circulation)
- For radial artery—locate first the ulnar artery and check for collateral flow

- Locate radial (or posttibial) artery by palpation.
  The appropriate limb is immobilized by securing to a board splint (or by assistant).
- Prepare site with appropriate antiseptic, e.g.,
  Betadine alcohol
- Using an Angiocath (20–24 gauge, 3–4 cm
  length) puncture the artery (anterior and posterior walls) at an angle of 30–45 degrees, and
  remove stylet (Fig. 8)
- Slowly withdraw catheter until pulsatile blood
  return is noted (may have to repeat above
  procedure several times)
- The catheter is then advanced up the arterial
  lumen to its hub
- A T-connector and three-way stopcock are
  attached (previously flushed with solution containing saline and heparin 1–2 units/ml) to the
  hub, and the saline:heparin solution run
  through at $\sim$ 1–3 ml/hr, continuous infusion
- A transducer can be connected to the system to
  continuously monitor the MAP
- Secure the catheter in place by suturing or
  securely taping (sterile tapes)
- N.B. In premature infants, identification and
  insertion into artery can be facilitated by use of
  bright light source, e.g., otoscope, to "transil-
  luminate" appropriate vessel, while dimming
  background

Complication

- Hemorrhage, infection, thromboembolism, and
  ischemia or gangrene are possible (and preventable) complications

Thoracentesis for Pleural Effusion

Indications

- May be diagnostic and therapeutic in management of pleural effusion

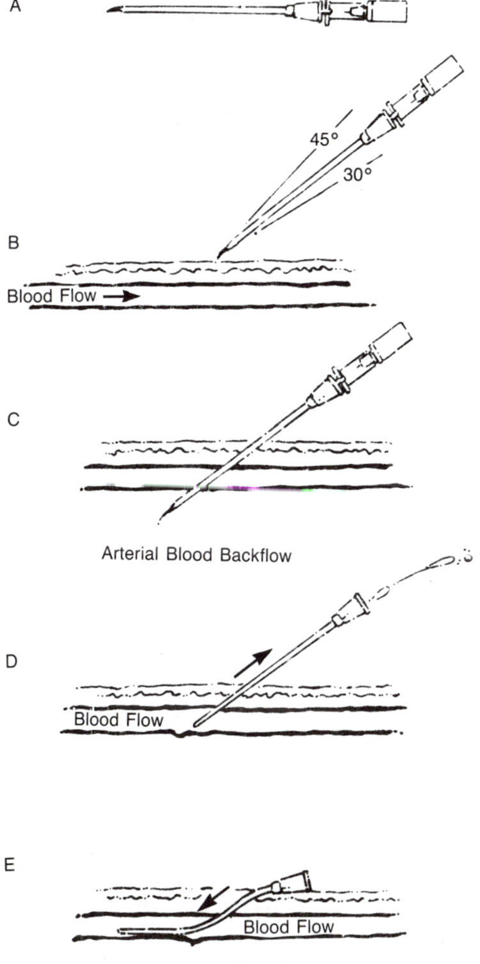

Figure 8 Percutaneous insertion of arterial catheter. (From Hughes WT, Buescher ES. Pediatric procedures. 2nd ed. Philadelphia: W.B. Saunders, 1980:83.)

Technique

- Positioning important
- Cooperative child should be leaning forward against pillow or embracing backrest of chair
- Infant may be held against chest of assistant
- Check fluid position with percussion for dullness and chest x-ray or ultrasound guidance if small amount of fluid
- Skin sterilized with Betadine and alcohol; then 1% Xylocaine (without epinephrine) used to infiltrate skin, muscle, and pleura at site
- 18 gauge needle or Angiocath attached via tubing to three-way stopcock and 20 cc syringe
- Needle inserted along posterior axillary line at anesthetized site corresponding to fluid level (sixth to seventh interspace appropriate usually), just above edge of rib to avoid intercostal vessels running along lower edge of ribs. Insertion of needle at other sites may be elected as dictated by location of fluid collection (e.g., loculations).
- Needle advanced until click of pleural penetration felt
- Fluid aspirated slowly via syringe and three-way stopcock, in aliquots of 100–500 ml if collection large
- Send fluid to appropriate labs for testing

Complications

- Infection
- Pneumothorax, hemothorax
- Pulmonary edema secondary to too rapid removal of large volumes of pleural fluid

HEMATOLOGIC PROCEDURES

Bone Marrow Aspiration and Biopsy

Indications

- For diagnosis of metastatic malignant disease,

metabolic "storage" disorders, leukemia, myeloproliferative disorders, aplastic or hypoplastic bone marrow disorders

Technique

- Sites
    1. <1 mo of age: tibia is preferred location
    2. >1 mo of age: posterior (or anterior) iliac crest preferable
    3. Sternal punctures are never performed in children
- Needles
    1. Reusable Salah or Klima aspiration needles usually used
    2. Disposable 18–21 gauge bone marrow aspiration needles are also available
    3. Occasionally an 18 or 21 gauge lumbar puncture needle may be used
    4. For biopsy a Jamshidi needle is preferable
- Position the patient either on his abdomen with a pillow or cushion under the pelvis or on his L or R side ("lumbar puncture" position)
- In older children aspiration may be performed using a local anesthetic. In younger children and infants, sedation may also be required, or general anesthesia used instead.
- After appropriate skin cleansing, 1–2% Xylocaine is used to anesthetize the skin down to the periosteum
- Insert the aspiration needle, with stylet in place, perpendicular to the skin, down to the periosteum. Using a to-and-fro motion, keeping your palm firmly over the needle and stylet, advance the needle with firm, steady pressure until a "grating" feeling is noted (a decrease in resistance).
- The obturator is removed and a 12 cc syringe attached to the needle hub. Apply strong suction for a few seconds, and aspirate ~ 0.2 ml of bone marrow.

- The syringe is then carefully removed from the needle and 6–10 slides smeared for appropriate staining
- The needle is removed, and pressure firmly applied to site for ~ 5 min or until bleeding ceases
- Apply a dry dressing
- For trephine biopsy, make a 1–2 mm incision with a scalpel blade over the iliac crest and then repeat above procedure using a biopsy needle
- Withdraw the stylet and advance the needle about 0.5 cm using a screwdriver motion
- Roll the needle to and fro to "break" the biopsy specimen from the surrounding tissue, and remove the needle
- The biopsy specimen is then removed from within the needle, using the stylet, and placed in appropriate fixative solution

GASTROENTEROLOGY PROCEDURES

Nonretention Enemas

Indications

- These are rectally administered solutions intended to be expelled within a few minutes after administration along with bowel contents. Generally administered to relieve constipation, to prevent involuntary escape of feces during surgery, or to promote visualization of bowel for diagnostic procedures, e.g., colonoscopy.

Technique

- Various solutions can be used, depending on need (e.g., saline, hypertonic phosphate). For appropriate volumes, see Table 4 (not indicated for disposables, e.g., Fleet).
- For saline enemas, the appropriate volume is

slowly run through a rectal tube, which is inserted into the lower rectum (after lubrication). The solution bag should not be elevated higher than 10–15 cm above the rectum.
- The buttocks may be held together after removal of the rectal catheter, to prolong retention of the fluid
- Prepackaged, disposable solutions (e.g., Fleet) are of much smaller volume, and need to be squeezed into the rectum

Complications

- Bowel perforation
- Transient bacteremia

TABLE 4 Maximal Volumes of Enemas to Be Administered Rectally*

Age	Volume
0–3 mo	30–100 ml
3–12 mo	100–250 ml
1–6 yr	250–500 ml
6–12 yr	500–1000 ml

* N.B. The volumes are guidelines only. In certain circumstances, e.g., encopresis, larger volumes may be recommended (see appropriate section).

LABORATORY PROCEDURES

CSF Cell Count

- Use a dry, clean Fuchs-Rosenthal counting chamber
- Place ½–1 drop of undiluted CSF on chamber A—place a coverslip over top. CSF should cover the entire chamber without overflowing. There should be no bubbles under the coverslip.
- In a separate test tube, place three drops of CSF and one drop of Fujiwara stain. Mix. Place mixture to cover chamber B.

- Examine side A under 40X objective
  1. Count number of RBCs in five large squares (the four corners and one in the center)
  2. Repeat by counting number of WBCs
  3. If count done from side B, multiply result by 4/3
  4. If more than three WBC seen, do differential from side B
- Notes
  1. Each big square contains 16 small squares
  2. Each five big squares = 80 small squares = 1 mm^3 = × 10^6/L
  3. If sample heavily blood stained, dilute CSF to 1:20 with sterile normal saline (1 part CSF plus 19 parts saline). After counting number of RBCs in five big squares, multiply the results by 20.
  4. If—
     - 0–25 cells are seen in one small square, count all five big squares
     - 25–50 cells are seen in one small square, count one big square and multiply by 5
     - >50 cells are seen in one small square, count one small square and multiply by 80

Gram Stain

- Make a thin smear of material to be studied
- Air dry
- Heat fix by passing slide through Bunsen flame two to three times
- Cover with crystal violet (or gentian violet) × 1 min
- Rinse with water
- Cover with Gram's iodine × 1 min
- Rinse with water
- Flush with 95% ethanol, acetone, or acid-alcohol until washings are colorless; not to exceed 10 sec

- Counterstain by flooding slide with safranin (or carbol-fuchsin) × 1 min
- Rinse with water
- Blot gently—leave to dry
- Place a drop of oil over stained field
- Examine using oil immersion (100X) objective

Tzank Smear

- Unroof vesicle with scalpel or needle
- Scrape base of lesion with scalpel blade (No. 10 or 15) without inducing bleeding
- Place material on a slide and make a thin smear
- Fix dry
- Stain with Giemsa
- Examine for multinucleated giant cells (herpes)

KOH Preparation

Indication

- Preliminary confirmation of suspected fungal infection

Technique

- Scrape scales from affected skin with side of scalpel blade onto black paper. If indicated, also pluck 5–10 hairs or take nail clippings or scrapings of subungual debris.
- Transfer some material to a microscope slide, apply 1–2 drops of 10% KOH (dissolves keratin), apply coverslip (wait 15–30 min), and examine under medium power. A positive test will show hyphae.
- Send the black paper containing the remainder of the collected scales to the lab for fungal culture (culture takes up to 1 mo).

Stool Smear

Technique

- Place small drop of feces on glass slide
- Place single drop of normal saline on edge of coverslip and, using this edge, agitate the drop of stool and mix it with the saline
- Lower coverslip over specimen and examine by microscope
- Look for fat, starch, meat fibers, WBC, yeast, and parasites
    1. Neutral fats: 1 drop of stool and 2 drops Sudan red stain on slide; mix with 2 drops saline; then place coverslip and examine slide under microscope. Red stained droplets = fat globules.
    2. Fatty acid crystals: best seen with polarizing attachment on microscope
    3. Leukocytes suggest bacterial infection or inflammatory bowel disease
    4. Erythrocytes suggest (amebic) colitis
    5. Parasites: examine stool smear-slide under low power to locate and under high power to identify. Add 1 drop 1% potassium iodide stain to 1 drop of stool on slide, for easier species identification

Reducing Substances in Stool (To Detect Carbohydrate Malabsorption)

Technique

- Dilute small amount of liquid stool with twice its volume of water in a test tube, or
- If to detect sucrose (which is not a reducing sugar): add 1 N HCl, instead of H_2O, to stool; boil mixture very briefly.
    1. In another tube, add 15 drops of stool mixture, then one Clinitest tablet, and compare color of resulting solution with Clinitest chart after reaction has ended

  2. Value <0.25% is normal; >0.5% suggests
     carbohydrate malabsorption
  3. Stool should be liquid to warrant performing
     test

Examination for Pinworms (Enterobiasis)

Technique

- Cellophane-tape specimen should be obtained
  before patient bathes, in AM
    1. Put piece of tape, sticky side out, on end of
       wooden tongue depressor
    2. Gently apply taped end of stick to perianal
       area
    3. On a glass slide, put 1 drop xylol; then
       apply the piece of tape (sticky side down),
       and search for ova under the microscope

V

LABORATORY REFERENCE VALUES

LABORATORY REFERENCE VALUES

The laboratory reference values section outlines the reference values for common and uncommon laboratory investigations at the Hospital for Sick Children. Depending on the individual test, these values are often age-specific, and this variation is noted. When possible, reference values are listed in the International System of Units (SI) units and in traditional units. There are often methodologic differences between laboratories (especially for uncommon investigations); it is important to obtain reference values from the laboratory where the test is done.

Reasons for ordering specific tests and interpretations of laboratory results have been kept to a minimum. However, when results can be altered by nonpathologic causes or by other factors (e.g., hemolysis), a comment is made.

Tests such as hormonal stimulation tests or tolerance tests are listed in their appropriate sub-specialty areas of the manual. For therapeutic drug concentrations see p 880.

HEMOGLOBIN, HEMATOCRIT, RBC COUNT, RETICULOCYTES[†]

	Hemoglobin (g/L)	Hematocrit	RBC Count ($\times$ 10^{12}/L)	Reticulocytes ($\times$ 10^9/L)
Birth				
28 wk gestation	110–170	0.30–0.40	3.0–4.5	
34 wk gestation	120–180	0.35–0.50	3.0–5.0	
38 wk gestation	140–200	0.40–0.55	3.5–5.5	
40 wk gestation	150–250*	0.52–0.79*	3.5–6.0	200–300
2 days	150–250*	0.46–0.74*	3.5–6.0	<5.0
2 wk	140–200	0.40–0.74*	3.5–6.0	<5.0
1 mo	115–180	0.35–0.54	3.5–5.5	
2 mo	90–135	0.27–0.40	3.5–5.5	
3–6 mo	100–140	0.30–0.42	3.5–5.0	5.0–250.0
1–5 yr	110–140	0.33–0.42	4.0–5.0	10.0–100.0
6–14 yr	120–160	0.36–0.48	4.5–5.5	10.0–100.0

* If a capillary value is close to the upper limit of normal, a VENOUS sample should be obtained. The venous hemoglobin value should be less than 220 g/L. The venous hematocrit value should be less than 0.65.

† See p 731 for conversion of SI to traditional units.

1. Hemoglobin: 120 g/L = 12.0 g/dl
2. Hematocrit: 0.36 = 36%
3. RBC count: $4.0 \times 10^{12}/L = 4.0 \times 10^{6}/mm^3$
4. Reticulocytes: $\dfrac{\text{Reticulocytes } (\times 10^9/L)}{\text{RBC count } (\times 10^{12}/L) \times 10}$ = Reticulocytes (% of RBC count)

   e.g., $\dfrac{10.0 \ (\times 10^9/L)}{4.0 \ (\times 10^{12}/L) \times 10}$ = 0.25%

RED BLOOD CELL INDICES

	MCV*	MCH†	MCHC‡
Birth			
28–37 wk gestation	120	-	
38–40 wk gestaton	110	-	
1 wk	110	-	
1 mo	90	24–34	320–360
2 mo	80	24–34	
3–12 mo	70	24–31	
Older	80–94	24–31	

* MCV = Mean Corpuscular Volume (fl)
† MCH = Mean Corpuscular Hemoglobin (pg)
‡ MCHC = Mean Corpuscular Hgb Concentration (g/L)

PLATELET COUNT

All ages: $150.0–450.0 \times 10^9/L$

ESR

All ages: 1–10 mm/hr

WHITE BLOOD CELL COUNT AND DIFFERENTIAL ($\times$ 10^9/L)

	Birth	1 Wk	2 Wk	3–12 Mo	2–5 Yr	6–10 Yr	Older
Total WBC	20.0–40.0	5.0–21.0	5.0–20.0	5.0–15.0	5.0–12.0	4.0–10.0	
Differential							
Polymorphs	6.0–26.0	1.5–10.0	1.0–9.5	1.5–8.5	1.5–8.5	1.5–8.0	2.0–7.5
Bands	0–4.5	0–0.8	0	0	0	0	0
Eosinophils	0.02–0.85	0.07–1.1	0.07–1.0	0.05–0.7	0.02–0.5	0–0.5	0–0.5
Basophils	0–0.6	0–0.2	0–0.2	0–0.2	0–0.2	0–0.2	0–0.2
Lymphocytes	2.0–11.0	2.0–17.0	2.0–17.0	4.0–10.5	2.0–8.0	1.5–7.0	1.5–4.0
Monocytes	0.4–3.1	0.3–2.7	0.2–2.4	0.05–1.1	0–0.8	0–0.8	0–0.8

NOTE: WBC formerly reported as /mm^3: e.g., 20.0 $\times$ 10^9/L = 20,000/mm^3. WBC differential counts reported now in SI units as absolute numbers ($\times$ 10^9/L); previously reported as a percentage of the total WBC count.

HEMOGLOBIN ELECTROPHORESIS

Hgb F	40 wk gestation	60–95%
	2 mo	30–55
	3 mo	15–30
	4 mo	5–15
	6 mo	2–5
	1 yr	0.2–2.0
Hgb A$_2$	>1 yr	1.2–3.2%

COAGULATION VALUES (for Full Term Newborns and Older)

Antithrombin III (AT-III)	<1 mo	40–70%
	≥3 mo	80–120%
Factors V, VIII, XIII		50–150%
Factors VII, IX, X, XI, XII	<1 mo	20–70%
	≥9 mo	50–150%
Fibrinogen	<6 mo	1.5–4.0 g/L (150–400 mg/dl)
	≥6 mo	2.0–4.0 g/L (200–400 mg/dl)

Note: Fibrinogen is an acute phase reactant

Ivy bleeding time		2–7 min
Partial thromboplastin time (PTT)	<1 mo	25–60 sec
	6 mo	25–45 sec
	≥9 mo	25–40 sec
Prothrombin time (PT)	<1 mo	10–16 sec
	≥1 mo	10–12 sec
Ristocetin cofactor		60–150%
von Willebrand factor		60–150%

BLOOD

Agent or Test	Reference Values			Notes
	SI Units	Traditional Units		

Acid-base (blood gases)

		Arterial	Venous		Notes
pH	Newborn	7.33–7.49	–		Normal values for capillary gas levels range from venous to arterial, depending on how arterialized the sample site is
	1 day	7.25–7.43	–		
	2 days–adult	7.35–7.45	7.32–7.42		
PCO_2	Birth–2 yr	26–41 mmHg	–		
	2 yr–adult	33–46	40–50		
PO_2 (room air)	Newborn	65–76 mm Hg	–		
	Child–adult	80–100	25–47		

		Actual bicarbonate	Base excess	
	Newborn	17–24 mmol/L	– 10 to – 2 mmol/L	mEq/L
	2 mo–2 yr	16–24	– 7 to 0	
	Child	18–25	– 3 to + 3	
	Adult	18–29	– 3 to + 3	

BLOOD

Agent or Test	Reference Values		Notes
	SI Units	Traditional Units	
Acid phosphatase (total)			
p-npp at 37° C			Source: Spleen, liver, prostate, osteoclasts, red blood cells, platelets
Newborn	7–20 U/L		
2–13 yr	6–15		
>13 yr	up to 11		
Adrenocorticotropic hormone (ACTH)			
Day 1	<88 pmol/L	<400 pg/ml	For adequate interpretation, cortisol should be measured in same sample
Over first few weeks of life the adrenals mature and values decrease to the following: Child and adult (0900 hr—diurnal variation)	<22 pmol/L	<100 pg/ml	
Alanine aminotransferase (ALT, formerly SGPT)			
At 37° C, with pyridoxal phosphate			Source: Liver, skeletal muscle, kidney, heart
<1 yr	<60 U/L		
1 yr–adult	<40		

BLOOD

Agent or Test	Reference Values		Notes
	SI Units	Traditional Units	
Albumin			
0–1 yr	32–48 g/L	3.2–4.8 g/dl	
child and adult	33–58	3.3–5.8	
Aldosterone			
<1 yr; free diet; varied time of day	166–2900 pmol/L	6–104 ng/dl	Varies widely depending on the time of day, posture, and sodium and potassium intake
1–4 yr; free diet; varied time of day	<940	<34	For adequate interpretation, serum sodium and potassium should be measured in same
5–15 yr; free diet; varied time of day	<600	<22	sample, along with 24-hr urine sodium collection. In hypo-
>15 yr; normal salt; ambulant; at noon	220–420	8–15	kalemic hypertension, serum potassium should be normal be-
>15 yr; low salt diet	550–1220	20–44	fore aldosterone is measured. Drugs, such as diuretics (e.g., furosemide, spironolactone), pur-gatives, and liquorice derivatives (e.g., carbenoxolone) interfere with results; should be discon-tinued 3 wk prior to testing.

BLOOD

Agent or Test	Reference Values		Notes
	SI Units	Traditional Units	
Alkaline phosphatase			
Kodak method, p-npp at 37° C			Source: Bone, liver, kidney, intestinal mucosa
Male			Isoenzymes exist for bone, liver, and intestine
<1 yr	175–600 U/L		
1–8 yr	175–400		
9–11 yr	180–475		
12–15 yr	200–630		
16–17 yr	100–455		
18–19 yr	80–210		
>19 yr	60–150		
Female			
<1 yr	185–555 U/L		
1–2 yr	185–520		
3–8 yr	185–425		
9–13 yr	160–500		
14–15 yr	90–400		
16–18 yr	45–140		
>18 yr	25–100		

BLOOD

Agent or Test	Reference Values		Notes
	SI Units	Traditional Units	
Alpha-1-antitrypsin	0.9–2.1 g/L	90–210 mg/dl	Alpha-1-antitrypsin is an acute phase reactant Protease inhibitor (PI) typing: MM—normal (89% of population) MS—normal variant (8%) MZ—heterozygous for deficiency (2.5%) SS and SZ—each <0.2% ZZ—homozygous for deficiency (0.01%)
Alpha-1-antitrypsin clearance See p 786			
Alpha-fetoprotein Adult normal	<5 µg/L	<5 rg/ml	Very high levels at birth
Aluminum	<560 nmol/L	<15 µg/L	

BLOOD

Agent or Test	Reference Values		Notes
	SI Units	Traditional Units	
Amino acids			Purpose: Screening is done by chromatography to detect genetic-metabolic disease. If screen is abnormal, quantitative values should be obtained. Reference values are age dependent and should be interpreted by a specialist in metabolic diseases.
Ammonium (NH_4^+)			
Newborn	<100 μmol/L	<180 μg/dl, as NH_4^+	
Child and adult	<60	<108	
Amylase			
<1 yr, poorly defined; lower than in older child			
1 yr–adult	20–140 U/L		Source: Pancreas, salivary glands

BLOOD

Agent or Test	Reference Values		Notes
	SI Units	Traditional Units	
Androstenedione			
Poorly defined in children			Source: Ovaries, adrenals. Until
Male 1–5 mo	<2.8 nmol/L	<80 ng/dl	puberty in females, and from 5
5 mo–adrenarche	<1.6	<45	mo of age to puberty in males,
adult	1.7–5.2	50–150	an adrenal-specific androgen
Female birth–adrenarche	<1.6	<45	In females, values are higher
adult	1.7–7.0	50–200	during the luteal phase of the cycle than during the follicular phase, but should still be within the range shown
Antihyaluronidase			
See p 790			
Antistreptolysin O (ASO)			
See p 790			
Aspartate aminotransferase (AST, formerly SGOT)			
37° C with pyridoxal phosphate			Source: Cardiac and skeletal
<1 yr	<110 U/L		muscle, liver, kidney, erythro-
1–10 yr	<45		cytes
11–20 yr	<36		

BLOOD

Agent or Test	Reference Values		Notes
	SI Units	Traditional Units	
Beta-1-C globulin			
See C3 COMPLEMENT (p 743)			
Beta-human chorionic gonadotropin			
See HUMAN CHORIONIC GONADOTROPIN			
Beta-hydroxybutyrate			
See 3-HYDROXYBUTYRATE (p 758)			
Bicarbonate (actual)			
See ACID-BASE (p 735)			
Bile salts (radioimmunoassay for glycocholate)			
Fasting	<1.3 μmol/L		
2 hr pc	<5.5		
Bilirubin (direct)			
1 mo–adult	0–7 μmol/L	0–0.4 mg/dl	
Bilirubin (total)			
Premature			In general, "physiologic hyperbili-
<24 hr	17–100 μmol/L	1–6 mg/dl	rubinemia" clears at approxi-
1–2 days	100–140	6–8	mately 1 wk of age for term neo-
3–5 days	170–200	10–12	nates and at 2 wk for prematures
1 mo–adult	<17	<1	

BLOOD

Agent or Test	Reference Values		Notes
	SI Units	*Traditional Units*	
Term			
<24 hr	34–100 μmol/L	2–6 mg/dl	
1–2 days	100–120	6–7	
3–5 days	70–200	4–12	
1 mo–adult	<17	<1	
Blood gases			
See ACID-BASE (p 735)			
Blood urea nitrogen (BUN)			
See UREA (p 774)			
C3 complement (beta-1-C globulin)			
0–1 yr	0.6–1.7 g/L	60–170 mg/dl	C3 is an acute phase reactant
1 yr–adult	0.8–1.8	80–180	
C4 complement			
0–6 mo	0.07–0.26 g/L	7–26 mg/dl	C4 is an acute phase reactant
6 mo–adult	0.10–0.40	10–40	
Calcium (ionized, free)			
>1 mo–adult	1.0–1.35 mmol/L	4.0–5.4 mg/dl	Acidosis increases free calcium whereas alkalosis decreases it (for a given total calcium)

BLOOD

Agent or Test	Reference Values		Notes
	SI Units	Traditional Units	
Calcium (total)			Prolonged venous stasis (e.g., prolonged use of a tourniquet) alters the result
Premature (birth–7 days)	1.75–2.5 mmol/L	7–10 mg/dl	
Term (birth–7 days)	1.8–3.0	7.2–12	
Child	2.25–2.74	9–11	
Adult	2.12–2.62	8.5–10.5	Serum calcium levels less than the aforementioned range may be normal if hypoalbuminemia is present. Adjusted calcium should be in the normal range.

For SI units: Adjusted Ca (mmol/L) = Calcium (mmol/L) − $\dfrac{\text{Albumin (g/L)}}{40}$ + 1.0

For traditional units: Adjusted Ca (mg/dl) = Calcium (mg/dl) − Albumin (g/dl) + 4.0

Carboxyhemoglobin

Expressed as fraction of total hemoglobin

Newborn (nonsmoking mother)	<0.05	
Nonsmokers	<0.05	

BLOOD

Agent or Test	Reference Values		Notes
	SI Units	Traditional Units	
Carcinoembryonic antigen (CEA)			
Adult	<3 μg/L		
Carnitine			
Total	60–70 μmol/L		
Free	40–50 μmol/L		
Carotene	0.9–3.7 μmol/L	50–200 μg/dl	
Ceruloplasmin			
Child >6 mo–adult	180–450 mg/L	18–45 mg/dl	Ceruloplasmin is an acute phase reactant
CH$_{50}$—total hemolytic complement	$\geq$1:12		Sample must be sent on ice immediately to laboratory
Chloride			
Premature infant	95–110 mmol/L	mEq/L	
Term infant	96–106		
Child	99–111		
Adult	98–106		

745

BLOOD

Agent or Test	Reference Values		Notes
	SI Units	Traditional Units	
Cholesterol			
<3 mo	<4.53 mmol/L	<175 mg/dl	Values are based on fasting states (before feeds in babies; after a 12 hr fast in older children)
3 mo–2 yr	<4.91	<190	
2–5 yr	3.00–5.30	115–205	
Male			
5–9 yr	3.23–4.89 mmol/L	125–190 mg/dl	
10–14 yr	3.21–5.22	125–200	
15–19 yr	3.05–4.94	120–190	
Female			
5–9 yr	3.39–5.09 mmol/L	130–195 mg/dl	
10–14 yr	3.23–5.30	125–205	
15–19 yr	3.05–5.35	120–205	
Cholinesterase-pseudocholinesterase			
Cholinesterase	620–1370 U/L		
Dibucaine no.	77–83 (heterozygote 45–70) (homozygote 15–30)		
Fluoride no.	56–68		
Chloride no.	4–15		
Scoline no.	87–92		

Agent or Test	Reference Values		Notes
	SI Units	Traditional Units	
Chorionic gonadotropin			
See HUMAN CHORIONIC GONADOTROPIN (p 758)			
Complement			
See C3, C4, CH_{50} (p 743 and 745)			
Copper			
Child >6 mo–adult	10.5–23.0 μmol/L	67–146 μg/dl	
Cortisol			Result at 2000 hr is <50% of the 0800 hr value in 88% of cases
Poorly defined during first weeks of life			Diurnal variation of cortisol may not develop until about 1 yr of age
Child 1–17 yr, in hospital			In Cushing's disease or syndrome, cortisol levels may be normal, but diurnal variation lost
0800–0900 hr	190–740 nmol/L	7–27 μg/dl	Other steroids produced in congenital adrenal hyperplasia or tumors crossreact with cortisol assay; only poor diurnal variation may be evident
2000 hr	30–300	1–11	Stress or shock can elevate cortisol levels
Healthy adult, 0800 hr	190–525	7–19	

BLOOD

Agent or Test	Reference Values		Notes
	SI Units	Traditional Units	
Creatine kinase (CK) Kodak method at 37° C. Values are for healthy school children with no restriction of physical activity.			Source: Skeletal and cardiac muscle, smooth muscle, brain Elevated CK levels occur after physical activity and intramuscular injections Blacks have significantly higher levels of CK than whites Bed rest for several days may drop CK levels by 20–30%
Male			
11 days–1 yr	<390 U/L		
1–12 yr	<255		
13–14 yr	<300		
15–16 yr	<570		
17+	<435		
Female			
11 days–1 yr	<390 U/L		
1–6 yr	<230		
7–14 yr	<215		
15–16 yr	<180		
17+	<170		

BLOOD

Agent or Test	Reference Values		Notes
	SI Units	Traditional Units	
Creatine kinase isoenzymes			
Child over 4 yr and adult (as fraction of total CK)			Source: CK-BB (predominantly brain); CK-MB (cardiac muscle, type II skeletal muscle fibers); CK-MM (skeletal muscle, cardiac muscle)
CK-MM	0.94–1.0		
CK-MB	0–0.06		Purpose: To help differentiate skeletal from cardiac muscle disease or trauma. CK-MB is not specific for myocardial damage in first weeks or months after birth
CK-BB	0		
Creatinine			
<5 yr	<44 μmol/L	<0.5 mg/dl	Low concentrations occur in patients with small muscle mass (as with muscle disease or severe malnutrition)
5–6 yr	<53	<0.6	
6–7 yr	<62	<0.7	
7–8 yr	<71	<0.8	
8–9 yr	<80	<0.9	
9–10 yr	<88	<1.0	
>10 yr	<106	<1.2	
Creatinine clearance			
See p 778			

BLOOD

Agent or Test	Reference Values		Notes
		Traditional Units	
Dehydroepiandrosterone sulfate (DHAS, DHEA-S)			Source: Adrenal glands
Male			
1–5 mo	<4 μmol/L	<1500 ng/ml	
6 mo–7 yr	<0.5	<180	
8–9 yr	<3	<1100	
10–12 yr	<6	<2200	
13–19 yr	3–12	1100–4400	
Female			
1–5 mo	<4 μmol/L	<1500 ng/ml	
6 mo–7 yr	<1.0	<350	
8–9 yr	<3	<1100	
10–12 yr	<8	<3000	
13–19 yr	1–12	350–4400	
DHAS			
See DEHYDROEPIANDROSTERONE SULFATE			
1,25-Dihydroxyvitamin D		40–150 pmol/L	

Agent or Test	Reference Values		Notes
	SI Units	Traditional Units	
Erythrocyte sedimentation rate (ESR)			
See p 731			
Estradiol			
Poorly defined in children			
Male			
Birth	<370 pmol/L	<100 pg/ml	
1 yr–adrenarche	<92	<25	
Adrenarche through puberty (rising to adult levels)			
Adult	<165	<45	
Female			
Birth–adrenarche (as in males)			
Adrenarche through puberty (rising to adult levels)			
Adult			
Follicular phase	110–183 pmol/L	30–50 pg/ml	
Luteal phase	550–845	150–230	
Treated with synthetic estrogens	<165	<45	

BLOOD

Agent or Test	Reference Values		Notes
	SI Units	Traditional Units	
FEP			
See FREE ERYTHROCYTE PROTOPORPHYRIN (p 753)			
Ferritin			
<1 yr	10–300 µg/L	ng/ml	
>1 yr	16–300		
α-Fetoprotein			
See ALPHA-FETOPROTEIN (p 739)			
Folate			
RBC folate	>270 nmol/L	>120 ng/ml	
Serum folate	>4 nmol/L	>1.8 ng/ml	
Follicle stimulating hormone (FSH)			
Male			
0–4 mo	<30 IU/L (most<12 IU/L)	mIU/ml	
4 mo–2 yr	<5		
2–11 yr	<7		
11 yr–adult	<14		

BLOOD

Agent or Test	Reference Values		Notes
	SI Units	Traditional Units	
Follicle stimulating hormone (continued)			
Female			
0–6 mo	<75 IU/L	mIU/ml	
6 mo–2 yr	<15 (most <10)		
2–10 yr	<7		
Puberty—rising to adult level	<18		
Adult			
Follicular and luteal values	<18		
Ovulatory value	<25		
Free erythrocyte protoporphyrin (FEP, zinc protoporphyrin)	<1.40 μmol/L of RBC	<80 μg/dl of RBC	Purpose: Investigation of lead poisoning, congenital erythropoietic porphyria, erythro-hepatic protoporphyria Increased FEP occurs in iron deficiency anemia and anemia of chronic disease

753

BLOOD

Agent or Test	Reference Values		Notes
	SI Units	Traditional Units	
Galactosemia screen			Purpose: Qualitative test of RBC galactose-1-phosphate uridyl transferase activity. A blood transfusion within 3 mo prior to this test may invalidate the results. Other screening tests may be available (depending on the center) that may not be invalidated by RBC transfusion, but results of these may be falsely negative if the child was not ingesting galactose–containing foods when the blood was taken.
Galactose-1-phosphate uridyl transferase			
Normal*	300–470 U/kg Hgb	18.3–28.6 Beutler and Baluda units/g Hgb	Purpose: Quantitative assessment of RBC galactose-1-phosphate uridyl transferase activity
Galactosemia, heterozygote*	140–220	8.5–13.4	

Agent or Test	Reference Values		Notes
	SI Units	Traditional Units	
Galactosemia, homo-zygote	0–40	0–2.4	*Duarte variant enzyme (a normal variant) may distort these ranges. A blood transfusion within 3 mo prior to this test may invalidate the result.
Gamma-glutamyl transferase (GGT)			
Kodak method at 37° C			Source: Liver, pancreas
<1 mo	<385 U/L		
1–2 mo	<225		
2–4 mo	<135		
4–7 mo	<75		
7 mo–15 yr	<45		
>15 yr	Male <75		
	Female <55		
Gases			
See ACID-BASE (p 735)			
Gastrin			
Fasting	<50 ng/L	pg/ml	
Globulin, beta-1-C			
See C3 COMPLEMENT (p 743)			

BLOOD

Agent or Test	Reference Values		Notes
	SI Units	Traditional Units	
Globulins			
By electrophoresis			
α_1	1–3 g/L	0.1–0.3 g/dl	
α_2 Birth–6 mo	2–7	0.2–0.7	
>6 mo	4–11	0.4–1.1	
β Birth–6 mo	3–6	0.3–0.6	
>6 mo	3–12	0.3–1.2	
γ Birth	6–12	0.6–1.2	
1–6 mo	2–7	0.2–0.7	
6 mo–2 yr	2–9	0.2–0.9	
>2 yr	4–14	0.4–1.4	
Glucose (fasting)			
Premature infant	>2.5 mmol/L	>45 mg/dl	
Term infant	>2.5	>45	
Child <3 yr	2.5–5.0	45–90	
Child >3 yr	2.8–6.1	50–110	
Adolescent–adult	3.3–6.1	60–110	
Glucose-6-phosphate dehydrogenase (G-6-PD)			
Newborn	1.6–2.8 IU/ml RBC	160–280 IU/100 ml RBC	
>2 mo	1.2–1.8	120–180	

BLOOD

Agent or Test	Reference Values		Notes
	SI Units	Traditional Units	
Gonadotropins			
See FOLLICLE STIMULATING HORMONE (p 752), LUTEINIZING HORMONE (p 764)			
Growth hormone			
After stimulation (by sleep, exercise, arginine, insulin, l-dopa or propranolol) peak value			Children with values between 5 and 8 may be normal, but require careful follow-up
should be:	>5 µg/L	>5 ng/ml	
and preferably:	>8		
Haptoglobin	0.5–2.0 g/L	50–200 mg/dl	Haptoglobin is an acute phase reactant
Hemoglobin (plasma)	<30 mg/L	<3 mg/dl	

BLOOD

Agent or Test	Reference Values		Notes
	SI Units	Traditional Units	
Hemoglobin A$_{1C}$ (glycosylated hemoglobin)			
Expressed as fraction of total hemoglobin			Abnormal or variant hemoglobins and hemoglobin F may interfere with the test
Healthy nondiabetic	0.040–0.060		
Diabetic with average control	0.09–0.100		
Human chorionic gonadotropin, beta subunit (β-HCG)			
Nonpregnant adult	<5 U/L		
3-Hydroxybutyrate (β-hydroxybutyrate)			
During documented hypoglycemia			
Expected values	1.5–2.0 mmol/L		
17-Hydroxyprogesterone			
Normal	<10 nmol/L	<3.3 µg/L	Cord blood and samples from neonates <24 hr old are not satisfactory
In most children 1–8 yr	<4	<1.3	Elevated values are seen in very sick newborns (up to 40 nmol/L)

BLOOD

Agent or Test	Reference Values		Notes
	SI Units	Traditional Units	
25-Hydroxyvitamin D			
Winter	20–60 nmol/L	8–24 ng/ml	Values exceeding these are not necessarily diagnostic of vitamin D toxicity, nor are lower levels diagnostic of deficiency. Levels may be increased in deficient patients after exposure to ultraviolet radiation.
Summer	25–80	10–32	
Immunoglobulins			
IgG			
0–6 mo	2–8 g/L	200–800 mg/dl	
6 mo–1 yr	2–10	200–1000	
1–2 yr	4–12	400–1200	
2–5 yr	4–12	400–1200	
5–10 yr	6–15	500–1500	
Adult	6–15	500–1500	

BLOOD

Agent or Test	Reference Values		Notes
	SI Units	Traditional Units	
IgA			After 10 years values for IgA and IgM increase to reach adult levels
0–6 mo	0.08–0.7 g/L	8–70 mg/dl	
6 mo–1 yr	0.11–0.9	11–90	Lower limit of IgA increases progressively in infants from approximately 0.01 g/L at 1 mo to 0.08 g/L at 6 mo
1–2 yr	0.15–1.2	15–120	
2–5 yr	0.22–1.6	22–160	
5–10 yr	0.35–2.4	35–240	
Adult	0.70–3.1	70–310	
IgM			
0–6 mo	0.2–1.0 g/L	20–100 mg/dl	
6 mo–1 yr	0.3–1.5	30–150	
1–2 yr	0.4–1.7	40–170	
2–5 yr	0.4–2.0	40–200	
5–10 yr	0.4–2.5	40–250	
Adult	0.5–3.5	50–350	
IgE (values are stated as < mean + 1 standard deviation)			Upper limit of IgE increases progressively in infants from approximately 5.5 μg/L at 6 wk to 17.5 μg/L at 6 mo. After 10 years the values decline to adult levels
0–6 mo	<17.5 μg/L	<7.3 kU/L	
6 mo–1 yr	<31	<13	
1–2 yr	<55	<23	
2–5 yr	<115	<48	
5–10 yr	<204	<85	
Adult	<98	<41	

BLOOD

Agent or Test	Reference Values		Notes
	SI Units	Traditional Units	
Insulin			
Fasting	<145 pmol/L	<20 mU/L	Reference values may be higher in obese patients. Hemolysis and insulin antibodies may lower values.
Intralipid			
See LIPID (p 762)			
Iron			
Newborn	4–28 μmol/L	20–160 μg/dl	Hemolysis elevates the result
4 mo–1 yr	5–13	30–70	
>1 yr	9–27	50–150	
Toxicity (1 yr and older)	>53	>300	
Iron-binding capacity (IBC)			
Newborn	11–31 μmol/L	60–175 μg/dl	
>1 yr	45–72	250–400	
Lactate			
Venous	1–2 mmol/L	9–18 mg/dl	Delayed separation of serum from RBC, and hemolysis both elevate the result

BLOOD

Agent or Test	Reference Values		Notes
	SI Units	Traditional Units	
Lactate dehydrogenase (LDH)			
At 30° C			Source: Highest concentrations in heart, liver, skeletal muscle, erythrocytes, kidney
Adult	45–85 U/L		Elevated in hemolyzed samples. Values are poorly defined and higher in children, and method dependent.
Lead	0–1.45 μmol/L blood	0–30 μg/dl blood	The concentration of lead in whole blood is 75 times greater than in serum or plasma
Lipid			
During supplementation, values should not exceed	1.0 g/L		Purpose: Monitoring for toxicity when exogenous intravenous lipids are administered
Lipoproteins			
By electrophoresis			Purpose: Investigation and classification of hyperlipidemia
See also CHOLESTEROL (p 746) TRIGLYCERIDES (p 772)			

BLOOD

| | Reference Values | | |
Agent or Test	SI Units	Traditional Units	Notes
Plasma HDL-Cholesterol			
Male			
5–9 yr	0.98–1.91 mmol/L	38–74 mg/dl	
10–14 yr	0.96–1.91	37–74	
15–19 yr	0.78–1.63	30–63	
Female			
5–9 yr	0.93–1.89 mmol/L	36–73 mg/dl	
10–14 yr	0.96–1.81	37–70	
15–19 yr	0.91–1.91	35–74	
Plasma LDL-Cholesterol			
Male			
5–9 yr	1.63–3.34 mmol/L	63–129 mg/dl	
10–14 yr	1.66–3.41	64–132	
15–19 yr	1.60–3.36	62–130	
Female			
5–9 yr	1.76–3.62 mmol/L	68–140 mg/dl	
10–14 yr	1.76–3.52	68–136	
15–19 yr	1.53–3.54	59–137	

Agent or Test	Reference Values		Notes
	SI Units	Traditional Units	
Luteinizing hormone (LH) (2nd Int. reference preparation)			Values rise through puberty to adult values
Male			
0–3 mo	<45 IU/L	mIU/ml	
4 mo–2 yr	<13		
2–6 yr	<8		
6–10 yr	<14		
Adult	<20		
Female			
1–6 mo	<40 IU/L	mIU/ml	
6 mo–2 yr	<14		
2–8 yr	<12		
8–12 yr	3–25		
Adult			
Follicular and luteal value	<90		
Ovulatory value	<200		
Magnesium			
Newborn	0.75–1.15 mmol/L	1.5–2.30 mEq/L	
Child	0.70–0.95	1.4–1.9	
		1.3–2.0	

BLOOD

Agent or Test	Reference Values		Notes
	SI Units	Traditional Units	
Methemoglobin In SI expressed as fraction of total hemo-globin	<0.03	<3%	
5'-Nucleotidase	0–14 U/L		Source: Liver
Osmolality	275–295 mmol/kg water	mOsm/kg water	May be lower in first 5 days after birth
Parathyroid hormone	10–55 ng/L	pg/ml	Immunoassay is PTH ''intact'' molecule type (Nichols)
Phenylalanine	<110 μmol/L	<1.8 mg/dl	
Phenylalanine/tyrosine ratio Normal ratio Equivocal Hetero/homozygote	<1.0 1.0–1.2 >1.2		Purpose: Determination of heterozygosity for phenylketo-nuria

BLOOD

Agent or Test	Reference Values		Notes
	SI Units	Traditional Units	
Phosphate			
Birth–1 mo	1.62–3.10 mmol/L	5.0–9.6 mg/dl	Reported values vary widely,
1–4 mo	1.55–2.62	4.8–8.1	especially during first month of
4 mo–1 yr	1.30–2.20	4.0–6.8	life
1–4 yr	1.16–2.10	3.6–6.5	Hemolysis causes an elevated
4–8 yr	1.16–1.81	3.6–5.6	value
9–14 yr	1.07–1.71	3.3–5.3	
>14 yr	0.87–1.52	2.7–4.7	

PI type

See ALPHA-1-ANTITRYPSIN (p 739)

Porphyrins

Purpose: Investigation of lead poisoning, erythrohepatic protoporphyria, and congenital erythropoietic porphyria—see FREE ERYTHROCYTE PROTOPORPHYRIN (p 753)
Investigation of acute intermittent porphyria—see UROPORPHYRINOGEN-I-SYNTHETASE (p 774)

BLOOD

Agent or Test	Reference Values		Notes
	SI Units	Traditional Units	
Potassium			
Premature infants	4.5–6.5 mmol/L	nEq/L	Hemolysis elevates values
Term infants	5.0–6.5		
2 days–2 wk	4.0–6.4		
2 wk–3 mo	4.0–6.2		
3 mo–1 yr	3.7–5.6		
1–16 yr	3.5–5.2		
Prolactin			
Birth (mean)	280 μg/L	ng/ml	Level drops to
Level drops after birth–4 wk			adult level by 12 wk
4 wk (mean)	75		of age (term); and
Adult range	0–30		by 20 wk (premature)

Protein

See TOTAL PROTEIN (p 772),
ALBUMIN (p 737), GLOBULINS (p 756)

Protoporphyrin, free erythrocyte

See FREE ERYTHROCYTE
PROTOPORPHYRIN (p 753)

BLOOD

Agent or Test	Reference Values		Notes
	SI Units	Traditional Units	
Pseudocholinesterase			
See CHOLINESTERASE (p 746)			
Pyruvate			
Venous	80–150 μmol/L	0.7–1.32 mg/dl, as pyruvic acid	Delayed separation of serum from RBC, and hemolysis both elevate the result
Pyruvate kinase			
Newborn	1.2–2.1 IU/ml RBC		
Older	1.0–1.4		
Renin			
Plasma renin activity			Normal values vary with method, sodium intake, time of day, posture, and age
Normal salt intake: <3 mo wide range; values as high as: (particularly high in premature infants)	14.00 ng/L/sec	50 ng/ml/hr	Antihypertensive medication may alter results; if possible, medication should be discontinued 1–3 wk prior to test
3 mo–1 yr	<4.20	<15	
1–4 yr	<2.80	<10	
4–15 yr	<1.70	<6	
Adult			
Supine, after 1–12 hr rest	<0.56	<2.0	
At 1200 hr, ambulant	<1.11	<4.0	

BLOOD

Agent or Test	Reference Values		Notes
	SI Units	Traditional Units	
Serum glutamic oxaloacetic transaminase (SGOT)			
See ASPARTATE AMINO-TRANSFERASE (AST), p 741			
Serum glutamic pyruvate transaminase (SGPT)			
See ALANINE AMINOTRANSFERASE (ALT), p 736			
Sodium			
Premature infant	132–140 mmol/L	mEq/L	
Term infant	133–142		
Child	135–143		
Adult	135–145		
Testosterone			
Male			
1–15 days	<6.6 nmol/L	<190 ng/dl	During puberty, levels correlate with pubertal stage or bone age rather than chronologic age
1–3 mo	<12.1	<350	
3–5 mo	<6.9	<200	
5–7 mo	<2.1	<60	During puberty, levels increase to adult values
7 mo–onset of puberty	<1.0	<30	
Adult	12.0–38.0	350–1100	

Agent or Test	Reference Values		Notes
	SI Units	Traditional Units	
Female			
Birth–onset of puberty	<1.0 nmol/L	<30 ng/dl	Levels during luteal phase are higher on average than in follicular phase
Puberty—levels increase to adult values. Levels are higher in girls experiencing anovulatory cycles, but still within normal range.			Levels may rise to 3.3 nmol/L (95 ng/dl) during estrogen or progesterone therapy
Adult	0.7–2.4	20–70	
Thyroid-stimulating hormone (TSH)			
Cord blood	<30 mU/L	μU/ml	
Rises shortly after birth to peak	<50		
Child >4 days of age	<5		
Adult	<5		

BLOOD

Agent or Test	Reference Values		Notes
	SI Units	Traditional Units	
Thyroxine (T_4)			
Levels rise shortly after birth to peak at 24 hr and then fall at 3 days to:	115–280 nmol/L	9–22 μg/dl	Premature infants have much lower values—the more premature, the lower the value
4 days–3 wk	100–245	8–19	In patients with normal thyroid
3 wk–2 mo	90–205	7–16	function, low T_4 values can
2 mo–1 yr	65–180	5–14	occur with absent or low levels
1 yr–childhood	65–165	5–13	of thyroxine-binding globulin
Adult	50–155	4–12	(TBG), hypoproteinemia, drugs (e.g., phenytoin), or severe hemolysis. In patients with normal thyroid function, high T_4 values can occur with high levels of TBG, as during pregnancy or while receiving contraceptive or estrogen therapy.
Thyroxine-binding globulin (TBG)			
Adult	10–28 mg/L	μg/ml	Values in children are ill defined, slightly higher than adult values

BLOOD

Agent or Test	Reference Values		Notes
	SI Units	Traditional Units	
Total protein			
0–6 mo	45–75 g/L	4.5–7.5 g/dl	
6 mo–2 yr	54–75	5.4–7.5	
Child and adult	53–85	5.3–8.5	
Triglycerides			
Male			
0–5 yr	0.34–1.13 mmol/L	30–100 mg/dl	
5–9 yr	0.32–0.96	28–85	
10–14 yr	0.37–1.25	33–111	
15–19 yr	0.43–1.61	38–143	
Female			
0–5 yr	0.34–1.13 mmol/L	30–100 mg/dl	
5–9 yr	0.36–1.42	32–126	
10–14 yr	0.44–1.35	39–120	
15–19 yr	0.41–1.42	36–126	

Agent or Test	Reference Values		Notes
	SI Units	Traditional Units	
Triiodothyronine (T_3) Do not confuse with T_3RU			T_3 assay has a low sensitivity for diagnosing hypothyroidism
Birth	<1.0 nmol/L	<70 ng/dl	
Rises rapidly after birth to a value at 3 days of:	0.8–5.4	50–350	
6 days–1 yr	1.4–4.6	90–300	
1 yr–childhood	1.4–4.1	90–270	
Adults	1.4–3.4	90–220	
Triiodothyronine resin uptake test (T_3RU) Do not confuse with T_3	0.25–0.35	25–35%	A synthetic resin and patient's TBG (thyroxine-binding globulin) compete for radioactive T_3 T_3RU >0.35 (>35%) indicates FEWER available binding sites in serum, as in hyperthyroidism (sites occupied by T_4) or absence or deficiency of TBG T_3RU <0.25 (<25%) indicates MORE available binding sites, as in hypothyroidism (little T_4 available to occupy sites) or increased TBG (e.g., during estrogen therapy or pregnancy)

BLOOD

Agent or Test	Reference Values		Notes
	SI Units	Traditional Units	
Urate (formerly URIC ACID)			
Child or adult female	120–360 μmol/L	2.0–6.0 mg/dl, as uric acid	
Adult male	180–420	3.0–7.0	
Urea (formerly BLOOD UREA NITROGEN, BUN)			
Newborn	2.9–10.0 mmol/L	8–28 mg/dl, as urea nitrogen	
1–2 yr	1.8–5.4	5–15	
2–16 yr	2.9–7.1	8–20	
Uric acid			
See URATE			
Uroporphyrinogen-I-synthetase	5.2–15.5 nmol/s/L RBC		Source: Erythrocytes Purpose: Investigation of acute intermittent porphyria
Vitamin A	0.70–2.10 μmol/L	20–60 μg/dl	
Vitamin B$_{12}$	150–670 pmol/L	200–900 pg/ml	
Vitamin D			
See 25-HYDROXYVITAMIN D (p 759), 1,25-DIHYDROXYVITAMIN D (p 750)			

Agent or Test	Reference Values		Notes
	SI Units	Traditional Units	
Vitamin E			
	7.0–12.0 μmol/L	0.3–0.5 mg/dl	
Zinc			
0–1 yr	11.5–22.2 μmol/L	75–145 μg/dl	
2–10 yr	10.7–20.0	70–130	
11–18 yr	10.0–19.0	65–124	
Adult	9.2–18.4	60–120	

URINE

Agent or Test	Reference Values		Notes
	SI Units	Traditional Units	
Amino acids, screen See METABOLIC STUDY (p 780)			
Bilirubin			Normally absent
Cadmium	<0.01 μmol/L		
Calcium	<0.1 mmol/kg body wt/day	<4 mg/kg body wt/day	
Related to creatinine	<0.56 μmol/μmol creatinine	<0.2 mg/mg creatinine	

URINE

Agent or Test	Reference Values		Notes
	SI Units	Traditional Units	
Catecholamines			
Norepinephrine	95 percentile (100th percentile)	95th percentile (100th percentile)	Drugs such as methyldopa, apresoline, quinidine,
0–2 yr	280 (375) μmol/mol creatinine	420 (558) μg/g creatinine	epinephrine or norepinephrine-related drugs like L-dopa, and
2–4 yr	80 (150)	120 (224)	renal function test dyes may
5–9 yr	60 (90)	90 (135)	interfere with catecholamine
10–19 yr	55 (60)	82 (92)	excretion and affect the results
Adult	76 (90)	114 (135)	
Epinephrine	95th percentile (100th percentile)	95th percentile (100th percentile)	
0–2 yr	45 (150) μmol/mol creatinine	75 (246) g/g creatinine	
2–4 yr	35 (60)	57 (97)	
5–9 yr	20 (40)	35 (66)	
10–19 yr	20(70)	34(110)	
Adult	14(50)	23(81)	

URINE

Agent or Test	Reference Values		Notes
	SI Units	Traditional Units	
Dopamine	95th percentile (100th percentile)	95th percentile (100th percentile)	
0–2 yr	2220 (3480) μmol/mol creatinine	3000 (4708) μg/g creatinine	
2–4 yr	1130 (2230)	1533 (3020)	
5–9 yr	770 (990)	1048 (1342)	
10–19 yr	400 (510)	545 (692)	
Adult	400 (580)	535 (781)	
Copper			
Normal	<0.6 μmol/day	<40 μg/day	
Coproporphyrin			
See PORPHYRINS (p 783)			
Cortisol (urine "free" cortisol)			
	nmol/day	μg/day	Most sensitive screen for increased cortisol production
4 mo–10 yr	<74	<27	
11–20 yr	<152	<55	
Adult	50–220	18–80	
	μmol/mol creatinine	μg/g creatinine	
4 mo–10 yr	11–55	35–176	
11–20 yr	<14	<44	
Adult	4–19	13–60	

Agent or Test

Creatinine clearance
Age-related reference ranges for creatinine clearance corrected for body surface area are shown in Figure 1. Note that SI units are printed in red.

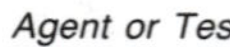

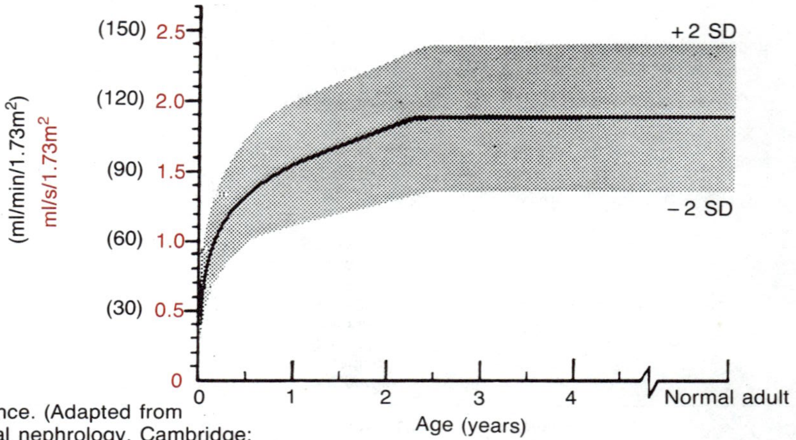

Figure 1   Creatinine clearance. (Adapted from McCrory WW. Developmental nephrology. Cambridge: Harvard University Press, 1972:98.)

URINE

Agent or Test	Reference Values		Notes
	SI Units	Traditional Units	
Dinitrophenylhydrazine (DNPH) test See METABOLIC STUDY (p 780)			
Glycosaminoglycuronoglycans See MUCOPOLYSACCHARIDE SCREEN (p 781)			
Hemoglobin			Normally absent; may be positive after exercise and during infectious or febrile states. Myoglobinuria may give a false positive result.
Homovanillic acid (HVA)	95th percentile (100th percentile)	95th percentile (100th percentile)	
0–1 yr	20 (48) mmol/mol creatinine	32 (77) mg/g creatinine	
2–4 yr	14 (37)	23 (60)	
5–9 yr	9 (21)	14 (34)	
10–19 yr	8 (27)	13 (43)	
Adult	5 (6)	3 (10)	
Ketones			Normally absent, but may be positive in febrile or toxic states or during fasting periods

URINE

Agent or Test	Reference Values		Notes
	SI Units	*Traditional Units*	
Mercury			
Random specimen	<0.05 µmol/L	<0.01 mg/L	
Dental fillings may elevate excretion to:	0.4	0.08	
Metabolic study			Purpose: The following screening tests are performed to detect metabolic disease: a. Two-dimensional amino acid chromatography—aminoaciduria b. Cyanide nitroprusside test—cystinuria, homocystinuria, glutathionemia, certain defects of tubule transport c. DNPH (dinitrophenylhydrazine) test—detects ketoacids in cases of PKU, MSUD, methionine malabsorption, tyrosinemia. Also detects ketones in normal subjects after a prolonged fast. For method see p 466. Cyanide nitroprusside and DNPH test results are normally negative

URINE

Agent or Test	Reference Values		Notes
	SI Units	Traditional Units	
Metanephrines (metanephrine and normetanephrine)			Medications like hydrocortisone and phenobarbital can cause false positive results, whereas propranolol and theophyllines can cause false negative results with certain laboratory techniques
<2 yr	<2.8 mmol/mol creatinine	<4.6 mg/g creatinine	
2–10 yr	<1.9	<3	
10–15 yr	<1.2	<2	
Adult	<0.6	<1	
Mucopolysaccharide screen (glycosamino-glycuronoglycans)			Normally not detectable A normal result does not rule out all mucopolysaccharidoses
Myoglobin			Normally not detectable Reacts like hemoglobin by dipstick. Confirmatory tests are available.

URINE

Agent or Test	Reference Values		Notes
	SI Units	Traditional Units	
Nitroprusside test			
See METABOLIC STUDY (p 780)			
Organic acids			Gas chromatography—mass spectrometry results need to be interpreted by a specialist in metabolic diseases Most diagnostic if urine is collected when patient is ill
Osmolality			
Infant	50–600 mmol/kg water	mOsm/kg water	Values should be interpreted in conjunction with serum osmolality and clinical state of patient
Child and adult: maximum (dehydration)	800–1400		
Child and adult: minimum (water diuresis)	40–80		
Oxalate			
	<8.1 μmol/kg body wt/day	<0.73 mg/kg body wt/day, as anhydrous oxalic acid	

URINE

Agent or Test	Reference Values		Notes
	SI Units	Traditional Units	
Porphobilinogen screen			
See PORPHYRINS			
Porphyrins			Screening tests are of value only during an acute attack
Child: ranges poorly defined			Urine porphobilinogen may be increased between (as well as during) attacks of acute intermittent porphyria
Adult			
Coproporphyrin	0–380 nmol/day	0–250 μg/day	
Protoporphyrin	Not detected		
Uroporphyrin	<36 nmol/day	<30 μg/day	Porphyrinuria may also occur in lead poisoning, liver disease, and conditions of increased erythropoiesis
Porphobilinogen	<13.3 μmol/day	<3 mg/day	
Potassium			Varies widely, depending on intake
Protein (quantitative)			
Over 1 yr of age	<0.10 g/m^2/day		
Protoporphyrin			
See PORPHYRINS			

URINE

Agent or Test	Reference Values		Notes
	SI Units	Traditional Units	
Reducing substances			Qualitative test (Clinitest tablet) detects reducing substances such as glucose, galactose, fructose, lactose, pentoses, and homogentisic acid. Only glucose is detected by glucose-specific dipsticks (Clinistix).
Sodium			
Infant	6–10 mmol/m^2 of body surface/day (approx. 0.3–3.5 mmol/day)	mEq/m^2/day	Urinary sodium should be interpreted in relation to serum sodium
		mEq/day	
Child	40–180 mmol/day		
Adult	80–200 mmol/day		
Specific gravity			
Child >6 mo and adult	>1.020 (after fluid deprivation)		
Urate			
	<60 μmol/kg body wt/day	<10 mg/kg body wt/day, as uric acid	
Related to creatinine	<0.67 μmol/μmol	<1 mg/mg creatinine,	

URINE

Agent or Test	Reference Values		Notes
	SI Units	Traditional Units	
Urinalysis, routine			
See p 458			
Urobilin and urobilinogen			Normally not detectable Urobilin is the oxidation product of unstable urobilinogen Increased in severe hemolytic jaundice and some liver disorders
Uroporphyrin			
See PORPHYRINS (p 783)			
Vanillylmandelic acid (VMA) 24 hr collection	95th percentile (100th percentile)	95th percentile (100th percentile)	Nonspecific elevations occur in fever, asthma, chronic anemia, or after surgery
0–1 yr	12 (16) μmol/day	2.3 (3.1) mg/day	
2–4 yr	15 (20)	3.0 (4.0)	
5–9 yr	18 (44)	3.5 (8.7)	
10–19 yr	30 (39)	6.0 (7.7)	
Adult	34 (41)	6.8 (8.1)	

URINE

Agent or Test	Reference Values		Notes
	SI Units	Traditional Units	
"Spot VMA"			Less satisfactory than 24 hr collection
	95th percentile (100th percentile)	95th percentile (100th percentile)	
0–1 yr	11 (34) mmol/mol creatinine	19 (59) mg/g creatinine	
2–4 yr	6.5 (12)	11 (21)	
5–9 yr	5 (5.5)	8 (9)	
10–19 yr	5 (8)	8 (14)	
Adult	3.5 (5)	6 (8)	

FECES

Agent or Test	Reference Values		Notes
	SI Units	Traditional Units	
Alpha-1-antitrypsin clearance			
	<22 ml/day		Falsely low values when lesion(s) is in the esophagus, stomach, or upper small bowel as low pH environment degrades alpha-1-antitrypsin Collection must be free of urine Serum alpha-1-antitrypsin re-quired during the collection

FECES

Agent or Test	Reference Values		Notes
	SI Units	Traditional Units	
Chymotrypsin			
37° C ATEE substrate	30–750 U/g		
Coproporphyrin			
See PORPHYRINS (p 788)			
Fat			
Fecal fat (fraction of intake)			Three or 5 day stool collection required
Premature infant	<0.20		Accurate account of dietary fat necessary during the period of stool collection
Term infant	<0.15		
>3 mo	<0.10		Regular fat study measures only the amount of LONG chain fatty acids in the stool
Occult blood			Qualitative study
			Detected when there is 4 ml whole blood per 100 g feces (i.e., 6 mg Hgb per g feces)

FECES

Agent or Test	Reference Values		Notes
	SI Units	Traditional Units	
Porphyrins Adult values (values poorly defined in children)			Fecal porphyrin may be elevated after GI bleeding
Coproporphyrin	<11 μmol/kg wet weight of stool	<700 μg/100 g wet weight of stool	Fecal porphyrins useful in porphyria variegata (protocopro-
Protoporphyrin	<27 μmol/kg wet weight of stool	<1500 μg/100 g wet weight of stool	porphyria) or hereditary copro- porphyria
			Normal values in acute intermit- tent porphyria or cutaneous hepatic porphyria (cutanea tarda)
Protoporphyrin See PORPHYRINS			

CEREBROSPINAL FLUID

Agent or Test	Reference Values		Notes
	SI Units	Traditional Units	
Glucose When blood glucose is normal	2.1–3.6 mmol/L	38–65 mg/dl	CSF glucose should be roughly ⅔ the blood glucose

CEREBROSPINAL FLUID

Agent or Test	Reference Values		Notes
	SI Units	Traditional Units	
Proteins			
CSF total protein			Excessively high protein levels
Premature	0.15–1.3 g/L	15–130 mg/dl	(>5 g/L) can occur if spinal
Term	0.40–1.2	40–120	canal is blocked
<1 mo	0.20–0.7	20–70	
>1 mo	0.15–0.4	15–40	
CSF IgG			
Normal	<0.1 of CSF total protein		

VIRAL AND OTHER TITERS

- N.B. Only changes in titer ($\geq$ four-fold increase or decrease over time) are diagnostic of recent infection (or reactivation)
- Adenovirus[1] —complement fixation
  < 1:2 negative; $\geq$ 1:64 high
- Antihyaluronidase $\geq$ 1:300 suggestive of recent streptococcal infection
- Antistreptolysin O (ASO) $\geq$ 300 Todd units suggestive of recent streptococcal infection
- *Chlamydia trachomatis*[1]—immunofluorescence < 1:8 negative; $\geq$ 1:64 high
- Cytomegalovirus (CMV)[1,2]—latex agglutination < 1:2 negative; $\geq$ 1:32 high
- Epstein-Barr virus (EBV)
  1. Heterophile antibody (sheep cell) when absorbed by beef red blood cells and not absorbed by guinea pig kidney $\geq$ 1:56 suggestive of recent infection
  2. Immunofluorescence
     - Antibody to VCA (viral capsid antigen) $\geq$ 1:640 suggestive of recent infection (false positive reactions can occur in connective tissue diseases or malignant disease)
     - Antibody to EA (early antigen)
       < 1:20 negative or old infection;
       $\geq$ 1:20 recent infection or reactivation
- Herpes simplex [1,2,3]—complement fixation
  < 1:2 negative; $\geq$ 1:64 high
- Influenza A and B[1] —complement fixation
  < 1:2 negative; $\geq$ 1:64 high
- Measles[1]—complement fixation
  < 1:2 negative; $\geq$ 1:64 high
- Mumps[1] —complement fixation
  < 1:2 negative; $\geq$ 1:64 high
- *Mycoplasma pneumoniae*—complement fixation $\geq$ 1:32 suggestive of recent infection
- Parainfluenza[1] —complement fixation
  < 1:2 negative; $\geq$ 1:64 high

- Respiratory syncytial virus[1] —complement fixation < 1:2 negative; ≥ 1:64 high
- Rubella[2]—latex agglutination < 1:2 negative; ≥ 1:64 possibility of recent infection; ≥ 1:20 considered rubella immune
- Toxoplasmosis[2]—complement fixation > 1:8 suggestive of exposure
  Indirect fluorescent antibody > 1:256 suggestive of exposure
- Varicella zoster—immunofluorescence ≥ 1:8 considered immune to V-Z

1. Negative: No previous exposure
    High: Suggestive of recent infection or reactivation
    Titers in between are suggestive of previous exposure

2. Neonates may have titers equal to, or one dilution higher, than maternal titers. Serum titers in neonates suspected of having congenital infection must be interpreted in conjunction with the maternal antibody titers.

3. In absence of CSF infection, antibody levels in serum are 200 or more times greater than in CSF

VI

FORMULARY

FORMULARY

See also Quick Guide to Resuscitation Drugs (inside front cover) and Emergency Drug Doses Table (p 656)

The formulary has been compiled in alphabetical order by generic name. The section comprising pages 798 to 852 contains dosages for children. The section comprising pages 856 to 868 contains dosages for neonates. The following is a limited list of common trade names and synonyms with their corresponding generic names:

Adrenaline—epinephrine
Advil—ibuprofen
Albuterol—Salbutamol
Aldactazide—Novospirozine
Aldactone—spironolactone
Aldomet—methyldopa
Alupent—orciprenaline
Amicar—aminocaproic acid
Amoxil—amoxicillin
Amphojel—aluminum hydroxide
Ancef—cefazolin
Antepar—piperazine
Apresoline—hydralazine
Aspirin—acetylsalicylic acid
Atarax—hydroxyzine
Ativan—lorazepam
Atrovent—ipratropium bromide
Augmentin—amoxicillin and potassium clavulanate
Bactrim—co-trimoxazole
Beclovent—beclomethasone
Benadryl—diphenhydramine
Bentyl—dicyclomine
Bentylol—dicyclomine
Berotec—fenoterol
Bicarbonate—sodium bicarbonate
Catapres—clonidine
Ceclor—cefaclor
Cefobid—cefoperazone
Cephulac—lactulose
Charcoal—activated charcoal
Chlor-Tripolon—chlorpheniramine

Citro-Mag—magnesium citrate
Claforan—cefotaxime
Clavulin—amoxicillin and potassium clavulanate
CM-3—cardiac cocktail
Cordarone—amiodarone
Corgard—nadolol
Corticotropin—ACTH
Cotazym—pancrelipase
Coumadin—warfarin
Cromoglycate Sodium— cromolyn sodium
Cuprimine— penicillamine
Cylert—pemoline
DDAVP—desmopressin
Decadron— dexamethasone
Demerol—meperidine
Depakene—valproic acid
Desferal—deferoxamine
Dextrose—glucose
Diamox—acetazolamide
1,25-Dihydroxycholecalciferol- calcitriol
Dilantin—phenytoin
Dimetane—brompheniramine
Diodoquin—iodoquinol
Diphenylhydantoin—phenytoi
Ditropan—oxybutynin
Diuril—chlorothiazide
Divalproex—valproic acid
Dramamine—dimenhydrinate

Dulcolax—bisacodyl
Eltroxin—levothyroxine
Entacyl—piperazine
Epival—valproic acid
Fer-In-Sol—ferrous sulfate
Fivent—cromolyn sodium
Flagyl—metronidazole
Fortaz—ceftazidime
Gamma benzene
  hexachloride—lindane
Gantrisin—sulfisoxazole
Gelusil—aluminum and
  magnesium hydroxide
Gravol—dimenhydrinate
Haldol—haloperidol
Hismanal—astemizole
HydroDiuril—
  hydrochlorothiazide
Hyperstat—diazoxide
Imodium—loperamide
Imuran—azathioprine
Inderal—propranolol
Indocid—indomethacin
INH—isoniazid
Intal—cromolyn sodium
Iron—ferrous sulfate, iron
  dextran
Isoptin—verapamil
Isuprel—isoproterenol
Kayexalate—sodium poly-
  styrene sulfonate
Keflex—cephalexin
Keflin—cephalothin
Kwell—lindane
Kwellada—lindane
Lanoxin—digoxin
Largactil—chlorpromazine
Lasix—furosemide
Loniten—minoxidil
Lytic Cocktail—cardiac cocktail
Maalox—aluminum and magnesium
  hydroxide
Macrodantin—nitrofurantoin macro-
  crystals
Magnesium Rougier—magnesium
  glucoheptonate
Mandol—cefamandole
Maxeran—metoclopramide
Mefoxin—cefoxitin
Metaproterenol—orciprenaline
Milk of Magnesia— magnesium
  hydroxide

Minipress—prazosin
Mogadon—nitrazepam
Motrin—ibuprofen
Mucomyst—acetylcysteine
Mycostatin—nystatin
Myochrysine—gold sodium thiomalate
Mysoline—primidone
Nalcrom—cromolyn sodium
Naprosyn—naproxen
Narcan—naloxone
NegGram—nalidixic acid
Nembutal—pentobarbital
Neo-Synephrine—phenylephrine
Pavulon—pancuronium
Pediazole—erythromycin ethyl-
  succinate and sulfisoxazole
Pentothal—thiopentone
Persantine—dipyridamole
Phenergan—promethazine
Phytonadione—vitamin K_1
Pitressin—vasopressin
Priscoline—tolazoline
Pronestyl—procainamide
Questran—
  cholestyramine
Racemic Epinephrine—
  epinephrine
Resonium Calcium—
  calcium polystyrene sul-
  fonate
Ritalin—methylphenidate
Rivotril—clonazepam
Rocaltrol—calcitriol
Rynacrom—cromolyn
  sodium
Salazopyrin—
  sulfasalazine
Scabanca—benzyl
  benzoate
Seldane—terfenadine
Septra—co-trimoxazole
Solu-Cortef—
  hydrocortisone
Solu-Medrol—
  methylprednisolone
Somophyllin-12— theophylline
Sudafed—
  pseudoephedrine
Sulcrate—sucralfate
Synthroid—levothyroxine
Tagamet—cimetidine
Tapazole—methimazole

Tegretol—carbamazepine
Tempra—acetaminophen
Tensilon—edrophonium
Theo-Dur—theophylline
Thiopental—thiopentone
Thorazine—
  chlorpromazine
Thyroxine—levothyroxine
TMP-SMX—co-trimoxazole
Tofranil—imipramine
Tolectin—tolmetin
Tylenol—acetaminophen
Urecholine—bethanechol

Valium—diazepam
Vanceril—beclomethasone
Ventolin—salbutamol
Vermox—mebendazole
Vibramycin—doxycycline
Vira-A—vidarabine
Vitamin B_6—pyridoxine
Xylocaine—lidocaine
Yodoxin—iodoquinol
Zantac—ranitidine
Zarontin—ethosuximide
Zinacef—cefuroxime
Zovirax—acyclovir

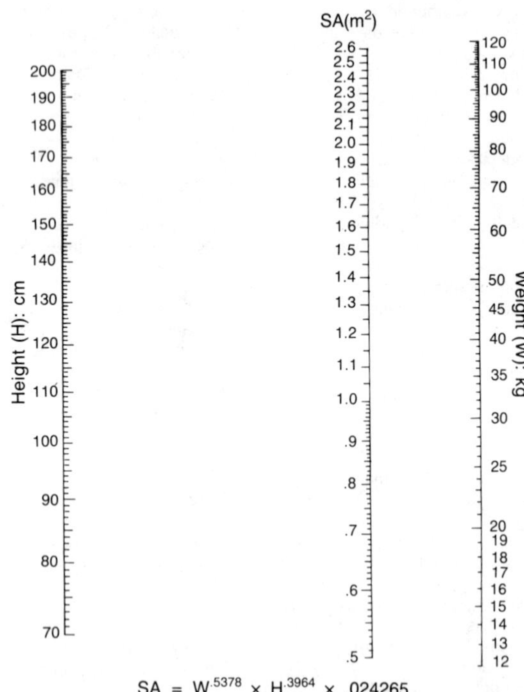

$$SA = W^{.5378} \times H^{.3964} \times .024265$$

To use the nomogram, a ruler is aligned with the height and weight on the two lateral axes.
The point at which the center line is intersected gives the corresponding value for surface area.

Figure 1 **A,** Body surface area nomogram for children and adults (From Haycock GB, Schwartz GJ, Wisotsky DH. J Pediatr 1978; 93: 62–66.)

Approximation of Surface Area (M²) to Weight (kg)

Weight Range	Approximate Surface Area
1 to 5 kg	$M^2 = (0.05 \times kg) + 0.05$
6 to 10 kg	$M^2 = (0.04 \times kg) + 0.10$
11 to 20 kg	$M^2 = (0.03 \times kg) + 0.20$
21 to 40 kg	$M^2 = (0.02 \times kg) + 0.40$

From Behrman RE, Vaughan VC. Nelson's textbook of pediatrics. 12th ed. Philadelphia: W.B. Saunders, 1983:26.

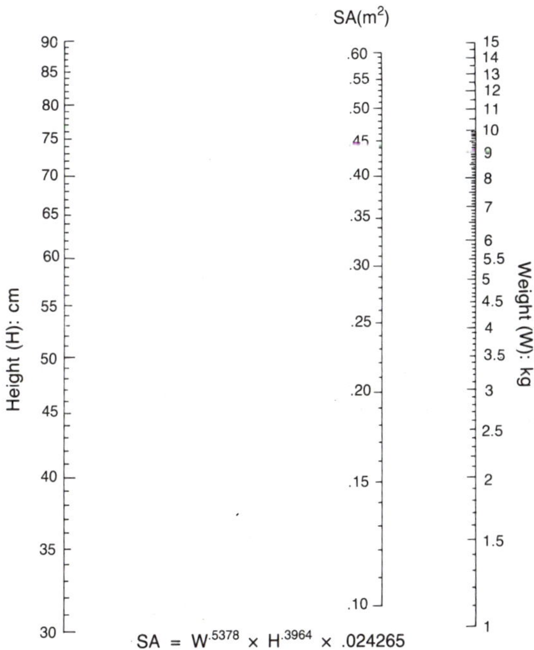

To use the nomogram, a ruler is aligned with the height and weight on the two lateral axes. The point at which the center line is intersected gives the corresponding value for surface area.

Figure 1 *B,* Body surface area nomogram for infants (From Haycock GB, Schwartz GJ, Wisotsky DH. J Pediatr, 1978; 93: 62–66.)

Drug Dosage Guidelines in Children

Drug	Dose	Comments
Acetaminophen (Tempra, Tylenol)	40–60 mg/kg/day PO or per rectum $\div$ q4–6h Max: 65 mg/kg/day	Optimal single antipyretic dose = 10–15 mg/kg.
Acetazolamide (Diamox)	*Glaucoma*: 15 mg/kg/day PO $\div$ tid–qid Max: 1.5 g/day *Epilepsy*: 8–30 mg/kg/day PO $\div$ tid–qid Max: 1.0 g/day *Urinary alkalinization*: 5 mg/kg/dose PO or IV	IM administration not recommended.
Acetylcysteine (Mucomyst)	*Cystic fibrosis*: 2 ml 20% sol^n by inhalation prn up to qid *Acetaminophen overdose*: loading: 140 mg/kg PO diluted in 3 vol of soft drink; then 70 mg/kg PO q4h $\times$ 17 doses	Use in reducing sputum viscosity currently controversial. May cause airway irritation when given by inhalation. If vomiting occurs within an hour of PO administration, repeat the dose.
Acetylsalicylic acid (Aspirin)	*JRA, pericarditis, rheumatic fever*: 60–100 mg/kg/day PO $\div$ qid *Kawasaki disease*: 100 mg/kg/day PO $\div$ qid until defervescence $\times$ 36 hr; then 5–10 mg/kg/day PO qam	Not recommended for fever during viral illness. Monitoring of serum drug concentrations is recommended during high dose therapy.
ACTH	*Infantile spasms*: 40–80 IU/day IM or SC once daily or $\div$ bid	

MAXIMAL DOSAGES ARE PRINTED IN RED

Drug	Dose	Comments
Activated charcoal	1 g/kg PO or NG 0.5 g/kg PO or NG q6h for repeat doses	Mix appropriate amount in 120–240 ml fluid.
Acyclovir (Zovirax)	*Varicella in immunocompromised host:* 1500 mg/m^2/day IV ÷ q8h *Herpes simplex:* <12 yr: 750 mg/m^2/day IV ÷ q8h ≥12 yr: 30 mg/kg/day IV ÷ q8h	Increase dosing interval to q12h in moderate, and to q24–48h in severe renal impairment.
Adrenaline	See Epinephrine	
Albumin	0.5–1 g/kg/dose IV prn Max: 6 g/kg/day	
Allopurinol (Zyloprim)	10 mg/kg/day PO ÷ tid–qid Max: 600 mg/day	Decrease daily dose to 67% in mild and 50% in moderate renal impairment. In severe renal impairment give 3 mg/kg q2–3 days.
Aluminum hydroxide (Amphojel) Aluminum and magnesium hydroxide (Gelusil ES, Maalox TC)	Infant: 2–5 ml PO q1–2h Child: 5–15 ml PO after meals and hs Adult: 15–45 ml PO after meals and hs	Antacid products with high buffering capacity preferred.

MAXIMAL DOSAGES ARE PRINTED IN RED

Drug Dosage Guidelines in Children

Drug	Dose	Comments
Amikacin	15–30 mg/kg/day IV or IM ÷ q8h	Increase dosing interval to q12h in mild and moderate, q24–48h in severe renal impairment. Monitoring of serum drug concentrations is recommended.
Aminocaproic acid (Amicar)	*Hemophilia prior to dental extractions*: 200 mg/kg/day PO ÷ q6h × 7–10 days after procedure Max: 30 g/day *Hemophilia acute hemorrhage*: 400 mg/kg/day PO or IV ÷ q6h	Decrease dose to 50 mg/kg once daily in severe renal impairment.
Aminophylline	See Theophylline	Contains 80% theophylline. See theophylline for dosages and multiply by 1.25 for aminophylline equivalent.
5-Aminosalicylic acid	Older child and adult: 1200–2400 mg/day PO ÷ tid–qid Max: 4 g/day	
Amiodarone (Cordarone)	Loading: 10 mg/kg/day PO once daily or ÷ bid × 7–10 days Maint: 5 mg/kg/day PO once daily	Continuous ECG monitoring during first 3 days of loading. Hospitalize during loading period. Reduce digoxin dose by 50%. Monitor thyroid, liver, lung, and eye function.

MAXIMAL DOSAGES ARE PRINTED IN RED

Drug	Dose	Comments
Amoxicillin (Amoxil)	20–50 mg/kg/day PO ÷ q8h Max: 4 g/day	
Amoxicillin and potassium clavulanate (Clavulin, Augmentin)	20–50 mg amoxicillin/kg/day PO ÷ q8h Max: 4 g amoxicillin/day	
Amphotericin B	Initial dose 0.25–0.5 mg/kg/day IV once daily Increase by 0.25 mg/kg/day up to 0.5–1.0 mg/kg/day once daily or q2 day Max: 1.0 mg/kg/dose or 70 mg/dose, whichever is less, given once daily or once every 2 days	Infuse at a concentration of $\leq$0.1 mg/ml in D5W over 4–6 hr. Monitor serum potassium. Premedication with meperidine–diphenhydramine–hydrocortisone may be useful.
Ampicillin	*Meningitis*: 200–300 mg/kg/day IV ÷ q6h *Other*: 50–100 mg/kg/day IV or IM ÷ q6h Max: 10 g/day	Increase dosing interval to q12–16h in severe renal impairment.
Astemizole (Hismanal)	<6 yr: 0.2 mg/kg/day PO once daily 6–12 yr: 5 mg PO once daily >12 yr: 10 mg PO once daily	Administer on an empty stomach.

MAXIMAL DOSAGES ARE PRINTED IN RED

Drug Dosage Guidelines in Children

Drug	Dose	Comments
Atropine	*Preop*: 0.01–0.02 mg/kg/dose IM or PO 30–60 min preop Max: 0.6 mg/dose; minimum 0.1 mg/dose *AV block, asystole, sinus bradycardia*: 0.02 mg/kg IV or ETT q20 min prn Max: 1 mg/dose; minimum 0.1 mg/dose *Cholinergic crisis*: 0.05 mg/kg IV; repeat q5 min until secretions dry Max: 2 mg/dose	
Azathioprine (Imuran)	*Renal transplant*: Post transplant 2–3 mg/kg/day IV or PO ÷ once daily or bid	Decrease dose to 75%, or increase dosing interval to q36h in severe renal impairment.
Beclomethasone (Beclovent, Vanceril)	3–5 yr: 1 puff bid–tid 6–14 yr: 2 puffs bid–qid; max: 10 puffs/day >14 yr: 2 puffs tid–qid; max: 20 puffs/day	1 puff = 50 μg
Benzyl benzoate (Scabanca)	Apply to skin of trunk and extremities; allow to dry; then apply a second time. Wash off 24 hr later.	Cream 25%; lotion 14%

MAXIMAL DOSAGES ARE PRINTED IN RED

Drug	Dose	Comments
Bethanechol (Urecholine)	*Urinary retention*: 0.3–0.6 mg/kg/day PO ÷ q6–8h 0.075–0.2 mg/kg/day SC ÷ q6–8h *GE reflux*: 0.4 mg/kg/day PO ÷ qid (before meals and hs) Max: 50 mg/dose	
Bisacodyl (Dulcolax)	0.3 mg/kg/dose PO <6 yr: 5 mg per rectum or 2.5 ml microenema >6 yr: 10 mg per rectum or 5 ml microenema	Takes 6–8 hr to work if given PO and 15–60 min if given per rectum. Do not break or chew tablets, or administer with milk or antacid.
Bretylium	Initial dose: 5 mg/kg IV Subsequent doses: 10 mg/kg IV q15–30 min prn Max: 30 mg/kg/total dose	For treatment of ventricular tachycardia and recurrent ventricular fibrillation. Cardiac monitoring required.
Brompheniramine (Dimetane)	0.35–0.5 mg/kg/day PO ÷ tid–qid	

MAXIMAL DOSAGES ARE PRINTED IN RED

Drug Dosage Guidelines in Children

Drug	Dose	Comments
Calcitriol (Rocaltrol, 1,25-Dihydroxy-cholecalciferol)	*Hypo PTH, vitamin D resistant rickets, dialysis:* Initial: 0.015–0.025 μg/kg/day PO ÷ bid Maint: increase as needed gradually to 0.5–1 μg/day PO	Monitor serum calcium. To achieve a rise in serum calcium requires at least 3 days of therapy at the increased dosage.
Calcium carbonate (Os-Cal)	*Calcium deficiency and hyperphosphatemia prophylaxis in renal patients:* Infant: 125 mg elemental Ca^{++} PO tid Child: 250 mg elemental Ca^{++} PO tid	Titrate dose according to serum PO_4.
Calcium chloride	*Cardiac arrest, hyperkalemia:* 10 mg/kg/dose = 0.1 ml of 10% sol^n/kg/dose q10–20 min IV prn Max: 1 g/dose = 10 ml 10% sol^n/dose	Irritating to veins. Each ml contains 100 mg $CaCl_2$ = 0.68 mmol of calcium.
Calcium gluconate	*Hyperkalemia:* 50 mg/kg/dose = 0.5 ml of 10% sol^n/kg/dose IV *Cardiac arrest:* 30 mg/kg/dose = 0.3 ml of 10% sol^n/kg/dose IV q10–20 min prn Max: 2 g/dose = 20 ml 10% sol^n/dose *Hypocalcemic seizures or tetany:* See p 116	Each ml contains 100 mg calcium gluconate = 0.23 mmol of calcium.

MAXIMAL DOSAGES ARE PRINTED IN RED

Drug	Dose	Comments
Calcium polystyrene sulfonate (Resonium Calcium)	*Acute hyperkalemia:* 1 g/kg/day PO ÷ tid–qid Maint: 500 mg/kg/day PO ÷ tid–qid	Moisten powder with water, honey, or jam for PO use. Exchanges ∼1.6 mmol potassium/g of resin.
Captopril	↑*BP*: initial: 0.45 mg/kg/day PO ÷ tid Maint: 0.3–0.6 mg/kg/day PO ÷ tid *CHF*: 1.5–6 mg/kg/day PO ÷ tid Max: 6 mg/kg/day	Increase dosing interval to q12–48h in moderate and to q48–108h in severe renal impairment.
Carbamazepine (Tegretol)	Initial: 10 mg/kg/day PO once daily or ÷ bid Maint: up to 20–30 mg/kg/day ÷ tid Max: 1.2 g/day	Increase dose gradually over 2–4 wk. Monitoring of serum drug concentration is recommended. Chewable tablets must be thoroughly chewed.
Cardiac cocktail (CM-3)	0.1 ml/kg IM 20–60 min pre-exam No supplementary doses Max: 2 ml/dose	Contains meperidine 25 mg/ml, chlorpromazine 6.25 mg/ml, promethazine 6.25 mg/ml. Reduce dose in patients with CNS impairment.
Cefaclor (Ceclor)	40 mg/kg/day PO ÷ q8h Max: 2 g/day	Decrease dose to 30–50% in moderate and to 20–30% in severe renal impairment.

MAXIMAL DOSAGES ARE PRINTED IN RED

Drug Dosage Guidelines in Children

Drug	Dose	Comments
Cefazolin (Ancef)	50–150 mg/kg/day IV or IM ÷ q8h Max: 6 g/day	Increase dosing interval to q12–36h in moderate and to q24–72h in severe renal impairment.
Cefoperazone (Cefobid)	100–150 mg/kg/day IV or IM ÷ q8–12h Max: 10 g/day	Monitor PT and PTT.
Cefotaxime (Claforan)	*Meningitis*: 200 mg/kg/day IV or IM ÷ q4–6h *Other*: 100–200 mg/kg/day IV or IM ÷ q4–6h Max: 10 g/day	Increase dosing interval to q8–12h in moderate and to q12–24h in severe renal impairment.
Cefoxitin (Mefoxin)	80–160 mg/kg/day IV or IM ÷ q4–6h Max: 12 g/day	Increase dosing interval to q8–24h in moderate or q24–48h in severe renal impairment.
Ceftazidime (Fortaz)	*Cystic fibrosis*: 200 mg/kg/day IV or IM ÷ q6h *Other*: 50–150 mg/kg/day IV or IM ÷ q8h Max: 6 g/day	Increase dosing interval to q12–24h in moderate and to q24–48h in severe renal impairment.
Ceftriaxone	*Meningitis*: Load: 75 mg/kg IV Then: 100 mg/kg/day IV ÷ q12h Max: 4 g/day *Other*: 50–75 mg/kg/day IV ÷ q12–24h Max: 2 g/day	

MAXIMAL DOSAGES ARE PRINTED IN RED

Drug	Dose	Comments
Cefuroxime (Zinacef)	*Meningitis*: 225 mg/kg/day IV or IM ÷ q8h *Other*: 75 mg/kg/day IV or IM ÷ q8h Max: 9 g/day	Increase dosing interval to q8–48h in moderate and to q24–72h in severe renal impairment.
Cephalexin (Keflex)	25–50 mg/kg/day PO ÷ qid Max: 3 g/day	Increase dosing interval to q6–8h in moderate and to q8–12h in severe renal impairment.
Cephalothin (Keflin)	75–125 mg/kg/day IV or IM ÷ q4–6h Max: 10 g/day	Increase dosing interval to q8–12h in severe renal impairment.
Chloral hydrate	*Sedation*: 25 mg/kg/dose PO hs *Hypnotic*: 50 mg/kg/dose PO 20–45 min prior to procedure Max: 1 g/dose	Decrease dose in patients with CNS impairment.
Chloramphenicol	50–100 mg/kg/day PO or IV ÷ q6h Max: 4 g/day	Monitoring of serum drug concentrations is recommended. Do not use palmitate in infants <1 yr old or in CF patients.

MAXIMAL DOSAGES ARE PRINTED IN RED

FORMULARY

Drug Dosage Guidelines in Children

Drug	Dose	Comments
Chloroquine	*Malaria prophylaxis*: 5 mg base/kg/dose PO once weekly 1–2 wk prior to, during, and for 6 wk after exposure Max: 300 mg base/wk *Malaria*: 10 mg base/kg PO stat, then 5 mg base/kg/dose PO 6, 24, and 48 hr later Max stat dose: 600 mg base Max subsequent doses: 300 mg base	250 mg chloroquine phosphate = 150 mg base
Chlorothiazide (Diuril)	20–40 mg/kg/day PO once daily or ÷ bid	
Chlorpheniramine (Chlor-Tripolon)	0.35 mg/kg/day PO ÷ q6–12h	

MAXIMAL DOSAGES ARE PRINTED IN RED

Drug	Dose	Comments
Chlorpromazine (Largactil, Thorazine)	*Antineoplastic emesis prophylaxis*: 0.3–0.5 mg/kg/dose IV q4–6h prn Max: <5 yr: 40 mg/day 5–12 yr: 75 mg/day *Nausea and vomiting*: 2 mg/kg/day PO, IM or IV ÷ q4–6h 4 mg/kg/day per rectum ÷ q6–8h *Afterload reduction*: 0.1–0.25 mg/kg/dose IV *Severe agitation and acute psychosis*: 0.5 mg/kg/dose PO; then 0.5–2 mg/kg/dose q2h PO until controlled or side effects occur	Has alpha blocking properties and may cause profound hypotension. Monitor BP after IV therapy. IV rate not to exceed 0.5 mg/min. Administer diphenhydramine concurrently during antineoplastic emesis prophylaxis to prevent extrapyramidal reactions.
Cholestyramine (Questran)	0.24–1.1 g/kg/day PO ÷ bid–tid	May alter absorption of other drugs.
Cimetidine (Tagamet)	20 mg/kg/day PO or IV ÷ q6h or tid with meals and qhs Max: 2400 mg/day	Increase dosing interval to q8h in moderate and to q12–24h in severe renal impairment.

MAXIMAL DOSAGES ARE PRINTED IN RED

FORMULARY

Drug Dosage Guidelines in Children

Drug	Dose	Comments
Clindamycin	10–30 mg/kg/day PO ÷ q6h 25–50 mg/kg/day IM or IV ÷ q6–8h Max: 2 g/day PO 4 g/day IM or IV	IV rate not to exceed 1200 mg/hr.
Clonazepam (Rivotril)	≤30 kg: initial dose 0.05 mg/kg/day PO ÷ bid or tid. Gradually increase daily dose by 0.05 mg/kg/day q3 days if needed to a max of 0.2 mg/kg/day. >30 kg: initial dose 1.5 mg/day PO ÷ tid. Gradually increase daily dose by 0.5–1 mg/day q3 days up to max of 20 mg/day PO ÷ tid.	Reduce dose in liver impairment.
Cloxacillin	50–200 mg/kg/day PO, IV or IM ÷ q6h Max: 12 g/day IV or 4 g/day PO	
Codeine	Pain: 2–3 mg/kg/day PO, IM or SC ÷ q4–6h Max: 5 mg/kg/day, 1.5 mg/kg/dose Cough: 0.8–1.2 mg/kg/day PO ÷ q4–6h Antidiarrheal: 2 mg/kg/day PO or IM ÷ q6h	May cause constipation or CNS depression. Dose is cumulative and may cause respiratory depression. Maximal dose should not be given for longer than 24 hr.
Cortisone	See p 853	

MAXIMAL DOSAGES ARE PRINTED IN RED

Drug	Dose	Comments
Co-trimoxazole (Septra, Bactrim)	*Bacterial infection*: 5–10 mg TMP/kg/day PO or IV ÷ q12h *Pneumocystis carinii*: 20 mg TMP/kg/day PO or IV ÷ q6h *Prophylaxis*: OM or UTI: 3–5 mg TMP/kg/day PO once daily Pneumocystis or asplenia: 5 mg TMP/kg/day PO once daily	Increase dosing interval to q12–24h in moderate and to q24–48h in severe renal impairment. Contains trimethoprim (TMP) and sulfamethoxazole in a ratio of 1 to 5.
Cromolyn sodium or cromoglycate sodium (Intal, Fivent, Rynacrom, Nalcrom)	1% inhalation sol^n (Intal): 2 ml/dose tid–qid via nebulizer Metered dose inhaler (Fivent): 2 puffs cid (1 mg/puff) Spincap (Intal): 60–80 mg/day via inhalation ÷ tid–qid Oral (Nalcrom): 400 mg/day ÷ qid with meals Nasal (Rynacrom): 1–2 squeezes into each nostril up to 6x/day Nasal insufflation (Rynacrom cartridges): 40 mg/day ÷ qid	

MAXIMAL DOSAGES ARE PRINTED IN RED

Drug Dosage Guidelines in Children

Drug	Dose	Comments
Dantrolene sodium	*Malignant hyperthermia*: 1 mg/kg/dose IV push q2–5 min until symptoms subside or max total dose of 10 mg/kg is reached	
Deferoxamine (Desferal)	*Iron intoxication*: 10–15 mg/kg/hr IV × 4 hr; then 2–5 mg/kg/hr IV 90 mg/kg IM (max 1 g/dose); then 40 mg/kg/dose IM q4–6h Max: 120 mg/kg/day or 8 g/day, whichever is less	Use IM route only if IV site not available. Continuous IV infusion rate not to exceed 15 mg/kg/hr. Therapeutic regimen is complex; contact poison center for details
Desmopressin (DDAVP)	*Diabetes insipidus*: 5–20 µg/day intranasally once daily or ÷ bid	
Dexamethasone (Decadron)	See p 854	
Dextromethorphan	1 mg/kg/day PO ÷ q6–8h	

MAXIMAL DOSAGES ARE PRINTED IN RED

Drug	Dose	Comments
Diazepam (Valium)	*Pre x-ray*: >30 kg: 0.2 mg/kg/dose PO × 1 dose only *Sedation*: 0.1 mg/kg/dose IV 0.1–0.8 mg/kg/day PO ÷ q6h *Status epilepticus*: 0.1–0.3 mg/kg/dose IV q10 min prn × 3 doses or 0.3–0.5 mg/kg/dose per rectum × 1 dose Max: ≤5 yr: 5 mg/dose >5 yr: 10 mg/dose	May cause hypotension and apnea when given IV. Be prepared to resuscitate. Administer IV at a rate not to exceed 2 mg/min.
Diazoxide (Hyperstat)	*Hypertensive crisis*: 1–2 mg/kg/dose IV q15 min prn Max total dose: 8 mg/kg or 4 doses *Hyperinsulinemic hypoglycemia*: 12–15 mg/kg/day PO ÷ q6–8h	Give IV undiluted as fast as possible. Larger doses may cause hypotension. For hypertensive crisis, upon reaching maximal total dose, consider use of nitroprusside.
Dicloxacillin	12–25 mg/kg/day PO ÷ q6h Max: 2 g/day	

MAXIMAL DOSAGES ARE PRINTED IN RED

Drug Dosage Guidelines in Children

Drug	Dose	Comments
Digoxin (Lanoxin)	*Digitalization*: divide total dose in 3 equal doses—1st stat, 2nd in 6 hr, 3rd in another 8 hr Term newborn—2 yr: PO: 0.05 mg/kg/total dose IV: 0.035 mg/kg/total dose >2 yr: PO: 0.04 mg/kg/total dose IV: 0.03 mg/kg/total dose Maximal total dose = 1.5 mg *Maint*: Term newborn—2 yr: PO: 0.01 mg/kg/day ÷ bid IV: 0.007 mg/kg/day ÷ bid >2 yr: PO: 0.008 mg/kg/day ÷ bid Max: 0.25 mg/day	IM administration not recommended. Begin maintenance dose 24 hr after 1st digitalization dose. Caution in patients with hypokalemia. Decrease maintenance dose to 50–75% in severe renal impairment. Reduce dose during concurrent administration of amiodarone or quinidine. Monitoring of serum drug concentrations is recommended.
Dimenhydrinate (Gravol, Dramamine)	5 mg/kg/day PO, IM, IV, or per rectum ÷ q6h Max: 300 mg/day	
Diphenhydramine (Benadryl)	*Antihistamine*: 5 mg/kg/day PO, IM or IV ÷ q6h *Anaphylaxis*: 1–2 mg/kg/dose IV Max: 300 mg/day 50 mg/dose	

MAXIMAL DOSAGES ARE PRINTED IN RED

Drug	Dose	Comments
Dipyridamole (Persantine)	5 mg/kg/day PO ÷ bid	
Dobutamine	2–20 μg/kg/min IV Max: 40 μg/kg/min	See drug infusion table (p 682). Should be used in critical care areas only.
Docusate (Colace)	5 mg/kg/day PO ÷ q6–8h or once daily 50–100 mg docusate sodium drops to enema solution per rectum prn	
Dopamine	*Renal vasodilation*: (dopaminergic): 2–5 μg/kg/min IV *Inotropic effect*: (beta-adrenergic): 5–20 μg/kg/min IV *Vasoconstrictive effect*: (alpha-adrenergic): >20 μg/kg/min IV Max: 25 μg/kg/min	See drug infusion table (p 682). Should be used in critical care areas only. Should be given through a central venous line, although in an emergency setting the drug may be administered peripherally for a short period, preferably through a separate line.
Doxycycline (Vibramycin)	5 mg/kg/day PO or IV ÷ q12h Max: 200 mg/day	Not recommended for children $\leq$8 yr of age.

MAXIMAL DOSAGES ARE PRINTED IN RED

815

Drug Dosage Guidelines in Children

Drug	Dose	Comments
Edrophonium (Tensilon)	*Test for myasthenia gravis*: 0.05 mg/kg/dose IV; if no response in 1 min, give 1 mg increments Max total dose: 10 mg or 0.2 mg/kg, whichever is less	When using this drug, atropine and equipment for resuscitation should be available.
Epinephrine (Adrenaline)	*Croup*: 0.05 ml/kg/dose of racemic epinephrine 2.25% inhalation sol^n diluted in 3 ml of 0.9% NaCl via nebulizer prn up to max of q1h Usual dose: 0.5 ml regardless of weight Max: 0.5 ml/dose *Status asthmaticus, cardiac arrest, anaphylaxis*: 0.01 mg/kg/dose IV, SC, or ETT q10–20 min prn (= 0.01 ml/kg of 1:1,000 or 0.1 ml/kg of 1:10,000) Max: 1.0 ml of 1:1,000 SC, 1.0 mg/dose IV or ETT 0.1–1.0 μg/kg/min IV as continuous infusion	1:1,000 = 1 mg/ml 1:10,000 = 0.1 mg/ml For SC injection 1:1,000 preferred. SC injection not suitable for cardiac arrest. Minimum dose in cardiac arrest is 1 ml of 1:10,000. Continuous IV infusion should be used in critical care areas only.

MAXIMAL DOSAGES ARE PRINTED IN RED

Drug	Dose	Comments
Erythromycin	Base (E-Mycin): 40 mg/kg/day PO ÷ q6h Estolate (Ilosone): 20–40 mg/kg/day PO ÷ q6–12h Ethylsuccinate (EES): 40 mg/kg/day PO ÷ q6h Ethylsuccinate and sulfisoxazole (Ped azole): 50 mg erythromycin/kg/day and 150 mg sulfisoxazole/kg/day PO ÷ q6–8h Gluceptate (Ilotycin): 20–50 mg/kg/day IV ÷ q6h Lactobionate (Erythrocin): 20–40 mg/kg/day IV ÷ q6h Stearate (Erythrocin): 20–40 mg/kg/day PO ÷ q6h Ointment (Ilotycin): Ophthalmic prophylaxis: 0.5–1 cm each conjunctival sac Ophthalmic infections: 3–6 times daily Max: 2 g/day PO, 4 g/day IV	Base is used in cystic fibrosis. 5 ml Pediazole = 200 mg erythromycin and 600 mg sulfisoxazole Gluceptate and lactobionate for IV use.

MAXIMAL DOSAGES ARE PRINTED IN RED

Drug Dosage Guidelines in Children

Drug	Dose	Comments
Ethambutol	15–25 mg/kg/day PO once daily Max: 1500 mg/day	The higher dose of 25 mg/kg/day should be used for a maximum of 60 days only. Ophthalmic testing (including color testing) recommended before and throughout treatment. Increase dosing interval to q24–36h in moderate and to q48h in severe renal impairment.
Ethosuximide (Zarontin)	Initial dose: 15 mg/kg/day PO once daily or ÷ bid Increase gradually q3 days to maximum of 40 mg/kg/day or 1.5 g/day, whichever is less	Monitoring of serum drug concentrations is recommended.
Fenoterol (Berotec)	0.04 mg/kg/day PO ÷ tid–qid 0.03 mg/kg/dose in 2–3 ml NS by inhalation qid prn 1–2 puffs q4–6h prn Max: 15 mg/day PO, 4 mg/day via inhalation	
Ferrous sulfate (Fer-In-Sol)	Treatment: 6 mg elemental Fe/kg/day PO ÷ tid Prophylaxis: 0.5–2 mg elemental Fe/kg/day PO once daily or ÷ bid–tid	300 mg tab = 60 mg elemental Fe 75 mg/0.6 ml drops = 15 mg elemental Fe/0.6 ml

MAXIMAL DOSAGES ARE PRINTED IN RED

Drug	Dose	Comments
Flucloxacillin	25–100 mg/kg/day PO ÷ q6h Max: 4 g/day	
Flucytosine	50–150 mg/kg/day PO ÷ q6h	Increase dosing interval to q12h in moderate and to q24–48h in severe renal impairment.
Furosemide (Lasix)	1–2 mg/kg/dose PO; increase to 3–6 mg/kg/dose PO q6–8h if needed 0.5–2 mg/kg/dose IV Max: 6 mg/kg/dose PO or IV	Slow IV push no faster than 20 mg/min.
Fusidic acid	≤1 yr: 1 ml/kg/day PO ÷ tid 1–5 yr: 5 ml PO tid 6–12 yr: 10 ml PO tid >12 yr: 15 ml PO tid	5 ml suspension = 246 mg fusidic acid

MAXIMAL DOSAGES ARE PRINTED IN RED

FORMULARY

Drug Dosage Guidelines in Children

Drug	Dose	Comments
Gentamicin	7.5 mg/kg/day IV or IM ÷ q8h Max initial dose: 100 mg IV or IM 1–2 mg/dose once daily intrathecally or intraventricularly	Monitoring of serum drug concentrations is recommended. Increase dosing interval to q12h in mild to moderate and to q24–48h in severe renal impairment. Monitoring of intraventricular drug concentrations is recommended if given by intraventricular route.
Glucagon	*Glucagon stimulation test*: 0.03 mg/kg IM Max: 1 mg *Hypoglycemia*: Infants: 0.5 mg IM or IV Children: 1.0 mg IM or IV	1 unit = 1 mg
Glucose	*Hypoglycemia*: 0.5–1 g/kg (1–2 ml/kg of 50% dextrose) IV	In young children, dilute 50% glucose 1:1 with sterile water (to a 25% solution) to avoid damage to soft tissues.
Gold sodium thiomalate (Myochrysine)	Week 1: 0.25 mg/kg IM once weekly Week 2: 0.5 mg/kg IM once weekly Then: 1.0 mg/kg IM once weekly or monthly Max: 50 mg/dose	Monitor CBC and urinalysis weekly. Rarely, coagulopathy may occur following the second injection.

MAXIMAL DOSAGES ARE PRINTED IN RED

Drug	Dose	Comments
Golytely	Older child: 240 ml PO q10 min until rectal effluent is clear Max: 4 L	
Griseofulvin	Microsize preparation: 15 mg/kg/day PO once daily Max: 1 g/day Ultramicrosize preparation: 5–10 mg/kg/day PO once daily Max: 660 mg/day	

MAXIMAL DOSAGES ARE PRINTED IN RED

Drug Dosage Guidelines in Children

Drug	Dose	Comments
Haloperidol (Haldol)	*Gilles de la Tourette*: Initial dose: 0.25 mg PO once daily Increase daily dose by 0.25 mg/day every 5–14 days prn Max: 7 mg/day *Severe agitation or acute psychosis*: 0.5 mg/dose PO then 0.01–0.1 mg/kg/dose PO q2h until symptoms controlled or side effects occur or 0.25 mg/dose IM then 0.005–0.05 mg/kg/dose IM q2h until symptoms controlled or side effects occur	This drug can cause extrapyramidal reactions—careful follow-up is required.
Heparin	Initial dose: 50–75 units/kg IV bolus Maint: 10–25 units/kg/hr via continuous IV infusion	Maintain PTT 1½–2½ times normal. Antidote = protamine sulfate.
Hydralazine (Apresoline)	Initial dose: 0.15–0.8 mg/kg/dose IV q4–6h or 1.5 μg/kg/min IV Maint: 0.75–7 mg/kg/day PO ÷ q6h Max: 200 mg/day or 7 mg/kg/day, whichever is less	Associated with development of drug induced lupus.

MAXIMAL DOSAGES ARE PRINTED IN RED

Drug	Dose	Comments
Hydrochlorothiazide (HydroDiuril)	2–4 mg/kg/day PO ÷ q12h	For hydrochlorothiazide in combination with spironolactone, see Novospirozine (p 834).
Hydrocortisone (Solu-Cortef)	See p 854	
Hydroxychloroquine (Plaquenil)	6 mg/kg/day PO once daily Max: 400 mg/day	To be taken with food. Ophthalmologic evaluation every 4 mo.
Hydroxyzine (Atarax)	2 mg/kg/day PO ÷ tid–qid Max: 400 mg/day	
Ibuprofen (Motrin, Advil)	40–50 mg/kg/day PO ÷ tid–qid Max: 2400 mg/day	
Imipramine (Tofranil)	*Enuresis:* ≥5 yr: 10–50 mg PO qhs ≥12 yr: up to 75 mg PO qhs Max: 2.5 mg/kg/day *Depression:* Initial: 0.5 mg/kg/dose PO qhs × 2 nights; then increase daily dose by 0.5 mg/kg/day (÷ bid–tid) every 3 days prn Max: 5 mg/kg/day (3.5 mg/kg/day in older adolescent)	Monitoring of serum drug concentrations during chronic therapy for depression is recommended. Monitor ECG when using doses larger than 3.5 mg/kg/day.

MAXIMAL DOSAGES ARE PRINTED IN RED

Drug Dosage Guidelines in Children

Drug	Dose	Comments
Indomethacin (Indocid)	1.5–3 mg/kg/day PO ÷ tid with meals Max: 200 mg/day	
Iodoquinol (Diodoquin, Yodoxin)	*Asymptomatic intestinal amebiasis*: 30–40 mg/kg/day PO ÷ tid × 20 days Max: 1.95 g/day	
Ipecac syrup	9–12 mo: 10 ml PO—no repeat 1–10 yr: 15 ml PO—can repeat once after 20 min >10 yr: 30 ml PO—can repeat once after 20 min	Do not give to patient with decreased level of consciousness. Contact poison center re treatment of patients <9 mo old.
Ipratropium bromide (Atrovent)	2 puffs (40 μg) tid–qid Inhalation solution: 250 μg in 3 ml NS q4–8h	
Iron dextran	Total dose elemental iron (mg) = (wt [kg] × desired increase in Hb [g/L] × 0.25) + (wt [kg] × 10) Give IM or IV divided over several days Max: <5 kg: 0.5 ml/day IM or IV <10 kg: 1 ml/day IM or IV <50 kg: 2 ml/day IM or IV >50 kg: 5 ml/day IM or 2 ml/day IV	Use only if oral route is not feasible. Be prepared to resuscitate during intravenous therapy. IV rate not to exceed 50 mg/min. Administer IM by Z-track technique. 1 ml contains 50 mg of elemental iron.

MAXIMAL DOSAGES ARE PRINTED IN RED

Drug	Dose	Comments
Isoniazid (INH)	10–20 mg/kg/day PO ÷ q12–24h Max: 500 mg/day (CNS disease) 300 mg/day (non-CNS disease)	Pyridoxine supplementation in adolescents and adults.
Isoproterenol (Isuprel)	*Asthma*: 0.1 μg/kg/min IV Max: 1 μg/kg/min IV 15–30 mg/day SL ÷ q6–8h prn 0.25–0.5 ml of 1:200 inhalation sol^n in 2 ml NS via nebulizer q3–4h 1–2 puffs q4–6h prn *CHF*: 0.05–0.5 μg/kg/min IV; increase by 0.1 μg/kg/min until effect achieved *Bradycardia or sinus arrest*: Bolus 3 μg/kg IV; then 0.05–0.5 μg/kg/min IV Max: 1 μg/kg/min IV	Monitor for tachycardia and arrhythmias. See drug infusion table (p 682). Should be used IV in critical care areas only.
Ketoconazole	*Antifungal*: 5–10 mg/kg/day PO once daily or ÷ q12h Max: 400 mg/day	

MAXIMAL DOSAGES ARE PRINTED IN RED

Drug Dosage Guidelines in Children

Drug	Dose	Comments
Lactulose (Cephulac)	*Constipation*: Initial dose 5–10 ml/day PO once daily *Hepatic encephalopathy*: <1 yr: 2.5 ml PO bid Max: 2.5 ml PO qid Older children and adolescents: 10–30 ml PO tid	For constipation, double daily dose until stool produced. When using in hepatic encephalopathy: 1. Decrease or discontinue if severe diarrhea develops. 2. Hypernatremia or hypokalemia may occur. 3. Treatment is effective if stool is mushy and stool pH <5.5.
Levothyroxine (Eltroxin, Synthroid)	1–6 mo: 7–12 μg/kg/day PO once daily 6–12 mo: 6–8 μg/kg/day PO once daily 1–5 yr: 4–6 μg/kg/day PO once daily 5–10 yr: 3–5 μg/kg/day PO once daily 10–20 yr: 2–3 μg/kg/day PO once daily	Adjust dose according to clinical state and thyroid function tests.
Lidocaine (Xylocaine)	*Ventricular arrhythmias*: Initial dose: 1 mg/kg/dose IV or ETT; may repeat once after 5 min Max: 100 mg/dose Subsequent infusion: 20–50 μg/kg/min IV Max: 4 mg/min	Monitoring of serum drug concentrations is recommended. Reduction of dose may be required if therapy continues longer than 24 hr. Should be used in critical care areas only.

MAXIMAL DOSAGES ARE PRINTED IN RED

Drug	Dose	Comments
Lindane (Kwellada, Kwell, gamma benzene hexachloride)	*Scabies*: Apply cream or lotion in a thin layer to skin below the neck and leave on overnight. Bathe in 8–12 hr. *Pediculosis capitis*: Work shampoo into dry hair for 4 min. Add water and work into hair another 4 min. Rinse. Repeat treatment in 7 days.	Consider use of an alternative scabicide in child <2 yr because of possible CNS toxicity.
Loperamide (Imodium)	0.08–0.24 mg/kg/day PO ÷ bid–tid Max: 16 mg/day	Following the first treatment day give 0.1 mg/kg/dose (max: 2 mg/dose, 16 mg/day) only after a loose stool.
Lorazepam (Ativan)	*Preop*: 0.05 mg/kg/dose PO *Status epilepticus*: 0.05 mg/kg/dose IV; may repeat once Max: 4 mg/dose, 8 mg/12 hr	Dilute injection with equal parts of NS or D5W. Administer IV at a rate not to exceed 2 mg/min.
Magnesium citrate (5%) (Citro-Mag)	*Cathartic*: 4 ml/kg/dose PO Max: 200 ml/dose	Solution contains 50 g/L. Caution in renal failure patients—magnesium may be absorbed.

MAXIMAL DOSAGES ARE PRINTED IN RED

Drug Dosage Guidelines in Children

Drug	Dose	Comments
Magnesium glucoheptonate (Magnesium Rougier)	*Hypomagnesemia*: 20–40 mg elemental Mg^{++}/kg/day PO ÷ tid	100 mg magnesium glucoheptonate = 5 mg elemental magnesium. Large doses may cause diarrhea. Caution in renal failure patients.
Magnesium hydroxide (Milk of Magnesia)	*Cathartic*: 0.5 ml/kg/dose PO = 40 mg/kg/dose PO	Caution in renal failure patients.
Magnesium sulfate	*Cathartic*: 250 mg/kg/dose PO *Hypomagnesemia*: 10 mg elemental Mg^{++}/kg/dose IV = 1.0 ml 10% $MgSO_4$/kg/dose = 0.42 mmol/kg/dose Then 10 mg elemental Mg^{++}/kg/day = 1.0 ml 10% $MgSO_4$/kg/day via continuous IV infusion	Caution in renal failure patients.
Mannitol	*Test for oliguria*: 0.2 g/kg/dose IV over 10 min × 1 dose *Cerebral edema*: 0.2–0.5 g/kg/dose IV over 10–30 min = 1.0–2.5 ml/kg IV of 20% solution	For further information on use of mannitol for cerebral edema see p 478.

MAXIMAL DOSAGES ARE PRINTED IN RED

Drug	Dose	Comments
Mebendazole (Vermox)	*Pinworm*: >2 yr: 100 mg PO once daily × 1; then repeat in 2 wks *Other nematodes*: >2 yr: 200 mg/day PO ÷ bid × 3 days	Not for use in children <2 yr.
Meperidine (Demerol)	*Pain*: 6 mg/kg/day PO, IM, SC, or IV ÷ q4–6h *Preop*: 1–2 mg/kg/dose IM, PO, or SC, 60 min preop Max: 100 mg/dose or 2 mg/kg/dose IV, IM, or SC, whichever is less or 4 mg/kg/dose PO	May cause constipation or CNS depression. Dose is cumulative and may cause respiratory depression.
Methicillin	150–200 mg/kg/day IM, or IV ÷ q6h	
Methimazole (Tapazole)	Initial dose: 0.4–0.7 mg/kg/day PO ÷ q8h Increase up to 1.5 mg/kg/day if no improvement within 2–3 wk Maint: 0.2 mg/kg/day PO ÷ q8h or once daily	
Methyldopa (Aldomet)	Initial dose: 10 mg/kg/day PO ÷ tid–qid Increase dose gradually over several days until desired effect achieved Max: 4 g/day or 65 mg/kg/day, whichever is less	Increase dosing interval to q9–18h in moderate and to q12–24h in severe renal impairment.

MAXIMAL DOSAGES ARE PRINTED IN RED

FORMULARY

Drug Dosage Guidelines in Children

Drug	Dose	Comments
Methylene blue	*Methemoglobinemia*: 1–2 mg/kg/dose IV as a 1% solution over 5 min; may repeat after 1 hr if cyanosis persists Max total dose: 7 mg/kg	
Methylphenidate (Ritalin)	0.25–1 mg/kg/day PO as a single morning dose or divided bid given in morning and at noon Max: 60 mg/day or 2 mg/kg/day, whichever is less	May cause decreased growth and rarely hallucinations. Consider discontinuation during school holidays and weekends. Sustained release tablets are available.
Methylprednisolone (Solu-Medrol)	See p 854	
Metoclopramide (Maxeran)	*Small bowel intubation*: 0.1 mg/kg/dose PO, IM or IV *Antineoplastic emesis prophylaxis*: 0.5–2 mg/kg/dose IV or PO q3–4h prn Max initial dose: 20 mg Max: 10 mg/kg/day *Delayed gastric emptying*: <5 yr: 0.5 mg/kg/day PO ÷ tid with meals 5–14 yr: 2.5–5 mg PO tid before meals >14 yr: 5–10 mg PO tid before meals	May alter absorption of other drugs.

MAXIMAL DOSAGES ARE PRINTED IN RED

Drug	Dose	Comments
Metronidazole (Flagyl)	*Symptomatic intestinal or invasive amebiasis:* 50 mg/kg/day PO ÷ tid × 5–10 days Max: 2.25 g/day *Giardiasis:* 15 mg/kg/day PO ÷ tid × 7 days Max: 750 mg/day or <25 kg: 35 mg/kg/day PO once daily × 3 days 25–40 kg: 50 mg/kg/day PO once daily × 3 days >40 kg: 2 g/day PO once daily × 3 days *Anaerobes:* 15–30 mg/kg/day PO ÷ q8h 30 mg/kg/day IV ÷ q6h Max: 4 g/day IV; 2 g/day PO *Trichomonas vaginalis:* >13 yrs: 2 g PO stat	Avoid alcohol—may cause Antabuse-like effect. When treating amebiasis, one must use a lumenicidal agent in addition (e.g., iodoquinol). When treating *Trichomonas vaginalis*, partner must also be treated.
Mineral oil	1 ml/kg/dose PO qhs >6 yr: 10–60 ml/dose PO qhs	Caution regarding aspiration—may cause lipoid pneumonia. Avoid in children <1 yr old.

MAXIMAL DOSAGES ARE PRINTED IN RED

Drug Dosage Guidelines in Children

Drug	Dose	Comments
Minoxidil (Loniten)	Initial dose: 0.2 mg/kg/day PO ÷ bid or once daily Max: 5 mg/dose Maint: Increase dosage gradually to obtain desired effect to 0.25–1.4 mg/kg/day Max: adolescent 100 mg/day, child 50 mg/day	
Morphine	*Pre x-ray*: 0.05 mg/kg/dose IV; may repeat × 1 in 15–20 min prn Max: 5 mg/dose *Preop*: 0.05–0.2 mg/kg/dose IM 30–60 min preop Max: 10 mg/dose *Pain*: 0.15–0.3 mg/kg/dose PO, IV, IM or SC q4h prn 0.1–1 μg/kg/min via continuous IV, or SC infusion	No dosing limit for palliative care.
Nabilone	See p 874	
Nadolol (Corgard)	*Hypertension*: 1 mg/kg/day PO once daily Increase daily dose by 1 mg/kg/day q3–4day Max: 4 mg/kg/day or 320 mg/day, whichever is less	To convert from propranolol to nadolol, use ⅔ of the daily propranolol dose.

MAXIMAL DOSAGES ARE PRINTED IN RED

Drug	Dose	Comments
Nalidixic acid (NegGram)	55 mg/kg/day PO ÷ q6h Max: 4 g/day	Do not use if creatinine clearance is less than 10 ml/min/1.73m^2.
Naloxone (Narcan)	0.03 mg/kg/dose IV If no response, may give up to 0.1 mg/kg/dose Repeat as needed q5–10 min	
Naproxen (Naprosyn)	10–20 mg/kg/day PO ÷ bid Max: 1.0 g/day	
Neomycin	*Infection*: 50–100 mg/kg/day PO ÷ q6–8h *Hepatic encephalopathy*: 20–30 mg/kg/day PO ÷ q6h Max: 2 g/day	
Neostigmine	*Myasthenia gravis*: test dose: 0.04 mg/kg/dose IM × 1 or 0.02 mg/kg/dose IV × 1 Treatment: 0.01–0.04 mg/kg/dose IM, IV, or SC q2–3h prn Max: 10 mg/day IM, IV, or SC 2 mg/kg/day PO ÷ q3–4h *Curare antagonism*: 0.02–0.08 mg/kg/dose IV together with atropine Max: 2.5 mg/dose IV	

MAXIMAL DOSAGES ARE PRINTED IN RED

FORMULARY

Drug Dosage Guidelines in Children

Drug	Dose	Comments
Nifedipine	*Hypertension:* Initial dose: 0.5 mg/kg/day PO ÷ q8h Increase to: 1–1.5 mg/kg/day PO	
Nitrazepam (Mogadon)	Initial dose: 0.25 mg/kg/day PO once daily or ÷ tid Increase gradually prn to 1.2 mg/kg/day	Reduce dose in liver impairment.
Nitrofurantoin macrocrystals (Macrodantin)	3–8 mg/kg/day PO ÷ q6h Max: 400 mg/day	
Nitroglycerin	0.5–10 μg/kg/min via continuous IV infusion	Should be used in critical care areas only. See drug infusion table (p 682).
Nitroprusside	0.5–8 μg/kg/min via continuous IV infusion Max: cumulative dose: 2.5 mg/kg/day	Caution regarding cyanide toxicity. See drug infusion table (p 682). Should be used with D5W. Should be used in critical care areas only.
Norepinephrine	0.02–0.1 μg/kg/min via continuous IV infusion	Should be administered through central line to avoid skin necrosis. See drug infusion table (p 682). Should be used in critical care areas only.
Novospirozine	2–4 mg of each component/kg/day PO ÷ bid	Contains equal amounts of hydrochloro- thiazide and spironolactone.

MAXIMAL DOSAGES ARE PRINTED IN RED

Drug	Dose	Comments
Nystatin (Mycostatin)	400,000–2,400,000 units/day PO ÷ q4–6h	
Orciprenaline (Alupent, metaproterenol)	0.9–2.0 mg/kg/day PO ÷ tid–qid Max: 20 mg/dose PO 0.01–0.03 ml of inhalation sol^n/kg/dose in 3 ml NS q4–6h by inhalation Max: 1.0 ml/dose	
Oxybutynin (Ditropan)	*Enuresis*: 5 mg/day PO qhs *Neurogenic bladder*: 10–15 mg/day PO ÷ bid–tid	Not recommended for children <5 yr.
Pancrelipase (Cotazym)	Infants: 1 regular cap or ⅓ tsp powder/120 ml formula Child or adult: regular cap: 6/meal, 2/snack ECS: 3/meal, 1/snack	1 regular cap = 8,000 units lipase 1 tsp powder = 24,000 units lipase 1 ECS = 8,000 units lipase ECS not to be used in children who cannot swallow capsule as mucosal ulceration may result. ECS usually preferred in older children. Titrate dose to stool fat content.

MAXIMAL DOSAGES ARE PRINTED IN RED

Drug Dosage Guidelines in Children

Drug	Dose	Comments
Pancuronium (Pavulon)	*Muscle paralysis for mechanical ventilation:* 0.1 mg/kg/dose IV q30 min prn *Prevention of fasciculation associated with succinylcholine:* 0.006–0.01 mg/kg/dose IV	If succinylcholine used for intubation, decrease initial pancuronium dose by 33%. Should be used in critical care or operating areas only.
Paraldehyde	200–400 mg/kg/dose (0.2–0.4 ml of undiluted paraldehyde/kg/dose) per rectum q4–8h Give as a 30–50% sol^n in oil or normal saline Max: 10 g/dose (10 ml of undiluted paraldehyde/dose) per rectum 100–150 mg/kg/dose (2–3 ml of a 5% sol^n/kg/dose) IV over 15–20 min; then 20 mg/kg/hr (0.4 ml of a 5% sol^n/kg/hr) as a continuous IV infusion	Do not administer in polyvinyl chloride plastic. Administer IV via a syringe pump with non-PVC tubing as 5% solution in normal saline. Undiluted paraldehyde contains 1 g/ml.
Pemoline (Cylert)	Initial dose: 37.5 mg/day PO as a single AM dose Increase daily dose by 18.75 mg at weekly intervals until desired response is obtained Max: 3 mg/kg/day or 150 mg/day, whichever is less	Not recommended for children <6 yr. Consider discontinuation during school holidays. Tablets: 18.75 mg, 37.5 mg, 75 mg.

MAXIMAL DOSAGES ARE PRINTED IN RED

Drug	Dose	Comments
Penicillamine (Cuprimine, Depen)	*Juvenile rheumatoid arthritis:* Initial dose: 3–5 mg/kg/day PO once daily Max: 250 mg/day Increase to max of 15 mg/kg/day PO ÷ bid–tid at 2–3 mo intervals Max: 1 g/day	Monitor CBC, urinalysis q1–2 wk. Administer on empty stomach.
Penicillin G (Benzylpenicillin)	100,000–400,000 units/kg/day IM or IV ÷ q4–6h Max: 20 million units/day IM or IV	600 mg $\sim$1 million units. Increase dosing interval to q8–12h in moderate and to q12–16h in severe renal impairment. 1 million units of penicillin G contains $\sim$1.7 mmol of either Na^+ or K^+.
Penicillin G benzathine (Bicillin)	*Rheumatic heart disease prophylaxis:* 1.2 million units IM once monthly *Streptococcal pharyngitis:* <27 kg: 600,000 units IM × 1 dose >27 kg: 1.2 million units IM × 1 dose *Syphilis (primary or secondary of less than 1 year's duration:* 50,000 units/kg IM × 1 dose Max: 2.4 million units/dose	

MAXIMAL DOSAGES ARE PRINTED IN RED

Drug Dosage Guidelines in Children

Drug	Dose	Comments
Penicillin G procaine	25,000–50,000 units/kg/day IM once daily or ÷ q12h Max: 4.8 million units/day	
Penicillin V	*Infection*: 15–50 mg/kg/day PO ÷ q6–8h Max: 3 g/day *Prophylaxis in asplenics*: >5 yr: 250 mg PO bid *Rheumatic fever prophylaxis*: >5 yr: 125–250 mg PO bid	250 mg ~ 400,000 units
Pentobarbital (Nembutal)	*Preop*: 2–4 mg/kg/dose PO in >8 yr 3–4 mg/kg/dose per rectum in <8 yr 60–120 min preop Max: 120 mg/dose PO or per rectum *Pre x-ray*: <15 kg: 6 mg/kg/dose IM or per rectum >15 kg: 5 mg/kg/dose IM or per rectum 20–30 min pre x-ray Max: 200 mg/dose	For pre x-ray, if initial dose is not effective, may give supplementary dose 1–1½ hr later of 2 mg/kg for ≤15 kg or 2.5 mg/kg for >15 kg.

MAXIMAL DOSAGES ARE PRINTED IN RED

Drug	Dose	Comments
Phenobarbital	*Status epilepticus*: 20 mg/kg IV loading dose *Epilepsy*: <3 mo: 5–6 mg/kg/day PO once daily or ÷ bid >3 mo: 3–5 mg/kg/day PO once daily or ÷ bid Adolescent: 2–4 mg/kg/day PO once daily or ÷ bid Max: 200 mg/day	Administer IV at a rate not to exceed 60 mg/min. Monitoring of serum drug concentrations is recommended.
Phenylephrine (Neo-Synephrine)	*Hypotension*: 0.1 mg/kg/dose IM q1–2h prn 5–20 μg/kg/dose IV q10–15 min prn or 0.1–0.5 μg/kg/min as continuous IV infusion Max initial infusion rate: 4 μg/min *SVT*: 0.01–0.1 mg/kg IV push *Hypercyanotic spell*: 0.1–0.5 μg/kg/min as continuous IV infusion	For SVT and hypercyanotic spells, the end-point dosage should be based on a successful result or a 50% increase in blood pressure over baseline.

MAXIMAL DOSAGES ARE PRINTED IN RED

Drug Dosage Guidelines in Children

Drug	Dose	Comments
Phenytoin (Dilantin)	Status epilepticus: 20 mg/kg IV loading dose Max: 1 g/dose *Epilepsy*: 0.5–3 yr: 7–9 mg/kg/day PO ÷ bid–tid 4–6 yr: 6.5 mg/kg/day PO ÷ bid–tid 7–9 yr: 6 mg/kg/day PO ÷ bid–tid 10–16 yr: 3–5 mg/kg/day PO ÷ bid–tid *Arrhythmia*: Loading: 1) 15 mg/kg/dose IV over 1 hr; simultaneously give 3 mg/kg/dose PO × 1 dose; then 6 hr later give 2 mg/kg/dose PO × 1 dose; start PO maintenance 6 hr later or 2) 5 mg/kg/dose PO q6h × 4 doses; then 2.5 mg/kg/dose PO q6h × 4 doses Maint: 5–6 mg/kg/day PO ÷ bid	IV push rate no faster than 50 mg/min. Monitoring of serum drug concentrations is recommended. Monitor for hypotension during infusion.
Piperacillin	200–300 mg/kg/day IV ÷ q4–6h Max: 24 g/day	Increase dosing interval to q8h in severe renal impairment.
Piperazine (Entacyl, Antepar)	*Roundworm*: 75 mg/kg/day PO ÷ bid–tid × 2 days Max: 3.5 g/day	

MAXIMAL DOSAGES ARE PRINTED IN RED

Drug	Dose	Comments
Potassium chloride	*Potassium replacement*: 2–3 mmol/kg/day IV or PO as starting dose *Digoxin toxicity*: 0.3 mmol/kg/dose IV	Administer well mixed IV at maximal rate of 0.5–1 mmol/kg/hr. Should be given under ECG control at maximal doses. Central line is necessary for administration of solutions containing ≥60 mmol of KCl/L.
Potassium iodide	*Thyrotoxicosis*: 2–4 mg/kg/day PO ÷ bid–tid	Give as Lugol's solution (5% iodine + 10% potassium iodide).
Prazosin (Minipress)	↑*BP*: initial dose: 30–40 µg/kg/day PO ÷ tid–qid; increase until desired effect is reached *CHF*: first dose: 5 µg/kg/dose PO; then 40–100 µg/kg/day PO ÷ q6h	
Prednisone	See p 855	

MAXIMAL DOSAGES ARE PRINTED IN RED

Drug Dosage Guidelines in Children

Drug	Dose	Comments
Primidone (Mysoline)	**0–8 yr** Starting dose: 125 mg PO qhs Increase on day 7 to: 125 mg PO bid Increase on day 14 to: 125 mg PO tid Increase on day 21 to: 10–25 mg/kg/day PO ÷ tid–qid **>8 yr** Starting dose: 250 mg PO qhs Increase on day 7 to: 250 mg PO bid Increase on day 14 to: 250 mg PO tid Increase on day 21 to: 750–1500 mg/day PO ÷ tid–qid	Monitoring of serum drug concentrations of primidone and phenobarbital is recommended.
Procainamide (Pronestyl)	15–60 mg/kg/day PO ÷ q4–6h Max: 500 mg/dose PO Loading dose: 12 mg/kg/hr IV for a maximum of 75 min Then 20–80 μg/kg/min by continuous IV infusion	Monitoring of serum drug concentrations of procainamide and NAPA is recommended. May be associated with SLE. IV loading dose should be switched to maintenance infusion rate prior to 75 min if arrhythmia reverts or QRS prolonged 50% over baseline.

MAXIMAL DOSAGES ARE PRINTED IN RED

Drug	Dose	Comments
Promethazine (Phenergan)	*Antihistamine:* 0.1 mg/kg/dose PO q6h and 0.5 mg/kg/dose PO qhs *Emesis:* 0.25–0.5 mg/kg/dose IM, PO, or per rectum q4–6h prn	
Propantheline (Pro-Banthine)	1.5 mg/kg/day PO ÷ q6h or 2.5 mg/kg/dose PO qhs	
Propranolol (Inderal)	*↑BP:* 0.5–4.0 mg/kg/day PO ÷ tid–qic *Arrhythmia:* 0.01–0.15 mg/kg/dose IV q6–8h prn Max: 3 mg/dose IV *Tetralogy spells:* 0.05–0.10 mg/kg/dose IV over 10 min Maint: 2–8 mg/kg/day PO ÷ tid–qid	Monitor heart rate. IV propranolol should be given only under ECG monitoring at a rate not to exceed 1 mg/min.
Propylthiouracil	Initial dose: 150 mg/m^2/day PO ÷ q8h or 10 mg/kg/day PO ÷ q8h Maint: usually 1/3–1/2 initial dose once patient is euthyroid	Administer on an empty stomach. May depress bone marrow.

MAXIMAL DOSAGES ARE PRINTED IN RED

Drug Dosage Guidelines in Children

Drug	Dose	Comments
Protamine sulfate	1 mg IV for every 100 units of heparin administered in the previous 3–4 hr at a rate not to exceed 5 mg/min Max: 50 mg/dose	Actual protamine neutralization factor for each heparin lot is listed on heparin label.
Pseudoephedrine (Sudafed)	4 mg/kg/day PO ÷ q6h	Use with caution in children <2 yr old.
Pyrantel pamoate (Combantrin)	*Pinworm or roundworm*: 11 mg/kg/dose PO × 1 dose only *Hookworm*: 11 mg/kg/day PO as a single daily dose × 3 days Max: 1 g/dose	For pinworm repeat dose after 2 wk.
Pyrazinamide	30 mg/kg/day PO ÷ q12h or once daily	
Quinidine	15–60 mg/kg/day of quinidine base PO ÷ q6h	Quinidine bisulfate = 65% quinidine base Quinidine sulfate = 80% quinidine base Quinidine gluconate = 60% quinidine base Slow release preparations are available. For patients also receiving digoxin, monitor digoxin levels and reduce digoxin dose accordingly. Monitoring of serum drug concentrations is recommended.

MAXIMAL DOSAGES ARE PRINTED IN RED

Drug	Dose	Comments
Quinine	*Malaria*: 25 mg/kg/day PO ÷ tid × 3 days Max: 650 mg/dose	Adult dose is 600 mg or 650 mg, depending on formulation available.
Ranitidine (Zantac)	1.25–1.9 mg/kg/day IV ÷ q6–12h 2.5–3.8 mg/kg/day PO ÷ q12h Max: 300 mg/day except in Zollinger-Ellison syndrome	Decrease dose to 25–50% in severe renal impairment.
Ribavirin	A sol^n containing 20 mg/ml is added to the reservoir of the SPAG-2 Give by inhalation for 12–18 hr/day for 3–7 days	Use small particle aerosol generator (SPAG-2).
Rifampin	*TB*: 10–20 mg/kg/day PO once daily or ÷ q12h Max: 600 mg/day *H. influenzae prophylaxis*: 20 mg/kg/day PO once daily × 4 days Max: 600 mg/day *Meningococcal prophylaxis*: 20 mg/kg/day PO ÷ q12h × 2 days Max: 1200 mg/day	May discolor urine, sweat, saliva, tears.

MAXIMAL DOSAGES ARE PRINTED IN RED

Drug Dosage Guidelines in Children

Drug	Dose	Comments
Salbutamol, albuterol (Ventolin)	0.3–0.6 mg/kg/day PO ÷ tid–qid Max: 4 mg PO qid 0.01–0.03 ml of 0.5% inhalation sol^n/kg/dose in 3 ml NS q1–4h by inhalation (In severe cases give initial dose of 0.03 ml/kg followed by 0.01 ml/kg [max 0.33 ml] q20 min) Max: 1.0 ml/dose 0.5–1 μg/kg/min IV; increase by 1 μg/kg/min q15 min up to 10 μg/kg/min 1–2 puffs q4–6h prn; max: 8 puffs/day	Limit nebulized salbutamol to qid for outpatients. IV use should be used in critical care areas only. May cause profound hypokalemia. 1 puff = 100 μg
Sodium bicarbonate	*Resuscitation*: Initial dose: 2–3 mmol/kg IV Subsequent doses: 1–2 mmol/kg IV q10–20 min prn according to blood gases	Use 8.4% concentration in children, 4.2% concentration in prematures and newborns.
Sodium polystyrene sulfonate (Kayexalate)	1 g/kg/dose PO q6h prn 1 g/kg/dose per rectum q2–6h prn	Administer rectally in appropriate volume of tap water, D10W, or equal parts tap water and 2% methylcellulose. Moisten resin with water, honey, or jam for PO use. Exchanges ~1 mmol (1 mEq) potassium/g.

MAXIMAL DOSAGES ARE PRINTED IN RED

Drug	Dose	Comments
Sorbitol (70%)	*Cathartic*: 1.5–2.0 ml/kg PO Max: 150 ml/dose	
Spectinomycin	30–40 mg/kg IM × 1 dose Max: 4 g/dose	
Spironolactone (Aldactone)	1–4 mg/kg/day PO once daily or ÷ bid, tid, or qid	For spironolactone in combination with hydrochlorothiazide, see Novospirozine (p 834)
Steroids	See p 853	
Streptomycin	20–40 mg/kg/day IM ÷ q12h Max: 2 g/day	
Succinylcholine	1–2 mg/kg/dose IV × 1 only Do not repeat	Contraindications: malignant hyperthermia and hyperkalemia. Should be used in critical care and operating areas only.
Sucralfate (Sulcrate)	Adolescents and adults: 1 g/dose PO qid (1 hr AC + qhs)	

MAXIMAL DOSAGES ARE PRINTED IN RED

847

Drug Dosage Guidelines in Children

Drug	Dose	Comments
Sulfasalazine (Salazopyrin)	40–60 mg/kg/day PO ÷ bid-qid Max: 4 g/day	Begin with ⅓ of recommended dose and increase gradually q2 days to maximum required dose.
Sulfisoxazole (Gantrisin)	120–150 mg/kg/day PO ÷ q4–6h Max: 6 g/day	Increase dosing interval to q8–12h in moderate, q12–24h in severe renal impairment.
Terfenadine (Seldane)	3–6 yr: 30 mg/day PO ÷ bid 7–12 yr: 60 mg/day PO ÷ bid >12 yr: 120 mg/day PO ÷ bid	
Tetracycline	25–50 mg/kg/day PO ÷ q6h Max: 3 g/day PO 15–25 mg/kg/day IM ÷ q8–12h 20–30 mg/kg/day IV ÷ q8–12h Max: 2 g/day IM or IV	Not recommended for children ≤8 yr. Do not administer PO with milk or antacids.

MAXIMAL DOSAGES ARE PRINTED IN RED

Drug	Dose	Comments

Theophylline	*Intravenous*
	For patients not currently receiving theophylline:
	  Loading dose: 6 mg/kg IV, then
	  2–6 mo: 0.4 mg/kg/hr IV
	  6–11 mo: 0.7 mg/kg/hr IV
	  1–9 yr: 1.0 mg/kg/hr IV
	  9–12 yr: 0.8 mg/kg/hr IV
	  12–16 yr: 0.7 mg/kg/hr IV
	  >16 yr (nonsmoker): 0.6 mg/kg/hr IV
	  Cardiac decompensation, cor pulmonale,
	  liver dysfunction: 0.2 mg/kg/hr IV
	Oral
	Max maintenance dose prior to serum
	  concentration monitoring:
	  6–52 wk: (0.2 × [age in wk] + 5) mg/kg/day
	  PO ÷ q6–8h
	  1–9 yr: 24 mg/kg/day PO ÷ q8–12h
	  9–12 yr: 20 mg/kg/day PO ÷ q12h
	  12–16 yr: 18 mg/kg/day PO ÷ q12h
	  >16 yr: 14 mg/kg/day PO ÷ q12h
	Max: 900 mg/day PO
		Dose according to ideal body weight. Administer IV at a rate not to exceed 20 mg/min. If giving theophylline by bolus q6h, multiply hourly rate by 6 for appropriate age group. Monitoring of serum drug concentrations is recommended.
		
		Max oral doses should be attained in a stepwise fashion to prevent intolerance in patients not converted from IV therapy (start at 50% of recommended dose). These doses are for sustained release products, e.g., Theo-Dur, Somophyllin-12. Monitoring of serum drug concentrations is recommended.

MAXIMAL DOSAGES ARE PRINTED IN RED

FORMULARY

Drug Dosage Guidelines in Children

Drug	Dose	Comments
Thiopentone (Pentothal, thiopental)	*Seizures*: Loading dose: 3–5 mg/kg IV Then 2–4 mg/kg/hr by continuous IV infusion	May cause hypotension in patients with hypovolemia. Monitoring of serum drug concentrations is recommended. Should be used in critical care areas only.
Ticarcillin	200–300 mg/kg/day IV ÷ q4–6h Max: 24 g/day	Increase dosing interval to q12–24h in moderate, q24–48h in severe renal impairment.
Tobramycin	7.5 mg/kg/day IV or IM ÷ q8h Max initial dose: 100 mg	Increase dosing interval to q12h in mild to moderate, q24–48h in severe renal impairment. Monitoring of serum drug concentrations is recommended.
Tolmetin (Tolectin)	20–40 mg/kg/day PO ÷ tid–qid Max: 2 g/day	
Trimethoprim	4 mg/kg/day PO ÷ q12h Max: 200 mg/day	Increase dosing interval to q18h in moderate, q24h in severe renal impairment.
Valproic acid (Depakene)	Initial dose: 15 mg/kg/day PO once daily or ÷ q8–12h. Each week increase dose by 5–10 mg/kg/day up to 30–60 mg/kg/day PO ÷ tid–qid Max: 60 mg/kg/day	An enteric coated preparation, divalproex (Epival), dissociates into valproic acid in GI tract; it may have better GI tolerance. Monitoring of serum drug concentrations is recommended.

MAXIMAL DOSAGES ARE PRINTED IN RED

Drug	Dose	Comments
Vancomycin	*Pseudomembranous colitis*: 50 mg/kg/day PO ÷ q6h Max: 500 mg/day *Meningitis*: 60 mg/kg/day IV ÷ q6h Max: 4 g/day *Other*: 40 mg/kg/day IV ÷ q6h Max: 2 g/day	Parenteral preparation is used for oral dosing. Increase dosing interval to q6–72h in mild, q3–8 days in moderate, q8 days in severe renal impairment. Monitoring of serum drug concentrations is recommended.
Vasopressin (Pitressin)	*UGI (variceal) bleeding*: 0.2–0.3 unit/kg/dose IV over 20 min Repeat in 1–2 hr if bleeding continues	
Verapamil (Isoptin)	0–2 yr: 0.1–0.2 mg/kg/dose IV 2–15 yr: 0.1–0.3 mg/kg/dose IV Repeat in 30 min if needed Max: 10 mg/dose IV 4–10 mg/kg/day PO ÷ tid–qid	Avoid use in early postcardiosurgical period, in severe CHF, or in presence of beta-blockers. Use IV under ECG monitoring
Vidarabine (Vira-A)	15–30 mg/kg/day IV	Infuse daily dose over 12–24 hr.

MAXIMAL DOSAGES ARE PRINTED IN RED

Drug Dosage Guidelines in Children

Drug	Dose	Comments
Vitamin K_1 (phytonadione)	*Anticoagulant overdose*: Infants: 1–2 mg/dose IV, SC, or IM q4–8h prn Children: 5–10 mg/dose IV, SC, or IM q4–8h prn *Vitamin K deficiency*: 2.5–25 mg/day PO	Administer IV at a rate not to exceed 1 mg/min; PO, IM, or SC route preferred.
Warfarin (Coumadin)	Day 0: 0.2 mg/kg PO Max: 10 mg/dose Day 1: PT$\leq$14: 0.2 mg/kg PO PT>14: 0.1 mg/kg PO Day 2: PT<16: 0.2 mg/kg PO 16$\leq$PT<19: 0.1 mg/kg PO PT$\geq$19: hold dose Day 3: PT<19: 0.1 mg/kg PO PT$\geq$19: 0.08 mg/kg PO	Monitor PT daily. Adjust dose to maintain PT between 16–19. Adjust dose only after 2 days therapy on same dose. Then, increase or decrease dose by 20%. If PT$\geq$24 anytime, hold dose and repeat PT daily until PT<24. Restart warfarin at 20% less than previous dose.
Zinc	*Supplementation*: 0.5–1 mg/kg/day PO ÷ bid–tid *Acrodermatitis enteropathica*: 10–45 mg/day PO ÷ bid–tid	

MAXIMAL DOSAGES ARE PRINTED IN RED

STEROIDS

I. Equivalents

Drug	Relative Glucocorticoid Activity	Glucocorticoid/ Mineralocorticoid Ratio	Approximate Equivalent Dose (Glucocorticoid Effect)
Hydrocortisone	1.0	33	20 mg
Cortisone acetate	0.8	27	25 mg
Prednisone	4.0	100	5 mg
Methylprednisolone	5.0	300	4 mg
Dexamethasone	30.0	∞	0.75 mg
Fludrocortisone	10.0	2.4	—

II. Specific indications

Cortisone acetate
Hypoadrenalism: 25 mg/m^2/day PO ÷ tid. In stress, use 3 × this replacement dose.

STEROIDS

Dexamethasone (Decadron)

Extubation (if previous difficulties with extubation): 1–2 mg/kg/day PO, IV or IM ÷ q6h beginning 24 hr prior to extubation and continuing 4–6 hr afterwards.

↑ICP: initial dose: 0.2–0.4 mg/kg IV; max: 10 mg; subsequent dose: 0.3 mg/kg/day IV or IM ÷ q6h. May be useful in cerebral tumors and malaria but not head injuries.

Hydrocortisone (Solu-Cortef)

Acute asthma: 4–6 mg/kg/dose IV q4–6h

Anaphylaxis: 5–10 mg/kg IV

Hypoadrenalism:

Maintenance: 20 mg/m²/day PO ÷ tid or 12 mg/m²/day IV ÷ q6h

In acute adrenal crisis or before surgery, give 50-100 mg/m² IV stat followed by 50-100 mg/m²/day IV ÷ q6h.

In CAH, administer half the daily dose at bedtime to suppress A.M. surge of ACTH.

Methylprednisolone (Solu-Medrol)

Pulse therapy (rheumatology, immunology): 10–30 mg/kg in 50–100 ml D5W IV over 1 hr Max: 1 g

Acute asthma: 0.5–1 mg/kg/dose IV q6h

Prednisone
Asthma: 5–15 mg/dose q alt day PO up to 1 mg/kg/dose q alt day PO
Nephrotic syndrome: See p 442
JRA: Life threatening complications: 1–2 mg/kg/day PO in divided doses
Nonlife threatening: 0.5–1 mg/kg/day PO
Inflammatory bowel disease: 1 mg/kg/day PO; Max: 60 mg/day
Initial anti-inflammatory dose: 1–2 mg/kg/day PO
Dosages must be individualized as per response

Fludrocortisone (Florinef)
Salt losing hypoadrenalism: 0.05–0.15 mg/day PO ÷ q12h

III. *Discontinuation of steroids* (for patients taking steroids for ≥ 10 days): Halve therapy q48h until physiologic replacement achieved (equivalent of 20–25 mg hydrocortisone/m^2/day); then halve dose every 10–14 days

IV. *Topical steroids*: See p 102

NEONATAL DRUG DOSAGE GUIDELINES

Drug	Dose	Comments
Acetaminophen (Tempra; Tylenol)	10–15 mg/kg/dose PO or per rectum q4–6h Max: 60 mg/kg/day	
Acyclovir (Zovirax)	*H. Simplex infections*: 15–30 mg/kg/day IV ÷ q8h	Decrease dose in renal impairment. Higher doses may be required in H. Zoster infections.
Albumin	0.5–1.0 g/kg IV	25% albumin to be diluted to 5% strength, e.g., 4 ml 25% albumin + 16 ml D5W.
Amikacin	<2 kg: 0–7 days: 15 mg/kg/day IV or IM ÷ q12h >7 days: 22.5 mg/kg/day IV or IM ÷ q8h >2 kg: 0–7 days: 20 mg/kg/day IV or IM ÷ q12h >7 days: 30 mg/kg/day IV or IM ÷ q8h	Decrease dose in renal impairment. Monitoring of serum drug concentrations is recommended.

Drug	Dose	Comments
Ampicillin	<2 kg: 0–7 days: *Meningitis:* 100 mg/kg/day IV ÷ q12h *Other:* 50 mg/kg/day IV ÷ q12h >7 days: *Meningitis:* 150 mg/kg/day IV ÷ q8h *Other:* 75 mg/kg/day IV ÷ q8h >2 kg: 0–7 days: *Meningitis:* 150 mg/kg/day IV ÷ q8h *Other:* 75 mg/kg/day IV ÷ q8h >7 days: *Meningitis:* 200 mg/kg/day IV ÷ q6h *Other:* 100 mg/kg/day IV ÷ q6h	Decrease dose in severe renal impairment.
Atropine	*Resuscitation:* 0.01–0.02 mg/kg/dose IV, IM, SC or ETT q20 min prn	ETT route to be used only if IV access not possible.

NEONATAL DRUG DOSAGE GUIDELINES

Drug	Dose	Comments
Caffeine	Load: 10 mg/kg PO or IV Maint: 2.5 mg/kg/dose PO or IV once daily	Monitoring of serum drug concentrations recommended.
Calcium gluconate	*Resuscitation:* 1.5 ml/kg/dose of a 2% sol^n = 30 mg/kg/dose q10–20 min prn *Maint:* 200–400 mg/kg/day IV	Avoid extravasation. Preferable to use a central line when giving a 10% sol^n. Administer at a rate not to exceed 10 mg/min. 10% sol^n: 1 ml = 100 mg of calcium gluconate = 0.23 mmol of calcium.
Calcium lactate	For infants <2000 g, receiving >50% of daily requirements as breast milk, starting at 2 wks of age, supplement as follows: <1000 g 40 mg q2h PO 1000–1250 g 60 mg q2h PO 1250–1500 g 70 mg q2h PO 1500–1800 g 120 mg q3h PO	Give after feeds. Discontinue when infant reaches 1800 g or 35 weeks post conception.
Cefotaxime (Claforan)	0–7 days: 100 mg/kg/day IV ÷ q12h >7 days: 150 mg/kg/day IV ÷ q8h	Decrease dose in renal impairment.

Drug	Dose	Comments
Chloramphenicol	<2 kg: 25 mg/kg/day IV as single daily dose >2 kg: 0–7 days: 25 mg/kg/day IV as single daily dose >7 days: 50 mg/kg/day IV ÷ q12h	Monitoring of serum drug concentrations is recommended.
Chlorothiazide (Diuril)	10–20 mg/kg/day PO ÷ q12h	
Cimetidine (Tagamet)	≤7 days: 10–15 mg/kg/day PO or IV ÷ q4–6h Infants <1 yr: 20 mg/kg/day PO or IV ÷ q4–6h	Decrease dose in renal impairment.
Clindamycin	<2 kg: 0–7 days: 10 mg/kg/day IV ÷ q12h >7 days: 15 mg/kg/day IV or PO ÷ q8h >2 kg: 0–7 days: 15 mg/kg/day IV ÷ q8h >7 days: 20 mg/kg/day IV or PO ÷ q6h	Do not administer PO to infants <7 days old.

NEONATAL DRUG DOSAGE GUIDELINES

Drug	Dose	Comments
Cloxacillin	<2 kg: 0–7 days: 50 mg/kg/day PO or IV ÷ q12h >7 days: 75 mg/kg/day PO or IV ÷ q8h >2 kg: 0–7 days: 75 mg/kg/day PO or IV ÷ q8h >7 days: 100 mg/kg/day PO or IV ÷ q6h	Higher doses should be used when treating CNS infections
Dexamethasone (Decadron)	*Subglottic stenosis or inflammation:* 0.5–1.0 mg/kg/dose IV or PO up to 3 doses/day	Do not use for longer than 1 day.
Diazepam (Valium)	*Seizure:* 0.1–0.2 mg/kg/dose IV	Administer at a rate not to exceed 0.05 mg/kg/min.

Drug	Dose	Comments
Digoxin (Lanoxin)	*Digitalization*: divide total dose into 3 equal doses—1st stat, 2nd in 6 hr, 3rd in another 8 hr Preterm (<37 wk): PO: 0.02 mg/kg/total dose IV: 0.015 mg/kg/total dose Term (>37 wk): PO: 0.05 mg/kg/total dose IV: 0.035 mg/kg/total dose *Maint Dose:* Preterm: PO: 0.004 mg/kg/day ÷ q12h IV: 0.003 mg/kg/day ÷ q12h Term: PO: 0.01 mg/kg/day ÷ q12h IV: 0.007 mg/kg/day ÷ q12h	Do not administer IM. When digitalizing to terminate tachycardia, the dose is divided ½, ¼, ¼. Oral digitalization may be poorly absorbed in severe uncompensated heart failure. Decrease maintenance dose in renal impairment. Monitoring of serum drug concentrations is recommended.
Dopamine	*Renal*: 2–5 µg/kg/min IV *Inotropic*: 5–20 µg/kg/min IV *Vasoconstrictive*: >20 µg/kg/min IV	Neonates may be less sensitive to dopamine. Should be used in critical care areas only. See drug infusion table p 682.
Epinephrine	*Resuscitation*: 0.1 ml/kg/dose of 1:10,000 IV, ETT, or SC	1:10,000 = 0.1 mg/ml

NEONATAL DRUG DOSAGE GUIDELINES

Drug	Dose	Comments
Erythromycin estolate (Ilosone)	<2 kg: 0–7 days: 20 mg/kg/day PO ÷ q12h >7 days: 30 mg/kg/day PO ÷ q8h >2 kg: 0–7 days: 20 mg/kg/day PO ÷ q12h >7 days: 30–40 mg/kg/day PO ÷ q8h	
Erythromycin gluceptate (Ilotycin)	20–40 mg/kg/day IV ÷ q6h	
Furosemide (Lasix)	1–2 mg/kg/dose IV or PO	Slow IV push.
Gentamicin	Preterm infants ≤1 kg: 3.5 mg/kg/day IV or IM once daily Preterm infants >1 kg + fullterm infants 0–7 days: 5 mg/kg/day IV or IM ÷ q12h Fullterm infants >7 days: 7.5 mg/kg/day IV or IM ÷ q8h	Decrease dose in renal impairment. Monitoring of serum drug concentrations is recommended.
Glucagon	1.0–1.5 mg/day IV as a continuous infusion	Dilute in D5W or D10W.
Glucose	Initial dose: 1–2 ml/kg of a 10% glucose solution (100–200 mg/kg) IV; then 5–7 mg/kg/min IV as a continuous infusion	See page 395 for further information.

Drug	Dose	Comments
Heparin	*Maint of indwelling lines:* 1 unit/ml run at 1–2 ml/hr *Thrombosis:* 50–100 units IV, then 20–30 units/kg/hr IV as a continuous infusion	Desired PTT = 60–80 sec
Hydralazine (Apresoline)	1.7–3.5 mg/kg/day IV ÷ q4–6h	
Indomethacin (Indocid)	*Patent ductus arteriosus:* 0.2 mg/kg/dose IV q8h Max: 3 doses	Reduce doses of aminoglycosides and digoxin to half until good urine output returns.
Insulin	0.01–0.02 units regular insulin/kg/hr IV as a continuous infusion	Titrate infusion rate according to blood glucose.
Isoproterenol (Isuprel)	0.05–1.0 μg/kg/min IV as a continuous infusion	Stop or slow if heart rate >200/min. Should be used in critical care areas only.
Morphine	*Pain:* 0.1–0.2 mg/kg/dose IV then 0.01–0.02 mg/kg/hr IV as a continuous infusion	

NEONATAL DRUG DOSAGE GUIDELINES

Drug	Dose	Comments
Naloxone (Narcan)	0.01–0.02 mg/kg/dose q5–10 min as necessary	Neonatal strength (0.02 mg/ml) may be given undiluted.
Novospirozine	2–4 mg of each component/kg/day PO ÷ q12h	Contains equal amounts of hydrochlorothiazide and spironolactone.
Pancuronium (Pavulon)	0.05–0.1 mg/kg/dose IV	Repeat as necessary. Should be used in critical care areas only.
Paraldehyde	150 mg/kg/hr (3 ml of a 5% sol^n/kg/hr) IV over 2 hr once daily 300 mg/kg (0.3 ml of undiluted paraldehyde/kg) × 1 PO 300 mg/kg (0.3 ml of undiluted paraldehyde/kg) × 1 per rectum diluted in oil or normal saline to make a 30–50% sol^n	Make a 5% solution by adding 1.75 ml of paraldehyde to D5W to make a total volume of 35 ml in a syringe. Change syringe every 3–4 hr. Undiluted paraldehyde contains 1 g/ml.

Drug	Dose	Comments
Penicillin G (Benzylpenicillin)	<2 kg: 0–7 days: *Meningitis*: 100,000 units/kg/day IV ÷ q12h *Other*: 50,000 units/kg/day IV ÷ q12h >7 days: *Meningitis*: 150,000 units/kg/day IV ÷ q8h *Other*: 75,000 units/kg/day IV ÷ q8h >2 kg: 0–7 days: *Meningitis*: 150,000 units/kg/day IV ÷ q8h *Other*: 50,000 units/kg/day IV ÷ q8h >7 days: *Meningitis*: 200,000 units/kg/day IV ÷ q6h *Other*: 100,000 units/kg/day IV ÷ q6h	Decrease dose in severe renal impairment.
Phenobarbital	Load: preterm (<37 wk): 10–20 mg/kg IV; may repeat dose of 5–10 mg/kg IV up to max total dose of 25 mg/kg term (>37 wk): 10–20 mg/kg IV; may repeat dose of 10 mg/kg IV up to max total dose of 30 mg/kg Maint: 4–6 mg/kg/day IV or PO once daily	Administer undiluted at a rate not to exceed 1 mg/kg/min. Monitoring of serum drug concentrations is recommended.

NEONATAL DRUG DOSAGE GUIDELINES

Drug	Dose	Comments
Phenytoin (Dilantin)	Load: 20 mg/kg IV Maint: 4–8 mg/kg/day PO or IV once daily or ÷ bid	Monitor for hypotension during infusion. Administer undiluted at a rate not to exceed 1 mg/kg/min. Poorly absorbed orally in the infant. Monitoring of serum drug concentrations is recommended.
Piperacillin	<2 kg: 0–7 days: 150 mg/kg/day IV ÷ q12h >7 days: 225 mg/kg/day IV ÷ q8h >2 kg: 0–7 days: 225 mg/kg/day IV ÷ q8h >7 days: 300 mg/kg/day IV ÷ q6h	Decrease dose in severe renal impairment.
Propranolol (Inderal)	*Resuscitation:* 0.01–0.10 mg/kg/dose IV *Other:* 0.5–1.0 mg/kg/day PO ÷ q6h	
Prostaglandin E_1	0.05–0.1 μg/kg/min IV as a continuous infusion	May cause apnea. Should be used in critical care areas only.
Pyridoxine (vitamin B_6)	50–100 mg/dose IV	With EEG monitoring.
Sodium bicarbonate	Dose = wt. (kg) × 0.3 × base deficit IV 1–3 mmol/kg IV over 5 min in mild asphyxia 3–5 mmol/kg IV over 5 min in severe asphyxia	4.2% = 0.5 mmol/ml 8.4% = 1 mmol/ml Dilute 8.4% 1:1 with sterile water or D5W or use 4.2% undiluted.

Drug	Dose	Comments
Sodium polystyrene sulfonate (Kayexalate)	1 g/kg/dose PO or per rectum	Mix in water or D5W. Exchanges approx. 1 mmol K^+/g.
Spironolactone (Aldactone)	2–4 mg/kg/day PO ÷ q12h	For spironolactone in combination with hydrochlorothiazide, see Novospirozine.
Theophylline	Loading dose: 5 mg/kg/dose IV Maint: 1.6–3.2 mg/kg/day IV ÷ q12h	Monitoring of serum theophylline and caffeine concentrations is recommended.

Tobramycin	Preterm infants ≤1 kg:
	  3.5 mg/kg/day IV or IM once daily
	Preterm infants >1 kg + fullterm infants 0–7 days: 5 mg/kg/day IV or IM ÷ q12h
	Full term infants >7 days:
	  7.5 mg/kg/day IV or IM ÷ q8h
		Decrease dose in renal impairment. Monitoring of serum drug concentrations is recommended.

Tolazoline (Priscoline)	1–2 mg/kg IV bolus then 0.5–2 mg/kg/hr IV as a continuous infusion	Watch for hypotension. Emergency release–investigational agent. Should be used in critical care areas only.

NEONATAL DRUG DOSAGE GUIDELINES

Drug	Dose			Comments
	Wt (g)	Postconceptual Age (wk)	Dosage	
Vancomycin	<800 or	<27	27 mg/kg/dose IV q36h	Decrease dose in renal impairment.
	800–1200 or	27–30	24 mg/kg/dose IV q24h	Monitoring of serum drug
	1200–2000 or	31–36	18 mg/kg/dose IV q12h	concentrations is recommended.
			or 27 mg/kg/dose IV q18h	
	>2000 or	>37	22.5 mg/kg/dose IV q12h	
Vitamin K$_1$ (phytonadione)	*Hemorrhagic Disease of the Newborn:* Prophylaxis: 0.5–1.0 mg IM or SC at birth Treatment: 1 mg/dose IM or IV			Administer IV at a rate not to exceed 1 mg/min.

DRUG INTERACTIONS

This chart lists the effects on the primary drug only. Therefore, when checking the interaction between two drugs, be sure to look under both drugs. As well, please note that this list is not comprehensive.

Primary Drug	Plus Secondary Drug Causes		
	↑ 1° Drug Effect or Toxicity	↓ 1° Drug Effect	Other
Aminoglycosides	Amphotericin B, cephalosporins, furosemide, polymixins—nephrotoxicity Ethacrynic acid, furosemide—ototoxicity	Carbenicillin and ticarcillin inactivate gentamicin in vitro; therefore use separate IV lines.	
Anticoagulants (oral)	Acetaminophen, acute alcohol intoxication, allopurinol, amiodarone, chloral hydrate, chloramphenicol, cimetidine, danazol, diazoxide, disulfiram, ethacrynic acid, influenza vaccine, INH, metronidazole, nalidixic acid, quinidine, sulfinpyrazone, sulfonamides, tetracyclines, thyroid hormones, vitamins A and E	Chronic alcohol abuse, barbiturates, carbamazepine, cholestyramine, oral contraceptives, griseofulvin, rifampin, spironolactone, vitamin C.	ASA, NSAID, dipyrida-mole—↑ risk of bleeding

DRUG INTERACTIONS

Primary Drug	Plus Secondary Drug Causes		
	↑ 1° Drug Effect or Toxicity	↓ 1° Drug Effect	Other
Barbiturates	Chloramphenicol, phenytoin, valproic acid	Pyridoxine, rifampin	
Benzodiazepines	Acetaminophen, cimetidine, oral contraceptives (with IV diazepam), INH, valproic acid	Antacids, caffeine, oral contraceptives (with IV lorazepam), rifampin	Valproic acid + clonazepam—may precipitate absence status. Alcohol—↑ CNS depression.
Beta-adrenergic blockers	Chlorpromazine, cimetidine, oral contraceptives, hydralazine	Barbiturates, indomethacin, rifampin, smoking	Clonidine—paradoxical ↑ BP Diazoxide, ether, enflurane, halothane— ↓ BP Nifedipine, verapamil—CHF, AV conduction defect, sinus node arrest
Carbamazepine	Cimetidine, erythromycin, INH, lithium	Phenytoin	
Cimetidine	Carbamazepine	Antacids	

Primary Drug	Plus Secondary Drug Causes		
	↑ 1° Drug Effect or Toxicity	↓ 1° Drug Effect	Other
Contraceptives (oral)		Ampicillin, barbiturates, carbamazepine, phenytoin, primidone, rifampin, tetracycline	
Corticosteroids		Antacids, barbiturates, phenytoin, rifampin	
Digoxin	Amiodarone, diazepam, erythromycin, nifedipine, quinidine, tetracycline, thiazides, verapamil	Alcohol, antacids, cholestyramine, cyclophosphamide, hydralazine, nitroprusside, penicillamine, prednisone, rifampin, sulfasalazine, vincristine	Amphotericin B, furosemide—↑ digoxin toxicity (2° to hypokalemia)
Dopamine			IV phenytoin, tolazoline—↓ BP
Methotrexate	Penicillins, probenecid, salicylates, sulfonamides		

DRUG INTERACTIONS

Primary Drug	Plus Secondary Drug Causes		
	↑ 1° Drug Effect or Toxicity	↓ 1° Drug Effect	Other
Neuromuscular blocking agents	Alkylating agents, aminoglycosides, amphotericin B, clindamycin, diazepam, ethacrynic acid, furosemide, quinidine, thiazides		Theophylline + pancuronium—arrhythmia
Phenytoin	Acute alcohol intoxication, anticoagulants, chloramphenicol, cimetidine, oral contraceptives, dexamethasone, imipramine, INH, sulfonamides, valproic acid	Chronic alcohol abuse, carbamazepine, diazoxide, folic acid, influenza vaccine, pyridoxine, theophylline	Valproic acid—↑seizures Phenobarbital—may ↑ or ↓ phenytoin effect Dopamine + IV phenytoin—↓ BP
Primidone		Carbamazepine, phenytoin	
Quinidine	Amiodarone, cimetidine	Barbiturates, phenytoin, primidone, rifampin	

Primary Drug	Plus Secondary Drug Causes		
	↑ 1° Drug Effect or Toxicity	↓ 1° Drug Effect	Other
Spironolactone			Cyclopropane, enflurane, ether, halothane, isoflurane, nitrous oxide—↓ BP Captopril, potassium salts—↑ K$^+$
Theophylline	Allopurinol, propranolol, cimetidine, erythromycin, influenza vaccine, viral illness	Barbiturates, phenytoin, smoking	
Valproic acid	Antacids, salicylates	Carbamazepine	Clonazepam—may precipitate absence status Phenytoin—↑ seizures
Verapamil			Beta-adrenergic blockers—CHF, bradycardia

CHEMOTHERAPY ANTIEMETICS

Emetic Potential	Antiemetic Combinations	
High Cis-platinum,[2] oral CCNU, IV BCNU, high-dose Ara-C, daunomycin, melphalan, ifosphamide, moderate to high dose cyclophosphamide, nitrogen mustard, actinomycin D, mitoxantrone, doxorubicin, amsacrine	*First line:*[1] *IV metoclopramide* 　and *IV diphenhydramine*[3] *Second line:*[1] *IV chlorpromazine* 　and *IV diphenhydramine*[3] *Third line:*[1] *PO nabilone* *Fourth line:*[1] *Fifth line:*[1]	0.5 mg/kg/dose (max initial dose: 20 mg) prior to chemo; then q3h prn; may be increased up to 2 mg/kg/dose; total dose not to exceed 10 mg/kg/day 1 mg/kg/dose prior to chemo; then q3h prn Max: 50 mg/dose, 300 mg/day 0.3–0.5 mg/kg/dose prior to chemo; then q4–6h prn Give IV slowly (at a rate not to exceed 0.5 mg/min) Max: <5 yr 40 mg/day; >5 yr 75 mg/day As above <18 kg 0.5 mg prior to chemo; 0.5 mg at 4 hr and 8 hr 18–30 kg 1 mg prior to chemo; 1 mg at 4 hr >30 kg 1 mg prior to chemo; 1 mg at 4 hr and 8 hr PO nabilone, IV metoclopramide, and IV diphenhydramine[3] PO nabilone, IV chlorpromazine, and IV diphenhydramine[3]

Emetic Potential	Antiemetic Combinations	
Mild		
High-dose MTX, 5-fluorouracil, hydroxyurea, bleomycin, procarbazine	*First line:* IV dimenhydrinate	2 mg/kg/dose prior to chemo then q3–4h prn; max 75 mg/dose Max: 300 mg/day
	Second line: PO nabilone:	See previous page
Low or No		
6-MP, 6-thioguanine, MTX, VM 26, VP 16, vincristine, vinblastine, vindesine, IT MTX, IT Ara-C	None	

1   Some consultants in addition to these drugs start with methylprednisolone (300 mg/m^2/dose IV prior to chemo; then q4–6h prn; max 3 doses/day). Others do not start with methylprednisolone but add it to the protocol only if the other drugs are not working.
2   Start with second line drugs.
3   Diphenhydramine is given to prevent the extrapyramidal reactions caused by metoclopramide or chlorpromazine.

THE TRANSFER OF DRUGS AND OTHER CHEMICALS INTO HUMAN BREAST MILK

TABLE 1   Drugs That Are Contraindicated During Breast Feeding

Drug	Reported Sign or Symptom in Infant or Effect on Lactation
Amethopterin*	Possible immune suppression; unknown effect on growth or association with carcinogenesis
Bromocriptine	Suppresses lactation
Cimetidine†	May suppress gastric acidity in infant, inhibit drug metabolism, and cause CNS stimulation
Clemastine (Tavist)	Drowsiness, irritability, refusal to feed, high pitched cry, neck stiffness
Cyclophosphamide*	Possible immune suppression; unknown effect on growth or association with carcinogenesis
Ergotamine	Vomiting, diarrhea, convulsions (doses used in migraine medications)
Gold salts	Rash, inflammation of kidney and liver
Methimazole	Potential for interfering with thyroid function
Phenindione	Hemorrhage
Thiouracil	Decreased thyroid function; does not apply to propylthiouracil

* Data not available for other cytotoxic agents
† Drug is concentrated in breast milk
Modified from Committee on Drugs, American Academy of Pediatrics. The transfer of drugs and other chemicals into human breast milk. Pediatrics 1983; 72:375.

TABLE 2 Drugs That Require Temporary Cessation of Breast Feeding

Drug	Recommended Alteration in Breast Feeding Pattern
Metronidazole	Discontinue breast feeding 12–24 hr to allow excretion of dose
Radiopharmaceuticals	Radioactivity present in milk; consult nuclear medicine physician before performing diagnostic study so that radionuclide that has shortest excretion time in breast milk can be used; prior to study the mother should pump her breast and store enough milk in freezer for feeding the infant; after study the mother should pump her breast to maintain milk production but discard all milk pumped for the required time that radioactivity is present in milk.
Gallium-69 (^{69}Ga)	Radioactivity in milk present for 2 wk
Iodine-125 (^{125}I)	Risk of thyroid cancer, radioactivity in milk present for 12 days
Iodine-131 (^{131}I)	Radioactivity in milk present 2–14 days depending on study
Radioactive sodium	Radioactivity in milk 96 hr
Technetium-99m (^{99m}TC), ^{99m}Tc macroaggregates, ^{99m}Tc O$_4$	Radioactivity in milk 15 hr to 3 days

Modified from Committee on Drugs, American Academy of Pediatrics. The transfer of drugs and other chemicals into human breast milk. Pediatrics 1983; 72:375.

RECOMMENDATIONS FOR PROPHYLACTIC THERAPY IN THE PREVENTION OF ENDOCARDITIS IN CHILDREN

I Dental procedures, oropharyngeal surgery, instrumentation of respiratory tract

Children tolerant of penicillin

1. Aqueous penicillin G 50,000 u/kg IV or IM. Give 30–60 min prior to procedure. Follow with penicillin V 900 mg PO 6 hr later (600 mg for children under 27 kg)

OR

2. Penicillin V 2.1 g PO 60 min prior to procedure; then 900 mg PO 6 hr later. For children less than 27 kg use 900 mg and 600 mg, respectively

Children allergic to penicillin or on continuous penicillin prophylaxis for rheumatic fever

1. Erythromycin 20 mg/kg (max 1g) PO 60–90 min prior to procedure; then 10 mg/kg (max 500 mg) PO 6 hr later

OR

2. *Clindamycin 10 mg/kg (max 600 mg/dose) PO 60–90 min prior to procedure and 6 hr later

II Gastrointestinal and genitourinary procedures or instrumentation

Children tolerant of penicillin

1. Ampicillin 100 mg/kg IV 30–60 min prior to procedure and 6 hr later (max 12 g/24 hr). May use amoxicillin 50 mg/kg (max 1 g) instead of second dose of ampicillin

PLUS

2. Gentamicin[†] 2 mg/kg IM or IV over period of 30–60 min prior to procedure and 6 hr later (max 250 mg/24 hr)

Children allergic to penicillin

1. *Clindamycin 20 mg/kg (max 600 mg); one dose IV over period of 20–30 min prior to procedure

PLUS

2. Gentamicin[†] 2 mg/kg IM or IV over period of 30–60 min prior to procedure and 6 hr later (max 250 mg/24 hr)

III Surgical procedures on infected and contaminated tissues, including incision and drainage of abscesses when _Staphylococcus aureus_ is suspected

Children tolerant of penicillin

1. Cloxacillin 50 mg/kg IM or IV 30–60 min prior to procedure and 6 hr later (max 4 g/24 hr)

PLUS

2. Gentamicin[†] 2 mg/kg IM or IV over period of 30–60 min prior to procedure and 6 hr later (max 250 mg/24 hr)

Children allergic to penicillin or on continuous penicillin prophylaxis for rheumatic fever

1. [*]Clindamycin 20 mg/kg (max 600 mg); one dose IV over period of 20–30 min prior to procedure

PLUS

2. Gentamicin[†] 2 mg/kg IM or IV over period of 30–60 min prior to procedure and 6 hr later (max 250 mg/24 hr)

IV Children with prosthetic tissue or mechanical valves

1. [*]Clindamycin 20 mg/kg (max 600 mg); one dose IV over period of 20–30 min prior to procedure

PLUS

2. Gentamicin[†] 2.0 mg/kg IM or IV over period of 30–60 min prior to procedure and 6 hr later (max 250 mg/24 hr)

---

* American Heart Association recommends vancomycin (20 mg/kg, max 1 g) IV over 1 hr instead of clindamycin. DO NOT REPEAT THE DOSE OF VANCOMYCIN.

† The second dose of gentamicin should be reduced in renal impairment

Modified from a report of an American Heart Association Committee. Circulation 1984; 70:1123A–1127A.

THERAPEUTIC DRUG MONITORING

General Guidelines

- The elimination half-life of a drug is simply defined as the time taken for the serum concentration to fall to half its original value. This parameter is a useful index of dose requirements, dosage interval, and time to steady state, but the "normal" listed values are subject to interindividual variability.
- Routine drug level requests should not be submitted prior to attainment of steady state conditions (normally equivalent to a duration of constant therapy of five elimination half-lives) unless (1) failure of therapeutic response or (2) onset of toxicity is in question.
- If individualization of therapy is a critical factor in the acute phase of patient care, two blood samples drawn approximately one half-life apart (in the first dosage interval or during constant rate infusion) can provide useful information about maintenance dose requirements.
- The adequacy of oral therapy can be most reliably assessed by steady state trough level analysis.
- The time of sampling is less critical for patients receiving long term therapy, if the drug has a long elimination half-life and is given by regular intermittent dosing, or if constant rate infusions are employed.
- If lack of efficacy or suspicion of toxicity is transient, but occurs at a regular point of the dosage interval, TDM samples should be collected at these times.

- WHENEVER A SAMPLE IS SENT FOR MEASUREMENT OF SERUM DRUG CONCENTRATIONS, THE TIME THE DRUG WAS GIVEN AND THE TIME THE SAMPLE WAS TAKEN SHOULD BOTH BE CLEARLY MARKED ON THE REQUISITION.

Drug	Time to Steady State (Elimination Half-Life)			Ideal Sampling Time	Optimal Serum Concentration Range	Comments
	Neonates	Infants >1 mo	Children >1 yr			
Amikacin	24 hr* (6)	24 hr (1.5)	24 hr (1.5)	Peak: 60 min post IM, 30 min after finish of IV infusion	Peak: 20–30 mg/L	Half-life may be prolonged in patients with renal dys-function. Both clearance and volume of distribution may be increased in cystic fibrosis.
	* Prolonged in premature neonates to 36 hr			Trough: immediately prior to next dose	Trough: 2.5–10 mg/L	
Caffeine	14 days (3 days)	24 hr (2.5)		Trough: immediately prior to next dose	30–70 μmol/L (6–14 mg/L)	Half-life of up to 100 hr in premature neonates decreases gradually throughout infancy to reach normal adult values by approximately 9 mo of age

THERAPEUTIC DRUG MONITORING

Drug	Time to Steady State (Elimination Half-Life)			Ideal Sampling Time	Optimal Serum Concentration Range	Comments
	Neonates	Infants >1 mo	Children >1 yr			
Carbamazepine	30 days (12 hr)	30 days (10 hr)	30 days (8 hr)	Trough: immediately prior to next oral dose	17–50 μmol/L (4–12 mg/L)	Owing to enzyme auto-induction, half-life during chronic dosing may be considerably shorter than after first dose. Consequently, within the first 4–8 wk of therapy, dose may need to be increased to maintain therapeutic levels.
Chloramphenicol	72 hr (15)	48 hr (10)	24 hr (5)	Peak: 1 hr after finish of infusion Trough: immediately prior to next dose	Peak: 15–25 mg/L Trough: <10 mg/L	Careful monitoring is advisable to take account of the very unpredictable pharmacokinetics in pediatric patients
Cyclosporin	-	-	36 hr (6) This drug is rarely used in children less than 1 yr old	Trough: immediately before regular oral or IV dose; every 24 hr during acute phase	At present time, this requires definition on a local basis to take account of sample	Monitoring is considered mandatory to avoid extremely low or high levels, which may precipi-

Drug	Time to Steady State (Elimination Half-Life)			Ideal Sampling Time	Optimal Serum Concentration Range	Comments
	Neonates	Infants >1 mo	Children >1 yr			
Cyclosporin (cont'd)					matrix, analytical method, clinical indication, and time since transplantation	tate therapeutic failure or nephrotoxicity, respectively
Digoxin	10 days* (2.5)	7 days (1.5)	7 days (1.5)	Monitor routinely on day 5 of therapy; otherwise restrict to the following circumstances: Detection of noncompliance Clarification of poor response Confirmation of clinical suspicion of toxicity The levels should be drawn in the post distribution phase (8–24 hr after a dose)	1–2.5 nmol/L (0.8–2.0 µg/L)	Half-life may be prolonged in renal impairment. In neonates, serum level results may show interference with an endogenous digoxin-like substance (EDLS). In infants and children, the concentration-effect relationship is somewhat imprecise, particularly in renal and hepatic impairment, owing to cross reactivity of standard assays with digoxin metabolites.

* Prolonged in premature neonates to 12–14 days

883

THERAPEUTIC DRUG MONITORING

Drug	Time to Steady State (Elimination Half-Life)			Ideal Sampling Time	Optimal Serum Concentration Range	Comments
	Neonates	Infants >1 mo	Children >1 yr			
Ethosuximide	-	-	7 days (1.5)	Trough: immediately prior to next oral dose	280–710 μmol/L (40–100 mg/L)	Specific patients tolerate and may benefit from serum levels that are significantly higher than the "recommended maximum limit."
Gentamicin	24 hr* (7)	24 hr (4)	24 hr (1.5) * Prolonged in premature neonates to 36–48 hr	Peak: 60 min post IM; 30 min after finish of IV infusion. Trough: immediately prior to next dose Monitor *peak and trough* 48 hr after starting therapy and then 1–2 x weekly.	Peak: 5–10 mg/L Trough: <2 mg/L	Half-life may be prolonged in patients with renal dysfunction and may be reduced in patients with cystic fibrosis

Drug	Time to Steady State (Elimination Half-Life)			Ideal Sampling Time	Optimal Serum Concentration Range	Comments
	Neonates	Infants >1 mo	Children >1 yr			
Methotrexate	Not applicable Monitoring of high single doses only			Dependent upon specific chemotherapy protocol	Calcium leucovorin therapy normally continues until MTX levels are less than 0.1 μmol/L.	Refer to individual protocol for target levels at specific time points after initiation of high dose infusion. Concentrations are elevated by impairment to renal filtration or secretion.
Phenobarbital	14 days (5)	7 days (2.5)	10 days (3)	Trough: immediately prior to next oral dose.	65–130 μmol/L (15–30 mg/L)	Neonatal elimination half-life may be prolonged by birth asphyxia
Phenytoin	7 days	5 days	7 days	Daily during IV stabilization Weekly during initial oral therapy Q 3–6 monthly during chronic oral therapy	40–80 μmol/L* (10–20 mg/L) * Neonates may respond to lower levels	Half-life may be dose and concentration dependent, which makes time to steady state highly variable and unpredictable
	Approximate values only					

FORMULARY

THERAPEUTIC DRUG MONITORING

Drug	Time to Steady State (Elimination Half-Life)			Ideal Sampling Time	Optimal Serum Concentration Range	Comments
	Neonates >1 mo	Infants	Children >1 yr			
Primidone	No data available			Trough: immediately prior to next oral dose.	23–55 μmol/L (5–12 mg/L)	Phenobarbital is the major metabolite of primidone in vivo and therefore should also be monitored. The expected parent drug to metabolite ratio is from 1:4 to 1:2.
Quinidine		24 hr (4)	24 hr (4)	Trough: immediately prior to next oral dose.	7–18 μmol/L (2–6 mg/L)	Monitoring is particularly important in the presence of cardiac, hepatic, or renal impairment
Salicylate	7 days	7 days	7 days	Trough: immediately prior to next oral dose. Time to peak level is variable and is prolonged by the EC product	For anti-inflammatory effect: 1.1–2.2 mmol/L (150–300 mg/L)	A non-linear relationship may exist between dose and concentration due to "capacity limited" protein binding and hepatic metabolism.

Salicylate (Time to Steady State): Approximate values only. (Half lives may be dose and concentration dependent)

Drug	Time to Steady State (Elimination Half-Life)			Ideal Sampling Time	Optimal Serum Concentration Range	Comments
	Neonates	Infants >1 mo	Children >1 yr			
Theophylline	5 days (1 day)	36 hr (6)	24 hr (4)	Infusion therapy: —pre dose if currently receiving theophylline —6 and 24 hr after start —daily as required Intermittent oral or IV: immediately prior to next dose	Neonates with apnea of prematurity: 28–67 μmol/L (5–12 mg/L) Older infant and child with bronchospasm: 55–110 μmol/L (10–20 mg/L)	Theophylline is partially converted to caffeine in the neonatal period when ideally the concentration of both methylxanthines should be monitored. Half-life may be prolonged by deficiencies in cardiac output or hepatic function.
Tobramycin	Refer to gentamicin guidelines; the two aminoglycosides are identical in every pharmacokinetic aspect					
Valproic acid	10 days (2 days)	72 hr (15)	36 hr (8)	Trough: immediately prior to next oral dose	350–700 μmol/L (50–100 mg/L)	Half-life may be prolonged in patients with hepatic disease and may be shortened in patients receiving other anticonvulsant drugs

THERAPEUTIC DRUG MONITORING

Drug	Time to Steady State (Elimination Half-Life)			Ideal Sampling Time	Optimal Serum Concentration Range	Comments
	Neonates	Infants >1 mo	Children >1 yr			
Vancomycin	36 hr (7.5)	24 hr (4.0)	24 hr (2.5)	Monitor 48 hr after starting therapy Peak: 60 min after completion of IV infusion Trough: immediately prior to next dose	Peak: 25–40 mg/L Trough: 5–10 mg/L	Half-life may be prolonged in premature low birth-weight neonates and in patients with renal impairment

VII

INDEX

INDEX

An "f" following a page number indicates a figure,
"t" indicates a table. References to emergency conditions are in red
for ease of reference.

Barlow dislocation test, 539f
Beclomethasone, 802
Behavior, patterns of, birth through
  5 years, 189–193t
Behavioral pediatrics, 29–38
Benzodiazepines, 870
Benzyl benzoate, 802
Beta-adrenergic blockers, 870
Bethanechol, 803
Bile salts, 742
Biliary atresia, 648–649
Bilirubin, direct, 742
  total, 742–743
Bilirubinuria, test for, 461
Biopsy, bone marrow, 720–722
  liver, 168
  punch, 690
  renal, in nephrotic syndrome,
    441
  skin, 689–690
Birth control methods, 245–259
  and efficacy of, 245t
Bisacodyl, 803
Bites, animal, 315–316
  human, 316–317
  snake, 585–586
  spider, 588
Black widow spider bites, 588
Bladder aspiration, suprapubic,
  711–712, 712f
Bladder catheterization, 709–710
Bleeding. *See* Hemorrhage
Blood, occult, in feces, 787
  reference values, 729, 735–775
Blood collection, 686–689
Blood gas(es), abnormality,
    common patterns of, 143t
  acid-base values of, 735
  analysis, 591
  sampling, arterial, 716–717
Blood group compatibility,
    recipient-donor, 279t
Blood pressure, measurements, in
    boys and girls, 445–448f
  in infants, 449–450f
Blood products, clinical use of,
    280t
Bochdalek hernia, 640–641
Body louse, 91
Body surface area, nomogram for
    children and adults, 796f

nomogram for infants, 797f
  and weight, 797
Bone marrow aspiration and
  biopsy, 720–722
Bone(s), age, adult height related
  to, 220–222t
  infarction, and osteomyelitis,
    differentiation between, 266t
Bottle feeding, considerations in,
    491
  forms available for, 491
  preparation for, 491–492
Bowel disease, inflammatory,
    156–157
Bradycardia, sinus, 51–52, 51f
Brain abscess, 317–318
Breast development, female, 224f
Breast feeding, advantages of, 489
  contraindications to, 489–490
  problems in, 489
  treatment of, 490–491
Breast milk, drug transfer into,
    876–877t
Breath holding, syncope, and
    convulsions, differentiation of,
    468t
Bretylium, 803
Brompheniramine, 803
Bronchiolitis, clinical features of,
    599
  management in, 600
Brown recluse spider bites, 588
Bulimia, 5, 5–6t
Burns, corrosive, of upper
    gastrointestinal tract, 556–557
  thermal, area of, estimation of,
    567f
    hospital admission in, criteria
      for, 566t
    inpatient, management of,
      566–569, 568t
    outpatient, management of,
      566
    severity of, 565t
    water temperature producing,
      565, 565t

C

Cadmium, in urine, 775
Caffeine, 858, 881
Calcitriol, 804